Nutrition in Sport and Exercise

Nutrition in Sport and Exercise

Edited by **Pablo De Souza**

SYRAWOOD
PUBLISHING HOUSE
New York

Published by Syrawood Publishing House,
750 Third Avenue, 9th Floor,
New York, NY 10017, USA
www.syrawoodpublishinghouse.com

Nutrition in Sport and Exercise
Edited by Pablo De Souza

International Standard Book Number: 978-1-68286-219-3 (Hardback)

Printed in China.

Contents

Preface

To understand the dietary and nutritive requirements of individuals who are involved in sports, it is important to understand their metabolism. This book unfolds the innovative aspects of nutrition in sports through detailed discussions about concepts such as metabolic responses of athletes, dietary regimes, food supplements, etc. Also included in this book are revolutionizing theories and strategies for sports nutrition and their respective impacts on health and performance. Topics discussed in this book will be most useful for dieticians, health professionals and students.

After months of intensive research and writing, this book is the end result of all who devoted their time and efforts in the initiation and progress of this book. It will surely be a source of reference in enhancing the required knowledge of the new developments in the area. During the course of developing this book, certain measures such as accuracy, authenticity and research focused analytical studies were given preference in order to produce a comprehensive book in the area of study.

This book would not have been possible without the efforts of the authors and the publisher. I extend my sincere thanks to them. Secondly, I express my gratitude to my family and well-wishers. And most importantly, I thank my students for constantly expressing their willingness and curiosity in enhancing their knowledge in the field, which encourages me to take up further research projects for the advancement of the area.

Editor

1

Hydrolyzed collagen intake increases bone mass of growing rats trained with running exercise

Satoko Takeda[1], Jong-Hoon Park[2,3], Eriko Kawashima[4], Ikuko Ezawa[5] and Naomi Omi[1,6,7*]

Abstract

Background: Some studies have shown that dietary hydrolyzed collagen peptides (HC) effectively prevent age-related bone loss. However, it is not known whether the intake of HC also has positive effect on bone mass or strength when combined with exercise during growth phase.

Methods: We examined the effects of 11 weeks of HC intake and running exercise on bone mass and strength in growing rats. Rats were randomized into four groups, the 20% casein group (Casein20), the 40% casein group (Casein40), the 20% HC group (HC20), and the 40% HC group (HC40). Each group was further divided into exercise groups (Casein20 + Ex, Casein40 + Ex, HC20 + Ex, HC40 + Ex) and non-exercise group (Casein20, Casein40, HC20, HC40). In the HC intake groups, 30% of casein protein was replaced with HC. Exercise group rats were trained 6 days per week on a treadmill (25–30 m/min, 60 min) for 60 days. After being sacrificed, their bone mineral content (BMC) and bone strength were evaluated.

Results: Exercise and dietary HC effects were observed in the adjusted BMC of lumbar spine and tibia among the 20% protein groups ($p < 0.001$ for exercise; $p < 0.05$ for dietary HC, respectively). These effects were also noted in the adjusted wet weight and dry weight of femur among the 20% protein groups ($p < 0.001$, $p < 0.01$ for exercise; $p < 0.01$, $p < 0.001$ for dietary HC, respectively). On the other hand, in adjusted bone breaking force and energy, dietary HC effect was not significant. Among the 40% protein groups, similar results were obtained in the adjusted BMC, femoral weight, bone breaking force, and energy. There were no differences between the 20% protein groups and the 40% protein groups.

Conclusions: The present study demonstrated that moderate HC intake (where the diet contains 20% protein, of which 30% is HC) increased bone mass during growth period and further promoted the effect of running exercise. On the other hand, a higher HC intake (where the diet contains 40% protein, of which 30% is HC) had no more beneficial effect on bone mass than the moderate HC intake.

Keywords: Hydrolyzed collagen peptides, Bone mass, Bone strength, Physical exercise, Growing phase, Rats

Background

It is generally well accepted that physiologically mechanical loading, e.g., physical activity or exercise, plays important roles in having higher bone mass during growth period [1]. In addition, nutritional factors such as protein are essential for increasing bone formation [2]. Thus, for achieving peak bone mass during growing phase, not only mechanical loading but also sustaining adequate protein intake may be of significance. In particular, although young athletes involved in physical training have high protein intakes [3], the effects of protein intake and physical exercise on growing bone have not been well understood.

Type I collagen is the major structural protein, being the main extra cellular matrix protein for calcification. It is distributed throughout the whole body accounting for 25% of total body protein and for 80% of total conjunctive tissue in humans [4]. The synthesis of type I collagen also plays a role in further promoting osteoblast differentiation [5,6]. Collagen peptides, the enzymatic degradation products of collagens, have recently been shown to have several biological activities, and have been used as preservatives [7-9]. The intake of hydrolyzed collagen peptides (HC) in animal models has been shown to improve bone mineral density (BMD) and bone mineral content (BMC) [10], and

* Correspondence: ominaomi@taiiku.tsukuba.ac.jp
[1]Graduate School of Comprehensive Human Sciences, University of Tsukuba, Ibaraki, Japan
[6]Faculty of Health and Sport Sciences, University of Tsukuba, Ibaraki, Japan
Full list of author information is available at the end of the article

to increase the quantity of type I collagen in bone matrix of ovariectomized (OVX) rats [11]. Moreover, in patients with osteoporosis, oral intake of HC in addition to injection of calcitonin had a stronger inhibitory effect on bone resorption than the injection of calcitonin alone [12]. These results suggest that dietary collagen peptides would effectively prevent age-related bone loss. However, it has not been demonstrated whether the intake of HC also has positive effect on bone mass or strength in growing bone.

Some studies have investigated the effects of the intake level of protein on bone mass. Protein deficiency could decrease the secretion of insulin-like growth factor 1 (IGF-1) [13], which may prevent normal growth of bone mass. Recently, we also demonstrated that a low protein intake suppressed the acquisition of bone mass and the increase of bone strength during growth period [14]. Conversely, a high protein intake results in higher urinary calcium (Ca) excretion, which may lead to accelerated bone resorption [15]. Similarly, we demonstrated that a high protein intake suppressed the increase of bone strength during growth period in which treadmill running was performed [14]. However, these studies used only casein protein as a protein source of the diet; it is not known whether HC intake included in a high protein diet has positive effect on bone mass or strength when combined with running exercise during growth phase.

Accordingly, the aim of this study is to investigate 1) the effect of HC intake alone and HC intake combined with treadmill running exercise on bone mass and strength in growing rats, 2) whether the intake of a high protein diet containing HC has a positive effect on bone mass and strength of growing rats trained with running exercise.

Methods

Experimental animals and protocol

Fifty-nine male Wistar rats, 5 weeks of age were obtained from CLEA Japan, Inc (Tokyo, Japan). Rats were randomized into four groups, the 20% casein group (Casein20), the 40% casein group (Casein40), the 20% HC group (HC20), and the 40% HC group (HC40). Each group was further divided into exercise groups (Casein20 + Ex, Casein40 + Ex, HC20 + Ex, HC40 + Ex) and non-exercise groups (Casein20, Casein40, HC20, HC40) (n = 7 or 8 each). The experimental period was 11 weeks. The animals were individually housed at 23 ± 1°C and humidity of 50 ± 5% on an inverted 12/12 h light/dark cycle. All animals received food and water *ad libitum*. Body weight and food intake were measured at 48 h intervals throughout the experimental period. All experimental protocols in the present study were approved by the Committee on Animal Research at the University of Tsukuba.

Experimental diets

Each group received one of two levels of protein for its diet, 20% or 40% to total diet weight. Since the recommended dietary percentage of protein for growing animals is 17.9% [16], we used 20% protein as a moderate protein intake and 40% protein as a high protein intake. In the HC intake groups, 30% of casein protein was replaced with HC. Enzymatic HC was provided by JNC Corporation (Yokohama, Japan). The HC was of marine fish origin with a molecular weight of about 1 kDa. It was prepared with extraction by the enzymatic degradation. Then the extracted product was concentrated and dried. The product is powder with little taste and odor. All diets were controlled at 0.6% Calcium (Ca) and 0.6% Phosphate (P). These diet compositions are described in Table 1.

Exercise

Exercise group rats were trained 6 days per week on a treadmill (KN-73, Natsume, Tokyo). The running speed and time were gradually increased (10–25 m/min, 10–60 min). Regular training started on the second week, and the running speed was further increased (25–30 m/min). Finally, the rats ran for 60 consecutive minutes (27–30 m/min). The training period was 60 days. This running speed (30 m/min) corresponds to 60 ~ 70% VO_2max for rats [17]. To this training was added a warm-up session (15 m/min, 5 min) and a cool-down session (15 m/min, 5 min), making the total exercise time to 70 minutes.

Dissection

After 11 weeks (at 16 weeks of age), rats were fasted for 12 h and dissected. The femur, tibia and lumbar spine were collected, and cleaned of adjacent tissues. The length of femora was immediately measured, and stored at 4°C for later mechanical testing. The tibiae and lumbar spines were stored in 70% ethanol for bone mineral content assessment.

Bone mineral content

The BMC and area of lumbar spines and tibiae were analyzed by dual-energy X-ray absorptiometry (DXA: Aloka DCS-600R) [18].

Femoral weights, length and mechanical testing

Femoral length was measured with a precision caliper. The femoral breaking force and energy were measured by the three point bending method using a bone strength measuring apparatus (Iio Co., Japan) as described in a previous report [19]. Subsequently, the femora were dried at 100°C for 24 h in the electric furnace, and their dry weight were measured. Next, the dried femur were burned to ash at 600°C for 15 h, and their ash weight were measured. The data of femoral breaking force and

Table 1 Composition of experimental diets

Constituents	20% Protein		40% Protein	
	collagen(-) (0.6% Ca, 0.6% P)	collagen(+) (0.6% Ca, 0.6% P)	collagen(-) (0.6% Ca, 0.6% P)	collagen(+) (0.6% Ca, 0.6% P)
Glucose monohydrate	60.4	60.3	40.8	40.6
Casein (Vitamin free)	20.0	14.0	40.0	28.0
Hydrolyzed collagen	–	6.0	–	12.0
Cystine	0.2	0.2	0.2	0.2
Cottonseed oil	10.0	10.0	10.0	10.0
$CaCO_3$	1.4879	1.4777	1.4774	1.4734
KH_2PO_4	1.1424	0.9667	0.9666	1.0636
K_2HPO_4	1.4621	1.2373	1.2372	1.3613
Roughage	3.0	3.0	3.0	3.0
Choline chloride	0.2	0.2	0.2	0.2
Water soluble Vitamin mixture[a)]	0.1	0.1	0.1	0.1
Oil soluble Vitamin mixture	b)	b)	b)	b)
Ca P free salt mixture[c)]	2.0	2.0	2.0	2.0

[a)]The water soluble vitamin in mixture (in %): thiamine, 0.5; riboflavin, 0.5; pyridoxine, 0.5; calcium pantothenate, 2.8; nicotinamide, 2.0; inositol, 20.0; B12, 0.002; foric acid, 0.2; vitamin biotin, 0.01; and glucose monohydrate, 3.7.
[c)]The Calcium (Ca) Phosphorus (P) free salt mixture (in %): potassium chloride,57.7; sodium chloride,20.9;magnesium sulfate,anhydrous,17.9; copper(II)sulfate pentahydrate,0.078;sodium fluoride,0.113;cobalt(II)chloride,0.004;potassium Iodide,0.01; magnese(II)sulfate pentahydrate,0.06; hexaammonium heptamolybdate tetrahydrate,0.005; iron(II)sulfate heptahydrate,3.22;zinc sulfate heptahydrate,0.44.

energy were adjusted to the dry weight (the adjusted breaking force and energy) to exclude the influence of body mass.

Bone metabolic marker

Serum bone-specific alkaline phosphatase (BAP) activity, the bone mineralization parameters and tartrate-resistant acid phosphatase (TRAP) activity, and the bone resorption markers were determined as previously reported [20].

Statistical methods

The results are expressed as the mean ± standard error of the mean (SE) and were analyzed with SPSS (version 21.0 J; SPSS Inc., Chicago, IL, USA). The data were analyzed using a two-way analysis of variance (ANOVA). Moreover, *t*-test was performed on four pairs of 20% protein groups and 40% protein groups of the same diet and physical activity to assess significant difference between the moderate and the higher protein groups (Casein20 × Casein40, Casein20 + Ex × Casein40 + Ex, HC20 × HC40, HC20 + Ex × HC40 + Ex). Statistical significance was taken at the $p < 0.05$ level.

Results

Food intake and body weight

At the beginning of the experiment, body weight did not differ among the groups. In the food intake during experiment, exercise effect was obtained ($p < 0.001$), and was significantly lower in the exercise groups than in the sedentary groups. These effects were detected both among the 20% protein groups and the 40% protein groups (Table 2). Therefore, the body weight gain, the food efficiency, and the final body weight were significantly lower in the exercise groups than in the sedentary groups ($p < 0.001$, respectively). Dietary HC effect was not obtained in these data among the 20% protein groups, but the effect was obtained in the food intake, the body weight gain, the food efficiency, and the final body weight among the 40% protein groups ($p < 0.05$, $p < 0.01$, $p < 0.05$ and $p < 0.05$, respectively, casein groups > HC groups) (Table 2). The food intake was significantly higher in the Casein20, HC20, and HC20 + Ex groups than the Casein40 ($p < 0.01$), HC40 ($p < 0.01$) and HC40 + Ex groups ($p < 0.05$, respectively) (Table 2).

BMC

Exercise and dietary HC effects were obtained in the adjusted BMC of lumbar spine, tibia proximal metaphysis, and tibia diaphysis among the 20% protein groups ($p < 0.001$ for exercise, $p < 0.05$ for dietary HC, respectively). These adjusted BMC values were significantly higher in the exercise groups than those in the sedentary groups, and were also significantly higher in the HC groups than those in the casein groups. Among the 40% protein groups, similar results were obtained except for tibia diaphysis ($p < 0.01$ for exercise; $p < 0.05$ for dietary HC, respectively) (Figure 1). There were no differences between the 20% protein groups and the 40% protein groups.

Table 2 Body weight, body weight gain, food intake, energy intake, and food efficiency

		20% protein	Two-way ANOVA (p value)			40% protein	Two-way ANOVA (p value)		
			Exercise	Collagen	Interaction		Exercise	Collagen	Interaction
Initial body weight (g)									
Collagen(-)	EX(-)	115.3 ± 0.9	0.739	0.665	0.787	113.7 ± 2.1	0.759	0.218	0.240
	EX(+)	116.1 ± 1.5				115.5 ± 0.7			
Collagen(+)	EX(-)	116.3 ± 1.6				116.6 ± 1.2			
	EX(+)	116.4 ± 1.8				115.6 ± 0.6			
Final body weight (g)									
Collagen(-)	EX(-)	405.3 ± 5.5	<0.001	0.250	0.350	411.7 ± 8.8	<0.001	0.014	0.903
	EX(+)	342.0 ± 7.2				354.1 ± 8.5			
Collagen(+)	EX(-)	391.0 ± 8.5				391.5 ± 5.4			
	EX(+)	340.5 ± 7.3				335.7 ± 8.7			
Body weight gain (g/d)									
Collagen(-)	EX(-)	4.0 ± 0.1	<0.001	0.189	0.259	4.1 ± 0.1	<0.001	0.006	0.758
	EX(+)	3.1 ± 0.1				3.2 ± 0.1			
Collagen(+)	EX(-)	3.7 ± 0.1				3.7 ± 0.1			
	EX(+)	3.0 ± 0.1				3.0 ± 0.1			
Food intake (g/d)									
Collagen(-)	EX(-)	20.9 ± 0.2	<0.001	0.215	0.147	19.9 ± 0.2**	<0.001	0.019	0.712
	EX(+)	18.2 ± 0.4				17.9 ± 0.3			
Collagen(+)	EX(-)	20.2 ± 0.2				19.3 ± 0.2**			
	EX(+)	18.3 ± 0.3				17.5 ± 0.12*			
Food efficiency[1]									
Collagen(-)	EX(-)	0.19 ± 0.00	<0.001	0.224	0.784	0.20 ± 0.00**	<0.001	0.028	0.926
	EX(+)	0.17 ± 0.00				0.18 ± 0.00*			
Collagen(+)	EX(-)	0.18 ± 0.01				0.19 ± 0.00			
	EX(+)	0.16 ± 0.00				0.17 ± 0.01			

[1]Food efficiency was calculated by Body weight gain (g/d)/Food intake (g/d). EX(−): sedentary group, EX(+): exercise group.
Values are expressed as means ± SE. Data were analyzed by two-way ANOVA at the 5% level of significance. Interaction means Exercise-Collagen interaction.
*p < 0.05 and *p < 0.01 vs. respective 20% protein group.

Femoral weights and length

Exercise and dietary HC effects were obtained in the adjusted wet weight and dry weight of femur among the 20% protein groups ($p < 0.001$, $p < 0.01$ for exercise; $p < 0.01$, $p < 0.001$ for dietary HC, respectively). In the adjusted ash weight, exercise effect was obtained among the 20% protein groups ($p < 0.001$). Among the 40% protein groups, similar results were obtained for exercise ($p < 0.001$, respectively) and for dietary HC ($p < 0.01$, $p < 0.001$, $p < 0.01$, respectively) (Table 3). There were no differences between the 20% protein groups and the 40% protein groups. In femoral length, the exercise groups were lower than the sedentary groups in both the 20% protein groups and the 40% protein groups, and exercise effect was obtained among the 20% protein groups ($p < 0.01$) (Table 3). Dietary HC effect was not obtained in femoral length both among the 20% protein groups and the 40% protein groups.

Bone breaking force and energy of femur

Among the 20% protein groups, exercise effect was obtained in the adjusted femoral breaking force and energy ($p < 0.01$, respectively) and the exercise groups were significantly higher than those in the sedentary groups, whereas dietary HC effect was not significant (Table 4). Similarly, among the 40% protein groups, exercise effect was only obtained in the adjusted femoral breaking force and energy ($p < 0.01$ for adjusted breaking force; $p < 0.05$ for adjusted breaking energy), and dietary HC effect was not significant (Table 4). There were no differences in both the adjusted femoral breaking force and energy between the 20% protein groups and the 40% protein groups.

Bone metabolic marker

BAP activity did not differ among the 20% protein groups (Casein20: 38.70 ± 15.20U/L, Casein20 + Ex: 55.28 ±

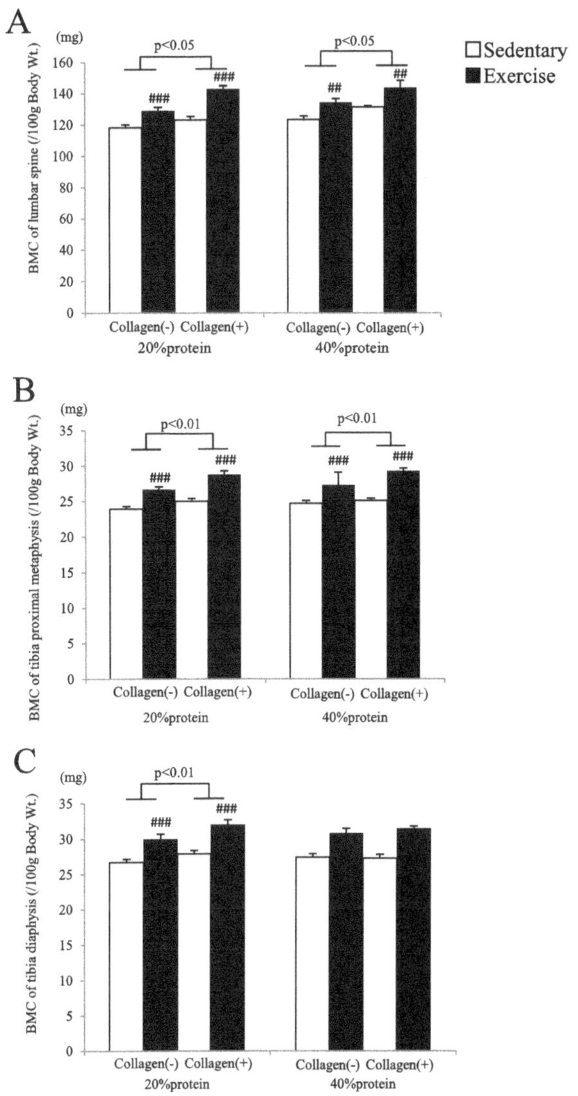

Figure 1 Adjusted bone mineral content of lumbar spine, tibia proximal metaphysis, and tibia diaphysis. Bone mineral content of lumbar spine **(A)**, tibia proximal metaphysis **(B)** and tibia diaphysis **(C)** adjusted to the 100 g body weight. The lumbar spine and tibia of each rat were isolated by dissection, and muscle and connective tissue were carefully removed. BMC was then measured by dual-energy X-ray absorptiometry. Vertical bars indicate the standard error. p value indicates statistical significant difference among dietary protein groups.

12.14U/L, HC20: 33.91 ± 8.91U/L, HC20 + Ex: 33.91 ± 10.16U/l). Similarly, among the 40% protein groups, there were no differences (Casein40: 35.75 ± 8.69U/l, Casein40 + Ex: 38.14 ± 10.01U/l, HC40: 33.31 ± 7.90U/l, HC40 + Ex: 37.66 ± 7.58U/l). Moreover, TRAP activity did not also differ among the 20% and 40% protein groups, respectively (Casein20: 19.39 ± 2.11U/L, Casein20 + Ex: 24.59 ± 3.36U/L, HC20: 17.75 ± 3.97U/L, HC20 + Ex: 18.81 ± 2.20U/L, Casein40: 19.65 ± 1.27U/L, Casein40 + Ex: 22.10 ± 4.47U/L, HC40: 20.47 ± 1.43U/L, HC40 + Ex: 21.75 ± 1.67U/L). In these two bone metabolic markers, there were no differences between the 20% protein groups and the 40% protein groups.

Discussion

We investigated the effects of HC intake and treadmill running exercise on bone mass and strength in growing male rats. This study demonstrated that HC intake increases bone mass in both trained and untrained growing rats. Although these results were shown in both moderate and high protein intake groups, the level of these beneficial effects on bone mass was similar for the two groups. The intake of a high protein diet containing HC may have no more beneficial effect on bone mass and strength on growing rats trained with running exercise than the intake of a moderate protein diet containing HC.

In the present study, we showed the effect of HC intake and treadmill running exercise on adjusted BMC of lumbar spine and tibia. The adjusted BMC was higher in the exercise groups (Casein20 + Ex, Casein40 + Ex, HC20 + Ex, and HC40 + Ex) than in the sedentary groups (Casein20, Casein40, HC20, and HC40). Especially in the trained HC intake groups (HC20 + Ex, HC40 + Ex), those effects were strongly observed. Guillerminet et al. [21] had shown that the BMD for OVX mice fed with the diet including HC (porcine origin) was significantly higher as compared to OVX mice fed on a standard AIN-93N diet. Mizoguchi et al. [22] had also shown that the HC (marine fish origin) intake increased the level of serum osteocalcin (OC), a well-known marker of osteogenesis, along with the BMD and the bone strength of femur in OVX rats. The levels of serum hydroxyproline and glycine of the HC intake group were increased in those cases. These results suggest that dietary HC intake increases the level of serum amino acid (hydroxyproline and glycine), the important components of bone, which then increases the BMD and bone strength. Moreover, *in vitro* study, hydrolyzed collagens (bovine, porcine, and fish origin, respectively having a molecular weight of 2 or 5 kDa) in osteoblasts had significant and dose-dependent increase in ALP activity, a well-known marker of osteogenesis [23]. These results suggest that dietary hydrolyzed collagen may increase bone formation. Although, our result did not show the difference of bone formation marker, we cautiously postulated that the beneficial effect of HC intake in this study could have acted on bone during growth phase since we assessed the bone markers by end-point experiment when being already adult bone. Taken together, these results suggest that HC intake has a beneficial effect on bone mass in growing rats and this effect is more beneficial for rats participating in treadmill running exercise.

Our study also investigated whether the intake of a high protein diet containing HC has positive effects on bone mass and strength of growing rats trained with

Table 3 Femoral weights and length

		20% protein	Two-way ANOVA (p value)			40% protein	Two-way ANOVA (p value)		
			Exercise	Collagen	Interaction		Exercise	Collagen	Interaction
Wet weight (g)									
Collagen(-)	EX(-)	0.9860 ± 0.0010	0.189	0.116	0.888	1.0127 ± 0.0206	0.326	0.570	0.271
	EX(+)	0.9633 ± 0.0290				0.9712 ± 0.0107			
Collagen(+)	EX(-)	1.0191 ± 0.0215				1.0020 ± 0.0159			
	EX(+)	0.9910 ± 0.0145				1.0044 ± 0.0319			
Wet weight (g/100g Body Wt.)									
Collagen(-)	EX(-)	0.2434 ± 0.0026	<0.001	0.006	0.633	0.2461 ± 0.0045	<0.001	0.001	0.191
	EX(+)	0.2796 ± 0.0077				0.2772 ± 0.0037			
Collagen(+)	EX(-)	0.2605 ± 0.0032				0.2560 ± 0.0035			
	EX(+)	0.2918 ± 0.0057				0.2988 ± 0.0066			
Dry weight (g)									
Collagen(-)	EX(-)	0.6363 ± 0.0088	0.013	0.152	0.540	0.6401 ± 0.0126	0.327	0.207	0.508
	EX(+)	0.6031 ± 0.0110				0.6202 ± 0.0075			
Collagen(+)	EX(-)	0.6450 ± 0.0142				0.6475 ± 0.0082			
	EX(+)	0.6247 ± 0.0088				0.6436 ± 0.0199			
Dry weight (g/100g Body Wt.)									
Collagen(-)	EX(-)	0.1570 ± 0.0021	0.001	<0.001	0.851	0.1556 ± 0.0028	<0.001	<0.001	0.365
	EX(+)	0.1751 ± 0.0027				0.1769 ± 0.0021			
Collagen(+)	EX(-)	0.1649 ± 0.0021				0.1654 ± 0.0016			
	EX(+)	0.1838 ± 0.0028				0.1915 ± 0.0040			
Ash weight (g)									
Collagen(-)	EX(-)	0.3981 ± 0.0109	0.193	0.572	0.686	0.4040 ± 0.0125	0.726	0.442	0.751
	EX(+)	0.3793 ± 0.0117				0.3972 ± 0.0037			
Collagen(+)	EX(-)	0.3998 ± 0.0128				0.4086 ± 0.0071			
	EX(+)	0.3899 ± 0.0108				0.4083 ± 0.0175			
Ash weight (g/100g Body Wt.)									
Collagen(-)	EX(-)	0.0982 ± 0.0016	<0.001	0.095	0.896	0.0982 ± 0.0027	<0.001	0.005	0.688
	EX(+)	0.1101 ± 0.0026				0.1134 ± 0.0024			
Collagen(+)	EX(-)	0.1022 ± 0.0016				0.1044 ± 0.0012			
	EX(+)	0.1147 ± 0.0034				0.1215 ± 0.0034			
Ash weight (g/Dry weight)									
Collagen(-)	EX(-)	0.6252 ± 0.0069	0.553	0.396	0.985	0.6310 ± 0.0033	0.223	0.577	0.540
	EX(+)	0.6287 ± 0.0042				0.6413 ± 0.0094			
Collagen(+)	EX(-)	0.6200 ± 0.0044				0.6313 ± 0.0038			
	EX(+)	0.6237 ± 0.0083				0.6347 ± 0.0037			
Length (cm)									
Collagen(-)	EX(-)	3.710 ± 0.014	0.004	0.216	0.109	3.696 ± 0.015	0.084	0.851	0.082
	EX(+)	3.623 ± 0.023				3.646 ± 0.009			
Collagen(+)	EX(-)	3.699 ± 0.017				3.668 ± 0.010			
	EX(+)	3.675 ± 0.018				3.669 ± 0.023			

Table 3 Femoral weights and length *(Continued)*

		20% protein	Exercise	Collagen	Interaction	40% protein	Exercise	Collagen	Interaction
Long Width (cm)									
Collagen(-)	EX(-)	0.440 ± 0.005	0.848	0.266	0.722	0.441 ± 0.005	1.000	0.035	0.3391
	EX(+)	0.438 ± 0.004				0.436 ± 0.003			
Collagen(+)	EX(-)	0.444 ± 0.006				0.446 ± 0.005			
	EX(+)	0.445 ± 0.005				0.451 ± 0.006			
Short Width (cm)									
Collagen(-)	EX(-)	0.352 ± 0.004	0.169	0.328	0.591	0.348 ± 0.005	0.121	0.385	0.746
	EX(+)	0.345 ± 0.003				0.344 ± 0.002			
Collagen(+)	EX(-)	0.346 ± 0.004				0.353 ± 0.003			
	EX(+)	0.343 ± 0.003				0.346 ± 0.005			

Values are expressed d as means ± SE. Data were analyzed by two-way ANOVA at the 5% level of significance. Interaction means Exercise-Collagen interaction.

running exercise. Although the adjusted BMC of lumbar spine and tibia were significantly higher in the HC groups than in the casein groups among both the 20% protein groups and the 40% protein groups, the dietary HC effect had no dose-dependent increase. In the previous study, we had shown that a high protein, two times the 20% moderate casein intake, had no positive effect on bone mass and strength in growing rats [14]. Moreover, in this study, the intake of a high protein diet containing HC also had no more beneficial effect than a moderate protein diet containing HC on bone mass and strength in growing rats. These results suggest that the beneficial effect of HC intake on increasing bone mass may have been limited.

Interestingly, the beneficial effect of HC intake was not observed on bone strength. Seventy percent of bone strength depends on its density and 30% depends on its quality [24]. The bone quality is determined by the degree

Table 4 Breaking force and energy of the femoral diaphysis

		20% protein	Two-way ANOVA (p value)			40% protein	Two-way ANOVA (p value)		
			Exercise	Collagen	Interaction		Exercise	Collagen	Interaction
Breaking force (×10^6 dyn)									
Collagen(-)	EX(-)	29.358 ± 1.396	0.574	0.523	0.068	27.864 ± 1.105	0.757	0.708	0.547
	EX(+)	26.702 ± 0.928				29.132 ± 1.994			
Collagen(+)	EX(-)	26.618 ± 1.358				29.222 ± 1.101			
	EX(+)	28.037 ± 0.803				28.816 ± 1.255			
Breaking force (×10^6 dyn/100g Body Wt.)[1]									
Collagen(-)	EX(-)	7.234 ± 0.329	0.001	0.909	0.082	6.766 ± 0.227	0.002	0.274	0.605
	EX(+)	7.741 ± 0.231				8.343 ± 0.179			
Collagen(+)	EX(-)	6.798 ± 0.31				7.455 ± 0.254			
	EX(+)	8.237 ± 0.218				8.591 ± 0.352			
Breaking energy (×10^5 erg)									
Collagen(-)	EX(-)	20.301 ± 1.598	0.458	0.919	0.182	17.202 ± 1.778	0.492	0.195	0.145
	EX(+)	19.430 ± 1.116				20.546 ± 1.048			
Collagen(+)	EX(-)	18.203 ± 1.704				21.499 ± 1.280			
	EX(+)	21.231 ± 1.480				20.290 ± 1.982			
Breaking energy (×10^5 erg/100d Body Wt.)[1]									
Collagen(-)	EX(-)	4.987 ± 0.37	0.002	0.886	0.269	4.191 ± 0.436	0.010	0.070	0.190
	EX(+)	5.758 ± 0.221				5.833 ± 0.296			
Collagen(+)	EX(-)	4.644 ± 0.407				5.496 ± 0.376			
	EX(+)	6.202 ± 0.389				6.047 ± 0.569			

Values are expressed as means ± SD. Data were analyzed by two-way ANOVA at the 5% level of significance. Interaction means Exercise-Collagen interaction.
[1]Breaking force and energy adjusted to the 100g body weight to exclude the influence of body mass.

of bone mineralization, microdamage accumulation, bone size, collagen crosslinks formation and bone turnover rate [25]. Thus, the reason for the same level of bone strength between the casein groups and the HC intake groups despite the higher level of bone mass in the HC intake groups than in the casein intake groups might be in the bone quality difference. Mizoguchi et al. had investigated that mineral and collagen derived from fish-skin supplementation tend to improve bone strength in OVX rats [26]. On the other hand, there are very few studies investigating the effect of HC intake on bone strength during growth phase. Our data suggest that the effect of HC intake may change in different bone statuses. More investigation is necessary to discuss the effect of HC intake on bone quality and strength.

Our study had several limitations. The food intake and final body weight were significantly lower in the exercise groups than in the sedentary groups. Moreover, among the 40% protein groups, these data were significantly lower in the HC intake groups than in the casein intake groups. Growth of bone is considerably influenced by body mass [27]. Therefore, we were unable to precisely describe the relation of weight-related growth and benefits of physical exercise. Moreover, we had investigated the effect of HC intake by exchanging a part of casein with HC (30% of protein was HC). Therefore, the amount of carbohydrate and essential amino acids were different between 20% protein diet and 40% protein diet. This may have had some effect on the results of our previous study. Further research is needed to assess the effect of HC intake in conditions where the amount of other nutrition is adjusted.

In summary, the present study demonstrated that moderate HC intake (where the diet contains 20% protein, of which 30% is HC) increased bone mass during growth periods and further promoted the effect of running exercise. On the other hand, a high protein diet containing HC (where the diet contains 40% protein, of which 30% is HC) had no more beneficial effect on bone mass than the moderate protein intake. These results could be of potential interest for new nutritional support in the increasing effect of physical exercise on bone mass during growth.

Competing interests

The authors declare no competing interests.

Authors' contributions

ST conceived of the study and carried out: 1) study design, 2) data collection, 3) data analysis, 4) statistical analysis and 5) preparing manuscript. JHP assisted in 1) data analysis and 2) preparing the manuscript. EK assisted in 1) study design and 2) data collection. IE assisted in coordination and helped to draft the manuscript. NO procured grant funding and assisted in: 1) study design, 2) data collection and analysis, and 3) preparing the manuscript. All authors read and approved the final manuscript.

Acknowledgements

The authors are grateful to all of the members of the Exercise and Nutrition Laboratory at the University of Tsukuba for their kind cooperation in the anatomy work. PARK, JH is supported by Japan Society for the Promotion of Science (JSPS).

Author details

[1]Graduate School of Comprehensive Human Sciences, University of Tsukuba, Ibaraki, Japan. [2]Center for Disease Biology and Integrative Medicine, University of Tokyo, Tokyo, Japan. [3]Department of Physical Education, Konkuk University, Seoul, South Korea. [4]Yokohama Research Center, JNC Corporation, Yokohama, Japan. [5]Japan Women's University, Tokyo, Japan. [6]Faculty of Health and Sport Sciences, University of Tsukuba, Ibaraki, Japan. [7]Institute of Health and Sports Sciences, Graduate School of Comprehensive Human Sciences, University of Tsukuba, Tsukuba, Ibaraki 305-8574, Japan.

References

1. Hind K, Burrows M: **Weight-bearing exercise and bone mineral accrual in children and adolescents: a review of controlled trials.** *Bone* 2007, **40**(1):14–27.
2. Chevalley T, Bonjour JP, Ferrari S, Rizzoli R: **High-protein intake enhances the positive impact of physical activity on BMC in prepubertal boys.** *J Bone Miner Res* 2008, **23**(1):131–142.
3. Carlsohn A, Cassel M, Linne K, Mayer F: **How much is too much? A case report of nutritional supplement use of a high-performance athlete.** *Br J Nutr* 2011, **25**:1–5.
4. Oishi Y, Fu ZW, Ohnuki Y, Kato H, Noguchi T: **Molecular basis of the alteration in skin collagen metabolism in response to in vivo dexamethasone treatment: effects on the synthesis of collagen type I and III, collagenase, and tissue inhibitors of metalloproteinases.** *Br J Dermatol* 2002, **147**(5):859–868.
5. Takeuchi Y, Nakayama K, Matsumoto T: **Differentiation and cell surface expression of transforming growth factor-beta receptors are regulated by interaction with matrix collagen in murine osteoblastic cells.** *J Biol Chem* 1996, **271**(7):3938–3944.
6. Takeuchi Y, Suzawa M, Kikuchi T, Nishida E, Fujita T, Matsumoto T: **Differentiation and transforming growth factor-beta receptor down-regulation by collagen-alpha2beta1 integrin interaction is mediated by focal adhesion kinase and its downstream signals in murine osteoblastic cells.** *J Biol Chem* 1997, **272**(46):29309–29316.
7. Gaffney PJ, Edgell TA, Dawson PA, Ford AW, Stocker E: **A pig collagen peptide fraction. A unique material for maintaining biological activity during lyophilization and during storage in the liquid state.** *J Pharm Pharmacol* 1996, **48**(9):896–898.
8. Khare SD, Krco CJ, Griffiths MM, Luthara HS, David CS: **Oral administration of an immunodominant human collagen peptide modulates collagen-induced arthritis.** *J Immunol* 1995, **155**(7):3653–3659.
9. Ku G, Kronenberg M, Peacock DJ, Tempst P, Banquerigo ML, Braun BS, Reeve JR Jr, Brahn E: **Prevention of experimental autoimmune arthritis with a peptide fragment of type II collagen.** *Eur J Immunol* 1993, **23**(3):591–599.
10. Wu J, Fujioka M, Sugimoto K, Mu G, Ishimi Y: **Assessment of effectiveness of oral administration of collagen peptide on bone metabolism in growing and mature rats.** *J Bone Miner Metab* 2004, **22**(6):547–553.
11. Nomura Y, Oohashi K, Watanabe M, Kasugai S: **Increase in bone mineral density through oral administration of shark gelatin to ovariectomized rats.** *Nutrition* 2005, **21**(11–12):1120–1126.
12. Adam M, Spacek P, Hulejová H, Galiánová A, Blahos J: **Postmenopausal osteoporosis. Treatment with calcitonin and a diet rich in collagen proteins.** *Cas Lek Cesk* 1996, **135**(3):74–78.
13. Yahya ZA, Bates PC, Millward DJ: **Responses to protein deficiency of plasma and tissue insulin-like growth factor-I levels and proteoglycan synthesis rates in rat skeletal muscle and bone.** *J Endocrinol* 1990, **127**(3):497–503.
14. Takeda S, Kobayashi Y, Park JH, Ezawa I, Omi N: **Effect of different levels of dietary protein and physical exercise on bone mineral density and bone strength in growing male rats.** *J Nutr Sci Vitaminol* 2012, **58**(4):240–246.
15. Jenkins DJ, Kendall CW, Vidgen E, Augustin LS, Parker T, Faulkner D, Vieth R, Vandenbroucke AC, Josse RG: **Effect of high vegetable protein diets on urinary calcium loss in middle-aged men and women.** *Eur J Clin Nutr* 2003, **57**(2):376–382.

16. Reeves PG, Nielsen FH, Fahey GC Jr: **AIN-93 purified diets for laboratory rodents: final report of the American Institute of Nutrition ad hoc writing committee on the reformulation of the AIN-76A rodent diet.** *J Nutr* 1993, **123**(11):1939–1951.
17. Wheeler DL, Graves JE, Miller GL, Vander-Griend RE, Wronski TJ, Powers SK, Park HM: **Effects of running in the torisional strength, morphometry, and bone mass of the rat skeleton.** *Med Sci Sports Exerc* 1995, **27**(4):520–529.
18. Omi N, Tsukahara N, Ezawa I: **Effect of milk on bone metabolism in growing male and female rats.** *J Home Econ Jpn* 2001, **52**(8):689–698.
19. Ezawa I, Okada R, Nozaki Y, Ogata E: **Breaking-properties and ash contents of the femur of growing rat fed a low calcium diet.** *J Jpn Soc Food Nutr* 1979, **32**(5):329–335.
20. Omi N, Goseki M, Oida S, Sasaki S, Ezawa I: **The nutritional evaluation of globin on maintenance of bone metabolism in ovariectomized osteoporotic rats.** *J Nutr Sci Vitaminol* 1994, **40**(5):443–457.
21. Guillerminet F, Fabien-Soulé V, Even PC, Tomé D, Benhamou CL, Roux C, Blais A: **Hydrolyzed collagen improves bone status and prevents bone loss in ovariectomized C3H/HeN mice.** *Osteoporos Int* 2012, **23**(7):1909–1919.
22. Mizoguchi T, Tamura K, Yoshida T, Nagasawa S, Terashima N, Horosawa N, Yagasaki H, Matahira Y, Ito M: **Mineral and collagen derived from fish-skin supplementation improves bone metabolism in overiectomized rats part II.** *J Jpn Dent Mater* 2006, **25**(2):192.
23. Guillerminet F, Beaupied H, Fabien-Soulé V, Tomé D, Benhamou CL, Roux C, Blais A: **Hydrolyzed collagen improves bone metabolism and biomechanical parameters in ovariectomized mice: an in vitro and in vivo study.** *Bone* 2010, **46**(3):827–834.
24. NIH Consensus Development Panel: **Osteoporosis prevention, diagnosis, and therapy.** *JAMA* 2001, **285**(6):785–795.
25. Saito M, Fujii K, Marumo K: **Degree of mineralization-related collagen crosslinking in the femoral neck cancellous bone in cases of hip fracture and controls.** *Calcif Tissue Int* 2006, **79**(3):160–168.
26. Mizoguchi T, Tamura K, Yoshida T, Nagasawa S, Terashima N, Horosawa N, Yagasaki H, Matahira Y, Ito M: **Mineral and collagen derived from fish-skin supplementation improves bone metabolism in overiectomized rats.** *J Jpn Dent Mater* 2005, **24**(5):398.
27. Huang TH, Hsieh SS, Liu SH, Chang FL, Lin SC, Yang RS: **Swimming training increases the post-yield energy of bone in young male rats.** *Calcif Tissue Int* 2010, **86**(2):142–153.

Sports drink consumption and diet of children involved in organized sport

Dona L Tomlin[1], Shannon K Clarke[1], Meghan Day[2], Heather A McKay[3] and Patti-Jean Naylor[1*]

Abstract

Background: Organized sport provides one option for children to be physically active. However, there is a paucity of information about the relationship between children's participation in organized sport and their diet, and specifically their sports drink consumption. Therefore, the relationship between sports participation in children and the consumption of sports drinks, sugar-sweetened beverages (SSBs) and other components of diet was examined.

Methods: A cross-sectional descriptive study was conducted using baseline data from the Action Schools! BC Dissemination study cohort (n = 1421; 9.90 (0.58) y; 736 girls, 685 boys). The differences between the dietary behaviours of children participating in organized sport (sport) versus those that did not participate (non-sport) was examined. A modified Physical Activity Questionnaire for Older Children (PAQ-C) was used to measure physical activity levels and participation in organized sport. A Food Frequency Questionnaire (FFQ) and 24-hour dietary recall were used to assess eating behaviour and macronutrient intake (including protein, fat, and carbohydrate as well as sugar, fibre and total calories). Fruit, vegetable and beverage quantities were hand-tallied from the dietary recall. Fruit, vegetable and beverage frequency was assessed using the FFQ. Analysis of covariance (ANCOVA) was used to analyse differences between groups and a chi-square test of association was use to determine if participation in sport was significantly associated with the proportion of children consuming sports drinks and SSBs, and with gender.

Results: Children involved in sport had a lower body mass index (BMI) and were more physically active than children in the non-sport group ($p < 0.01$). Only a small number (n = 20/1421) of children consumed sports drinks and no difference in consumption of sports drink between sport and non-sport participants ($p > .05$) was observed. However, children involved in organized sport consumed more total calories, fat, fibre, fruit, vegetables and non-flavoured milk ($p < 0.01$) than non-sport children.

Conclusions: Children involved in organized sport were more physically active, consumed a healthier diet than non-participants and on average had lower BMI's despite consuming more calories. As consumption of sports drinks among this age group was low, this may be an ideal time to begin educating children and their parents about the appropriate consumption of sports drinks and the perils of consuming too many SSBs, specifically.

Keywords: Organized sport, Children, Diet, Physical activity, Sugar-sweetened beverage, Sports drink

Background

The continued challenge of escalating levels of childhood obesity levels in Canada and around the world demands innovative approaches to healthy eating and physical activity [1]. A healthy diet is a necessary ingredient to promote normal maturation, healthy growth, injury prevention and overall health during the crucial years of growth and development [2]. However, the relationship between nutrition, physical activity, sport, weight management, fitness and health is complex. For example, in theory, children who participate in sport require the highest levels of nutrition to meet the energy demands of their activities. Still, there are limited data that describe the association between sport participation and eating behaviours (including beverage consumption) in children.

Although research that addresses this issue in children is limited, athletic adolescents appear to consume a

* Correspondence: pjnaylor@uvic.ca
[1]School of Exercise Science, Physical and Health Education, University of Victoria, Victoria, BC, Canada
Full list of author information is available at the end of the article

healthier diet than their non-athletic counterparts [3-5]. Only one study on pre-adolescents [6] was found in the literature and it addressed physical activity rather than sport, demonstrating that increased levels of physical activity in 8–10 year old African-American girls were associated with lower BMI, higher carbohydrate consumption and lower fat intake.

Within the diets of many children and youth, consumption of sugar sweetened beverages (SSBs) has been linked to their excess weight gain [7]. SSBs include carbonated beverages as well as other beverages that contain added caloric sweeteners. Many of these drinks contain few nutrients and excess consumption can also lead to dental erosion and decay [8]. Sports drinks are a specific category of SSBs. Although sports drinks may be helpful in replenishing blood glucose levels during and following high-intensity exercise and maintaining hydration during prolonged exercise in hot environments [9], excessive consumption may increase the risk of children and adolescents becoming overweight or obese [10].

There is limited evidence about the consumption of sports drinks by adolescents and specifically adolescent athletes. Importantly, to the best of our knowledge there are no published data that describe sports drink consumption in children nor specifically about children who participate in organized sport compared to those who do not. In light of the gaps in the literature and with 75% of Canadian children participating in organized sport [11], the purpose of this study was to examine the relationship between sports participation and consumption of sports drinks, SSBs, fruits, vegetables, milk and macronutrients (including protein, fat, and carbohydrate as well as sugar, fibre and total calories) in children.

Methods

Study design

A cross-sectional descriptive analysis was conducted using baseline data from the Action Schools! BC Dissemination study, a large cluster randomised controlled trial evaluating the effectiveness of a school-based physical activity and healthy eating intervention (n = 1494). Specifically, the relationship between participation in sport and both eating behaviours (sports drink, SSB, milk, fruit and vegetable consumption) and macronutrient intake (including protein, fat, and carbohydrate as well as sugar, fibre and total calories) in n = 1421 grade 4 and 5 children (9.90 (0.58) y; 736 girls and 685 boys) attending 30 schools across four regions of BC was examined. Baseline data were collected during the fall of 2005. The study was approved by the Clinical Research Ethics Board at the University of British Columbia and the Human Research Ethics Board at the University of Victoria.

Participants

Students were recruited in September 2005 via invitation/information letters sent home by the teachers. Written consent was obtained from parents/guardians; children gave verbal and written assent. In all, 1494 students consented to participate in the study at baseline. Of those, 1441 students were measured (n = 52 students were absent and n = 1 moved prior to being measured). The 1421 children who completed the question regarding their participation in organized sport that was part of the Physical Activity Questionnaire for Children (PAQ-C) were included in the analysis.

Measurement procedures

Descriptive characteristics

Stretched stature to the nearest 0.1 cm (Seca 214 Portable Stadiometer) and weight to the nearest 0.1 kg (Conair digital electronic scale) were each measured twice and the mean was used in the analysis. Body Mass Index (BMI) was calculated from height and weight as kg/m^2. Overweight/obesity was calculated using age and BMI [12].

Dietary measures

Two instruments were used to assess the diet of each participant. The EHSA Food Processor Nutrition and Fitness Software (v. 10.0, Salem, OR) was used to determine macronutrients (also including total calories, fibre and sugar) consumed from a validated 24-hour dietary recall [13]. As well, fruit, vegetables, milk, 100% fruit juice, sports drinks and SSBs (including flavoured milk, carbonated beverages, non-carbonated flavoured beverages, sweetened coffee and tea, and sports beverages) were hand-tallied from the dietary recall, with serving size determined using the Canadian Nutrient File [14]. Typical frequency of fruit, vegetable, milk and 100% fruit juice consumption was assessed using a targeted Food Frequency Questionnaire (FFQ) adapted from the US National Cancer Institute's National Institutes of Health: Eating at America's Table Study Quick Food Scan [15].

Physical activity

Physical activity and participation in organized sport was measured using a modified version of the PAQ-C [16]. The PAQ-C is a valid and reliable tool for assessing moderate-to-vigorous physical activity (PA) over the previous 7 days [16,17]. The physical activity score (PA score) ranges from 1 (low active) to 5 (high active) and was calculated from the mean score of nine questions related to frequency and intensity of PA. In addition, students were asked if they participated in organized sport outside of school and then to describe the sport activity and indicate the days they participate in that sport during the week. Those who reported participation in any organized sport and identified the sport and participation frequency were assigned to the 'sport' group and those who did not were assigned to the 'non-sport' group. Of the students who participated in the study, 886 fell into the sport group (441 girls, 445 boys) and 535 into the non-sport group (295 girls, 240 boys). 65.0% of boys and 59.9% of girls participated in sports ($\chi^2 = 3.87$, $p < 0.05$).

Statistical analyses

Data were analyzed using the Statistical Package for the Social Sciences (SPSS; v20.0, Chicago, IL). Descriptive summaries were generated and the differences in physical activity and dietary measures between sport and non-sport groups were initially analysed using one-way analysis of variance (ANOVA). As there were significant differences in the number of boys and girls between groups and in total caloric consumption, a one-way analysis of covariance (ANCOVA) was used to determine differences in diet between groups while adjusting for caloric intake and gender. A chi-square test of association was used to determine if participation in sport was significantly associated with the proportion of children consuming SSBs or sports drinks, or with gender.

Results

Descriptive characteristics

There was no difference in age ($p = 0.42$) between sport and non-sport groups. However, BMI was significantly lower in the sport group (Difference = 1.65 kg/m^2, $p < 0.01$) and fewer sport participants were overweight or obese ($p < 0.01$).

Physical activity

PA score was significantly higher ($p < 0.01$) in the sport versus non-sport group (Table 1).

Dietary measures

Results from the 24-hour dietary recall and FFQ are provided (Table 1). Total calories and gender differed significantly between groups. When controlling for these the sport group consumed significantly more fibre, vegetable and fruit servings (independently and together) and non-flavoured milk, but a similar amount of protein, carbohydrate and sugar compared with the non-sport group. From the FFQ, the sport group consumed fruit, vegetables, non-flavoured milk and 100% juice more frequently than the non-sport group. Consumption of SSBs or sports drinks did not differ significantly between the groups. Similar proportions of sport and non-sport participants reported SSB ($\chi^2 = .626$, $p = .429$) and sports drink ($\chi^2 = 1.38$, $p = .240$) consumption on the dietary recall.

Discussion

The profile of children participating in organized sport compared to those that were not provides new insight into the relationship between sport participation and children's consumption of sports drinks specifically, and aspects of their overall diet generally. Contrary to previous reports on adolescents no difference was found in consumption of sports drinks or SSBs between children participating in sport and those that were not. However, similar to previous reports, children involved in sport had, on average, lower BMIs, were more physically active and had a healthier diet profile (consumed more fruit, vegetables, non-flavoured milk and fibre). Each of these will be discussed in turn.

Descriptive characteristics

BMI is considered by some to be a reasonable measure of adiposity in children [18]. This study adds to a small body of literature that investigated the relationship between sport participation and BMI in children. Based on BMI, higher proportions of overweight and obesity were seen in this study (29.8% overweight or obese) compared to Canadian children measured in the 2004 Canadian Community Health Survey (CCHS; 25.8% overweight or obese) [19] but in the present study the sport group had lower BMI (18.31 versus 19.96 kg/m^2; $p < 0.01$) and lower rates of overweight/obesity (27.8 versus 33.3%; $p < 0.01$) than the non-sport group.

These findings align with a few studies that reported that organized sport participation in children was associated with lower BMI [6,20,21] while contradicting other findings that found no association between sport participation and weight status [22]. The different methods adopted across studies might partially explain these variable findings. One study used an overweight cut-off point [21] as was used in the present study, and another used an obesity cut-off point [22]. For analysis some studies calculated simple correlations [6,20] while the present study applied ANCOVA to evaluate group-based differences.

Physical activity

While 62.4% of children in the current study reported participation in organized sport, the Canadian Fitness and Lifestyle Research Institute (CFLRI) reported 75% sport participation among 5–17 year old Canadians [11]. This discrepancy may be because while the CFLRI results were based on parental reports, children involved in the current study self-reported their participation. The results are also consistent with previous findings that children involved in organized sport are more likely to be physically active than non-participating peers [22,23]. The PA score averages of 2.9 and 3.3 for non-sport and sport groups, respectively are similar to those reported in grade 4, 5 and 6 students in the United Kingdom [24] and 9–18 year olds in Canada [25].

Table 1 Descriptive characteristics and results of analysis of covariance (ANCOVA) of physical activity, dietary intake and beverage consumption for sport and non-sport children

	Non-sport group (295 girls, 240 boys)		Sport group (441 girls, 445 boys)		
Variables	**N**	**Mean (SD)**	**N**	**Mean (SD)**	**Significance**
Descriptive characteristics					
Age (years)	528	9.90 (0.60)	881	9.93 (.57)	$p = 0.42$
BMI (kg/m^2)	532	19.96 (3.97)	882	18.31 (3.29)	$p < 0.01$
% overweight/obese [a]	532	33.3%	882	27.8%	$p < 0.01$
Physical activity					
PAscore	491	2.9 (0.7)	807	3.3 (0.6)	$p < 0.01$
Dietary intake					
24 hour recall					
Calories (Kcal/d)	527	1837.3 (707.6)	870	1966.8 (755.0)	$p < 0.01$
Protein (g/d)	527	69.0 (30.9)	870	74.7 (33.0)	$P = 0.23$
Fat (g/d)	527	62.2 (37.2)	870	65.8 (38.0)	$p < 0.05$
Carbohydrate (g/d)	527	256.1 (101.1)	870	275.2 (105.8)	$p = 0.16$
Sugar (g/d)	527	110.8 (58.6)	870	122.0 (64.2)	$p = 0.11$
Fibre (g/d)	527	14.8 (7.6)	870	16.4 (8.8)	$p < 0.05$
Fruit servings/d	527	2.4 (2.5)	868	2.8 (2.8)	$p < 0.05$
Vegetable servings/d	527	1.8 (1.9)	868	2.1 (2.1)	$p < 0.05$
FV servings/d	527	4.2 (3.4)	868	4.9 (3.8)	$p < 0.01$
FFQ					
Fruit (times/d)	533	1.1 (0.7)	878	1.3 (0.7)	$p < 0.01$
Vegetable (times/d)	532	1.0 (0.6)	876	1.2 (0.7)	$p < 0.01$
Beverages					
24 hour recall					
Non-flavoured milk (mls/d)	527	296.2 (298.7)	868	350.8 (332.8)	$p < 0.05$
100% juice (mls/d)	527	170.1 (249.5)	868	201.0 (269.6)	$p = 0.11$
100% juice servings/d	527	1.4 (2.0)	868	1.6 (2.2)	$p = 0.11$
Sports drinks (mls/d)	5	412.0 (236.9)	15	338.3 (230.8)	$p = 0.92$
SSB - no 100% juice (mls/d)	527	216.9 (285.1)	868	206.9 (306.3)	$p = 0.11$
SSB - with 100% juice (mls/d)	527	387.0 (357.4)	868	407.9 (385.4)	$p = 0.88$
FFQ					
Milk (times/d)	535	1.3 (1.2)	885	1.5 (1.5)	$p < 0.05$
100% Juice (times/d)	535	0.8 (1.0)	882	0.9 (1.1)	$p < 0.05$

[a] – determined by Cole [12].
FV = Fruit and vegetable.
SSB = Sugar sweetened beverage.

Dietary measures

The healthier diet profile observed in the sport group was consistent with previous research on adolescent athletes who, on average, consumed significantly more health promoting foods such as milk and fruit [3,4,26] and, for boys, more vegetables as well [26]. The sport group had higher caloric intake, consuming more fruit, vegetables, fibre and non-flavoured milk than the non-sport group. Even so, less than 50% of the children in sport and non-sport groups met recommended guidelines for fruits and vegetables and the sport group consumed more fat. While these results support the notion that sport-involved children have healthier diets, clearly the diets of both groups have room for improvement.

SSB consumption by both sport and non-sport children in the study was slightly lower than the 450–534 g reported for 9–13 y olds in the CCHS [27]. As well, unlike other reports on adolescents, no differences in SSB or sports drink consumption was observed between those who were and were not involved in organized sport. Ranjit and colleagues noted a positive association between sports drink consumption and participation in organized physical activity and a negative association between soda consumption and organized activity in adolescents [10]. In other research, athletic adolescents were more likely to consume sports drinks than non-athletic adolescents [3]. It is possible that the younger cohort in the current study was not yet influenced by coaches and the media, or was not involved in high intensity training and sport competition (back-to-back training, multiple games or tournament play). It may also be that the younger students lacked the purchasing power of the older adolescents.

Strengths and limitations

One novel element of the study was that, to our knowledge, it is the first examination of sports drink consumption in this age group. A strength of the study was the relatively large sample size (n = 1421) of similar aged children. Also, two different instruments were used to assess diet and even though the dietary recall measured volume and the FFQ measured frequency, both instruments showed similar trends.

We also acknowledge that a cross-sectional study has a number of limitations. Self-report instruments were used to assess PA and diet. In an effort to mitigate this limitation, a questionnaire (PAQ-C) with well-established internal reliability and validity [16] was employed. The measure of organized sport did not address the quality of participation (e.g. intensity) or seasonal variations in level of participation. A single 24-hour dietary recall was used which, despite its common usage, has been criticized for not capturing usual patterns of food consumption [28]. This is especially true for food and beverages, like sports drinks, that may not be consumed daily. Finally, the cross-sectional nature of the data prohibits an evaluation of any causal relationships between variables.

Conclusions

This data suggest that pre-adolescent children involved in sport have healthier diets, physical activity and weight profiles (despite consuming more calories) than children not involved in organized sport. It also shows that at around age 10 years only a small proportion of children are consuming high calorie sports drinks. This speaks to the pre-adolescent period as a potential 'window-of-opportunity' when parents and coaches might exert a positive influence on children's behaviour regarding consumption of sports drinks and SSBs. Athletes and their parents should be educated about proper nutrition relative to their child's/athlete's level of training and competition; including the dangers of high 'empty' nutrient value of SSBs and sports drinks.

Abbreviations

ANOVA: One-way analysis of variance; ANCOVA: One-way analysis of covariance; BMI: Body mass index; FV: Fruit and vegetable; PA: Physical activity; PA Score: Physical activity score; SSB: Sugar-sweetened beverage.

Competing interests

The authors declare that they have no competing interests.

Authors' contributions

SC developed the research question, conducted the preliminary analysis and edited the manuscript. DT supported data collection, provided quality assurance and database management, conducted the secondary analyses, then wrote and edited the overall manuscript. PJN and HMK wrote the funding proposal, managed the implementation of the overall study and edited the manuscript. PJN helped develop the research question and also supervised the analysis of the data. MD worked with PJN and HMK to design the healthy eating component of the trial, including instrument selection and analysis and edited the manuscript. All authors read and approved the final manuscript.

Acknowledgements

We would like to thank the teachers and administrators who made recruitment and data collection possible and the children and parents that participated in the Action Schools! BC study. We would also like to thank the many undergraduate and graduate students that collected and entered the Action Schools! BC data. HAM was supported as a MSFHR (Senior) Scholar. We are grateful for the support from CIHR and the Heart and Stroke Foundation of Canada for funding for this project (OCO 74248; PJN & HAM, CO-PIs) as well as the BC Ministry of Health.

Author details

[1]School of Exercise Science, Physical and Health Education, University of Victoria, Victoria, BC, Canada. [2]BC Ministry of Health, 4th Floor, 1520 Blanshard Street, Victoria, BC, Canada. [3]Centre for Hip Health and Mobility, Vancouver Coastal Health Research Institute, VGH Campus. 302 - 2647Willow Street, Vancouver, BC, Canada.

References

1. Lobstein T, Baur L, Uauy R: **Obesity in children and young people: a crisis in public health.** *Obes Rev* 2004, **5**:4–85.
2. Meyer F, O'Connor H, Shirreffs SM: **Nutrition for the young athlete.** *J Sports Sci* 2007, **25**:73–S82.
3. Cavadini C, Decarli B, Grin J, Narring F, Michaud PA: **Food habits and sport activity during adolescence: differences between athletic and non-athletic teenagers in Switzerland.** *Eur J Clin Nutr* 2000, **54**(S1):16–20.
4. Croll JK, Neumark-Sztainer D, Story M, Wall M, Perry C, Harnack L: **Adolescents involved in weight-related and power team sports have better eating patterns and nutrient intakes than non – sport-involved adolescents.** *J Am Diet Assoc* 2006, **106**(5):709–717.
5. Ottevaere C, Huybrechts I, Béghin L, Cuenca-Garcia M, De Bourdeaudhuij I, Gottrand F, Hagströmer M, Kafatos A, Le Donne C, Moreno LA: **Relationship between self-reported dietary intake and physical activity levels among adolescents: the HELENA study.** *Int J Behav Nutr Phy* 2011, **8**(1):8.
6. Jago R, Baranowski T, Yoo S, Cullen K, Zakeri I, Watson K, Himes J, Pratt C, Sun W, Pruitt L: **Relationship between physical activity and diet among African-American girls.** *Obes Res* 2004, **12**(suppl 1):55S–63S.
7. Malik VS, Schulze MB, Hu FB: **Intake of sugar-sweetened beverages and weight gain: a systematic review.** *Am J Clin Nutr* 2006, **84**(2):274–288.
8. Milosevic A: **Sports drinks hazard to teeth.** *Br J Sports Med* 1997, **31**(1):28–30.
9. Rodrguez NR, DiMarco NM, Langley S: **Position of the American Dietetic Association, Dietitians of Canada, and the American College of Sports Medicine: Nutrition and athletic performance.** *J Am Diet Assoc* 2009, **109**(3):509–527.
10. Ranjit N, Evans MH, Byrd-Williams C, Evans AE, Hoelscher DM: **Dietary and activity correlates of sugar-sweetened beverage consumption among adolescents.** *Pediatrics* 2010, **126**(4):754–e761.

11. *Canadian Fitness and Lifestyle Research Institute.* Ottawa, Ontario, Canada: Canadian Fitness and Lifestyle Research Institute; 2013. http://72.10.49.94/media/node/1161/files/CFLRI_CANPLAY_2011-12_B2_EN.pdf.
12. Cole TJ, Bellizzi MC, Flegal KM, Dietz WH: **Establishing a standard definition for child overweight and obesity worldwide: international survey.** *BMJ* 2000, **320**(7244):1240.
13. Mullenbach V, Kushi LH, Jacobson C, Gomez-Marin O, Prineas RJ, Roth-Yousey L, Sinaiko AR: **Comparison of 3-day food record and 24-hour recall by telephone for dietary evaluation in adolescents.** *J Am Diet Assoc* 1992, **92**(6):743–745.
14. *Canadian Nutrient File.* Ottawa, Ontario, Canada: Health Canada; 2010. www.hc-sc.gc.ca/fn-an/nutrition/fiche-nutri-data/index-eng.php.
15. *National Cancer Institute.* Bethesda, MD, USA: National Institutes of Health; 2000. http://riskfactor.cancer.gov/diet/screeners/fruitveg/allday.pdf.
16. Crocker PRE, Bailey DA, Faulkner RA, Kowalski KC, McGrath R: **Measuring general levels of physical activity: preliminary evidence for the Physical Activity Questionnaire for Older Children.** *Med Sci Sports Exerc* 1997, **29**(10):1344–1349.
17. Kowalski KC, Crocker PRE, Faulkner RA: **Validation of the physical activity questionnaire for older children.** *Pediatric exercise science* 1997, **9**(2):174–186.
18. Dietz WH, Bellizzi MC: **Introduction: the use of body mass index to assess obesity in children.** *Am J Clin Nutr* 1999, **70**(1):123s–125s.
19. Shields M: **Overweight and obesity among children and youth.** *Health Rep* 2006, **17**(3):27–42.
20. Manios Y, Yiannakouris N, Papoutsakis C, Moschonis G, Magkos F, Skenderi K, Zampelas A: **Behavioral and physiological indices related to BMI in a cohort of primary schoolchildren in Greece.** *Am J Hum Biol* 2004, **16**(6):639–647.
21. Antonogeorgos G, Papadimitriou A, Panagiotakos D, Priftis K, Nicolaidou P: **Association of extracurricular sports participation with obesity in Greek children.** *J Sports Med Phys Fitness* 2011, **51**(1):121.
22. Trost SG, Pate RR, Saunders R, Ward DS, Dowda M, Felton G: **A prospective study of the determinants of physical activity in rural fifth-grade children.** *Prev Med* 1997, **26**(2):257.
23. *Canadian Fitness and Lifestyle Research Institute.* Ottawa, Ontario, Canada: Canadian Fitness and Lifestyle Research Institute; 2010. http://www.cflri.ca/media/node/101/files/CANPLAY2010-Bulletin2PALevels-EN.pdf.
24. Ernst M, Pangrazi R: **Effects of a physical activity program on children's activity levels and attraction to physical activity.** *Pediatr Exerc Sci* 1999, **11**:393–405.
25. Thompson AM, Baxter-Jones ADG, Mirwald RL, Bailey DA: **Comparison of physical activity in male and female children: does maturation matter?** *Med Sci Sports Exerc* 2003, **35**(10):1684–1690.
26. Ottevaere C, Huybrechts I, Béghin L, Cuenca-Garcia M, De Bourdeaudhuij I, Gottrand F, Hagströmer M, Kafatos A, Le Donne C, Moreno LA: **Relationship between self-reported dietary intake and physical activity levels among adolescents: the HELENA study.** *Int J of Behav Nutr Phy* 2011, **8**(1):8.
27. Garriguet D: **Overview of Canadians' eating habits.** *Health Rep* 2004, **2**:82–620.
28. Nelson M, Black AE, Morris JA, Cole TJ: **Between- and within-subject variation in nutrient intake from infancy to old age: estimating the number of days required to rank dietary intakes with desired precision.** *Am J Clin Nutr* 1989, **50**(1):155–167.

3

Effects of 8 weeks of Xpand® 2X pre workout supplementation on skeletal muscle hypertrophy, lean body mass, and strength in resistance trained males

Ryan P Lowery[1], Jordan M Joy[1], Joshua E Dudeck[1], Eduardo Oliveira de Souza[2], Sean A McCleary[1], Shawn Wells[3], Robert Wildman[3] and Jacob M Wilson[1*]

Abstract

Background: Xpand® 2X is a proprietary blend comprised of branched chain amino acids, creatine monohydrate, beta-alanine (CarnoSyn®), quercetin, coenzymated B-vitamins, alanyl-glutamine (Sustamine®), and natural nitrate sources from pomegranate and beet root extracts purported to enhance the neuromuscular adaptations of resistance training. However to date, no long-term studies have been conducted with this supplement. The purpose of this study was to investigate the effects of a multi-ingredient performance supplement (MIPS) on skeletal muscle hypertrophy, lean body mass and lower body strength in resistance-trained males.

Methods: Twenty resistance-trained males (21.3 ± 1.9 years) were randomly assigned to consume a MIPS or a placebo of equal weight and volume (food-grade orange flavors and sweeteners) in a double-blind manner, 30 minutes prior to exercise. All subjects participated in an 8-week, 3-day per week, periodized, resistance-training program that was split-focused on multi-joint movements such as leg press, bench press, and bent-over rows. Ultrasonography measured muscle thickness of the quadriceps, dual-energy X-ray absorptiometry (DEXA) determined lean body mass, and strength of the bench press and leg press were determined at weeks 0, 4, and 8 of the study. Data were analyzed with a 2 × 3 repeated measures ANOVA with LSD post hoc tests utilized to locate differences.

Results: There was a significant group-by-time interaction in which the MIPS supplementation resulted in a significant ($p < 0.01$) increase in strength of the bench press (18.4% vs. 9.6%) compared with placebo after 4 and 8 weeks of training. There were no significant group by time interactions between MIPS supplementation nor the placebo in leg press strength ($p = .08$). MIPS supplementation also resulted in a significant increase in lean body mass (7.8% vs. 3.6%) and quadriceps muscle thickness (11.8% vs. 4.5%) compared with placebo (group*time, $p < 0.01$).

Conclusions: These results suggest that this MIPS can positively augment adaptations in strength, and skeletal muscle hypertrophy in resistance-trained men.

Keywords: Pre-workout, Performance, Hypertrophy, Supplementation, Sports nutrition

* Correspondence: jmwilson@ut.edu
[1]Department of Health Sciences and Human Performance, The University of Tampa, Tampa, FL, USA
Full list of author information is available at the end of the article

Background

Sports nutrition scientists have attempted to augment training induced adaptations through a number of supplementation protocols, which generally attempt to enhance and/or speed skeletal muscle development. Research-supported interventions include the provision of the branched chain amino acids (BCAAs), creatine monohydrate, and several other amino acids and their byproducts [1]. Additionally, it has been postulated that a critical period for supplementation is prior (e.g., 30–60 minutes before) to the workout [2]. However, little research have been done on the effects of multi-ingredient pre-workout supplementation on long-term changes in skeletal muscle hypertrophy, lean body mass, and performance.

Multi-ingredient performance supplements (MIPS) may be comprised of ingredients such as BCAAs, creatine, beta-alanine, agmatine sulfate, taurine, creatinol-o-phosphate, and a combination of nitrate-containing compounds purported to enhance both acute performance and long-term neuromuscular adaptations [3-5]. Each of these ingredients has been studied individually for their positive effects on human performance adaptations. For example, pure creatine monohydrate, beta-alanine, and creatinol-o-phosphate have each been shown to enhance muscle adaptations [6,7]. In addition to supporting skeletal muscle hypertrophy, a vast array of nootropics, which have previously been demonstrated to augment preworkout performance including the combinations of glucuronolactone, tyrosine, caffeine, and *rhodiola rosea* are found within the MIPS [8-10]. Lastly, the MIPS contains agmatine sulfate, pomegranate and beet root extracts, which has been shown to enhance skeletal muscle blood flow [11]. However, information is lacking as to how resistance-training individuals will respond to the combination of these ingredients.

Therefore, the primary purpose of this study was to investigate the effects of 8 weeks of a MIPS in resistance-trained individuals during a periodized resistance training program on skeletal muscle hypertrophy, lean body mass, and strength relative to a placebo matched control.

Methods

Overview

Our study consisted of a randomized, double-blind, diet-controlled design, wherein a pre-workout supplemented and a placebo supplemented group were assigned to an 8-week periodized resistance training protocol. Muscle thickness, lean body mass, and strength were examined collectively at the end of weeks 0, 4, and 8 to assess the effects of the MIPS.

Subjects

Twenty-four resistance-trained males aged 21.3 ± 1.9 years with a respective average leg press and bench press of 3.40 ± 0.2 and 1.38 ± 0.9 times their bodyweight and a minimum of 1 year of resistance training experience were recruited for the study. Subjects could not participate if they were currently taking any medications including anti-inflammatory agents, any performance enhancing supplements, or if they smoked. Specifically, subjects could not have taken nutritional supplements for at least three months prior to data collection. Inclusion criteria included that subjects had previously been performing a minimum of 3 days per week resistance training. Each participant signed an informed consent approved by the University of Tampa Institutional Review Board before participating in the study.

Resistance training protocol

Our resistance training protocol was a modified combination from Kraemer et al. [12] and Montiero et al. [13]. These researchers found that a non-linear resistance-training program yielded greater results than a traditional or non-periodized program in athletes. The program was designed to train all major muscle groups using mostly compound movements for the upper and lower body (Table 1). The programmed, non-linear training split was divided into hypertrophy days consisting of 8–12 repetition maximum (RM) loads for 3 sets, with 60–120 seconds rest and strength days consisting of 2 to 5 RM loads for 3 sets for all exercises except the leg press and bench press which received 5 total sets. Subjects resistance-trained on Monday, Wednesday, and Friday of each week. Monday and Wednesday consisted of hypertrophy style training while Friday was dedicated to strength. Weights were progressively increased by 2–5% when the prescribed repetitions could be completed. All training sessions were closely monitored to ensure effort and intensity were maximal each training session. A research assistant worked individually with each subject to make sure full range of motion as well as rest intervals and repetition schemes were followed.

Table 1 Resistance training protocol

Monday	Wednesday	Friday
hyper - leg&chest	*hyper - back&delts*	*strength*
Leg Press	Pullups	Leg Press
Leg Curl	90° Bent Rows	Bench Press
Leg Extension	Shrugs	Leg Extension
Hyperextension	Shoulder Press	Close Grip Bench Press
Bench Press	Lateral Raise	
Dumbbell incline Bench Press	Reverse Laterals	
Close Grip Bench Press	Bicep curls	
Tricep cable extension		
Rep Scheme: 6 - 15	Rep Scheme: 6 - 15	Rep Scheme: 1 - 5

Strength, lean body mass, and muscle mass testing

Strength was assessed via 1-RM testing of the leg press and bench press. Lean Body Mass was determined on a Lunar Prodigy dual energy x-ray absorptiometry (DEXA) apparatus (software version, enCORE 2008, Madison, Wisconsin, U.S.A.). Skeletal muscle hypertrophy was determined via changes in quadriceps ultrasonography (determined by taking the combined muscle thickness of the *vastus lateralis* (VL) and *vastus intermedius* (VI) muscles. The reliability of measurements of muscle thickness by the same investigator was 0.98. These tests were performed at the end of weeks 0,4, and 8 in replacement of the heavy day in order to ensure full recovery (Friday).

Supplementation and diet control

Prior to the study, subjects were randomly assigned to consume Xpand® 2X (MIPS) or an isocaloric placebo of equal weight and volume (food-grade orange flavors and sweeteners) in a double-blind manner 30 minutes prior to exercise. On the non-training days, subjects were instructed to consume three equal servings spread evenly throughout the day with breakfast, lunch, and dinner. Two weeks prior to as well as throughout the study, subjects were placed on a diet consisting of 25% protein, 50% carbohydrates, and 25% fat by a registered dietitian who specializes in sport nutrition. Post study, analysis of the subjects recorded diets revealed diets consisted of 23% protein, 46% carbohydrates, and 31% fat, with no differences between groups. Subjects met as a group with the dietitian and were given individual meal plans at the beginning of the study as well as instructed not to consume any alcohol as it can dehydrate and impair the subjects' results. Upon completion of the study, all subjects' diets were analyzed to ensure compliance. Since the dietician worked weekly with the subjects, no subject's data had to be removed due to non-compliance. No adverse side effects were found in either group.

Statistical analysis

Repeated measures analysis of variance was performed to assess group, time, and group by time interactions. If any main effects were found, an LSD post hoc was employed to locate differences. An alpha priori of $p < 0.05$ was established. Statistica (StatSoft®, Tulsa, OK, USA) was used for all statistical analysis.

Results

MIPS supplementation contributed to a significant increase in quadriceps muscle thickness compared with placebo (group-by-time, $p < 0.01$). After 8 weeks of training, the MIPS contributed to quadriceps thickness increases of 11.8%, which was significantly greater than the increases resulting from the training alone in the placebo group of 4.5% ($p < 0.01$) (Figure 1). In addition, MIPS supplementation contributed to a significant increase in lean body mass (LBM) compared with placebo (group-by-time, $p < 0.01$). After 8 weeks of training, MIPS supplementation significantly contributed to a LBM increase of 7.8%, which was significantly greater than the increases resulting from the placebo group of 3.6% ($p < 0.01$) (Figure 2). The MIPS significantly contributed to an increase in bench press strength compared with placebo (group-by-time, $p < 0.05$). After 8 weeks of training, the MIPS contributed to bench press strength increases of 18.4%, which was significantly greater than the increases resulting from the training alone in the placebo group of 9.6% ($p < 0.01$) (Figure 3) in which the MIPS group increased 41.4%, while the placebo group increased 34.2%. Lastly, there was a trend toward an increase in leg press strength (group-by-time, $p = .08$).

Discussion

The primary purpose of this study was to investigate the effects of 8 weeks of a MIPS in resistance-trained individuals during a periodized resistance training program on skeletal muscle hypertrophy, lean body mass, and strength relative to a placebo matched control. The primary findings of this research were in congruence with our hypotheses that Xpand® 2X supplementation can improve adaptations in skeletal muscle hypertrophy, LBM, and strength.

Skeletal muscle hypertrophy and lean body mass

This MIPS contains a proprietary blend of ingredients reported previously to augment the accretion of skeletal muscle. For example, creatine monohydrate has been reported as the most effective ergogenic aid currently available regarding LBM and high-intensity exercise capacity, particularly in untrained individuals [14]. Creatine and its various forms have been thoroughly researched, yet to date no study has shown any form of creatine to be superior to creatine monohydrate, which was used in this study (23, 33). Supplementation with creatine can increase total resistance training volume via ATP resynthesis [14], and total training volume has been closely linked with skeletal muscle accretion. Additionally, creatine supplementation has been demonstrated to increase the activation of satellite cells and myonuclei in muscle following chronic resistance training [15]. Moreover it is conceivable that the osmotic pressure created by creatine that increases the hydration status of cells, resulting in potentially hypertrophic effects [16]. This mechanism of action is what causes creatine to increase strength, but can benefit almost every body system, including the brain, bones, muscles, and liver [17].

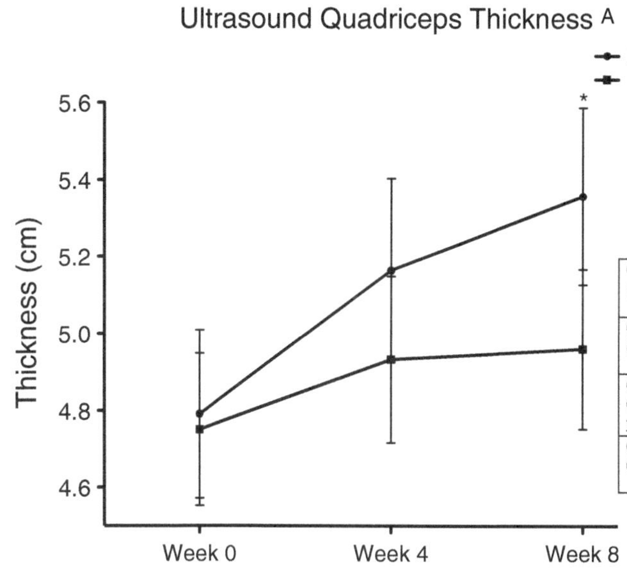

Quadriceps Hypertrophy

Quadriceps Ultrasound (CM) XPAND **A**	4.79 ± 0.78	5.16 ± 0.9	5.4 ± 0.8
Quadriceps Ultrasound (CM) Placebo	4.75 ± 0.53	4.9 ± 0.5	4.96 ± 0.8
Quadriceps Ultrasound (% Change) XPAND **A**		7.8 ± 4.2*	11.8 ± 2.6 *
Quadriceps Ultrasound (% Change) Placebo		3.8 ± 2.8	4.5 ± 3.1

A = Significant Treatment X Time Effect using a Repeated Measures ANOVA
* = Significantly different than corresponding Placebo using LSD Post Hoc

Figure 1 **Percent change ultrasound muscle hypertrophy.**

Lastly, long term studies have observed that those supplementing with creatine experience 200% increases in LBM compared to placebo [14].

Branched chain amino acids have previously been shown as efficacious in the accretion of skeletal muscle mass [2]. One BCAA of particular interest is leucine, which has been shown to increase muscle protein synthesis (MPS) without the presence of the other essential amino acids [18] Additionally, Karlsson et al. [19] found that supplementation with BCAAs during resistance exercise results in greater phosphorylation of ribosomal S6 kinase, a rate limiting enzyme in the signaling network responsible for regulation of protein synthesis in skeletal muscles. Moreover, BCAAs seem to decrease soreness after eccentric exercise [20] and, they prevent declines in both testosterone and power following an overreaching cycle [21].

Beta-Alanine supplementation has consistently been demonstrated to augment muscle carnosine concentrations in humans [22-25]. Harris et al. [22] concluded

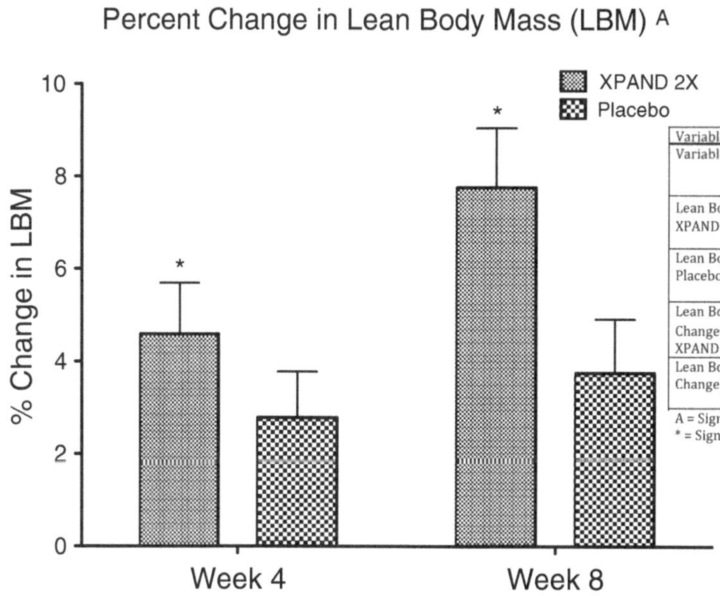

Lean Body Mass

Variable	Week 0	Week 4	Week 8
Variable	Week 0	Week 4	Week 8
Lean Body Mass (kg) **A** XPAND	58.47 ± 6.02	61.18 ± 5.45	62.96 ± 5.62
Lean Body Mass (Kg) Placebo	58.76 ± 6.32	60.24 ± 5.63	60.8 ± 5.81
Lean Body Mass (% Change) **A** XPAND		4.6 ± 1.1 % *	7.8 ± 1.3 % *
Lean Body Mass (% Change) Placebo		2.78 ± 1.0 %	3.76 ± 1.2

A = Significant Treatment X Time Effect using a Repeated Measures ANOVA
* = Significantly different than corresponding Placebo using LSD Post Hoc

Figure 2 **Percent change in lean body mass.**

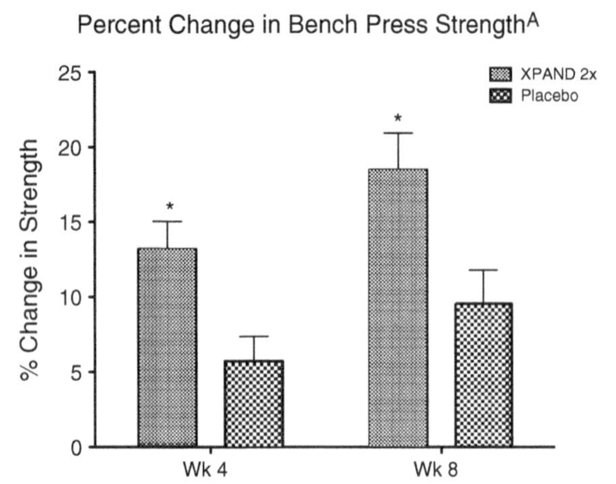

Figure 3 Percent change in bench press strength.

that carnosine plays an essential role as an intracellular buffer within the skeletal muscle of humans. More importantly, beta-alanine supplementation has been shown to enhance physical performance during high intensity exercise bouts while also delaying the onset of neuromuscular fatigue [26].

Agmatine is a derivative of the amino acid arginine. Agmatine has been studied for its impact on nitric oxide, wellbeing, and hormone status [27,28]. Agmatine has been noted to support nitric oxide (NO) production via stimulation of endothelial nitric oxide synthase (eNOS). [29-31]. This process is essential for the proper functioning of the polyamine biosynthetic pathways to occur [29-31]. The body's organs require polyamines for their growth, renewal, and metabolism. Polyamines also have a profound stabilizing effect on a cell DNA and are essential to the healthy function of the nervous system [29,30]. Therefore, these pathways, although not fully elucidated, play an important role in normal cell homeostasis.

Lastly, Creatinol-O-Phosphate (COP) is known primarily for its abilities as an intracellular buffer. Creatinol-O-Phosphate has been shown to assist in stabilizing intracellular and extracellular pH levels, ultimately prolonging anaerobic glycolysis in the presence of lactic acid [7]. Creatinol-O-Phosphate has also been shown to activate satellite cells in skeletal muscle, theoretically increasing their capacity for muscle growth [7]. To date this is the first study that we are aware of to analyze this specific combination of ingredients.

Strength

Strength is one of the most critical attributes underlying success in sport [32]. The collective results of the present study suggest that bench press strength following Xpand® 2X supplementation are optimized within the context of a periodized training split. Most of the individual ingredients found within the pre-workout matrix have been demonstrated to individually enhance a variety of strength measures. For example, creatine monohydrate has repeatedly been shown to augment strength [33]. In addition to creatine, this MIPS contains a number of nootropics including glucuronolactone, caffeine, and taurine, which can possibly decrease perceived exertion and augment intra-workout performance. For example, caffeine has been demonstrated to enhance strength acutely through an adenosine receptor antagonist mediated mechanism and subsequent central nervous system stimulation [34].

Research suggests that taurine might increase the mechanical threshold for skeletal muscle contraction, promote intracellular membrane stabilization, and increase membrane polarization [22]. Taurine has also been noted for its performance enhancing, antioxidant, and nerve conduction effects [22,35]. Moreover the combination of caffeine and taurine has previously been shown to augment performance to a greater degree than caffeine alone [36].

Conclusions

The collective results of our research indicate that Xpand® 2X (MIPS) supplementation results in significant increases in bench press strength, hypertrophy, and lean body mass in resistance-trained men. Therefore, coaches, trainers, and athletes may increase the benefits of their workouts by supplementing with MIPS prior to exercise. Future research should investigate if supplementation with MIPS would result in better adaptations than supplementation with each of the ingredients alone.

Competing interests
RPL, JMJ, JED, EOS, SAM, and JMW declare that they have no competing interests. SW and RW are employed by Dymatize®.

Authors' contributions
RPL, JMJ, JED, SAM, and JMW contributed in concept and design, data acquisition, analysis of data, and manuscript preparation. EOS was involved in concept and design, analysis of data, and manuscript preparation. SW and RW were involved in concept and design and manuscript preparation. All authors read and approved the final manuscript.

Author details
[1]Department of Health Sciences and Human Performance, The University of Tampa, Tampa, FL, USA. [2]Laboratory of Neuromuscular Adaptations to Strength Training, School of Physical Education and Sport, University of São Paulo, São Paulo, Brazil. [3]Dymatize® Enterprises, LLC. & Dymatize® Nutrition Sport Performance Institute (DNSPI), Dallas, Texas, USA.

References

1. Wilson JM: **Effects of amino acids and their metabolites on aerobic and anaerobic sports.** *Strength Condition J* 2012, **34**:33–48.

2. Cribb PJ, Hayes A: **Effects of supplement timing and resistance exercise on skeletal muscle hypertrophy.** *Med Sci Sports Exer* 2006, **38:**1918–1925.
3. Ormsbee MJ, Mandler WK, Thomas DD, Ward EG, Kinsey AW, Simonavice E, Panton LB, Kim JS: **The effects of six weeks of supplementation with multi-ingredient performance supplements and resistance training on anabolic hormones, body composition, strength, and power in resistance-trained men.** *J Int Soc Sports Nutr* 2012, **9:**49.
4. Shelmadine B, Cooke M, Buford T, Hudson G, Redd L, Leutholtz B, Willoughby DS: **Effects of 28 days of resistance exercise and consuming a commercially available pre-workout supplement, NO-Shotgun(R), on body composition, muscle strength and mass, markers of satellite cell activation, and clinical safety markers in males.** *J Int Soc Sports Nutr* 2009, **6:**16.
5. Spillane M, Schwarz N, Leddy S, Correa T, Minter M, Longoria V, Willoughby DS: **Effects of 28 days of resistance exercise while consuming commercially available pre- and post-workout supplements, NO-Shotgun (R) and NO-Synthesize(R) on body composition, muscle strength and mass, markers of protein synthesis, and clinical safety markers in males.** *Nutr Metab* 2011, **8:**78.
6. Hoffman J, Ratamess N, Kang J, Mangine G, Faigenbaum A, Stout J: **Effect of creatine and beta-alanine supplementation on performance and endocrine responses in strength/power athletes.** *Int J Sport Nutr Exer Metab* 2006, **16:**430–446.
7. Nicaise J: **Creatinol O-phosphate (COP) and muscular performance: a controlled clinical trial.** *Curr Therapeut Res Clin Exp* 1975, **17:**531–534.
8. Neri DF, Wiegmann D, Stanny RR, Shappell SA, McCardie A, McKay DL: **The effects of tyrosine on cognitive performance during extended wakefulness.** *Aviat Space Environ Med* 1995, **66:**313–319.
9. Costill DL, Dalsky GP, Fink WJ: **Effects of caffeine ingestion on metabolism and exercise performance.** *Med Sci Sports* 1978, **10:**155–158.
10. De Bock K, Eijnde BO, Ramaekers M, Hespel P: **Acute Rhodiola rosea intake can improve endurance exercise performance.** *Int J Sport Nutr Exer Metab* 2004, **14:**298–307.
11. de Nigris F, Williams-Ignarro S, Sica V, Lerman LO, D'Armiento FP, Byrns RE, Casamassimi A, Carpentiero D, Schiano C, Sumi D, *et al*: **Effects of a pomegranate fruit extract rich in punicalagin on oxidation-sensitive genes and eNOS activity at sites of perturbed shear stress and atherogenesis.** *Cardiovasc Res* 2007, **73:**414–423.
12. Kraemer WJ, Spiering BA, Volek JS, Martin GJ, Howard RL, Ratamess NA, Hatfield DL, Vingren JL, Ho JY, Fragala MS, *et al*: **Recovery from a national collegiate athletic association division I football game: muscle damage and hormonal status.** *J Strength Cond Res* 2009, **23:**2–10.
13. Monteiro AG, Aoki MS, Evangelista AL, Alveno DA, Monteiro GA, Picarro Ida C, Ugrinowitsch C: **Nonlinear periodization maximizes strength gains in split resistance training routines.** *J Strength Cond Res* 2009, **23:**1321–1326.
14. Buford TW, Kreider RB, Stout JR, Greenwood M, Campbell B, Spano M, Ziegenfuss T, Lopez H, Landis J, Antonio J: **International Society of Sports Nutrition position stand: creatine supplementation and exercise.** *J Int Soc Sports Nutr* 2007, **4:**6.
15. Dangott B, Schultz E, Mozdziak PE: **Dietary creatine monohydrate supplementation increases satellite cell mitotic activity during compensatory hypertrophy.** *Int J Sports Med* 2000, **21:**13–16.
16. Parise G, Mihic S, MacLennan D, Yarasheski KE, Tarnopolsky MA: **Effects of acute creatine monohydrate supplementation on leucine kinetics and mixed-muscle protein synthesis.** *J Appl Physiol* 2001, **91:**1041–1047.
17. Kraemer WJ, Volek JS: **Creatine supplementation. Its role in human performance.** *Clin Sports Med* 1999, **18:**651–666. ix.
18. Norton LE, Layman DK: **Leucine regulates translation initiation of protein synthesis in skeletal muscle after exercise.** *J Nutr* 2006, **136:**533S–537S.
19. Karlsson HK, Nilsson PA, Nilsson J, Chibalin AV, Zierath JR, Blomstrand E: **Branched-chain amino acids increase p70S6k phosphorylation in human skeletal muscle after resistance exercise.** *Am J Physiol Endocrinol Metab* 2004, **287:**E1–E7.
20. Jackman SR, Witard OC, Jeukendrup AE, Tipton KD: **Branched-chain amino acid ingestion can ameliorate soreness from eccentric exercise.** *Med Sci Sports Exerc* 2010, **42:**962–970.
21. Kraemer WJ, Ratamess NA, Volek JS, Hakkinen K, Rubin MR, French DN, Gomez AL, McGuigan MR, Scheett TP, Newton RU, *et al*: **The effects of amino acid supplementation on hormonal responses to resistance training overreaching.** *Metab: Clin Exper* 2006, **55:**282–291.
22. Harris RC, Tallon MJ, Dunnett M, Boobis L, Coakley J, Kim HJ, Fallowfield JL, Hill CA, Sale C, Wise JA: **The absorption of orally supplied beta-alanine and its effect on muscle carnosine synthesis in human vastus lateralis.** *Amino acids* 2006, **30:**279–289.
23. Hill CA, Harris RC, Kim HJ, Harris BD, Sale C, Boobis LH, Kim CK, Wise JA: **Influence of beta-alanine supplementation on skeletal muscle carnosine concentrations and high intensity cycling capacity.** *Amino acids* 2007, **32:**225–233.
24. Derave W, Ozdemir MS, Harris RC, Pottier A, Reyngoudt H, Koppo K, Wise JA, Achten E: **beta-Alanine supplementation augments muscle carnosine content and attenuates fatigue during repeated isokinetic contraction bouts in trained sprinters.** *J Appl Physiol* 2007, **103:**1736–1743.
25. Baguet A, Koppo K, Pottier A, Derave W: **Beta-alanine supplementation reduces acidosis but not oxygen uptake response during high-intensity cycling exercise.** *Eur J Appl Physiol* 2010, **108:**495–503.
26. Artioli GG, Gualano B, Smith A, Stout J, Lancha AH Jr: **Role of beta-alanine supplementation on muscle carnosine and exercise performance.** *Med Sci Sports Exer* 2010, **42:**1162–1173.
27. Horyn O, Luhovyy B, Lazarow A, Daikhin Y, Nissim I, Yudkoff M: **Biosynthesis of agmatine in isolated mitochondria and perfused rat liver: studies with 15N-labelled arginine.** *Biochem J* 2005, **388:**419–425.
28. Molderings GJ, Haenisch B: **Agmatine (decarboxylated L-arginine): physiological role and therapeutic potential.** *Pharmacol Therapeut* 2012, **133:**351–365.
29. Abe K, Abe Y, Saito H: **Agmatine suppresses nitric oxide production in microglia.** *Brain Res* 2000, **872:**141–148.
30. Gao Y, Gumusel B, Koves G, Prasad A, Hao Q, Hyman A, Lippton H: **Agmatine: a novel endogenous vasodilator substance.** *Life Sci* 1995, **57:**PL83–PL86.
31. Raasch W, Regunathan S, Li G, Reis DJ: **Agmatine, the bacterial amine, is widely distributed in mammalian tissues.** *Life Sci* 1995, **56:**2319–2330.
32. Wilson JM, Duncan NM, Marin PJ, Brown LE, Loenneke JP, Wilson SM, Jo E, Lowery RP, Ugrinowitsch C: **Meta-analysis of post activation Potentiation and power: effects of conditioning activity, volume, gender, rest periods, and training status.** *J Strength Cond Res* 2012, **27**(3):854.
33. Becque MD, Lochmann JD, Melrose DR: **Effects of oral creatine supplementation on muscular strength and body composition.** *Med Sci Sports Exer* 2000, **32:**654–658.
34. Goldstein ER, Ziegenfuss T, Kalman D, Kreider R, Campbell B, Wilborn C, Taylor L, Willoughby D, Stout J, Graves BS, *et al*: **International society of sports nutrition position stand: caffeine and performance.** *J Int Soc Sports Nutr* 2010, **7:**5.
35. Jia F, Yue M, Chandra D, Keramidas A, Goldstein PA, Homanics GE, Harrison NL: **Taurine is a potent activator of extrasynaptic GABA(A) receptors in the thalamus.** *J Neurosci* 2008, **28:**106–115.
36. Seidl R, Peyrl A, Nicham R, Hauser E: **A taurine and caffeine-containing drink stimulates cognitive performance and well being.** *Amino acids* 2000, **19:**635–642.

Effect of *Magnolia officinalis* and *Phellodendron amurense* (Relora®) on cortisol and psychological mood state in moderately stressed subjects

Shawn M Talbott[1*], Julie A Talbott[1] and Mike Pugh[2]

Abstract

Background: Magnolia (*Magnolia officinalis*) and Phellodendron (*Phellodendron amurense*) barks are medicinal plants commonly used as traditional remedies for reducing stress and anxiety. Modern dietary supplements are intended to induce relaxation and reduce stress as well as stress-related eating. Previous studies have shown the combination of Magnolia/Phellodendron (MP) to reduce both cortisol exposure and the perception of stress/anxiety, while improving weight loss in subjects with stress-related eating. Competitive athletes are "stressed" by their intense exercise regimens in addition to their normal activities of daily living and thus may benefit from a natural therapy intended to modulate baseline perceptions of stress and stress hormone exposure.

Methods: We assessed salivary cortisol exposure and psychological mood state in 56 subjects (35 men and 21 women) screened for moderate stress and supplemented with a standardized/patented MP combination (Relora®, Next Pharmaceuticals) or Placebo for 4 weeks.

Results: After 4 weeks of supplementation, salivary cortisol exposure was significantly ($p<0.05$) lower (−18%) in the Relora group compared to Placebo. Compared to Placebo, the Relora group had significantly better ($p<0.05$) mood state parameters, including lower indices of Overall Stress (−11%), Tension (−13%), Depression (−20%), Anger (−42%), Fatigue (−31%), and Confusion (−27%), and higher indices of Global Mood State (+11%) and Vigor (+18%).

Conclusion: These results indicate that daily supplementation with a combination of Magnolia bark extract and Phellodendron bark extract (Relora®) reduces cortisol exposure and perceived daily stress, while improving a variety of mood state parameters, including lower fatigue and higher vigor. These results suggest an effective natural approach to modulating the detrimental health effects of chronic stress in moderately stressed adults. Future studies should examine the possible performance and recovery benefits of Relora supplementation in athletes overstressed by the physical and psychological demands of training and competition.

Keywords: Stress, Cortisol, Vigor, Magnolia, Phellodendron, Mood, Relora

Background

The relationship between chronic psychological stress and reduced health is well established [1], with psychological stress having been shown to increase susceptibility to a wide range of diseases including anxiety, depression, diabetes, and obesity [2-4]. Even the "stress" of short-term sleep loss has significant implications for long-term health and well-being due to adverse systemic health effects including suppressed immune function, abdominal obesity, insomnia, depression, and generalized fatigue [5,6].

Interventions for stress and anxiety range from nutritional support to the use of antidepressant medications such as benzodiazepines and selective serotonin reuptake inhibitors [7,8]. A United States Patent (No. 6,582,735) has been granted for the use of an extract of *Magnolia officinalis* bark for stress related conditions involving elevated cortisol, such as control of body weight, sleep disturbances and restlessness [9].

Extracts of *Magnolia officinalis* bark and its active constituent, honokiol, have been studied in animal models

* Correspondence: smtalbott@supplementwatch.com
[1]SupplementWatch, 648 Rocky Knoll, Draper, UT 84020, USA
Full list of author information is available at the end of the article

with comparable anxiolytic activity to diazepam (a benzodiazepine anxiolytic used to treat anxiety), but without associated side effects such as sedation [10-13]. Berberine, a constituent of the *Phellodendron* extract, has also demonstrated a significant anxiolytic effect in rodent stress studies, including the elevated plus maze test and the forced swim test [14,15]. The combination of magnolia plus phellodendron appears to be even more effective in controlling stress/anxiety compared to either herb used separately [16-19].

The subject of this study, Relora® (Next Pharmaceuticals, Inc, Salinas, CA), is a proprietary dietary supplement formulation consisting of a blend of extracts of *Magnolia officinalis* bark and *Phellodendron amurense* bark standardized to honokiol and berberine, respectively. In previous studies, Relora has demonstrated efficacy for reducing stress and anxiety in animals [18,19] and enhancing feelings of well-being in human subjects [20,21]. One study also measured the effects of Relora on salivary cortisol, finding benefits in reducing cortisol and increasing dehydroandrostenedione (DHEA) levels in stressed subjects [20].

In this study, we report the effects of using the Relora combination of magnolia bark and phellodendron bark on salivary cortisol and psychological well-being of healthy subjects under moderate levels of perceived psychological stress. The current study employed a well-validated psychological assessment known as the Profile of Mood States (POMS) to assess mood state. A key objective of the study was to explore how 4 weeks of magnolia/phellodendron supplementation (Relora versus a placebo) affected cortisol, various moods, and overall stress levels under conditions of moderate psychological stress.

Methods

Dietary supplement

Relora® is a proprietary blend of a patented extract of the bark of *Magnolia officinalis* and an extract of the bark of *Phellodendron amurense* (US Patent Nos. 6,582,735 and 6,814,987). The product is standardized to "not less than 1.5% honokiol and 0.1% berberine." Subjects ingested 500 mg/day at breakfast (250 mg) and dinner (250 mg) in white opaque capsules or a look-alike placebo that was identical in size, shape and color.

Study design

This study was done in accordance with the Helsinki Declaration, as revised in 1983, for clinical research involving humans and all procedures, measurements, and informed consent processes were reviewed and approved by an external third-party review board (Aspire IRB; Santee, CA).

Subjects signed informed consent documents after the study details were explained. The study used a randomized placebo-controlled, double-blind design. Subjects were randomly assigned, through a random number generator, to either 500 mg/day containing supplement (250 mg of Relora®, consumed at breakfast and dinner) or a look-alike Placebo (250 mg of rice flour); bottles were labeled only with a pre-assigned random code. Subjects self-administered the allotted capsule twice daily in the morning with breakfast and in the evening with dinner for 4 weeks. Subjects were contacted weekly to remind them to take their capsules daily. Empty bottles were returned after the study for a count of any unused capsules (an indicator of missed doses). Compliance with these instructions was high (data not shown).

We screened 60 subjects for moderate levels of psychological stress, with 56 subjects completing the study. Sixty (60) subjects were randomized to receive Supplement (30 subjects) or look-alike Placebo (30 subjects) for 4 weeks. The 4-week duration was selected as more representative of persistent changes in mood state that may result from superior hormone balance, as opposed to short-term changes in emotions that may be more closely linked with stressors of daily living.

At Baseline (week 0) and Post-supplementation (week 4), we assessed body weight and body fat percentage (Tanita BDF-300A bioelectrical impedance analyzer), overall stress (Yale Stress Survey), psychological mood state (Profile of Mood States Survey) and salivary cortisol. Mood State (Vigor, Depression, Anger, Confusion, Fatigue, and Anxiety) was assessed using the validated Profile of Mood States (POMS) survey [22,23]. Cortisol exposure was assessed in pooled saliva samples collected at three time points during each collection day (morning, afternoon, and evening). The morning sample was collected upon waking at approximately 6am; the afternoon sample at approximately 2pm; and the evening sample immediately before bed at approximately 10pm to represent as much of a total daily "cortisol exposure" for each subject as possible. Cortisol circadian rhythm data will be reported elsewhere. Saliva samples were analyzed for free cortisol by enzyme immunoassay (EIA; Salimetrics, State College, PA, USA).

Fifty-six subjects (35 men & 21 women, age 28±11 years) completed the study, with two women in each group lost to follow up (did not return final surveys or saliva samples).

Mood assessment

We employed the Profile Of Mood States (POMS) questionnaire, to measure 6 primary psychological factors (tension, depression, anger, fatigue, vigor or confusion), plus the combined "global mood state" as an indication of subjective well-being. The POMS methodology has been used in nearly 3,000 studies and its validity is well established. The POMS profile uses 65 adjective-based intensity scales scored on a 0–4 hedonic scale (0 = not at all, 4 = extremely). The 65 adjective responses are categorized into the six mood factors (tension, depression, anger, fatigue, vigor or confusion), tabulated, scored and analyzed. The output of the POMS questionnaire is an assessment of the positive and negative moods of each subject at baseline and 4-weeks.

Data management and analysis

All questionnaires were completed at a central location and transcribed to a central database. Subjects that did not complete the questionnaires or submitted incomplete questionnaires were dropped from the study and not included in the study analysis (four subjects – two females from each group). Data was identified by subject number and examined for accuracy and completeness. Tabulated data was analyzed with JMP 8.0 (SAS Institute) using standard parametric paired t-tests and significance was assessed with a two-tailed alpha level set at 0.05.

Results

Over the course of the 4-week supplementation period, there were no adverse events or side effects reported. There were no significant changes in body weight or body fat percentage.

At week 4, salivary cortisol exposure was significantly ($p<0.05$) lower (−18%) in the Relora group (Figure 1).

Significantly better ($p<0.05$) mood state indices were observed in the Relora group for Overall Stress (−11%) and Global Mood State (−11%) compared to Placebo (Figure 2). Mood State subscales (Figure 3) were significantly better ($p<0.05$) in the Relora group compared to Placebo at week 4; Tension (−13%), Depression (−20%), Anger (−42%), Fatigue (−31%), Confusion (−27%), and Vigor (+18%).

Discussion

Antidepressant drugs are the most commonly prescribed class of medications in the United States and are used by athletes and non-athletes alike [24]. More than 10% of the American population is taking one or more antidepressant drugs, which represents 27 million individuals taking more than 120 million prescriptions and spending over $80 billion per year. According to a recent survey [25], large numbers of Americans feel an antidepressant drug would be helpful for; dealing with day-to-day stresses (83%); making things easier in relations with family and friends (76%); and helping people feel better about themselves (68%). However, because antidepressant drugs carry the United States Food and Drug Administration's most stringent "black box" warning (associated with serious life-threatening adverse effects), there is need for safe and effective natural approaches to reducing stress and anxiety.

In addition to a balanced diet, regular physical activity, and various stress management techniques, certain dietary supplements may be effective in naturally maintaining the normal balance between stress, cortisol, and emotional well-being. For example, there are numerous commercial examples of general-purpose "relaxation" and "calming" teas based on traditional herbal blends such as chamomile, fennel, lemon balm and others, while magnolia and phellodendron bark extracts have been specifically demonstrated as natural anxiolytic agents, [7-21,26]. As such, appropriate dietary supplements may be a safe and effective natural adjunct to diet/exercise/stress management techniques to bring stress response and cortisol levels back to within normal ranges in individuals suffering from chronic stress or in athletes suffering from overtraining syndrome.

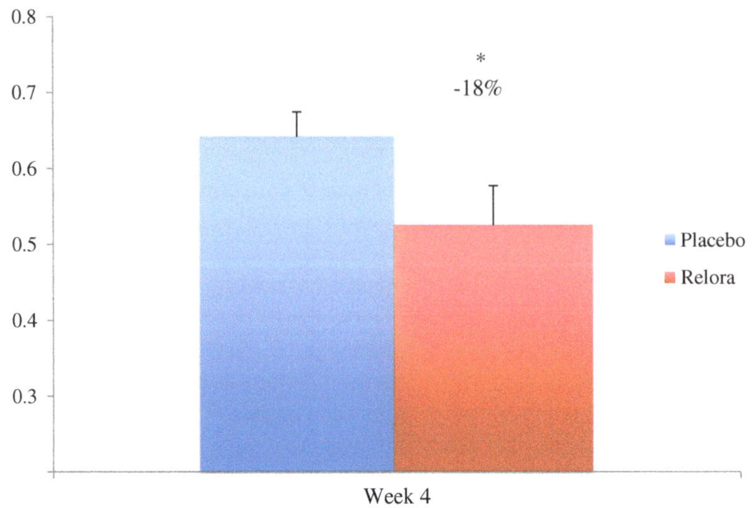

Figure 1 Salivary Cortisol (ug/ml). Salivary cortisol was 18% lower ($p<0.05$) in the Relora group compared to Placebo at Week 4 (0.525 ± 0.190 to 0.642 ± 0.353).

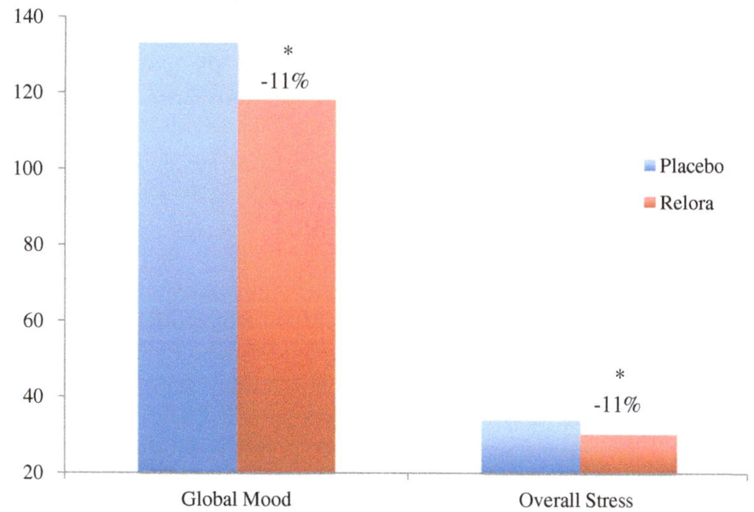

Figure 2 Global Mood State (POMS) and Overall Stress (Yale Stress Survey). Global Mood State was 11% better ($p<0.05$) in the Relora group compared to Placebo (118±18 to 133±30) – lower score is a "better" Global Mood State (POMS). Overall Stress (Yale Stress Survey) was 11% lower ($p<0.05$) in the Relora group compared to Placebo (30.2±5.2 to 33.9±7.4). The global mood state was calculated based on scoring (0-4 with 0 = not at all, 2 = moderately and 4 = extremely) answers to 58 of the 65 adjectives of the POMS (a lower number is a "better" global mood state). Global Mood State is the combined score of the 6 subscales of the POMS (McNair et al., [9]).

Magnolia bark *(Magnolia officinalis)* and Phellodendron bark (*Phellodendron amurense*) are traditional herbal medicines used since 100A.D. for treating "stagnation of Qi" in Chinese medicine [7,8,17], which is analogous to what we view in Western medicine as reduced psychological vigor or burnout. Magnolia bark extracts are rich in the phenolic compound, honokiol [12], while Phellodendron bark extracts are rich in berberine [14,15] – each of which contributes to the primary anti-stress, anti-anxiety, and cortisol-lowering effects of the plants [9-19,26]. Research has shown magnolia and phellodendron extracts and their primary bioactives (honokiol and berberine) to possess powerful "mental acuity" benefits [10,11,16] via their actions in modulating the activity of various neurotransmitters and related enzymes in the brain, including brain-derived neurotrophic factor, acetylcholine, choline acetyltransferase, and acetylcholinesterase.

Numerous animal studies have demonstrated that honokiol and berberine act as anxiolytic agents [9-19,26]. When compared to pharmaceutical agents such as Valium (diazepam), honokiol and berberine appear to be as effective in their anti-anxiety activity yet not nearly as powerful in their sedative ability [9,12,13]. These results have been demonstrated in numerous animal studies and suggest that

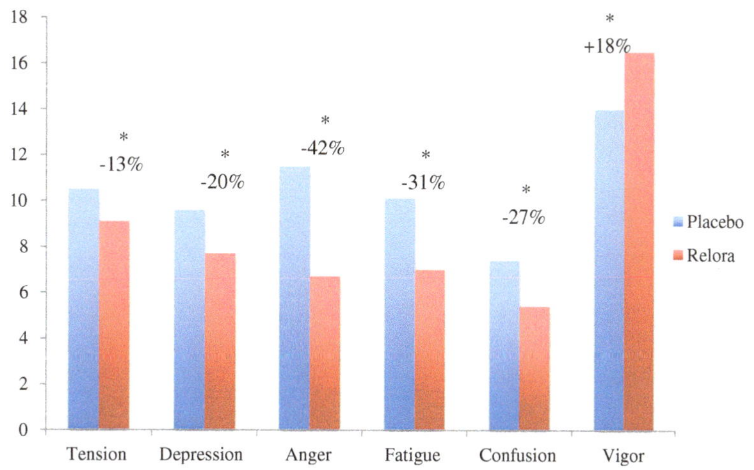

Figure 3 Profile of Mood States (POMS). Numerical scores for each of the 6 subscales of the POMS (McNair et al., [9]). The Relora group showed significantly improved mood state parameters compared to Placebo at Week 4 (* = $p<0,05$).

Relora, which is standardized to both honokiol (from magnolia bark) and berberine (from phellodendron), is an effective natural approach for controlling the detrimental effects of everyday stressors, without the tranquilizing side effects of pharmaceutical agents [14-19,26]. Previous human studies on Relora have shown similar anti-stress and anxiolytic benefits in moderately stressed subjects [20,21]. The results reported in this study expand on previous findings of simple "relaxation" benefits of Relora to demonstrate specific effects on psychological mood state parameters in moderately-stressed subjects, including benefits for Global Mood State (analogous to an assessment of overall well-being), Tension, Depression, Fatigue, and Vigor (the opposite psychological state from "Burnout"). The magnitude of benefit in stress hormone (cortisol) reduction (18%) and mood state improvement (11%-42%) is meaningful from the perspective of optimal mental and physical performance. For example, the 18% higher Vigor or the 20% lower Depression score observed in the Relora group, could reasonably be associated with subjects reporting "feeling good" (in the case on our moderately-stressed subjects) or "performing well" (in the case of over-stressed or over-trained athletes, which should be the subject of future studies).

Although our study was not conducted in competitive athletes, a number of our moderately stressed healthy subjects were recreational runners and cyclists who commented about feeling more "balanced" in their workouts when their stress levels were balanced. This is a logical individual perception based on a number of studies in elite-level and recreational athletes that have found a direct relationship between overall stress (physical training and psychological stress) and athletic performance, including both mental and physical performance parameters [27-31]. Competitive athletes tend to be characterized by an elevated Vigor score and lower Fatigue score compared to non-athletes [27]. However, in many intervention studies of athletes, a dose–response exists between training stress and mood state [28,29], so as overall physical "training stress" is elevated beyond a certain tipping point, psychological mood state becomes depressed. In addition, low Vigor scores and overall reduced psychological mood state have been identified as predictors of future athletic injury [30]. The most dramatic changes in psychological mood state are logically the result of intensified periods of training (e.g. increased training intensity and/or duration), which can be modulated positively or negatively by psychological stress (e.g. exams), competitive anxiety, social support network, sleep patterns, and recovery methods [27-31]. Based on the magnitude of the positive changes in cortisol levels and mood state parameters, we would recommend further athlete-specific studies to gauge the possible mental/physical performance benefits of Relora in enhancing post-exercise recovery and preventing over-training syndrome in competitive athletes.

Results from the current study indicate that daily supplementation with a combination of magnolia bark and phellodendron bark (Relora) reduces cortisol exposure and perceived stress, while improving a variety of mood state parameters. Compared to the Placebo group, salivary cortisol exposure was significantly lower (−18%) in the Relora group, while mood state parameters were significantly and meaningfully higher, including an 11% superior Global Mood State and 18% higher Vigor, with 13% lower Tension and 20% lower Depression indices. These results indicate that daily supplementation with a combination of Magnolia and Phellodendron (Relora) is an effective natural approach to the detrimental health effects of chronic stress.

Conclusions

The present study indicates a significant "anti-stress" benefit of magnolia/phellodendron bark (Relora) supplementation in moderately stressed non-athletes, and suggests a possible benefit for athletes to recover from "training stress" induced by the physical and psychological demands of competition and training. Future studies should examine the potential benefits of Relora in helping athletes to enhance post-exercise recovery and possibly to help prevent overtraining syndrome.

Competing interests

This study was funded by the manufacturer of Relora (Next Pharmaceuticals) and conducted by SupplementWatch. The authors of this paper have no direct financial relationship with Next Pharmaceuticals or with the Relora dietary supplement. ST and JT are employees of SupplementWatch. ST and MP are employees of MonaVie, which markets a dietary supplement containing Relora as one of several ingredients.

Authors' contributions

Each author contributed significantly to the successful carriage of this study. ST designed the study and drafted the manuscript. JT coordinated the IRB approval, subject visits, and sample inventory. MP participated in the study design and coordination of subject visits. All authors read and approved the manuscript.

Author details

[1]SupplementWatch, 648 Rocky Knoll, Draper, UT 84020, USA. [2]MonaVie, 10855 S River Front Parkway, South Jordan, UT 84095, USA.

References

1. Cohen S, Janicki-Deverts D, Miller GE: **Psychological stress and disease.** *JAMA* 2007, **14**. Oct 10;298:1685–7, 2007.
2. Dallman MF, la Fleur SE, Pecoraro NC, Gomez F, Houshyar H, Akana SF: **Minireview: glucocorticoids – food intake, abdominal obesity, and wealthy nations in 2004.** *Endocrinology* 2004, **145**:2633–2638.
3. Epel E, Lapidus R, McEwen B, Brownell K: **Stress may add bite to appetite in women: a laboratory study of stress-induced cortisol and eating behavior.** *Psychoneuroendocrinology* 2001, **26**:37–49.
4. Epel ES, McEwen B, Seeman T, Matthews K, Castellazzo G, Brownell KD, Bell J, Ickovics JR: **Stress and body shape: stress-induced cortisol secretion is consistently greater among women with central fat.** *Psychosom Med* 2000, **62**:623–632.

5. Szelenberger W, Soldatos C: **Sleep disorders in psychiatric practice.** *World Psychiatry* 2005, **4**:186–90.
6. Taheri S, Lin L, Austin D, Young T, Mignot E: **Short sleep duration is associated with reduced leptin, elevated ghrelin, and increased body mass index.** *PloS Med* 2004, **1**:e62.
7. Weeks BS: **Formulations of dietary supplements and herbal extracts for relaxation and anxiolytic action: Relarian.** *Med Sci Monit* 2009, **15**(11):RA256–62.
8. Lee YJ, Lee YM, Lee CK, Jung JK, Han SB, Hong JT: **Therapeutic applications of compounds in the Magnolia family.** *Pharmacol Ther* 2011, **130**(2):157–76.
9. Xu Q, Yi LT, Pan Y, Wang X, Li YC, Li JM, Wang CP, Kong LD: **Antidepressant-like effects of the mixture of honokiol and magnolol from the barks of Magnolia officinalis in stressed rodents.** *Prog Neuropsychopharmacol Biol Psychiatry* 2008, **32**(3):715–25.
10. Chiang J, Shen YC, Wang YH, Hou YC, Chen CC, Liao JF, Yu MC, Juan CW, Liou KT: **Honokiol protects rats against eccentric exercise-induced skeletal muscle damage by inhibiting NF-kappaB induced oxidative stress and inflammation.** *Eur J Pharmacol* 2009, **610**(1–3):119–27.
11. Harada S, Kishimoto M, Kobayashi M, Nakamoto K, Fujita-Hamabe W, Chen HH, Chan MH, Tokuyama S: **Honokiol suppresses the development of post-ischemic glucose intolerance and neuronal damage in mice.** *J Nat Med* 2012, **66**(4):591–9.
12. Kuribara H, Stavinoha WB, Maruyama Y: **Behavioural pharmacological characteristics of honokiol, an anxiolytic agent present in extracts of Magnolia bark, evaluated by an elevated plus-maze test in mice.** *J Pharm Pharmacol* 1998, **50**:819–26.
13. Kuribara H, Stavinoha WB, Maruyama Y: **Honokiol, a putative anxiolytic agent extracted from magnolia bark, has no diazepam-like side-effects in mice.** *J Pharm Pharmacol* 1999, **51**:97–103.
14. Peng WH, Lo KL, Lee YH, Hung TH, Lin YC: **Berberine produces antidepressant-like effects in the forced swim test and in the tail suspension test in mice.** *Life Sci* 2007, **81**(11):933–8.
15. Peng WH, Wu CR, Chen CS, Chen CF, Leu ZC, Hsieh MT: **Anxiolytic effect of berberine on exploratory activity of the mouse in two experimental anxiety models: interaction with drugs acting at 5-HT receptors.** *Life Sci* 2004, **75**(20):2451–62.
16. Li LF, Lu J, Li XM, Xu CL, Deng JM, Qu R, Ma SP: **Antidepressant-like effect of magnolol on BDNF up-regulation and serotonergic system activity in unpredictable chronic mild stress treated rats.** *Phytother Res* 2012, **26**(8):1189–94.
17. Maruyama Y, Kuribara H, Morita M, Yuzurihara M, Weintraub ST: **Identification of magnolol and honokiol as anxiolytic agents in extracts of saiboku-to, an oriental herbal medicine.** *J Nat Prod* 1998, **61**:135–8.
18. Sufka KJ, Roach JT, Chambliss WG Jr, Broom SL, Feltenstein MW, Wyandt CM, Zeng L: **Anxiolytic properties of botanical extracts in the chick social separation-stress procedure.** *Psychopharmacology (Berl)* 2001, **153**(2):219–24.
19. Qiang LQ, Wang CP, Wang FM, Pan Y, Yi LT, Zhang X, Kong LD: **Combined administration of the mixture of honokiol and magnolol and ginger oil evokes antidepressant-like synergism in rats.** *Arch Pharm Res* 2009, **32**(9):1281–92.
20. Garrison R, Chambliss WG: **Effect of a proprietary Magnolia and Phellodendron extract on weight management: a pilot, double-blind, placebo-controlled clinical trial.** *Altern Ther Health Med* 2006, **12**(1):50–54.
21. Kalman DS, Feldman S, Feldman R, Schwartz HI, Krieger DR, Garrison R: **Effect of a proprietary Magnolia and Phellodendron extract on stress levels in healthy women: a pilot, double-blind, placebo-controlled clinical trial.** *Nutr J* 2008, **7**:11.
22. McNair DM, Lorr M, Droppleman LF: *Manual for the Profile of Mood States.* San Diego, CA: Educational and Industrial Testing Services; 1971.
23. Leunes A: **Updated bibliography on the profile of mood states in sport and exercise psychology research.** *J Appl Sport Psychol* 2000, **12**(1):110–113.
24. Olfson M, Marcus SC: **National patterns in antidepressant medication treatment.** *Arch Gen Psychiatry* 2009, **66**(8):848–56.
25. Harman JS, Edlund MJ, Fortney JC: **Trends in antidepressant utilization from 2001 to 2004.** *Psychiatr Serv* 2009, **60**(5):611–6.
26. Li JM, Kong LD, Wang YM, Cheng CH, Zhang WY, Tan WZ: **Behavioral and biochemical studies on chronic mild stress models in rats treated with a Chinese traditional prescription Banxia-houpu decoction.** *Life Sci* 2003, **74**(1):55–73.
27. Berglund B, Safstrom H: **Psychological monitoring and modulation of training load of world-class canoeists.** *Med Sci Sports Exer* 1994, **26**(8):1036–1040.
28. Santhiago V, Da Silva AS, Papoti M, Gobatto CA: **Effects of 14-week swimming training program on the psychological, hormonal, and physiological parameters of elite women athletes.** *J Strength Cond Res* 2011, **25**(3):825–32.
29. Pierce EF Jr: **Relationship between training volume and mood states in competitive swimmers during a 24-week season.** *Percept Mot Skills* 2002, **94**(3 Pt 1):1009–12.
30. Lavallée L, Flint F: **The relationship of stress, competitive anxiety, mood state, and social support to athletic injury.** *J Athl Train* 1996, **31**(4):296–9.
31. Faude O, Meyer T, Urhausen A, Kindermann W: **Recovery training in cyclists: ergometric, hormonal and psychometric findings.** *Scand J Med Sci Sports* 2009, **19**(3):433–41.

The effect of protein timing on muscle strength and hypertrophy: a meta-analysis

Brad Jon Schoenfeld[1*], Alan Albert Aragon[2] and James W Krieger[3]

Abstract

Protein timing is a popular dietary strategy designed to optimize the adaptive response to exercise. The strategy involves consuming protein in and around a training session in an effort to facilitate muscular repair and remodeling, and thereby enhance post-exercise strength- and hypertrophy-related adaptations. Despite the apparent biological plausibility of the strategy, however, the effectiveness of protein timing in chronic training studies has been decidedly mixed. The purpose of this paper therefore was to conduct a multi-level meta-regression of randomized controlled trials to determine whether protein timing is a viable strategy for enhancing post-exercise muscular adaptations. The strength analysis comprised 478 subjects and 96 ESs, nested within 41 treatment or control groups and 20 studies. The hypertrophy analysis comprised 525 subjects and 132 ESs, nested with 47 treatment or control groups and 23 studies. A simple pooled analysis of protein timing without controlling for covariates showed a small to moderate effect on muscle hypertrophy with no significant effect found on muscle strength. In the full meta-regression model controlling for all covariates, however, no significant differences were found between treatment and control for strength or hypertrophy. The reduced model was not significantly different from the full model for either strength or hypertrophy. With respect to hypertrophy, total protein intake was the strongest predictor of ES magnitude. These results refute the commonly held belief that the timing of protein intake in and around a training session is critical to muscular adaptations and indicate that consuming adequate protein in combination with resistance exercise is the key factor for maximizing muscle protein accretion.

Background

Protein timing is a popular dietary strategy designed to optimize the adaptive response to exercise [1]. The strategy involves consuming protein in and around a training session in an effort to facilitate muscular repair and remodeling, and thereby enhance post-exercise strength- and hypertrophy-related adaptations [2]. It is generally accepted that protein should be consumed just before and/or immediately following a training session to take maximum advantage of a limited anabolic window [3]. Proponents of the strategy claim that, when properly executed, precise intake of protein in the peri-workout period can augment increases in fat-free mass [4]. Some researchers have even put forth the notion that the timing of food intake may have a greater positive effect on body composition than absolute daily nutrient consumption [5].

* Correspondence: brad@workout911.com
[1]Department of Health Science, Lehman College, Bronx, NY, USA
Full list of author information is available at the end of the article

A number of studies support the superiority of protein timing for stimulating increases in acute protein synthesis pursuant to resistance training when compared to placebo [6-9]. Protein is deemed to be the critical nutrient required for optimizing post-exercise protein synthesis. The essential amino acids, in particular, are believed primarily responsible for enhancing this response, with little to no contribution seen from provision of non-essential amino acids [10,11]. Borsheim et al. [10] found that a 6 g dose of essential amino acids (EAAs) consumed immediately post-exercise produced an approximate twofold increase in net protein balance compared to a comparable dose containing an approximately equal mixture of essential and non-essential amino acids, indicating a dose–response relationship up to 6 g EAAs. However, increasing EAA intake beyond this amount has not been shown to significantly heighten post-exercise protein synthesis [2]. There is limited evidence that carbohydrate has an additive effect on enhancing post-exercise muscle protein synthesis when combined with amino acid ingestion [12], with a majority of studies failing to demonstrate any such benefit [13-15].

Despite the apparent biological plausibility of the strategy, the effectiveness of protein timing in chronic training studies has been decidedly mixed. While some studies have shown that consumption of protein in the peri-workout period promotes increases in muscle strength and/or hypertrophy [16-19], others have not [20-22]. In a review of literature, Aragon and Schoenfeld [23] concluded that there is a lack of evidence to support a narrow "anabolic window of opportunity" whereby protein need to be consumed in immediate proximity to the exercise bout to maximize muscular adaptations. However, these conclusions were at least in part a reflection of methodological issues in the current research. One issue in particular is that studies to date have employed small sample sizes. Thus, it is possible that null findings may be attributable to these studies being underpowered, resulting in a type II error. In addition, various confounders including the amount of EAA supplementation, matching of protein intake, training status, and variations in age and gender between studies make it difficult to draw definitive conclusions on the topic. Thus, by increasing statistical power and controlling for confounding variables, a meta-analysis may help to provide clarity as to whether protein timing confers potential benefits in post-exercise skeletal muscle adaptations.

A recent meta-analysis by Cermak et al. [24] found that protein supplementation, when combined with regimented resistance training, enhances gains in strength and muscle mass in both young and elderly adults. However, this analysis did not specifically investigate protein timing per se. Rather, inclusion criteria encompassed all resistance training studies in which at least one group consumed a protein supplement or modified higher protein diet. The purpose of this paper therefore is to conduct a meta-analysis to determine whether timing protein near the resistance training bout is a viable strategy for enhancing muscular adaptations.

Methodology

Inclusion criteria

Only randomized controlled trials or randomized crossover trials involving protein timing were considered for inclusion. Protein timing was defined here as a study where at least one treatment group consumed a minimum of 6 g essential amino acids (EAAs) ≤ 1 hour pre- and/or post-resistance exercise and at least one control group did not consume protein < 2 hours pre- and/or post-resistance exercise. Resistance training protocols had to span at least 6 weeks and directly measure dynamic muscle strength and/or hypertrophy as a primary outcome variable. There were no restrictions for age, gender, training status, or matching of protein intake, but these variables were controlled via subgroup analysis using meta-regression.

Search strategy

To carry out this review, English-language literature searches of the PubMed and Google Scholar databases were conducted for all time periods up to March 2013. Combinations of the following keywords were used as search terms: "nutrient timing"; "protein supplementation"; "nutritional supplementation"; "protein supplement"; "nutritional supplement"; "resistance exercise"; "resistance training"; "strength training". Consistent with methods outlined by Greenhalgh and Peacock [25], the reference lists of articles retrieved in the search were then screened for any additional articles that had relevance to the topic. Abstracts from conferences, reviews, and unpublished dissertations/theses were excluded from analysis. A total of 34 studies were identified as potentially relevant to this review. To reduce the potential for selection bias, each of these studies were independently perused by two of the investigators (BJS and AAA), and a mutual decision was made as to whether or not they met basic inclusion criteria. Study quality was then assessed with the PEDro scale, which has been shown to be a valid measure of the methodologic quality of RCTs [26] and possesses acceptable inter-rater reliability [27]. Only those studies scoring ≥5 on the PEDro scale–a value considered to be of moderate to high quality [27]-were accepted for analysis. Any inter-reviewer disagreements were settled by consensus and/or consultation with the third investigator. Initial pre-screening revealed 29 potential studies that investigated nutrient timing with respect to muscular adaptations. Of these studies, 3 did not meet criteria for sufficient supplemental protein intake [28-30] and in another the timing of consumption was outside the defined post-workout range [31]. Thus, a total of 25 studies ultimately were deemed suitable for inclusion. Two of the studies were subsequently excluded because they did not contain sufficient data for calculating an effect size and attempts to obtain this information from the authors were unsuccessful [19,32], leaving a total 23 studies suitable for analysis. The average PEDro score of these studies was 8.7, indicating an overall high level of methodological quality. Table 1 summarizes the studies meeting inclusion criteria.

Coding of studies

Studies were read and individually coded by two of the investigators (BJS and AAA) for the following variables: Descriptive information of subjects by group including gender, body mass, training status (trained subjects were defined as those with at least one year resistance training experience), age, and stratified subject age (classified as either young [18–49 years] or elderly [50+ years];

Table 1 Summary of studies meeting inclusion criteria

Study	Subjects	Supplementation	Protein matched with control?	Anthropometric and/or body composition assessment method	Training protocol	Strength results	Body composition results
Antonio et al., [33]	19 untrained young women	18.3 g EAA or an equal dose of cellulose placebo taken (collectively) 20 minutes pre and post-exercise	No	DXA	Periodized progressive resistance training consisting of exercises for all major muscle groups performed 3 days/wk for 6 wks	Total weight lifted at the 12 RM intensity did not significantly change in either group	No significant body composition changes occurred in either group
Goddard et al., [34]	17 untrained older men (60–80 y)	12 g of essential amino acids and 72 g (total) of fructose and dextrose consumed immediately after exercise	No	Computed tomography (CT).	Progressive resistance training consisting of knee extensions preformed 3 days/ wk for 12 wks	Training produced a significant increase in 1RM strength and measures of maximal torque, no differences between groups	No significant differences in muscle CSA increase between groups
Rankin et al., [35]	13 untrained young men	Chocolate milk (providing a protein dose of 0.21 g/kg) or a CHO-electrolyte beverage (Gatorade) immediately after exercise	No	Dual X-ray absorptiometry (DXA) and multiple upper & lower body circumference measurements	Periodized progressive resistance training consisting of exercises for all major muscle groups performed 3 days/wk for 10 wks	1 RM strength increased in all exercises, with no significant difference between groups	No significant differences in fat reduction, mean mass gain, or circumference changes between groups
Andersen et al., [36]	22 untrained young men	25 g protein (combination of whey, casein, egg white, and glutamine) or 25 g maltodextrin immediately before and after exercise	No	Muscle biopsy	Periodized progressive resistance training consisting of lower body exercises performed 3 days/ wk for 14 wks	Squat jump height increased only in the protein group, whereas countermovement jump height and peak torque during slow isokinetic muscle contraction increased similarly in both groups.	The protein group showed hypertrophy of type I & II muscle fibers, whereas no significant change occurred in the CHO group
Bird et al., [37]	32 untrained young men	6 g EAA or 6% CHO solution + 6 g EAA or placebo during exercise	No	DXA and muscle biopsy	Progressive resistance training consisting of exercises for all major muscle groups performed 2 days/wk for 12 wks	Training caused a significant increase in 1RM in the leg press similarly in both treatment groups compared to placebo, isokinetic strength increased in all groups, with no differences between groups	CHO + EAA showed greater gains in fat-free mass compared to placebo, fat mass decreased in all groups without any significant difference between groups
Coburn et al., [38]	33 untrained young men	20 g whey + 6.2 g leucine or 26.2 g maltodextrin 30 minutes prior to and immediately after exercise	No	Magnetic resonance imaging (MRI)	Progressive resistance training consisting of knee extensions performed 3 days/ wk for 8 wks	Significantly greater 1 RM strength increase in the trained limb in the protein group compared to placebo	No significant body composition changes occurred in any of the groups, CSA increases did not differ between the protein and placebo groups
Candow, Burke, et al., [39]	27 untrained young men & women	Whey (1.2 g/kg) + sucrose (0.3 g/kg) or placebo (1.2 g/kg maltodextrin + 0.3 g/kg sucrose)	No	DXA	Progressive, periodized resistance training consisting of exercises for all major muscle	1 RM strength increases in the squat and bench press were significantly greater in the protein	Lean mass increase was significantly greater in the protein groups than placebo

Table 1 Summary of studies meeting inclusion criteria *(Continued)*

		Note that only the soy treatment was excluded from analysis.			groups performed 4 days/wk for 6 wks	groups than placebo	
Candow, Chilibeck, et al., [40]	29 untrained older men	Multi-ingredient supplement containing a protein dose of 0.3 g/kg immediately before exercise and a CHO-based placebo immediately after, or the reverse order of the latter, or placebo before & after exercise	No	Air-displacement plethysmography, ultrasound	Progressive resistance training consisting of exercises for all major muscle groups performed 3 days/wk for 12 wks	1 RM strength increases in the leg press & bench press occurred in all groups, no significant differences between groups	Lean mass and muscle thickness increased in all groups, no significant difference between groups
Cribb and Hayes, [16]	23 young recreational male bodybuilders	1 g/kg of a supplement containing 40 g whey isolate, 43 g glucose, and 7 g creatine monohydrate consumed either immediately before and after exercise or in the early morning and late evening	Yes	DXA and muscle biopsy	Progressive resistance training consisting of exercises for all major muscle groups performed 3 days/wk for 10 wks	Immediate pre-post supplementation caused greater increases in 1-RM in 2 out of 3 exercises	Significant increases in lean body mass and muscle CSA of type II fibers in immediate vs. delayed supplementation
Hartman et al., [41]	56 untrained young men	17.5 g protein within milk or a soy beverage, or CHO control immediately after exercise and again 1 hr after exercise *Note that only the soy treatment was excluded from analysis.*	No	DXA and muscle biopsy	Progressive resistance training consisting of exercises for all major muscle groups performed 5 days/wk for 12 wks	All groups experienced 1RM strength gains, but no between-group differences were seen	Type II muscle fiber area increased in all groups, but with greater increases in the milk group than in the soy and control groups, fat-free mass increased to a greater extent in the milk group compared to the soy & control groups
Hoffman et al., [42]	21 well-trained young men	42 g protein within a multi-ingredient supplement or a CHO placebo taken once in the morning and again after training	No	DXA	Progressive, periodized resistance training consisting of exercises for all major muscle groups performed 4 days/wk for 12 wks	1 RM bench press strength (but not squat strength) significantly increased in the protein group, while no measures of strength increased in the placebo group	No significant between-group or absolute changes in body composition occurred
Willoughby et al., [17]	19 untrained young men	20 g whey-dominant protein or 20 g dextrose consumed 1 hour before and after exercise	No	Hydrostatic weighing, muscle biopsy, surface measurements	Progressive resistance training consisting of exercise for all major muscle groups performed 4 days/wk for 10 wks	Protein supplementation caused greater increases in relative strength (maximal strength corrected for bodyweight) in bench press & leg press	Significant increase in total body mass, fat-free mass, and thigh mass with protein vs. carb supplementation
Eliot et al., [43]	42 untrained older men	35 g whey protein + CHO-electrolyte solution, or whey/CHO + 5 g creatine, or creatine-only, or CHO placebo	No	DXA and bioelectrical impedance	Progressive resistance training consisting of exercise for all major muscle groups performed	Not measured	No significant effects of any of the whey and/or creatine treatments were seen beyond body composition

Table 1 Summary of studies meeting inclusion criteria *(Continued)*

		Note that creatine treatments were excluded from analysis			3 days/wk for 14 wks		changes caused by training alone
Mielke et al., [44]	39 untrained young men	20 g whey protein + 6.2 g of leucine or 20 g maltodextrin 30 minutes before and immediately after exercise	No	Hydrodensitometry,	Dynamic constant external resistance (DCER) bilateral leg extension and bench press exercises were performed 3 days/ wk for 8 wks.	1 RM strength increased significantly in both groups without any between-group differences	No significant training-induced changes in body composition in either group,
Verdijk et al., [21]	28 untrained elderly men	10 g casein hydrolysate or placebo consumed immediately before and after exercise	No	DXA, CT, and muscle biopsy	Progressive resistance training consisting leg press and knee extension performed 3 days/ wk for 12 wks	1 RM leg press & leg extension strength increased, with no significant difference between groups	No significant differences in muscle CSA increase between groups
Hoffman et al., [20]	33 well-trained young men	Supplement containing 42 g protein (milk/ collagen blend) and 2 g carbohydrate consumed either immediately before and after exercise or in the early morning and late evening	Yes	DXA	Progressive resistance training consisting exercises for the major muscle groups peformed 4 days/ wk for 10 wks.	1 RM & 5 RM bench press & squat strength increased, with no significant difference between groups	No significant differences in total body mass or lean body mass between groups.
Hulmi et al., [18]	31 untrained young men	15 g whey isolate or placebo consumed immediately before and after exercise	No	MRI, muscle biopsy	Progressive, periodized total body resistance training consisting of exercises for all major muscle groups trained performed 2 days/ wk for 21 wks	Strength increased similarly in the protein & placebo group, but only the protein group increased isometric leg extension strength vs the control group	Significant increase in CSA of the vastus lateralis but not of the other quadriceps muscles in the protein group vs placebo
Josse et al., [45]	20 untrained young women	18 g protein within milk or an isocaloric maltodextrin placebo immediately after exercise and again 1 hr later	No	DXA	Progressive, periodized resistance training consisting of exercises for all major muscle groups performed 5 days/wk for 12 wks	1 RM strength increased similarly in both groups, but milk significantly outperformed placebo in the bench press	Lean mass increased in both groups but to a significantly greater degree in the milk group, fat mass decreased in the milk group only
Walker et al., [46]	30 moderately trained men and women	19.7 g of whey protein and 6.2 g leucine or isocaloric CHO placebo 30–45 minutes before exercising and the second packet 30–45 minutes after exercising.	No	DXA	Bodyweight-based exercises and running at least 3 days/wk, externally loaded training not specified	1 RM bench press strength increased significantly in the protein group only	Total mass, fat-free mass, and lean body mass increased significantly in the protein group only
Vieillevoye et al., [47]	29 untrained young men	15 g EAA + 15 g saccharose. or 30 g saccharose consumed with breakfast and immediately after exercise	No	Ultrasonography, 3-site skinfold assessment with calipers, 3-site circumference measurements	Progressive, periodized resistance training consisting of exercises for all major muscle groups performed 2 days/wk for 12 wks	Maximal strength significantly increased in both groups, with no between-group diffrerence	Muscle mass significantly increased in both groups with no differences between groups, muscle thickness of the gastrocnemius medialis significantly increased in the EAA group only

Table 1 Summary of studies meeting inclusion criteria *(Continued)*

Wycherly et al., [22]	34 untrained, older men & women w/ type 2 diabetes	21 g protein, 0.7 g fat, 29.6 g carbohydrate consumed either immediately prior to, or at least 2 h following exercise	Yes	DXA, waist circumference	Progressive resistance training consisting of exercises for all major muscle groups performed 3 days/wk for 16 wks	Not measured	Fat mass, fat-free mass, and waist circumference decreased with no significant differences between groups
Erskine et al., [48]	33 untrained young men	20 g whey protein or placebo consumed immediately before and after exercise	No	MRI	4-6 sets of elbow flexion performed 3 days/wk for 12 weeks	No significant differences in maximal isometric voluntary force or 1 RM strength between groups	No significant differences in muscle CSA between groups
Weisgarber et al., [49]	17 untrained young men and women	Whey protein dosed at 0.3 g/kg or isocaloric CHO immediately before, during, and after exercise	No	DXA and ultrasound	Progressive resistance training consisting of exercises for all major muscle groups performed 4 days/wk for 8 wks	1 RM strength in the chest press increased in both groups without any between-group difference	Significant increases in muscle mass were seen without any difference between groups

whether or not total daily protein intake between groups was matched; whether the study was an RCT or crossover design; the number of subjects in each group; blinding (classified as single, double, or unblinded); duration of the study; type of hypertrophy measurement (MRI, CT, ultrasound, biopsy, etc.) and region/muscle of body measured, if applicable; lean body mass measurement (i.e. DXA, hydrostatic weighing, etc.), if applicable, and; strength exercise (s) employed for testing, if applicable. Coding was cross-checked between coders, and any discrepancies were resolved by mutual consensus. To assess potential coder drift, 5 studies were randomly selected for recoding as described by Cooper et al. [50]. Per case agreement was determined by dividing the number of variables coded the same by the total number of variables. Acceptance required a mean agreement of 0.90.

Calculation of effect size

For each 1-RM strength or hypertrophy outcome, an effect size (ES) was calculated as the pretest-posttest change, divided by the pretest standard deviation (SD) [51]. The sampling variance for each ES was estimated according to Morris and DeShon [51]. Calculation of the sampling variance required an estimate of the population ES, and the pretest-posttest correlation for each individual ES. The population ES was estimated by calculating the mean ES across all studies and treatment groups [51]. The pretest-posttest correlation was calculated using the following formula [51]:

$$r = \left(s_1^2 + s_2^2 - s_D^2\right) / \left(2\, s_1 s_2\right)$$

where s_1 and s_2 are the SD for the pre- and posttest means, respectively, and s_D is the SD of the difference scores. Where s_2 was not reported, s_1 was used in its place. Where s_D was not reported, it was estimated using the following formula [52]:

$$s_D = \sqrt{\left(\left(s_1^2/n\right) + \left(s_2^2/n\right)\right)}$$

Statistical analyses

Meta-analyses were performed using hierarchical linear mixed models, modeling the variation between studies as a random effect, the variation between treatment and control groups as a random effect nested within studies, and group-level predictors as fixed effects [53]. The within-group variances were assumed known. Observations were weighted by the inverse of the sampling variance [51]. An intercept-only model was created, estimating the weighted mean ES across all studies and treatment groups. Second, a basic model was created which only included the class of the group (treatment or control) as a predictor. A full model was then created with the following predictors: the class of the group (treatment or control), whether or not the groups were protein matched, training status (experienced or novice), blinding (double, single, or none), gender (male, female, or mixed), age (young or old), body mass in kg, and the duration of the study in weeks. The full model was then reduced by removing one predictor at a time, starting with the most insignificant predictor [54]. The final model represented the reduced model with the lowest Akaike's Information Corrected Criterion (AICC) [55] and that was not significantly different ($P > 0.05$) from the full model when compared using a likelihood ratio test (LRT). Model parameters were estimated by the method of restricted maximum likelihood (REML) [56];

an exception was during the model reduction process, in which parameters were estimated by the method of maximum likelihood (ML), as LRTs cannot be used to compare nested models with REML estimates. Denominator df for statistical tests and CIs were calculated according to Berkey et al. [57]. The treatment/control classification variable was not removed during the model reduction process.

Separate analyses were performed for strength and hypertrophy. ESs for both changes in cross-sectional area (CSA) and FFM were pooled in the hypertrophy analysis. However, because resistance exercise is associated with the accretion of non-muscle tissue, separate sub-analyses on CSA and FFM were performed. Because the effect of protein timing might interact with whether the treatment and control groups were matched for total protein intake, an additional model was created that included an interaction term between the treatment/control classification variable and the protein match variable. Also, because the effect of protein timing might vary by training experience, a model was created that included an interaction term between the treatment/control classification variable and the training status variable. Adjustment for post hoc multiple comparisons was performed using a simulation-based procedure [58]. All analyses were performed using SAS Enterprise Guide Version 4.2 (Cary, NC). Effects were considered significant at $P \leq 0.05$. Data are reported as means (±SEs) and 95% CIs.

Results

Study characteristics

The strength analysis comprised 478 subjects and 96 ESs, nested within 41 treatment or control groups and 20 studies. The weighted mean strength ES across all studies and groups was 1.39 ± 0.24 (CI: 0.88, 1.90). The hypertrophy analysis comprised 525 subjects and 132 ESs, nested with 47 treatment or control groups and 23 studies. The weighted mean hypertrophy ES across all studies and groups was 0.47 ± 0.08 (CI: 0.31, 0.63).

Basic model

There was no significant difference between the treatment and control for strength (difference = 0.38 ± 0.36; CI: -0.34, 1.10; P = 0.30). The mean strength ES difference between treatment and control for each individual study, along with the overall weighted mean difference across all studies, is shown in Figure 1. For hypertrophy, the mean ES was significantly greater in the treatment compared to the control (difference = 0.24 ± 0.10; CI: 0.04, 0.44; P = 0.02). The mean hypertrophy ES difference between treatment and control for each individual study, along with the overall weighted mean difference across all studies, is shown in Figure 2.

Full model

In the full meta-regression model controlling for all covariates, there was no significant difference between the treatment and control for strength (difference = 0.28 ±

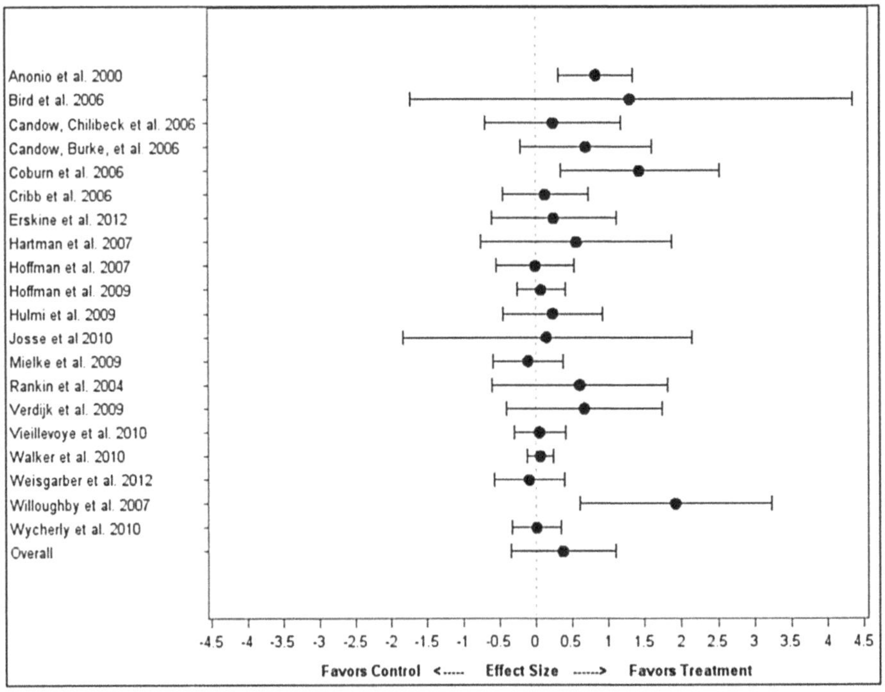

Figure 1 Impact of protein timing on strength by study.

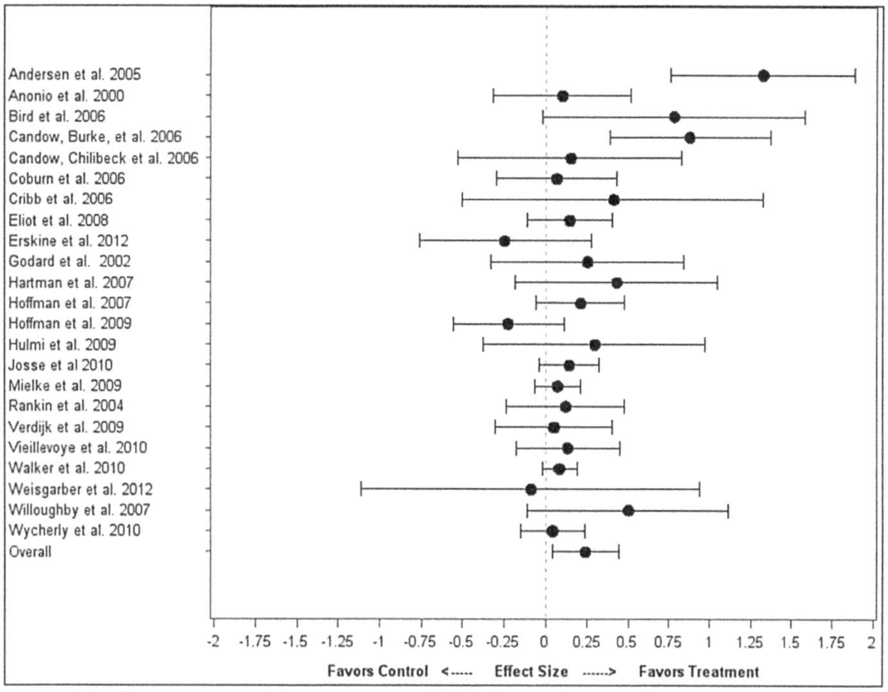

Figure 2 Impact of protein timing on hypertrophy by study.

0.40; CI: -0.52, 1.07; P = 0.49) or hypertrophy (difference =0.16 ± 0.11; CI: -0.07, 0.38; P = 0.18).

Reduced model: strength

After the model reduction procedure, only training status and blinding remained as significant covariates. The reduced model was not significantly different from the full model (P = 0.73). In the reduced model, there was no significant difference between the treatment and control (difference = 0.39 ± 0.36; CI: -0.34, 1.11; P = 0.29). The mean ES for control was 0.93 ± 0.31 (CI: 0.32, 1.54). The mean ES for treatment was 1.31 ± 0.30 (CI: 0.71, 1.92).

Reduced model: hypertrophy

After the model reduction procedure, total protein intake, study duration, and blinding remained as significant covariates. The reduced model was not significantly different from the full model (P = 0.87). In the reduced model, there was no significant difference between the treatment and control (difference = 0.14 ± 0.11; CI: -0.07, 0.35; P = 0.20). The mean ES for control was 0.36 ± 0.09 (CI: 0.18, 0.53). The mean ES for treatment was 0.49 ± 0.08 (CI: 0.33, 0.66). Total protein intake (in g/kg) was the strongest predictor of ES magnitude (estimate = 0.41 ± 0.14; CI: 0.14, 0.69; P = 0.004).

To confirm that total protein intake was mediator variable in the relationship between protein timing and hypertrophy, a model with only total protein intake as a covariate was created. The difference between treatment and control was not significant (difference = 0.14 ± 0.11; CI: -0.07, 0.35,; P = 0.19). Total protein intake was a significant predictor of ES magnitude (estimate = 0.39 ± 0.15; CI: 0.08, 0.69; P = 0.01). Figure 3 shows the total protein intake-adjusted ES's for each study, as well as the overall effect from the meta-regression with only total protein intake as a covariate.

Interactions

For strength, the interaction between treatment and training status was nearly significant (P = 0.051), but post hoc comparisons between treatment and control within each training status classification were not significant (adjusted P = 0.47 for difference within non-experienced groups, and adjusted P = 0.99 for difference within experienced groups). There was no significant interaction between treatment and whether groups were protein matched (P = 0.43). For hypertrophy, there was no significant interaction between treatment and training status (P = 0.63) or treatment and protein matching (P = 0.59).

Hypertrophy sub-analyses

Separating the hypertrophy analysis into CSA or FFM did not materially alter the outcomes. For FFM, there was no significant difference between treatment and control (difference = 0.08 ± 0.07; CI: -0.07, 0.24; P = 0.27). Total protein intake remained a strong predictor of ES

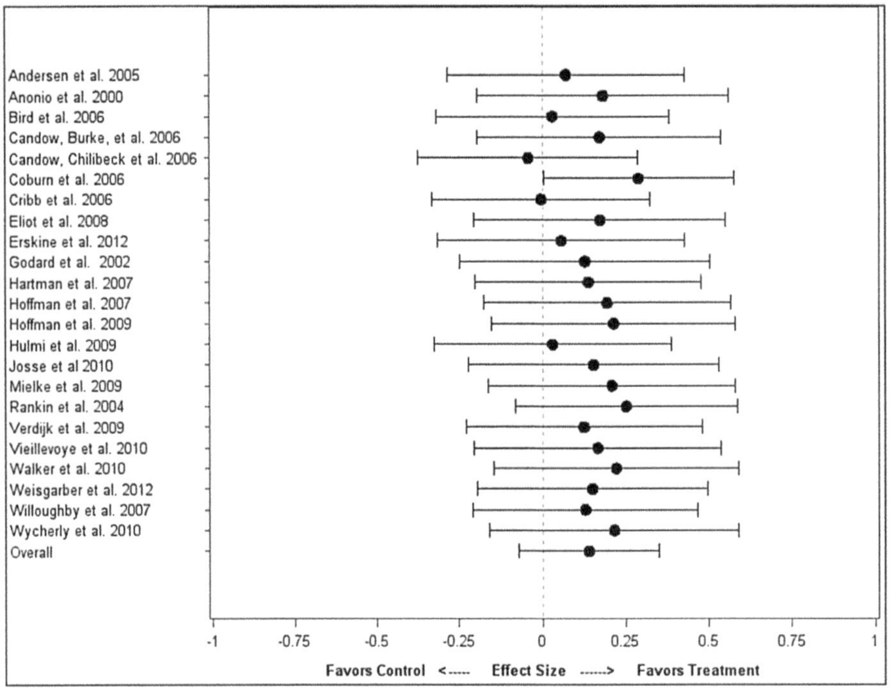

Figure 3 Impact of protein timing on hypertrophy by study, adjusted for total protein intake.

magnitude (estimate = 0.39 ± 0.07; CI: 0.25, 0.53; P < 0.001). For CSA, there was no significant difference between treatment and control (difference = 0.14 ± 0.16; CI: -0.17, 0.46; P = 0.37). Total protein intake was again a predictor of ES magnitude (estimate = 0.55 ± 0.24; CI: 0.08, 1.20; P = 0.02).

Discussion

This is the first meta-analysis to directly investigate the effects of protein timing on strength and hypertrophic adaptations following long-term resistance training protocols. The study produced several novel findings. A simple pooled analysis of protein timing without controlling for covariates showed a significant effect on muscle hypertrophy (ES = 0.24 ± 0.10) with no significant effect found on muscle strength. It is generally accepted that an effect size of 0.2 is small, 0.5 is moderate, and 0.8 and above is a large, indicating that the effect of protein timing on gains in lean body mass were small to moderate. However, an expanded regression analysis found that any positive effects associated with protein timing on muscle protein accretion disappeared after controlling for covariates. Moreover, sub-analysis showed that discrepancies in total protein intake explained the majority of hypertrophic differences noted in timing studies. When taken together, these results would seem to refute the commonly held belief that the timing of protein intake in the immediate pre- and post-workout period is critical to muscular adaptations [3-5].

Perceived hypertrophic benefits seen in timing studies appear to be the result of an increased consumption of protein as opposed to temporal factors. In our reduced model, the amount of protein consumed was highly and significantly associated with hypertrophic gains. In fact, the reduced model revealed that total protein intake was by far the most important predictor of hypertrophy ES, with a ~0.2 increase in ES noted for every 0.5 g/kg increase in protein ingestion. While there is undoubtedly an upper threshold to this correlation, these findings underscore the importance of consuming higher amounts of protein when the goal is to maximize exercise-induced increases in muscle mass. Conversely, total protein intake did not have an impact on strength outcomes and ultimately was factored out during the model reduction process.

The Recommended Dietary Allowance (RDA) for protein is 0.8 g/kg/day. However, these values are based on the needs of sedentary individuals and are intended to represent a level of intake necessary to replace losses and hence avert deficiency; they do not reflect the requirements of hard training individuals seeking to increase lean mass. Studies do in fact show that those participating in intensive resistance training programs need significantly more protein to remain in a non-negative nitrogen balance. Position stands from multiple scientific bodies estimate these requirements to be approximately double that of the RDA [59,60]. Higher levels of protein consumption appear to be particularly important during the early stages of intense resistance training. Lemon et al. [61] displayed that novice bodybuilders required a protein intake of 1.6-1.7 g/kg/day to remain in a non-negative nitrogen balance. The increased protein requirements in novice subjects have been attributed to changes in muscle protein synthetic rate and the need to sustain greater lean mass rather than increased fuel utilization [62]. There is some evidence that protein requirements actually decrease slightly to approximately 1.4 g/kg/day in well-trained individuals because of a greater efficiency in dietary nitrogen utilization [63], although this hypothesis needs further study.

The average protein intake for controls in the unmatched studies was 1.33 g/kg/day while average intake for treatment was 1.66 g/kg/day. Since a preponderance of these studies involved untrained subjects, it seems probable that a majority of any gains in muscle mass would have been due to higher protein consumption by the treatment group. These findings are consistent with those of Cermak et al. [24], who found that protein supplementation alone produced beneficial adaptations when combined with resistance training. The study by Cermak et al. [24] did not evaluate any effects regarding timing of intake, however, so our results directly lend support to the theory that meeting target protein requirements is paramount with respect to exercise-induced muscle protein accretion; immediate intake of dietary protein pre and/or post-workout would at best appear to be a minor consideration. The findings also support previous recommendations that a protein consumption of at least 1.6 g/kg/day is necessary to maximize muscle protein accretion in individuals involved in resistance training programs [61].

For the matched studies, protein intake averaged 1.91 g/kg/day versus 1.81 g/kg/day for treatment and controls, respectively. This level of intake for both groups meets or exceeds suggested guidelines, allowing for a fair evaluation of temporal effects. Only 3 studies that employed matched protein intake met inclusion criteria for this analysis, however. Interestingly, 2 of the 3 showed no benefits from timing. Moreover, another matched study actually found significantly greater increases in strength and lean body mass from a time-divided protein dose (i.e. morning and evening) compared with the same dose provided around the resistance training session [19]. However, this study had to be excluded from our analysis because it lacked adequate data to calculate an ES. The sum results of the matched-protein studies suggest that timing is superfluous provided adequate protein is ingested, although the small number of studies limits the ability to draw firm conclusions on the matter.

This meta-analysis had a number of strengths. For one, the quality of studies evaluated was high, with an average PEDro score of 8.7. Also, the sample was relatively large (23 trials encompassing 478 subjects for strength outcomes and 525 subjects for hypertrophy outcomes), affording good statistical power. In addition, strict inclusion/exclusion criteria were employed to reduce the potential for bias. Combined, these factors provide good confidence in the ability draw relevant inferences from findings. Another strength was the rigid adherence to proper coding practices. Coding was carried out by two of the investigators (BJS and AAA) and then cross-checked between coders. Coder drift was then assessed by random selection of studies to further ensure consistency of data. Finally and importantly, the study benefited from the use of meta-regression. This afforded the ability to examine the impact of moderator variables on effect size and explain heterogenecity between studies [64]. Although initial findings indicated an advantage conferred by protein timing, meta-regression revealed that results were confounded by discrepancies in consumption. This ultimately led to the determination that total protein intake rather than temporal factors explained any perceived benefits.

There are several limitations to this analysis that should be taken into consideration when drawing evidence-based conclusions. First, timing of the meals in the control groups varied significantly from study to study. Some provided protein as soon as 2 hours post workout while others delayed consumption for many hours. A recent review by Aragon and Schoenfeld [23] postulated that the anabolic window of opportunity may be as long as 4–6 hours around a training session, depending on the size and composition of the meal. Because the timing of intake in controls were all treated similarly in this meta-analysis, it is difficult to determine whether a clear anabolic window exists for protein consumption beyond which muscular adaptations suffer.

Second, the majority of studies evaluated subjects who were inexperienced with resistance exercise. It is well-established that highly trained individuals respond differently to the demands of resistance training compared with those who lack training experience [65]. In part, this is attributed to a "ceiling effect" whereby gains in muscle mass become progressively more difficult as a trainee gets closer to his genetic hypertrophic potential. There also is emerging evidence showing that regimented resistance exercise attenuates anabolic intracellular signaling in rodents [66] and humans [67], conceivably diminishing the hypertrophic response. Our sub-analysis failed to show an interaction effect between resistance training status and protein timing for either strength or hypertrophy. However, statistical power was low because only 4 studies using trained subjects met inclusion criteria. Future research should therefore focus on determining the effects of protein timing on muscular adaptations in those with at least 1 year or more of regular, consistent resistance training experience.

Third, in an effort to keep our sample size sufficiently large, we pooled CSA and FFM data to determine hypertrophy ES. FFM is frequently used as a proxy for hypertrophy, as it is generally assumed that the vast majority of the gains in fat free mass from resistance training are myocellular in nature. Nevertheless, resistance exercise also is associated with the accretion of non-muscle tissue as well (i.e. bone, connective tissue, etc.). To account for any potential discrepancies in this regard, we performed sub-analyses on CSA and FFM alone and the results essentially did not change. For FFM, the difference between treatment and control was not significant ($P = 0.27$), with a ES difference of −0.08. Protein intake again was highly significant, with an ES impact of ~0.2 per every 1 g/kg/day. For CSA, the difference between treatment and control was not significant ($P = 0.37$), with a ES difference of −0.14. Protein intake was again significant ($P = 0.02$) with an ES impact of ~0.33 per every 0.5 g/kg.

Finally and importantly, there was a paucity of timing studies that attempted to match protein intake. As previously discussed, our results show that total protein intake is strongly and positively associated with post-exercise gains in muscle hypertrophy. Future studies should seek to control for this variable so that the true effects of timing, if any, can be accurately assessed.

Practical applications

In conclusion, current evidence does not appear to support the claim that immediate (≤ 1 hour) consumption of protein pre- and/or post-workout significantly enhances strength- or hypertrophic-related adaptations to resistance exercise. The results of this meta-analysis indicate that if a peri-workout anabolic window of opportunity does in fact exist, the window for protein consumption would appear to be greater than one-hour before and after a resistance training session. Any positive effects noted in timing studies were found to be due to an increased protein intake rather than the temporal aspects of consumption, but a lack of matched studies makes it difficult to draw firm conclusions in this regard. The fact that protein consumption in non-supplemented subjects was below generally recommended intake for those involved in resistance training lends credence to this finding. Since causality cannot be directly drawn from our analysis, however, we must acknowledge the possibility that protein timing was in fact responsible for producing a positive effect and that the associated increase in protein intake is merely coincidental. Future research should seek to control for protein intake so that the true value regarding nutrient timing can be properly evaluated. Particular focus should be placed on carrying out these studies with well-trained subjects to better determine whether resistance training experience plays a role in the response.

Competing interests

The authors declare that they have no competing interests.

Authors' contributions

BJS and AAA performed the literature search, performed quality assessment, and coded the studies. JWK devised and carried out the statistical analysis. All authors took part in writing the manuscript. All authors read and approved the final manuscript.

Acknowledgement

This study was supported by a grant from Dymatize Nutrition, Dallas, TX.

Author details

[1]Department of Health Science, Lehman College, Bronx, NY, USA. [2]California State University, Northridge, CA, USA. [3]Weightology, LLC, Issaquah, WA, USA.

References

1. Phillips SM, Van Loon LJ. **Dietary protein for athletes: from requirements to optimum adaptation.** *J Sports Sci* 2011, **29**(Suppl 1):S29-38.
2. Kerksick C, Harvey T, Stout J, Campbell B, Wilborn C, Kreider R, *et al*: **International society of sports nutrition position stand: nutrient timing.** *J Int Soc Sports Nutr.* 2008 Oct 3, **5**:17.
3. Lemon PW, Berardi JM, Noreen EE: **The role of protein and amino acid supplements in the athlete's diet: does type or timing of ingestion matter?** *Curr Sports Med Rep* 2002 Aug, **1**(4):214–221.
4. Ivy J, Portman R: *Nutrient timing: The future of sports nutrition.* North Bergen, NJ: Basic Health Publications; 2004.
5. Candow DG, Chilibeck PD: **Timing of creatine or protein supplementation and resistance training in the elderly.** *Appl Physiol Nutr Metab* 2008 Feb, **33**(1):184–190.
6. Tipton KD, Elliott TA, Cree MG, Wolf SE, Sanford AP, Wolfe RR: **Ingestion of casein and whey proteins result in muscle anabolism after resistance exercise.** *Med Sci Sports Exerc* 2004 Dec, **36**(12):2073–2081.
7. Rasmussen BB, Tipton KD, Miller SL, Wolf SE, Wolfe RR: **An oral essential amino acid-carbohydrate supplement enhances muscle protein anabolism after resistance exercise.** *J Appl Physiol* 2000 Feb, **88**(2):386–392.
8. Tipton KD, Elliott TA, Ferrando AA, Aarsland AA, Wolfe RR: **Stimulation of muscle anabolism by resistance exercise and ingestion of leucine plus protein.** *Appl Physiol Nutr Metab* 2009 Apr, **34**(2):151–161.
9. Tipton KD, Ferrando AA, Phillips SM, Doyle D Jr, Wolfe RR: **Postexercise net protein synthesis in human muscle from orally administered amino acids.** *Am J Physiol* 1999 Apr, **276**(4 Pt 1):E628–E634.
10. Borsheim E, Tipton KD, Wolf SE, Wolfe RR: **Essential amino acids and muscle protein recovery from resistance exercise.** *Am J Physiol Endocrinol Metab* 2002 Oct, **283**(4):E648–E657.
11. Tipton KD, Gurkin BE, Matin S, Wolfe RR: **Nonessential amino acids are not necessary to stimulate net muscle protein synthesis in healthy volunteers.** *J Nutr Biochem* 1999 Feb, **10**(2):89–95.
12. Miller SL, Tipton KD, Chinkes DL, Wolf SE, Wolfe RR: **Independent and combined effects of amino acids and glucose after resistance exercise.** *Med Sci Sports Exerc* 2003 Mar, **35**(3):449–455.
13. Koopman R, Beelen M, Stellingwerff T, Pennings B, Saris WH, Kies AK, *et al*: **Coingestion of carbohydrate with protein does not further augment postexercise muscle protein synthesis.** *Am J Physiol Endocrinol Metab* 2007 Sep, **293**(3):E833–E842.
14. Staples AW, Burd NA, West DW, Currie KD, Atherton PJ, Moore DR, *et al*: **Carbohydrate does not augment exercise-induced protein accretion versus protein alone.** *Med Sci Sports Exerc* 2011 Jul, **43**(7):1154–1161.
15. Glynn EL, Fry CS, Timmerman KL, Drummond MJ, Volpi E, Rasmussen BB: **Addition of carbohydrate or alanine to an essential amino acid mixture**

does not enhance human skeletal muscle protein anabolism. *J Nutr* 2013 Mar, **143**(3):307–314.
16. Cribb PJ, Hayes A: **Effects of supplement timing and resistance exercise on skeletal muscle hypertrophy.** *Med Sci Sports Exerc* 2006 Nov, **38** (11):1918–1925.
17. Willoughby DS, Stout JR, Wilborn CD: **Effects of resistance training and protein plus amino acid supplementation on muscle anabolism, mass, and strength.** *Amino Acids* 2007, **32**(4):467–477.
18. Hulmi JJ, Kovanen V, Selanne H, Kraemer WJ, Hakkinen K, Mero AA: **Acute and long-term effects of resistance exercise with or without protein ingestion on muscle hypertrophy and gene expression.** *Amino Acids* 2009 Jul, **37**(2):297–308.
19. Burk A, Timpmann S, Medijainen L, Vahi M, Oopik V: **Time-divided ingestion pattern of casein-based protein supplement stimulates an increase in fat-free body mass during resistance training in young untrained men.** *Nutr Res* 2009 Jun, **29**(6):405–413.
20. Hoffman JR, Ratamess NA, Tranchina CP, Rashti SL, Kang J, Faigenbaum AD: **Effect of protein-supplement timing on strength, power, and body-composition changes in resistance-trained men.** *Int J Sport Nutr Exerc Metab* 2009 Apr, **19**(2):172–185.
21. Verdijk LB, Jonkers RA, Gleeson BG, Beelen M, Meijer K, Savelberg HH, *et al*: **Protein supplementation before and after exercise does not further augment skeletal muscle hypertrophy after resistance training in elderly men.** *Am J Clin Nutr* 2009 Feb, **89**(2):608–616.
22. Wycherley TP, Noakes M, Clifton PM, Cleanthous X, Keogh JB, Brinkworth GD: **Timing of protein ingestion relative to resistance exercise training does not influence body composition, energy expenditure, glycaemic control or cardiometabolic risk factors in a hypocaloric, high protein diet in patients with type 2 diabetes.** *Diab Obes Metab* 2010 Dec, **12**(12):1097–1105.
23. Aragon AA, Schoenfeld BJ: **Nutrient timing revisited: is there a post-exercise anabolic window?** *J Int Soc Sports Nutr* 2013 Jan 29, **10**(1):10–15. 5,2783.
24. Cermak NM, Res PT, de Groot LC, Saris WH, van Loon LJ: **Protein supplementation augments the adaptive response of skeletal muscle to resistance-type exercise training: a meta-analysis.** *Am J Clin Nutr* 2012 Dec, **96**(6):1454–1464.
25. Greenhalgh T, Peacock R: **Effectiveness and efficiency of search methods in systematic reviews of complex evidence: audit of primary sources.** *BMJ* 2005 Nov 5, **331**(7524):1064–1065.
26. Elkins MR, Herbert RD, Moseley AM, Sherrington C, Maher C: **Rating the quality of trials in systematic reviews of physical therapy interventions.** *Cardiopulm Phys Ther J* 2010 Sep, **21**(3):20–26.
27. Moseley AM, Herbert RD, Sherrington C, Maher CG: **Evidence for physiotherapy practice: a survey of the physiotherapy evidence database (PEDro).** *Aust J Physiother* 2002, **48**(1):43–49.
28. Esmarck B, Andersen JL, Olsen S, Richter EA, Mizuno M, Kjaer M: **Timing of postexercise protein intake is important for muscle hypertrophy with resistance training in elderly humans.** *J Physiol* 2001 Aug 15, **535**(Pt 1):301–311.
29. Holm L, Olesen JL, Matsumoto K, Doi T, Mizuno M, Alsted TJ, *et al*: **Protein-containing nutrient supplementation following strength training enhances the effect on muscle mass, strength, and bone formation in postmenopausal women.** *J Appl Physiol* 2008 Jul, **105**(1):274–281.
30. White KM, Bauer SJ, Hartz KK, Baldridge M: **Changes in body composition with yogurt consumption during resistance training in women.** *Int J Sport Nutr Exerc Metab* 2009 Feb, **19**(1):18–33.
31. Kerksick CM, Rasmussen CJ, Lancaster SL, Magu B, Smith P, Melton C, *et al*: **The effects of protein and amino acid supplementation on performance and training adaptations during ten weeks of resistance training.** *J Strength Cond Res* 2006 Aug, **20**(3):643–653.
32. Bemben MG, Witten MS, Carter JM, Eliot KA, Knehans AW, Bemben DA: **The effects of supplementation with creatine and protein on muscle strength following a traditional resistance training program in middle-aged and older men.** *J Nutr Health Aging* 2010 Feb, **14**(2):155–159.
33. Antonio J, Sanders MS, Ehler LA, Uelmen J, Raether JB, Stout JR: **Effects of exercise training and amino-acid supplementation on body composition and physical performance in untrained women.** *Nutrition* 2000 Nov-Dec, **16**(11-12):1043–1046.
34. Godard MP, Williamson DL, Trappe SW: **Oral amino-acid provision does not affect muscle strength or size gains in older men.** *Med Sci Sports Exerc* 2002 Jul, **34**(7):1126–1131.
35. Rankin JW, Goldman LP, Puglisi MJ, Nickols-Richardson SM, Earthman CP, Gwazdauskas FC: **Effect of post-exercise supplement consumption on adaptations to resistance training.** *J Am Coll Nutr* 2004 Aug, **23**(4):322–330.
36. Andersen LL, Tufekovic G, Zebis MK, Crameri RM, Verlaan G, Kjaer M, *et al*: **The effect of resistance training combined with timed ingestion of protein on muscle fiber size and muscle strength.** *Metabolism* 2005 Feb, **54**(2):151–156.
37. Bird SP, Tarpenning KM, Marino FE: **Independent and combined effects of liquid carbohydrate/essential amino acid ingestion on hormonal and muscular adaptations following resistance training in untrained men.** *Eur J Appl Physiol* 2006 May, **97**(2):225–238.
38. Coburn JW, Housh DJ, Housh TJ, Malek MH, Beck TW, Cramer JT, *et al*: **Effects of leucine and whey protein supplementation during eight weeks of unilateral resistance training.** *J Strength Cond Res* 2006 May, **20** (2):284–291.
39. Candow DG, Burke NC, Smith-Palmer T, Burke DG: **Effect of whey and soy protein supplementation combined with resistance training in young adults.** *Int J Sport Nutr Exerc Metab* 2006 Jun, **16**(3):233–244.
40. Candow DG, Chilibeck PD, Facci M, Abeysekara S, Zello GA: **Protein supplementation before and after resistance training in older men.** *Eur J Appl Physiol* 2006 Jul, **97**(5):548–556.
41. Hartman JW, Tang JE, Wilkinson SB, Tarnopolsky MA, Lawrence RL, Fullerton AV, *et al*: **Consumption of fat-free fluid milk after resistance exercise promotes greater lean mass accretion than does consumption of soy or carbohydrate in young, novice, male weightlifters.** *Am J Clin Nutr* 2007 Aug, **86**(2):373–381.
42. Hoffman JR, Ratamess NA, Kang J, Falvo MJ, Faigenbaum AD: **Effects of protein supplementation on muscular performance and resting hormonal changes in college football players.** *J Sports Sci Med* 2007, **6**:85–92.
43. Eliot KA, Knehans AW, Bemben DA, Witten MS, Carter J, Bemben MG: **The effects of creatine and whey protein supplementation on body composition in men aged 48 to 72 years during resistance training.** *J Nutr Health Aging* 2008 Mar, **12**(3):208–212.
44. Mielke M, Housh TJ, Malek MH, Beck T, Schmidt RJ, Johnson GO, *et al*: **The effects of whey protein and leucine supplementation on strength, muscular endurance, and body composition during resistance training.** *J Exerc Physiol Online* 2009, **12**:39–50.
45. Josse AR, Tang JE, Tarnopolsky MA, Phillips SM: **Body composition and strength changes in women with milk and resistance exercise.** *Med Sci Sports Exerc* 2010 Jun, **42**(6):1122–1130.
46. Walker TB, Smith J, Herrera M, Lebegue B, Pinchak A, Fischer J: **The influence of 8 weeks of whey-protein and leucine supplementation on physical and cognitive performance.** *Int J Sport Nutr Exerc Metab* 2010 Oct, **20**(5):409–417.
47. Vieillevoye S, Poortmans JR, Duchateau J, Carpentier A: **Effects of a combined essential amino acids/carbohydrate supplementation on muscle mass, architecture and maximal strength following heavy-load training.** *Eur J Appl Physiol* 2010 Oct, **110**(3):479–488.
48. Erskine RM, Fletcher G, Hanson B, Folland JP: **Whey protein does not enhance the adaptations to elbow flexor resistance training.** *Med Sci Sports Exerc* 2012 Sep, **44**(9):1791–1800.
49. Weisgarber KD, Candow DG, Vogt ESM: **Whey protein before and during resistance exercise has no effect on muscle mass and strength in untrained young adults.** *Int J Sport Nutr Exerc Metab* 2012 Jul, **4**.
50. Cooper H, Hedges L, Valentine J: *The handbook of research synthesis and meta-analysis.* 2nd edition. New York: Russell Sage Foundation; 2009.
51. Morris SB, DeShon RP: **Combining effect size estimates in meta-analysis with repeated measures and independent-groups designs.** *Psychol Methods* 2002 Mar, **7**(1):105–125.
52. *Technical guide: Data analysis and interpretation [online]. [Internet].: National Center for Education Statistics. [updated 17 Dec. 2007].* http://nces.ed.gov/programs/coe/guide/g3c.asp.
53. Hox JJ, de Leeuw ED, Hox JJ, de Leeuw ED: **Multilevel models for meta-analysis.** In *Reise SP, Duan N, editors. Multilevel modeling. Methodological advances, issues, and applications.* Edited by Duan N. Mahway, NJ: Lawrence Erlbaum Associates; 2003:90–111.
54. Burnham KP, Anderson DR: *Model selection and inference: A practical information-theoretic approach.* New York: Springer-Verlag; 2002.

55. Hurvich CM, Tsai CL: **Regression and time series model selection in small samples.** *Biometrika* 1989, **76**:297–307.
56. Thompson SG, Sharp SJ: **Explaining heterogeneity in meta-analysis: a comparison of methods.** *Stat Med* 1999 Oct 30, **18**(20):2693–2708.
57. Berkey CS, Hoaglin DC, Mosteller F, Colditz GA: **A random-effects regression model for meta-analysis.** *Stat Med* 1995 Feb 28, **14**(4):395–411.
58. Edwards D, Berry JJ: **The efficiency of simulation-based multiple comparisons.** *Biometrics* 1987 Dec, **43**(4):913–928.
59. Campbell B, Kreider RB, Ziegenfuss T, La Bounty P, Roberts M, Burke D, *et al*: **International society of sports nutrition position stand: protein and exercise.** *J Int Soc Sports Nutr* 2007 Sep 26, **4**:8.
60. American College of Sports Medicine, American Dietetic Association, Dietitians of Canada: **Joint position statement: Nutrition and athletic performance. american college of sports medicine, american dietetic association, and dietitians of canada.** *Med Sci Sports Exerc* 2000 Dec, **32**(12):2130–2145.
61. Lemon PW, Tarnopolsky MA, MacDougall JD, Atkinson SA: **Protein requirements and muscle mass/strength changes during intensive training in novice bodybuilders.** *J Appl Physiol* 1992 Aug, **73**(2):767–775.
62. Lemon PW: **Beyond the zone: protein needs of active individuals.** *J Am Coll Nutr* 2000 Oct, **19**(5 Suppl):513S–521S.
63. Moore DR, Del Bel NC, Nizi KI, Hartman JW, Tang JE, Armstrong D, *et al*: **Resistance training reduces fasted- and fed-state leucine turnover and increases dietary nitrogen retention in previously untrained young men.** *J Nutr* 2007 Apr, **137**(4):985–991.
64. van Houwelingen HC, Arends LR, Stijnen T: **Advanced methods in meta-analysis: multivariate approach and meta-regression.** *Stat Med* 2002 Feb 28, **21**(4):589–624.
65. Peterson MD, Rhea MR, Alvar BA: **Applications of the dose-response for muscular strength development: a review of meta-analytic efficacy and reliability for designing training prescription.** *J Strength Cond Res* 2005 Nov, **19**(4):950–958.
66. Ogasawara R, Kobayashi K, Tsutaki A, Lee K, Abe T, Fujita S, *et al*: **mTOR signaling response to resistance exercise is altered by chronic resistance training and detraining in skeletal muscle.** *J Appl Physiol* 2013 Jan, **31**.
67. Coffey VG, Zhong Z, Shield A, Canny BJ, Chibalin AV, Zierath JR, *et al*: **Early signaling responses to divergent exercise stimuli in skeletal muscle from well-trained humans.** *FASEB J* 2006 Jan, **20**(1):190–192.

6

Combined effect of branched-chain amino acids and taurine supplementation on delayed onset muscle soreness and muscle damage in high-intensity eccentric exercise

Song-Gyu Ra[1,2†], Teruo Miyazaki[3†], Keisuke Ishikura[4], Hisashi Nagayama[5], Shoichi Komine[1], Yoshio Nakata[6], Seiji Maeda[7], Yasushi Matsuzaki[8] and Hajime Ohmori[7*]

Abstract

Background: Previous studies have evaluated the effectiveness of branched-chain amino acid (BCAA) supplementation for preventing delayed onset muscle soreness (DOMS) and muscle damage induced by eccentric exercise, their findings have been inconclusive. Since taurine has anti-inflammatory and anti-oxidative effects, the present study investigated the combined effect of BCAA and taurine on DOMS and muscle damage.

Methods: Thirty-six untrained male subjects (22.5 ± 3.8 years) were assigned to four groups (placebo + placebo [placebo], BCAA + placebo, placebo + taurine, and BCAA + taurine [combined]) and given a combination of 3.2 g BCAA (or placebo) and 2.0 g taurine (or placebo), three times a day, for two weeks prior to and three days after eccentric elbow flexor exercises. DOMS and muscle damage in the biceps brachii were subjectively and objectively evaluated using the visual analogue scale (VAS), upper arm circumference (CIR), and blood parameters (creatine kinase, lactate dehydrogenase [LDH], aldolase, and 8-hydroxydeoxyguanosine [8-OHdG]).

Results: In the combined group, VAS and 8-OHdG two days after exercise, CIR two and three days after exercise and LDH from one to three days after exercise were significantly lower than the placebo group. The area under the curve from before exercise to four days later for CIR, LDH, and aldolase was also significantly lower in the combined group than in the placebo group.

Conclusion: A combination of 3.2 g BCAA and 2.0 g taurine, three times a day, for two weeks prior to and three days after exercise may be a useful nutritional strategy for attenuating exercise-induced DOMS and muscle damage.

Keywords: Double-blind study, Amino acids, Combined supplementation, BCAA, Taurine, DOMS

Introduction

The importance and benefits of regular exercise in maintaining overall health and preventing aging are well known. However, unaccustomed and sudden exercise results in dull pain in the skeletal muscle within hours or days after exercise, which is referred to as delayed onset muscle soreness (DOMS) [1]. DOMS is one of the symptoms of eccentric-exercise (ECC)-induced muscle damage. Muscle damage is characterized as disruption of the membrane by mechanical stress, infiltration of inflammatory cells to the injured tissue, and increased production of inflammatory cytokines [2]. Pain resulting from DOMS leads to a decrease in exercise performance and muscle strength gains for up to three weeks [3].

Branched-chain amino acids (valine, leucine, and isoleucine; BCAAs) are abundant and catabolized in the skeletal muscle, and they help to inhibit protein breakdown [4] and enhance protein synthesis [5]. BCAAs have been reported in many studies to attenuate DOMS and muscle damage induced by exercise [4,6-11]. Shimomura *et al.* reported that BCAA supplementation prior to squat

* Correspondence: ohmori@taiiku.tsukuba.ac.jp
†Equal contributors
[7]Faculty of Health and Sport Sciences, University of Tsukuba, Tsukuba, Ibaraki 305-8574, Japan
Full list of author information is available at the end of the article

exercises decreased DOMS within a few days after exercise [7,8]. Furthermore, the beneficial effects of BCAA supplementation on DOMS together with the inhibition of muscle damage was also observed for a training program involving trained long-distance runners [4] and in cycling exercise [9,10]. In contrast, a study by Jackman *et al.* found no attenuating effects of BCAA supplementation on DOMS in the quadriceps muscle with the knee extended or on inflammation during the recovery period following high-intensity knee extension exercise, but DOMS was attenuated when measured with the knee flexed [11]. Thus, the positive effects of BCAA supplementation on DOMS and muscle damage were weak in high-intensity exercise. Previous studies have evaluated the combined effects of various nutrients and BCAA supplements on DOMS and muscle damage. Stock *et al.* examined the combined effect of leucine supplementation and a carbohydrate beverage on DOMS and serum muscle damage markers during the recovery period following squat exercises; however, no significant effects were found before or after exercise [12]. Furthermore, the combination of protein (free-form amino acids including BCAA) and carbohydrate supplements given before and after ECC had no effect on muscle damage, loss of strength, or muscle soreness [13]. Therefore, combining BCAAs with other anti-inflammatory nutrients might be beneficial for alleviating DOMS and muscle damage.

Taurine (2-aminoethanesulfonic acid), which is abundant in skeletal muscle, has been reported to have many physiological and pharmacological actions, including membrane stabilization, anti-oxidation, osmoregulation, modulation of ion flux, and control of Ca^{2+} homeostasis, in addition to playing roles as a neurotransmitter and neuromodulator [14]. In particular, it was reported that taurine has a cytoprotective effect against free radical-mediated skeletal muscle injury induced by downhill running in rats [15,16]. The authors also confirmed that oral taurine administration in rats reduces exercise- and drug-induced oxidative stress [17,18]. Interestingly, a multi-nutrient supplement containing BCAA and taurine as well as some vitamin B and plant extracts improved inflammation and joint pain in middle-age individuals [19]. Therefore, we hypothesized that taurine might enhance the beneficial effect of BCAA on DOMS and muscle damage induced by exercise.

In the present study, we investigated by means of a randomized, placebo-controlled, double-blind trial whether a combination of BCAA and taurine supplements can provide an effective nutritional strategy for attenuating DOMS and muscle damage induced by high-intensity exercise in humans.

Methods

Subjects and amino acid treatment protocol

This randomized, placebo-controlled, double-blind trial was conducted with 36 male college volunteers who did not have any musculoskeletal disorders and had not partaken in any regular resistance training prior to the study (Table 1). The study was carried out in accordance with the Declaration of Helsinki and was approved by the Human Subjects Committee of the University of Tsukuba. All subjects provided written informed consent.

Subjects were randomly and equally divided into the following four groups ($n = 9$ per group): double-placebo control supplementation (PLCB); BCAA and placebo-2 supplementation (BA); taurine and placebo-1 supplementation (TAU); and BCAA and taurine supplementation (COMB). Subjects were orally administered two sachets containing a combination of BCAA (or placebo-1) and taurine (or placebo-2) after every meal for two weeks prior to exercise (Table 1 and Figure 1). We chose this timeframe because previous studies showed a significant increase in muscular taurine concentration following two weeks of taurine administration in rats [18,20], but not after one week in humans [21]. Since the present study was designed as a double-blind trial, the duration of BCAA supplementation prior to exercise was matched to the two-week duration of taurine supplementation. All subjects were instructed to fill out a supplemental checklist after every meal. The BCAA and taurine sachets contained 3.2 g (9.6 g/day) of a BCAA mixture (Ile: Leu: Val = 1:2:1; Aminofeel®, Seikatsu Bunkasya Co. Inc., Chiba, Japan) and 2.0 g (6.0 g/day) of taurine, respectively. The daily doses of BCAA and taurine were based on the doses used in previous studies, which examined the effectiveness of BCAA supplementation on DOMS [9,22] and plasma taurine levels [23]. The daily doses per body weight of BCAA and taurine were 145.7 ± 5.3 (109.5–181.5) and 95.5 ± 2.5 (80.3–116.5) mg/kg (mean ± standard error, range), respectively. The placebo-1 and -2 supplements were compounded to the same volume and color as the BCAA and taurine supplements, respectively, by using similar proportions of starch for the double-blind method (Table 1). Supplementation was continued in a double-blind manner until dinner on the third day after exercise. Evaluation using a visual analogue scale (VAS) and by assessing muscle damage markers was completed on the morning of the fourth day after exercise. No significant differences in physical parameters measured a week before starting supplementation were noted between the groups (Table 1). All subjects were sedentary men who were non-athletes. They were instructed to continue their normal activities and to abstain from any strenuous exercise for at least one month before the experiment. Moreover, they were instructed to continue their usual food intake, not to change the amount or frequency of dietary meat or seafood intake, and not to use any dietary supplements, anti-inflammatory drugs, or anything else that could affect muscle soreness and damage until the end of the study. They were also

Table 1 Grouping conditions and characteristics of subjects

	Supply condition		Physiological characteristics before experiment						
Group	BCAA	Taurine	Age (years)	Height (cm)	Body W. (kg)	Fat (%)	Muscle W. (kg)	MVC (Nm)	CIR (mm)
PLCB	Placebo-1	Placebo-2	22.2 ± 1.1	170.8 ± 1.9	67.5 ± 3.5	18.3 ± 1.9	51.9 ± 1.8	36.5 ± 3.0	257.4 ± 7.6
BA	3.2 g	Placebo-2	22.9 ± 1.1	176.7 ± 3.6	73.5 ± 4.3	20.1 ± 1.7	55.3 ± 2.4	41.9 ± 3.8	267.7 ± 7.9
TAU	Placebo-1	2.0 g	22.2 ± 0.8	173.7 ± 2.2	65.5 ± 2.7	17.3 ± 1.3	51.7 ± 1.7	39.1 ± 2.4	251.3 ± 7.4
COMB	3.2 g	2.0 g	23.1 ± 1.3	174.5 ± 1.8	61.5 ± 1.6	14.2 ± 1.0	50.0 ± 1.3	35.0 ± 2.6	243.4 ± 6.6

Footnote: Data are expressed as means ± S. E. *Abbreviation*: *PLCB*, double-placebo control group; *BA*, branched-chain amino acids and placebo-2 supplement group; *TAU*, taurine and placebo-1 supplement group; *COMB*, combined (taurine and BCAA) supplement group; *Placebo-1 and 2*, placebo of BCAA and taurine supplementation, respectively (3.2g or 2.0g starch mainly), *Body W.*, body weight; *Muscle W.*, muscle weight; *MVC*, maximal voluntary strength of isometric contraction; *CIR*, upper arm circumference.

instructed to abstain from stretching or massage therapy during the experimental period.

Exercise protocol

Figure 1 outlines the experimental protocol, including the time course corresponding to amino acid supplementation, exercise, and parameter measurement. On the day of exercise, all subjects assembled at our laboratory at 07:00 after fasting overnight. Following blood sampling, they ingested their assigned supplements 15 min prior to performing ECC. After the exercise at 10:00, subjects were supplied with jelly-type food (160 kcal/180 g; Nihon Pharmaceutical Co., Ltd., Toyama, Japan) to minimize protein catabolism due to fasting [24]. The exercise protocol, designed to induce soreness in the elbow flexors, was modified from a previously published method of voluntary ECC [25]. During the week prior to initiating amino acid supplementation, the maximal voluntary strength of isometric contraction (MVC) in the non-dominant arm of each subject was measured at 1.57 rad (90°) of elbow flexion.

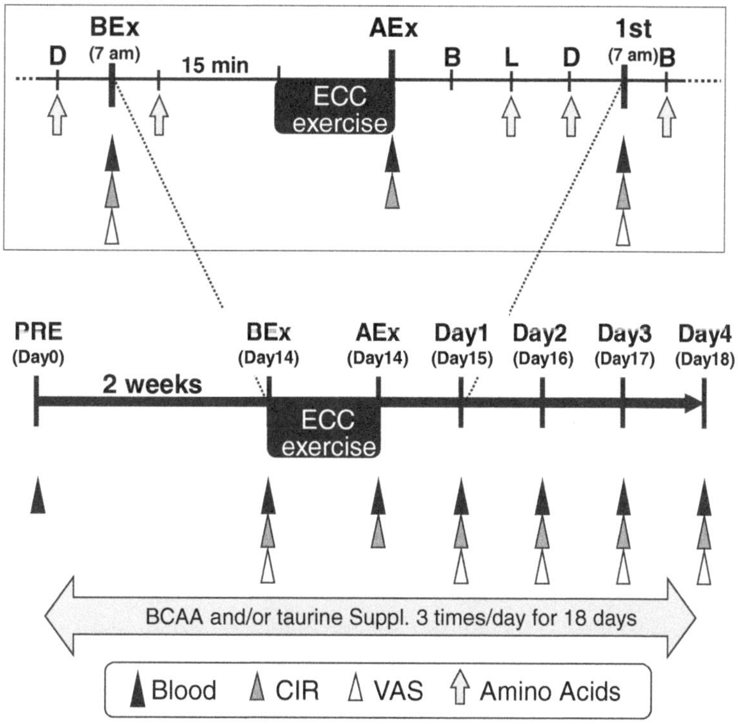

Figure 1 A schematic illustrating the experimental protocol and time course of the present study. Participants were supplied with two kinds of sachets consists of combination of BCAA (or placebo of BCAA) and taurine (or placebo of taurine) from 2 weeks before exercise to the end of the experiment. Participants were performed elbow extension as part of ECC in the non-dominant arm using dumbbell weight. Muscle soreness and damage were then monitored for 4 days after ECC. *Abbreviations*: *PRE*, prior to amino acid supplementation; *BEx*, before exercise; *AEx*, immediately after exercise; *Day1-Day4*, 1st to 4th days following exercise; *ECC*, 6 sets of 5 repetitions of eccentric elbow extensions at 90% of maximal isometric strength; *VAS*, visual analogue scale for delayed onset muscle soreness assessment; *CIR*, upper arm circumference; *Blood*, blood sampling; *Amino Acids*, combination of amino acids (BCAA and/or taurine) supplementation; *Suppl.*, supplementation; *B*, breakfast; *L*, lunch; *D*, dinner.

For the ECC protocol, subjects were seated on a bench with their arm positioned in front of their body and resting on a padded support, such that their shoulder was secured at a flexion angle of 0.79 rad (45°) and their forearm was maintained in the supinated position throughout the exercise. Subjects were repeatedly weight-loaded upon dumbbell lowering to achieve a 90% MVC (34.3 ± 1.3 Nm). Subjects performed six sets of five repetitions of elbow extension from the flexed position at 90° to the fully extended position slowly over 5 s, while maintaining a constant speed of movement by following a verbal metronome provided by the investigator. After each extension, the investigator returned the dumbbell to the starting position (90°) to prevent excess muscle activation induced by the weight. Subjects were permitted to rest for 3 s between repetitions and for 2 min between sets. The intensity of ECC at 90% MVC was determined on the basis of our preliminary experiments and likely induced natural muscle damage as all subjects found it difficult to lower the dumbbell at a constant speed during the later sets due to decreased muscle function. The subjects also required verbal encouragement from the investigator to maintain constant speed.

Blood parameters of muscle damage

Blood samples were collected from the antecubital vein at seven different time points: prior to amino acid supplementation, before exercise, immediately after exercise, at one to four days after exercise (Day1–4) (Figure 1). On the day of exercise, blood was collected before supplement intake, and exercise was started thereafter. Immediately after exercise, blood was collected again. In the four days following exercise, blood was collected at 07:00 before breakfast and amino acid intake. Serum was centrifuged for 30 min after the formation of a solid clot, and the plasma was immediately separated. The serum activities of creatine kinase (CK), lactate dehydrogenase (LDH), and aldolase were analyzed and used as parameters of muscle damage, as described in the Japan Society of Clinical Chemistry consensus methods. Serum levels of 8-hydroxydeoxyguanosine (8-OHdG), a marker of oxidative stress-induced DNA damage, were measured before exercise and on Day 2 after exercise by competitive enzyme-linked immunosorbent assay (Highly Sensitive 8-OHdG Check ELISA kit; Japan Institute for the Control of Aging, Fukuroi, Japan) after purification with a 10-kDa filter (Nanosep®; Pall Corporation, NY, US). Additionally, plasma taurine and BCAA concentrations were measured using an automatic amino acid analyzer (JLC-300V; JEOL, Tokyo, Japan) after de-proteination with a two-fold volume of 3% sulphosalicylic acid [26]. Plasma albumin concentrations were analyzed by the bromocresol green method (Albumin II-HA test Wako; Wako Pure Chemicals, Osaka, Japan).

Subjective assessments of muscle soreness

Subjective assessment of elbow flexor soreness in the biceps brachii muscle was surveyed using the VAS, which consisted of a 100-mm line with "no pain" at one end and "extreme pain" at the other end [25]. VAS scores were measured before exercise and on Days 1–4 with the arm in the extended position. Specifically, the exercised arm was placed on a table in the seated position and the investigator passively extended the elbow joint to test the perception of soreness. Because the degree of soreness in the extended arm position was influenced by the technique of the investigator, the same investigator performed all measurements to avoid inter-investigator measurement error. The test-retest reliability determined using an intraclass correlation coefficient (ICC) was 0.98.

Indirect marker of muscle damage via physical parameters

The upper arm circumference (CIR) was used as an indirect marker of muscle damage and measured before exercise, after exercise, and on Days 1–4 (Figure 1). CIR was measured at five points 3, 5, 7, 9, and 11 cm proximal to the elbow joint on a relaxed arm in the standing position using a constant-tension tape. To avoid daily variations in the measurement position, these sites on the upper arm were marked with a semi-permanent ink pen during the first testing session. CIR was measured in duplicate and the mean value of each point was used for analysis. The values immediately after exercise and on Days 1–4 were presented as the differences from the values before exercise. The test-retest reliability determined using an ICC for CIR was 0.99.

Statistical analysis

Data are expressed as means ± SE. The values of CK, LDH, aldolase, VAS, and CIR are presented as raw values and as the area under the curve (AUC) during the experimental period. The AUC was calculated as the sum of four or five trapezoid areas separated by each measurement time point. At each point, the effects of each supplement protocol on the measured outcomes were determined by one-way analysis of variance (ANOVA) followed by Tukey's test or the non-parametric Wilcoxon *post hoc* test. Significant differences between two points and between multiple points within the same group were analyzed using Student's paired t-test and repeated-measures ANOVA with Dunnett's *post hoc* multiple comparison test, respectively. Significant differences (two-tailed) were set at $P < 0.05$. Analysis was conducted using SPSS software version 18.0 for Windows (IBM, Chicago, IL).

Results

Plasma amino acid concentrations

Figure 2 shows the plasma concentrations of taurine, total BCAA, and individual BCAAs prior to amino acid

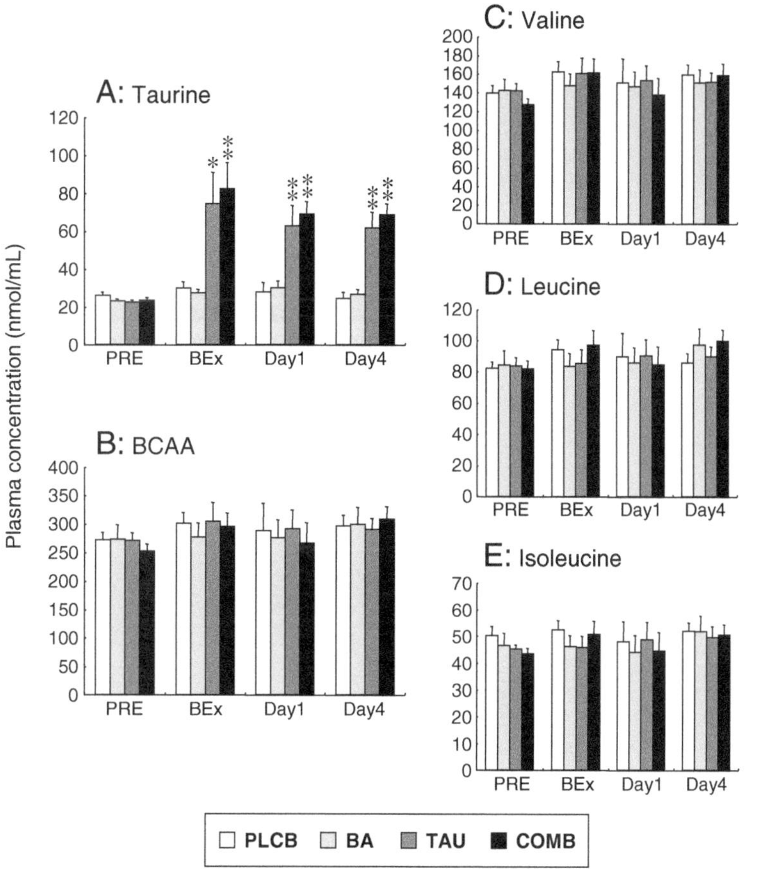

Figure 2 Plasma taurine (A), BCAA (B), valine (C), leucine (D) and isoleucine (E) concentrations. *Abbreviations: PLCB,* placebo supplementation group; *BA,* BCAA supplementation group; *TAU,* taurine supplementation group; *COMB,* combined (BCAA + taurine) supplementation group; *PRE,* prior to amino acid supplementation; *BEx,* before exercise; *Day1,* 1st day after exercise; *Day4,* 4th day after exercise. Data are expressed as means ± S.E. *$P < 0.05$, **$P < 0.01$ versus the PLCB and BA groups by one-way ANOVA.

supplementation, before exercise, and on Days 1 and 4. Prior to supplementation, there were no significant differences in plasma taurine concentration among the groups (Figure 2A). Before exercise and on Days 1 and 4, the plasma taurine concentration in the TAU and COMB groups was significantly increased compared with that in the PLCB and BA groups (Figure 2A). No significant differences in the plasma concentrations of total BCAA and individual BCAAs (valine, leucine, or isoleucine) were observed among the groups at any time points (Figure 2B-E).

The plasma albumin concentration (4.0–5.3 g/dL) in all subjects was within the normal range, and no significant differences were observed between the groups throughout the experimental period (data not shown).

Delayed onset muscle soreness following eccentric exercise

Figure 3A shows the VAS scores for subjective DOMS assessment. The VAS scores in all groups were significantly higher on Day 1 compared with before exercise. The VAS scores in the BA and COMB groups peaked on Day 1 while those in the PLCB and TAU groups peaked on Day 2. The increased VAS scores in all groups declined by Day 4. In the COMB group, the VAS scores on Day 2 were significantly lower than in the PLCB group.

Indirect marker of muscle damage

CIR as an indirect marker of muscle damage is shown in Figure 3B. CIR differences increased significantly and immediately after exercise in all groups and declined by Day 1. Thereafter, the CIR differences in all groups increased significantly until the end of the experimental period. In the COMB group, the CIR differences were lower than in the other groups throughout the experimental period, with significant differences on Days 2 and 3 compared with the PLCB group. Additionally, the AUC of the CIR differences in the COMB group was significantly lower than in the PLCB group. No significant differences in CIR were observed among the PLCB, BA, or TAU groups throughout the experimental period.

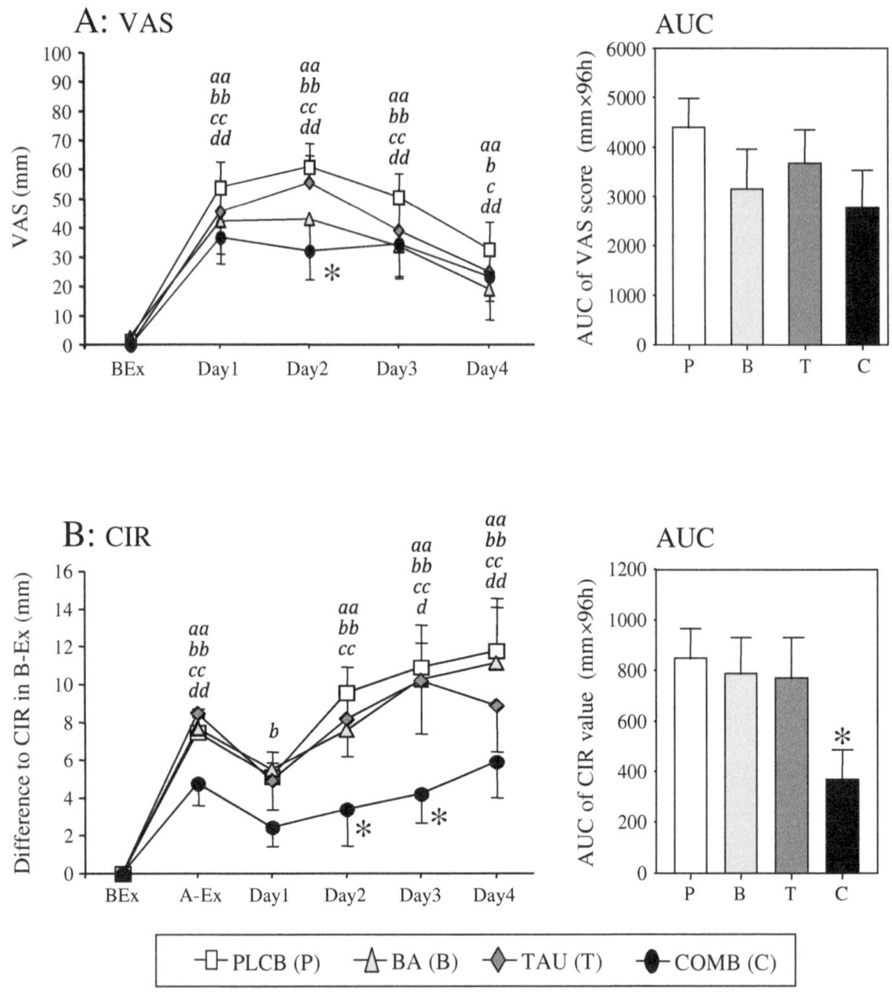

Figure 3 VAS score (A) and CIR (B) throughout the experiment. VAS score was used as subjectively assessment of muscle soreness in the exercised arm. CIR value as an indirect marker of muscle damage is presented as differences from the respective BEx. Both parameters were also shown as the AUC from BEx to Day4. *Abbreviations: VAS*, visual analog scale; *AUC*, area under the curve; *CIR*, upper arm circumference. Data are expressed as means ± S.E. *$P < 0.05$ versus the PLCB group by one-way ANOVA. ^{a,b,c,d} show the significant difference compared with the corresponding Pre in the PLCB, BCAA, TAU, and COMB groups, respectively, and single and double characters mean $P < 0.05$ and $P < 0.01$, respectively, by repeated measures ANOVA.

Blood parameters of muscle damage

The serum enzyme activities throughout the experimental period of CK, LDH, and aldolase, which serve as blood parameters of muscle damage, are presented in Figure 4. All serum markers remained unchanged in all groups until Day 1 and then increased from Day 2 to Day 4.

Serum CK activity in the PLCB, BA, and TAU groups was significantly higher on Days 3 and 4 compared with before exercise (Figure 4A). In the COMB group, a significant difference in CK activity compared with before exercise was found only on Day 4. Statistically significant differences among all groups was not found at any points throughout the experiment due to the large variance between individuals. Serum LDH activity from Day 1 to Day 3 and the AUC were significantly lower in the COMB group than in the PLCB group (Figure 4B). Similarly, serum aldolase activity in the COMB group was lower than in other groups, and a significant difference was noted only before exercise on Day 4 (Figure 4C). The AUC of aldolase was significantly lower in the COMB group than in the PLCB group.

Figure 5 shows serum 8-OHdG levels before exercise and on Day 2. Before exercise, there was no significant difference in serum 8-OHdG levels between any groups. Serum 8-OHdG levels in the PLCB, BA, and TAU groups were significantly increased on Day 2 compared with before exercise. On Day 2, 8-OHdG levels were significant lower in the COMB group than in the PLCB and BA groups.

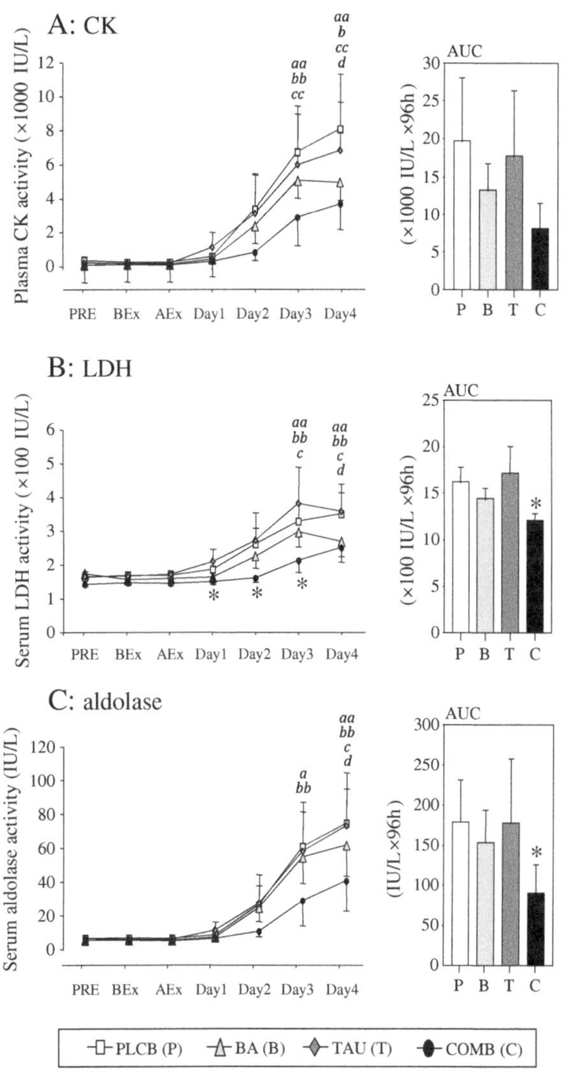

Figure 4 Serum activities of CK (A), LDH (B), and aldolase (C) throughout the experimental period. The AUC of these parameters calculated through the experimental period was also shown. *Abbreviations*: *CK*, creatine kinase; *LDH*, lactate dehydrogenase; *PLCB [P]*, placebo supplementation group; *BA [B]*, BCAA supplementation group; *TAU [T]*, taurine supplementation group; *COMB [C]*, combined (BCAA + taurine) supplementation group. Data are expressed as means ± S.E. $^{*}P < 0.05$ versus the PLCB group by one-way ANOVA. ^{a,b,c,d} show the significant difference compared with the corresponding Pre in the PLCB, BCAA, TAU, and COMB groups, respectively, and single and double characters mean $P < 0.05$ and $P < 0.01$, respectively, analyzed by repeated measures ANOVA.

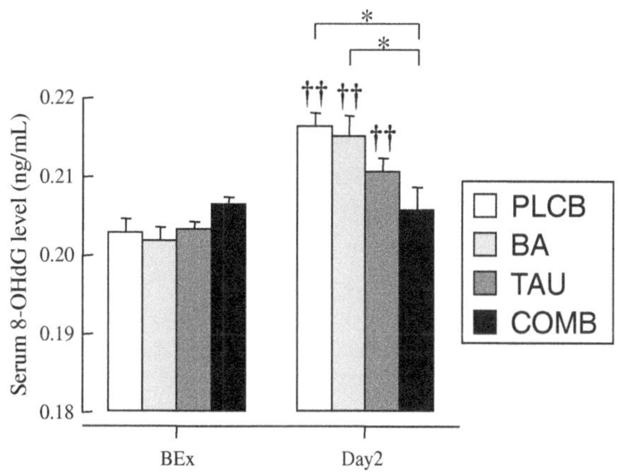

Figure 5 Serum 8-OHdG level at BEx and Day2. *Abbreviations*: *8-OHdG*, 8-hydroxydeoxyguanosine; *BEx*, before exercise; *Day2*, 2nd day after exercise. Data are shown as means ± S.E. $^{*}P < 0.05$ above the column with bar shows the significant difference analyzed by one-way ANOVA. $^{††}P < 0.01$ on the column without bar shows the significant difference compared to the respective values in the BEx by paired Student's *t*-test.

Discussion

Numerous studies have confirmed the effectiveness of BCAA supplementation on DOMS and muscle damage [4,7-11]. However, the attenuating effects of BCAA on the DOMS and muscle damage were occasionally limited, especially in case of intensive exercise. Consequently, more effective nutritional strategies need to be discovered. In the present study, the effects of BCAA supplementation combined with taurine on a highly intense ECC-induced DOMS and muscle damage were investigated via a randomized, placebo-controlled, and double-blind trial, because taurine was reported to decrease oxidative stress induced by ECC [16]. In ECC-induced DOMS and muscle damage, subjective and objective parameters including VAS scores, CIR, and serum levels of LDH and 8-OHdG were significantly improved by the combination of BCAA and taurine supplementation. This combined supplementation also tended to improve serum CK and aldolase activities, but not significantly. These parameters, especially serum CK activity, have a high degree of individual biological variability, and it is difficult to demonstrate a statistically significant difference between the small number of subjects [3]. Overall, the present study demonstrated that combined supplementation with BCAA and taurine is beneficial for reducing ECC-induced DOMS and muscle damage. However, it was impossible to determine whether the combined effects were due to the synergistic effect of both BCAA and taurine or the sum of the individual effects.

Compared with the effectiveness of BCAA supplementation on exercise-induced muscle soreness and damage reported in previous studies [4,7,9,22,25], BCAA supplementation alone was not sufficient to effectively inhibit muscle soreness and damage in the present study. This discrepancy might be due to differences in the exercise protocol (intensity and type) and the supplemental regimen (duration and dose). In a previous study by Shimomura *et al.*, the authors recognized that the intensity was low in a squatting exercise where subjects used only their body weight because the changes in the levels of serum muscle damage markers, including CK and myoglobin, were very small over the three days following exercise [7,8]. On the other hand, repeated arm extensions with weight loads of 90% MVC in the present study caused a significant increase in serum muscle damage markers in the placebo group, thereby implying higher exercise intensity. The present findings with this higher intensity suggest that a combination of BCAA and taurine taken during high-intensity exercise may prevent severe muscle soreness and damage that cannot be attenuated by BCAA alone.

In addition to exercise intensity, the amount of oral BCAA intake is one of the important factors for preventing exercise-induced muscle soreness and damage. Shimomura *et al.* suggested that the BCAA dose should be adjusted according to body mass to at least 92–100 mg/kg because the inhibitive effects of BCAA on DOMS and muscle damage were greater in females than in males [7,8]. The BCAA dose in the present study should be sufficient because daily BCAA supplementation at 9.6 g/day worked out to 145.67 ± 5.3 mg/kg. Furthermore, the overall BCAA intake was probably sufficient because amino acid supplementation was from two weeks before to three days after exercise throughout the whole experimental period. Therefore, both the amount per body mass and the duration of BCAA supplementation in the present study might be sufficient for attenuating DOMS and muscle damage.

However, plasma BCAA concentrations were not altered by the BCAA supplementation in the present study. The two-week duration of BCAA supplementation prior to exercise was used to match the duration of taurine supplementation because this study was a double-blind trial. Indeed, a previous study conducted with college swimmers found no differences in plasma BCAA concentration after supplementation with 12 g/day BCAA for two weeks [27]. Hamada *et al.* reported that the plasma BCAA concentration in healthy humans significantly and rapidly increased and peaked at 30 min after a single BCAA dose; however, the plasma concentration returned to the basal level within 1–2 h [28] because of transport to the skeletal muscle [24]. Since blood sampling in the present study was done before each BCAA supplementation, the plasma BCAA concentration should have already returned to the basal level by the sampling time.

Taurine content in the skeletal muscle is also thought to be important for preventing muscle damage; however, neither the optimal duration nor the total dose of taurine has been clarified. We previously confirmed in rats that two weeks of oral taurine administration significantly increases taurine concentration in both the skeletal muscle and plasma in a dose-dependent manner [20,26]. In the present study, oral taurine administration at 6.0 g/day for two weeks significantly increased the plasma taurine concentration. Therefore, we suggest that the taurine concentration in the skeletal muscle in the present study might have been increased in line with the plasma level. However, a previous study with humans reported that seven days of oral taurine supplementation (5.0 g/day) did not change the taurine concentration in the skeletal muscle or in the plasma [21]. This discrepancy between the present results and those of previous studies with humans might be due to differences in the supplemental protocol. Therefore, an effective protocol for taurine supplementation, including dose and duration, to increase muscle taurine concentration as well as plasma level should be clarified in the future. Interestingly, Galloway *et al.* demonstrated that BCAA concentration in the skeletal muscle after exercise was significantly increased by oral taurine administration for seven days [21]. Although the mechanism to increase the muscular BCAA pool is unclear, it is one of the possible reasons why taurine might enhance the inhibitive effect of BCAA on muscle damage induced by ECC.

Oxidative stress-induced muscle damage has been shown to be associated with muscle soreness, and exercise-induced free radicals cause oxidative damage to cellular DNA. Radák *et al.* confirmed that the levels of 8-OHdG, a product of DNA oxidation, in the biopsied quadriceps femoris muscle of humans were significantly increased after 24 h of ECC when DOMS was present, suggesting that DNA damage occurred at the time of developing muscle soreness [29]. In the present study, significantly increased serum 8-OHdG levels were observed in the PLCB, BA, and TAU groups on Day 2 when DOMS peaked. The increased levels of plasma 8-OHdG were significantly decreased by the combined supplementation and tended to be lower than those achieved by taurine supplementation alone. Since we also observed in our previous study that taurine treatment significantly inhibited hepatic 8-OHdG levels in response to drug-induced oxidative stress [17], taurine might play a protective role in anti-DNA oxidation associated with DOMS in the skeletal muscle. To our knowledge, there is no evidence that BCAAs can suppress exercise-induced DNA damage in the skeletal muscle. However, patients with liver cirrhosis showed that chronic oral BCAA therapy significantly decreased urinary 8-OHdG excretion, suggesting that BCAAs could reduce oxidative stress-induced DNA damage in the skeletal muscle [30]. This might be a possible reason for the combined effect of BCAA and taurine on DOMS and muscle damage through protecting against DNA damage.

In addition to oxidative stress, intramuscular inflammation has also been considered a possible cause of DOMS [31]. To attenuate DOMS, it is important to inhibit the acute inflammatory response triggered by pro-inflammatory cytokines released from inflammatory cells following exercise [32]. Indeed, polymorphonuclear leukocytes are activated after ECC-induced DOMS and muscle damage [33]. Within several hours after exercise, circulating neutrophils rapidly invade damaged muscle. Thereafter, neutrophils within the damaged muscle are replaced by macrophages over the next 24 h and these macrophages produce pro-inflammatory cytokines [4,6]. A previous study reported that BCAA decrease the levels of Th1-derived cytokines (interferon-γ and interleukin-2) after high-intensity exercise, including triathlon and long-distance running [22]. Furthermore, taurine is an important factor in the neutrophil-related inflammatory response because it scavenges hypochlorous acid excreted from activated neutrophils and forms the less toxic taurine-chloramine [16,17]. Consequently, the production of pro-inflammatory mediators, such as prostaglandin E2 (PGE2), nitric oxide, and cytokines, from macrophages and lymphocytes are suppressed [34]. In particular, PGE2 has been considered a critical inflammatory mediator because it is produced by macrophages, sensitizes muscle afferent nociceptors [35], and is associated with the production of bradykinin, a substrate known to mediate muscle pain [36]. Although taurine-chloramine and PGE2 were not measured in the present study, we speculate that taurine *per se* may suppress PGE2 production in the arachidonate cascade via phospholipase A2 and cyclooxygenase 2 [37], as both of these enzymes are activated by increased $[Ca^{2+}]i$ levels and oxidative stress [38]. Thus, taurine might synergistically enhance the beneficial effects of BCAA for reducing DOMS and muscle damage via an anti-inflammatory/immune response. However, this hypothesis requires verification.

In terms of the "no pain, no gain" theory, the requirement of exercise-induced muscle soreness and an inflammatory response for muscle hypertrophy remains controversial. In the present study, the combination of BCAA and taurine suppressed DOMS and the levels of serum marker of oxidative stress. The general consensus is that muscle hypertrophy is induced during the recovery from damages to the microstructure of the muscle fiber and extracellular matrix [39]. Because exercise-induced symptoms including the production of inflammatory cytokine (interleukin-6; IL-6, and fibroblast growth factor-2), oxidative stress and DOMS usually occur during recovery, these responses have been suggested to be necessary for exercise-induced muscle hypertrophy [40,41]. Therefore, even if DOMS and muscle damage were effectively attenuated by the combination of BCAA and taurine supplementation, there is a possibility that muscle hypertrophy can be also be suppressed, and previous reports have shown that supplementations of taurine or multi-nutrient including BCAA and taurine could attenuate the productions of reactive oxygen species [16] and IL-6 [19]. On the other hand, Flann *et al.* evaluated whether exercise-induced symptoms including muscle soreness and damage are necessary events for muscle remodeling in humans [42]. They showed that the volume and strength of the quadriceps muscle and the muscular mRNA expression of the myogenic insulin-like growth factor-IEa that contributes to muscle regeneration were caused independently of muscle soreness and increase serum CK levels. Thus, DOMS and inflammation are not always necessary for muscle hypertrophy to occur. Furthermore, if exercise-induced DOMS and inflammation are efficiently attenuated, subjects can avoid unnecessary pain.

Conclusion

This study confirmed that a combination of 3.2 g BCAA and 2.0 g taurine, three times a day, two weeks prior to and three days after exercise attenuates some subjective and objective markers of DOMS and muscle damage induced by high-intensity ECC, which could not have been influenced by BCAA or taurine supplementation alone. Therefore, combined supplementation with BCAA and taurine may be a useful strategy for attenuating DOMS and muscle damage and can help motivate beginners to continue an exercise program while assisting competitive athletes to train at higher intensity.

Abbreviations

AEx: Immediately after exercise; ANOVA: Analysis of variance; AUC: Area under the curve; BA: Branched-chain amino acid and placebo 2 supplementation group; BCAA: Branched-chain amino acid; BEx: Before exercise; CIR: Upper arm circumference; CK: Creatine kinase; COMB: Branched-chain amino acid and taurine supplementation; Day1–4: 1–4 days after the exercise; DOMS: Delayed onset muscle soreness; ECC: Eccentric exercise; ICC: Intraclass correlation coefficient; IL-6: Interleukin-6; LDH: Lactate dehydrogenase; MVC: Maximal voluntary strength of isometric contraction; PGE2: Prostaglandin E2; PLCB: double-placebo control supplementation group; PRE: Prior to amino acid supplementation; TAU: Taurine and placebo 1 supplementation; VAS: Visual analogue scale; 8-OHdG: 8-hydroxydeoxyguanosine.

Competing interests

The authors declare that they have no competing interests.

Authors' contributions

Significant manuscript writer: SGR, TM, and HO. Concept and design: SGR, TM, SM, YM, and HO. Data acquisition: SGR, TM, KI, HN, and SK. Data analysis and interpretation: SGR, TM, KI, HN, SK, YN, and HO. Statistical expertise: YN. Significant manuscript reviewer/reviser: SM, YM, and HO. All authors read and approved the final manuscript.

Acknowledgements

The authors would like to thank Dr. Masaharu Ito of Livence Co. Inc. (Tokyo, Japan), and Noriko Murakami and Norikazu Watanabe of Seikatsu Bunkasya Co. Inc. for their helpful discussion and assistance. The authors are also grateful to the Kasumigaura Research Agency for Adult Diseases (Ami, Japan) for the masked wrapping of amino acid powder for the double-blind study and to the Chemical Analysis Center, University of Tsukuba, for amino acids analysis.

This work was presented in part at the 12th International Congress on Amino Acids, Peptides and Proteins in August 2011, and at the 18th International Taurine Meeting in April 2012.

Declaration of funding sources
This study was supported in part by an educational grant from the Seikatsu Bunkasya Co. Inc. (Chiba, Japan).

Author details
[1]Graduate School of Comprehensive Human Sciences, University of Tsukuba, Tsukuba, Ibaraki 305-8574, Japan. [2]Research Fellow of the Japan Society for the Promotion of Sciences, Chiyoda-ku, Tokyo 102-0083, Japan. [3]Joint Research Center, Tokyo Medical University Ibaraki Medical Center, Ami, Ibaraki 300-0395, Japan. [4]Sports Research and Development Core, University of Tsukuba, Tsukuba, Ibaraki 305-8574, Japan. [5]School of Health and Physical Education, University of Tsukuba, Tsukuba, Ibaraki 305-8574, Japan. [6]Faculty of Medicine, University of Tsukuba, Tsukuba, Ibaraki 305-8574, Japan. [7]Faculty of Health and Sport Sciences, University of Tsukuba, Tsukuba, Ibaraki 305-8574, Japan. [8]Division of Gastroenterology and Hepatology, Department of Internal Medicine, Tokyo Medical University Ibaraki Medical Center, Ami, Ibaraki 300-0395, Japan.

References

1. Armstrong RB: **Initial events in exercise-induced muscular injury.** *Med Sci Sports Exerc* 1990, **22**:429–435.
2. Proske U, Morgan DL: **Muscle damage from eccentric exercise: mechanism, mechanical signs, adaptation and clinical applications.** *J Physiol* 2001, **537**:333–345.
3. Clarkson PM, Ebbeling C: **Investigation of serum creatine kinase variability after muscle-damaging exercise.** *Clin Sci (Lond)* 1988, **75**:257–261.
4. Matsumoto K, Koba T, Hamada K, Sakurai M, Higuchi T, Miyata H: **Branched-chain amino acid supplementation attenuates muscle soreness, muscle damage and inflammation during an intensive training program.** *J Sports Med Phys Fitness* 2009, **49**:424–431.
5. Buse MG, Reid SS: **Leucine. A possible regulator of protein turnover in muscle.** *J Clin Invest* 1975, **56**:1250–1261.
6. Negro M, Giardina S, Marzani B, Marzatico F: **Branched-chain amino acid supplementation does not enhance athletic performance but affects muscle recovery and the immune system.** *J Sports Med Phys Fitness* 2008, **48**:347–351.
7. Shimomura Y, Yamamoto Y, Bajotto G, Sato J, Murakami T, Shimomura N, Kobayashi H, Mawatari K: **Nutraceutical effects of branched-chain amino acids on skeletal muscle.** *J Nutr* 2006, **136**:529S–532S.
8. Shimomura Y, Inaguma A, Watanabe S, Yamamoto Y, Muramatsu Y, Bajotto G, Sato J, Shimomura N, Kobayashi H, Mawatari K: **Branched-chain amino acid supplementation before squat exercise and delayed-onset muscle soreness.** *Int J Sport Nutr Exerc Metab* 2010, **20**:236–244.
9. Coombes JS, McNaughton LR: **Effects of branched-chain amino acid supplementation on serum creatine kinase and lactate dehydrogenase after prolonged exercise.** *J Sports Med Phys Fitness* 2000, **40**:240–246.
10. Greer BK, Woodard JL, White JP, Arguello EM, Haymes EM: **Branched-chain amino acid supplementation and indicators of muscle damage after endurance exercise.** *Int J Sport Nutr Exerc Metab* 2007, **17**:595–607.
11. Jackman SR, Witard OC, Jeukendrup AE, Tipton KD: **Branched-chain amino acid ingestion can ameliorate soreness from eccentric exercise.** *Med Sci Sports Exerc* 2010, **42**:962–970.
12. Stock MS, Young JC, Golding LA, Kruskall LJ, Tandy RD, Conway-Klaassen JM, Beck TW: **The effects of adding leucine to pre and postexercise carbohydrate beverages on acute muscle recovery from resistance training.** *J Strength Cond Res* 2010, **24**:2211–2219.
13. White JP, Wilson JM, Austin KG, Greer BK, St John N, Panton LB: **Effect of carbohydrate-protein supplement timing on acute exercise-induced muscle damage.** *J Int Soc Sports Nutr* 2008, **5**:5.
14. Schaffer SW, Jong CJ, Ramila KC, Azuma J: **Physiological roles of taurine in heart and muscle.** *J Biomed Sci* 2010, **17**(Suppl 1):S2.
15. Dawson R Jr, Biasetti M, Messina S, Dominy J: **The cytoprotective role of taurine in exercise-induced muscle injury.** *Amino Acids* 2002, **22**:309–324.
16. Silva LA, Silveira PC, Ronsani MM, Souza PS, Scheffer D, Vieira LC, Benetti M, De Souza CT, Pinho RA: **Taurine supplementation decreases oxidative stress in skeletal muscle after eccentric exercise.** *Cell Biochem Funct* 2011, **29**:43–49.
17. Miyazaki T, Karube M, Matsuzaki Y, Ikegami T, Doy M, Tanaka N, Bouscarel B: **Taurine inhibits oxidative damage and prevents fibrosis in carbon tetrachloride-induced hepatic fibrosis.** *J Hepatol* 2005, **43**:117–125.
18. Miyazaki T, Matsuzaki Y, Ikegami T, Miyakawa S, Doy M, Tanaka N, Bouscarel B: **Optimal and effective oral dose of taurine to prolong exercise performance in rat.** *Amino Acids* 2004, **27**:291–298.
19. Dunn-Lewis C, Kraemer WJ, Kupchak BR, Kelly NA, Creighton BA, Luk HY, Ballard KD, Comstock BA, Szivak TK, Hooper DR, Denegar CR, Volek JS: **A multi-nutrient supplement reduced markers of inflammation and improved physical performance in active individuals of middle to older age: a randomized, double-blind, placebo-controlled study.** *Nutr J* 2011, **10**:90.
20. Yatabe Y, Miyakawa S, Miyazaki T, Matsuzaki Y, Ochiai N: **Effects of taurine administration in rat skeletal muscles on exercise.** *J Orthop Sci* 2003, **8**:415–419.
21. Galloway SD, Talanian JL, Shoveller AK, Heigenhauser GJ, Spriet LL: **Seven days of oral taurine supplementation does not increase muscle taurine content or alter substrate metabolism during prolonged exercise in humans.** *J Appl Physiol* 2008, **105**:643–651.
22. Bassit RA, Sawada LA, Bacurau RF, Navarro F, Martins E Jr, Santos RV, Caperuto EC, Rogeri P, Costa Rosa LF: **Branched-chain amino acid supplementation and the immune response of long-distance athletes.** *Nutrition* 2002, **18**:376–379.
23. Ishikura K, Miyakawa S, Yatabe Y, Takekoshi K, Omori H: **Effect of taurine supplementation on blood glucose concentration during prolonged exercise.** *Jpn J Phys Fitness Sports Med* 2008, **57**:475–484.
24. Shimomura Y, Fujii H, Suzuki M, Murakami T, Fujitsuka N, Nakai N: **Branched-chain alpha-keto acid dehydrogenase complex in rat skeletal muscle: regulation of the activity and gene expression by nutrition and physical exercise.** *J Nutr* 1995, **125**:1762S–1765S.
25. Nosaka K, Sacco P, Mawatari K: **Effects of amino acid supplementation on muscle soreness and damage.** *Int J Sport Nutr Exerc Metab* 2006, **16**:620–635.
26. Ishikura K, Miyazaki T, Ra SG, Endo S, Nakamura Y, Matsuzaka T, Miyakawa S, Ohmori H: **Effect of taurine supplementation on the alteration in amino acid content in skeletal muscle with exercise in rat.** *J Sport Sci Med* 2011, **10**:306–314.
27. Tang FC: **Influence of branched-chain amino acid supplementation on urinary protein metabolite concentrations after swimming.** *J Am Coll Nutr* 2006, **25**:188–194.
28. Hamada K, Koba T, Sakurai M, Matsumoto K, Higuchi T, Imaizumi K, Hayase H, Ueno H: **Effective dose of branched-chain amino acids on blood response in healthy men.** *J Jpn Soc Clin Nutr* 2005, **27**:1–10.
29. Radak Z, Pucsok J, Mecseki S, Csont T, Ferdinandy P: **Muscle soreness-induced reduction in force generation is accompanied by increased nitric oxide content and DNA damage in human skeletal muscle.** *Free Radic Biol Med* 1999, **26**:1059–1063.
30. Ohno T, Tanaka Y, Sugauchi F, Orito E, Hasegawa I, Nukaya H, Kato A, Matunaga S, Endo M, Tanaka Y, Sakakibara K, Mizokami M: **Suppressive effect of oral administration of branched-chain amino acid granules on oxidative stress and inflammation in HCV-positive patients with liver cirrhosis.** *Hepatol Res* 2008, **38**:683–688.
31. Szymanski DJ: **Recommendations for the avoidance of delayed onset muscle soreness.** *Strength Cond J* 2001, **23**:7–13.
32. Peake J, Nosaka K, Suzuki K: **Characterization of inflammatory responses to eccentric exercise in humans.** *Exerc Immunol Rev* 2005, **11**:64–85.
33. Croisier JL, Camus G, Deby-Dupont G, Bertrand F, Lhermerout C, Crielaard JM, Juchmes-Ferir A, Deby C, Albert A, Lamy M: **Myocellular enzyme leakage, polymorphonuclear neutrophil activation and delayed onset muscle soreness induced by isokinetic eccentric exercise.** *Arch Physiol Biochem* 1996, **104**:322–329.
34. Schuller-Levis GB, Park E: **Taurine: new implications for an old amino acid.** *FEMS Microbiol Lett* 2003, **226**:195–202.
35. Cheung K, Hume P, Maxwell L: **Delayed onset muscle soreness: treatment strategies and performance factors.** *Sports Med* 2003, **33**:145–164.
36. Murase S, Terazawa E, Queme F, Ota H, Matsuda T, Hirate K, Kozaki Y, Katanosaka K, Taguchi T, Urai H, Mizumura K: **Bradykinin and nerve growth factor play pivotal roles in muscular mechanical hyperalgesia after exercise (delayed-onset muscle soreness).** *J Neurosci* 2010, **30**:3752–3761.
37. Kudo I, Murakami M: **Phospholipase A2 enzymes.** *Prostaglandins Other Lipid Mediat* 2002, **68–69**:3–58.

38. Gijon MA, Spencer DM, Siddiqi AR, Bonventre JV, Leslie CC: **Cytosolic phospholipase A2 is required for macrophage arachidonic acid release by agonists that Do and Do not mobilize calcium. Novel role of mitogen-activated protein kinase pathways in cytosolic phospholipase A2 regulation.** *J Biol Chem* 2000, **275:**20146–20156.
39. Newham DJ, McPhail G, Mills KR, Edwards RH: **Ultrastructural changes after concentric and eccentric contractions of human muscle.** *J Neurol Sci* 1983, **61:**109–122.
40. Olwin BB, Hannon K, Kudla AJ: **Are fibroblast growth factors regulators of myogenesis in vivo?** *Prog Growth Factor Res* 1994, **5:**145–158.
41. Radak Z, Chung HY, Goto S: **Systemic adaptation to oxidative challenge induced by regular exercise.** *Free Radic Biol Med* 2008, **44:**153–159.
42. Flann KL, LaStayo PC, McClain DA, Hazel M, Lindstedt SL: **Muscle damage and muscle remodeling: no pain, no gain?** *J Exp Biol* 2011, **214:**674–679.

Thoracic aorta vasoreactivity in rats under exhaustive exercise: effects of Lycium barbarum polysaccharides supplementation

Zhifang Zhao[1†], Yan Luo[1†], Guanghua Li[1*], Lingqin Zhu[1], Yin Wang[1] and Xuehong Zhang[2]

Abstract

Background: Reduced arterial compliance is associated with an increased rate of morbidity and mortality in cardiovascular disease. Exercise is beneficial for compromised arterial compliance. However, the beneficial effects of exercise are lost with exhaustion. Lycium barbarum L. has been used in China for centuries to maintain good health. In this regard, the primary purpose of this study was to characterize the effects of the polysaccharides from Lycium barbarum (LBPs) on arterial compliance during exhaustive exercise.

Methods: A four-week swimming exercise program was designed for rats, and the blood levels of malondialdehyde (MDA), super oxide dismutase (SOD), nitric oxide(NO) and heat shock protein 70(HSP70) were detected. The tension of aorta rings was measured to evaluate the response of rats on noradrenaline (NA)-induced contractions.

Results: The rats administered LBPs showed longer swimming time until exhaustion than the control group of rats. Exercise-induced MDA elevation was repressed by LBPs supplementation. The LBPs-supplemented rats displayed a significant increase of SOD, NO, HSP70 than the non-supplemented rats. Additionally, LBPs significantly up-regulated the expression of eNOS and improved the endothelium-dependent vasodilatation of the aorta ring.

Conclusion: Our study proved that LBPs administration significantly inhibited the oxidative stress, and improved the arterial compliance.

Keywords: Lycium barbarum polysaccharides, Exhaustive exercise, Thoracic aorta, Vasoreactivity

Introduction

Arterial compliance, the inverse of arterial stiffness, is now recognized as an important determinant of cardiovascular morbidity and mortality [1]. Exercise can affect arterial compliance. It is well known that aerobic exercise reduces arterial stiffness. Moderate-intensity aerobic exercise at 65% of its maximal oxygen uptake lowers both central and peripheral arterial stiffness [2]. In addition, twelve weeks of aerobic exercise enhances vascular compliance (especially of the arms and legs) in obese male adolescents [3]. However, the beneficial effects of exercise are lost with exhaustion. For example, High-intensity strength exercise leads to a decrease in arterial compliance [4,5]. Twenty to forty hours of continuous mountain trail running decreases the large artery compliance [6]. Moreover, marathon runners have increased aortic stiffness compared to that of the control group [7]. In contrast, one-year of exercise fails to improve the arterial stiffness or function of heart failure with preserved ejection fraction (HFpEF) in patients [8]. The mechanism of different effects of exercise on arterial compliance remains unclear.

Lycium barbarum (also called Wolfberry, Fructus Lycii or Gouqizi), belonging to the plant family Solanaceae, has been widely used for 2000 years in traditional Chinese Medicine [9-11]. Polysaccharides (LBPs) which constitute more than 40% of the fruit extract are the major valuable and active ingredient in Lycium barbarum [12]. LBPs have been shown to exert a large variety of biological activities including eye-protective, anti-aging, antioxidant,

* Correspondence: ghlee0404@163.com
†Equal contributors
[1]Department of Physiology, School of Basic Medical Science, Ningxia Medical University, Yinchuan 750004, China
Full list of author information is available at the end of the article

immunoregulating, neuroprotective, cytoprotective and antitumor properties [13-17]. It has been reported that LBPs treatment prevented the increase of blood pressure in hypertension rats induced by the two-kidney, one clip method in vivo. LBPs-treated rats showed a significant decrease in the concentration of phenylephrine in isolated aortic rings as compared with non-treated hypertensive rats [18]. However, the effects of LBPs on arterial compliance in rats with exhaustive exercise have not been investigated. In the present study, we aimed to determine the effects of LBPs on the arterial compliance from lesions induced by exhaustive exercise.

Materials and methods

Animals

A total of 40 male Sprague Dawley rats (180 ± 20 g) were bred, five per cage, in light-and temperature-controlled conditions (12 hours light: 12 hours dark; 24.0 ± 0.2°C) and provided with standard laboratory diet and tap water ad libitum. The experimental procedures were approved by the animal ethics committee of the Ningxia Medical University and Use Committee in accordance with the guidelines of the Council of the Physiological Society of China.

After an adaptation period of one week, all animals were randomly divided into 4 groups (n = 10): control sedentary group (CS), swimming exercise group (SE), exhaustive swimming exercise group (ES), exhaustive swimming exercise with LBPs group (ES-LBP). The rats in ES-LBP group received 200 mg/kg/day by gavage for 28 days. In CS, SE, ES groups, the rats were given the same volume of isotonic saline solution by oral administration for 28 days. The dose of LBPs was chosen on the basis of preliminary experiments, which was safe and effective without undue toxicity in rats.

Exercise protocol

During the first week, rats were acclimated to swimming exercises for 5 days with increasing duration from 5 minutes on the first day to 60 minutes by the fifth day [19]. The rats in the control group were subjected to water immersion without exercises. The rats swam in a plastic tank (diameter, 60 cm; depth, 80 cm) filled with water at 32 ±1°C. After acclimation, rats were assigned to swim for 60 minutes per day, 5 days per week, for 4 weeks (between 8:00 am and 12:00 am). At the end of the training, the rats of the ES and ES-LBP groups were subjected to a swim to exhaustion with a load of 5% of their body weight strapped on their backs. The point of exhaustion was defined when a rat failed to rise to the surface of water, drown over 10 seconds and could not maintain coordination [20]. This exhaustion time was subsequently recorded.

Samples collection

All animals were anesthetized with urethane (1.5 g/kg) and sacrificed immediately after the exhaustive exercise. The chest was rapidly opened and the thoracic aorta was carefully isolated in order to preserve the vascular endothelium, which was then placed into modified cold Krebs' solution. The isolated vessel was cut into rings of approximately 3–4 mm wide for measuring isometric force. The rest of the aorta was frozen in liquid nitrogen immediately and stored at −80°C for the assay of endothelial NO synthase (eNOS) mRNA expression . Blood was collected from inferior vena cava in heparinized tube and centrifuged at 1,700×g for 10 minutes (at 4°C) to obtain plasma. The plasma was frozen at −80°C to measure the expression of malondialdehyde (MDA), super oxide dismutase (SOD), nitric oxide (NO) and heat shock protein 70(HSP70).

Assay of isometric force in Rat aorta rings

The isolated aortic rings were cleaned to remove the adherent tissues and hung in 10-ml organ bath with Krebs' solution at 37°C, pH 7.4, and containing 95% O_2 and 5% CO_2. The modified Krebs' solution was composed of the following components: 110 mM NaCl, 4.6 mM KCl, 2.5 mM $CaCl_2$, 24.8 mM $NaHCO_3$, 1.2 mM KH_2PO_4, 1.2 mM $MgSO_4$, and 5.6 g glucose. The tissue's isometric tension was measured with force transducers that connected with a BL-420E$^+$ biological function experimental system (Chengdu Technology and Market, Chengdu, China). The vessel rings were equilibrated for 1 hour with the tension of 2.0 g and pre-contracted with KCl (60 mM) to produce the maximal KCL-induced contractile plateau. Subsequently the cumulative dose–response curve for noradrenaline (NA) (10^{-10}-10^{-5}M) was obtained. The values of the NA-induced contraction were expressed as a percentage of maximal contraction induced by KCl.

Measurement of SOD, MDA and nitrite/nitrate (NOx) levels in plasma

The oxidative stress indices were measured to explore whether LBP could reduce exhaustive exercise-induced oxidative stress. The levels of SOD, MDA and NOx (NO^{2-} and NO^{3-}) were determined by using commercially available kits (Nanjing Jiancheng Bioengineering Institute, Nanjing, China) according to the manufacturer's instructions.

HSP70 determination

The plasma level of HSP70 was detected by a commercially available ELISA kit (Cusabio Biotechnology, Wuhan, China). The amount of HSP70 in plasma was estimated from the calibration curve ranging from 62.5 to 4000 pg/ml.

Table 1 GenBank accession code, primer sequences, and predicted size of the amplified product

Gene	Primer sequences	GenBank	bp
eNOS	Forward primer: 5'-CACACTGCTAGAGGTGCTGGAA-3'	NM_021838	109
	Reverse primer: 5'-TGCTGAGCTGACAGAGTAGTAC-3'		
β-actin	Forward primer: 5'-TCATGAAGTGTGACGTTGACATCCGT-3'		285
	Reverse primer: 5'-CCTAGAAGCATTTGCGGTGCAGGATG-3'		

RT-PCR analysis

Total RNA was prepared from the thoracic aorta using RNA AxyPrep Pure RNA isolation kit (AXYGEN, USA) according to the manufacturer's instructions. The purity and concentration of RNA was determined by spectrophotometry at 260 nm and 280 nm. Complementary DNA (cDNA) was synthesized using a reverse transcription kit (TransGen Biotechnology, Beijing). Quantitative PCR was performed using a quantitect SYBR green PCR kit (TransGen Biotechnology, Beijing) as follows: 35 cycles of denaturation at 94°C for 30 sec, annealing at 62°C for 30 sec and extension at 72°C for 30 sec. Primers used for the PCR were shown in Table 1. Relative gene expression levels were determined using the $2^{-\Delta\Delta Ct}$ method.

Statistical analysis

Results were presented as the mean ± SD. Two-way ANOVA was used to evaluate any differences between the two sets of dose–response curves. The remaining data were evaluated by one-way ANOVA and Student's t-test. The statistical analyses were performed by SPSS for Windows 11.5.0 software. P<0.05 was considered to indicate a statistically significant difference.

Results

Contractile response of vascular ring to NA

Vascular dysfunction is related to increased vasoconstriction and weakened diastolic function. Therefore, we are interested in determining whether there is any change in the vascular function by detecting the vascular reactivity of aortic rings to a physiological modulator, noradrenaline (NA). Cumulatively added NA (10^{-10}-10^{-5}M) caused concentration-dependent contractile responses in isolated aortic rings. We found that there was no significant difference between the SE and the CS group, while the ES group significantly increased the vasoconstrictive response to NA (P<0.01), LBPs treatment decreased the vasoconstrictive effect (P< 0.01) (Figure 1). Furthermore, the contractile responsiveness to NA of the SE group was significantly lower than that of the ES (P<0.01) and ES-LBP (P<0.01) groups (Figure 1).

Effects of LBPs on body weight and exhaustive exercise time in rats

After four weeks of swimming exercise, no significant difference was observed in body weight in either group (Table 2). However, as shown in Figure 2, LBPs prolonged the swimming time of rats compared with the ES group (P < 0.05), which was 77.07% higher.

Effects of LBPs on biochemical parameters after exhaustive exercise

It is well known that SOD can inhibit the oxidation of oxyamine by the xanthine–xanthine oxidase system. Therefore we evaluated the plasmic level of SOD. As shown in Figure 3a, the SOD level in the ES-LBP, SE groups significantly increased compared with that in the CS group (P<0.05 and P<0.01 respectively). However, the plasmic SOD level of exhaustive swimming rats was significantly lower than that of the ES-LBP and SE rats (P< 0.01). The results demonstrated that LBPs were able to increase antioxidant enzyme activities to attenuate the oxidative stress induced by exhaustive exercise.

Exhaustive exercise induces the generation of free radicals which may cause an increase in lipid peroxidation [21]. Measuring MDA is one of the most widely used approaches for evaluating oxidative damage to lipids. Figure 3b illustrates that the plasmic MDA levels of SE or ES-LBP rats significantly decreased compared with that of ES rats (P<0.05 and P< 0.01 respectively). This result indicates that LBPs can attenuate lipid peroxidation.

NO is an important vasodiator factor produced by vascular endothelial cells. We found that there was a significant increase in the SE group. As expected, the NO level

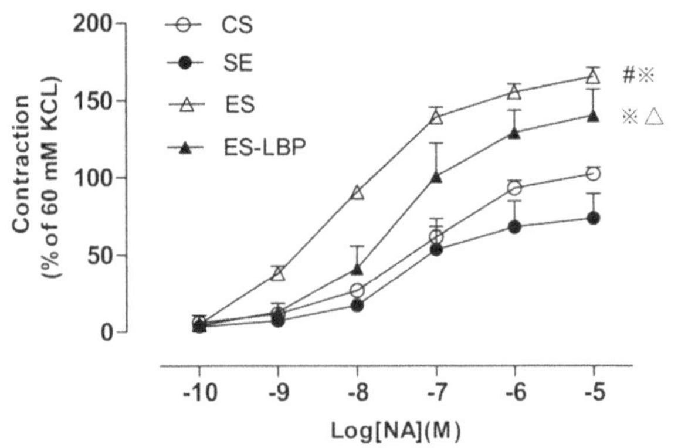

Figure 1 Contractile response of vascular ring to NA.
Dose-dependence of NA on contraction of the thoracic aorta rings separated from rats in CS SE, ES and ES-LBP groups. The contraction induced by 60 mM KCl was taken as 100%. Data are expressed as mean ± SD (n=10). #P<0.01 vs CS; ※P<0.01vs SE; △P<0.01 vs ES.

Table 2 Effects of LBP on body weight in rats

Group	Before experiment	One week	Two week	Three week	Four week
CS	191.67±26.90	204.83±13.43	264.08±12.31	304.44±9.97	346.58±15.55
SE	187.5±4.74	209.53±6.15	258.43±9.88	309.35±19.11	340.5±22.31
ES	191.2±10.77	210.67±10.91	263.5±14.05	304.58±17.12	329.13±15.06
ES-LBP	198.2±9.66	215.14±7.22	267.70±6.96	312.08±10.14	344.33±14.91

Effects of LBPs on body weight in rats. The values are expressed as mean ± SD (n=10).

was significantly reduced by exhaustive exercise. Further, we found this reduction induced by exhaustive exercise could be reversed by LBPs treatment (Figure 3c).

The expression of heat shock proteins (HSPs) is induced by hyperthermia ischemia, oxidative cytokine, muscular stress, glucose deprivation, alterations in calcium and pH [22]. HSP70 is a group of binding proteins with molecular weight of 70 KD, which is significantly increased by high-intensity exercise [23]. To determine the expression of HSP70 after exercise and supplement with LBPs, the plasmic level of HSP70, analyzed by ELISA, showed an immediate increase after both exercise sessions. As shown in Figure 3d, the HSP70 levels of SE or ES rats were increased. Furthermore, LBPs treatment induced a much higher increase in the ES group ($P< 0.01$).

Expression of eNOS mRNA

As the NO level can be up-regulated by LBPs, we therefore examined the effect of LBPs on the expression of eNOS in the aorta after exhaustive exercise. The expression of eNOS mRNA in aorta of four groups was shown in Figure 4. There were significant differences in the eNOS mRNA expression level among different groups. The eNOS expression was increased in both SE and ES-LBP groups ($P < 0.01$). However, the level of eNOS expression was significantly attenuated in rats after exhaustive exercise ($P < 0.01$). LBPs treatment significantly reversed the inhibition of the eNOS expression in rats from ES group ($p < 0.01$).

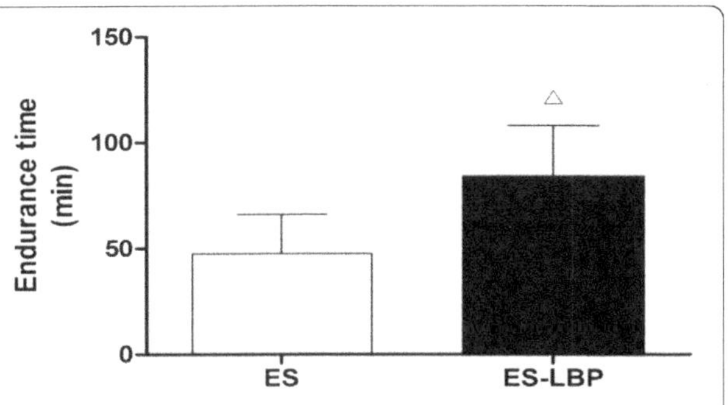

Figure 2 Effects of LBPs on exhaustive exercise time in the rats. LBPs supplementation significantly increased the time to fatigue compared to that of the ES. Data are mean ± SD (n =10). $^{\triangle}P < 0.01$ vs ES.

Discussion

The effects of LBPs on vascular vasoreactivity in exhaustive exercise rats were investigated. The major finding of this study was that the contraction induced by NA in thoracic aorta was increased in the presence of exhaustive exercise. Furthermore, supplementation with the LBPs for 4 weeks remarkably improved the vascular reactivity of ES-LBP rats compared to the ES rats (Figure 1). As the arterial compliance is judged by the responsiveness to NA, the results showed that the compliance or distensibility of aorta was increased in LBPs treated animals [24].

Arterial compliance, the inverse of arterial stiffness, is now recognized as an important determinant of cardiovascular morbidity and mortality [1], which can increase the workload placed on the myocardium. The changes in arterial compliance of exercise training rats depend on the exercise mode, intensity and duration. Twelve weeks of air board exercise leads to an increase in cardio-respiratory fitness and vascular compliance, which may reduce the risk of later development of cardiovascular disease [3] and improve coronary artery perfusion preventing ischemic events [25], and decline pulse pressure and wall stress [26]. Moreover, Nickel [27] showed that 30 minutes of moderate-intensity aerobic exercise transiently increased small arterial compliance after exercise, but not sustained. Extremely high volume exercise may be associated with decreases in cardiovascular function and large artery compliance [6]. Ahmadi et al. [28] recently reported that coronary artery calcification was associated with impaired aortic compliance.

The present study has confirmed these varying effects of exercise on arterial compliance. In SE rats, which were subjected to swimming exercise for four weeks, the attenuated contractile responses of aorta to NA were clearly observed, whereas in rats exposed to exhaustive swimming exercise, depressed vasodilator response was observed (Figure 1). This inhibition was completely reversed by the treatment of LBPs in the ES group. In isolated aortic rings of LBPs-treated rats, the responsiveness to phenylephrine was attenuated in comparison with non-treated hypertensive rats [18].

Generally, exhaustive exercise induced oxidative stress impaired endothelial function [29] that decreased artery

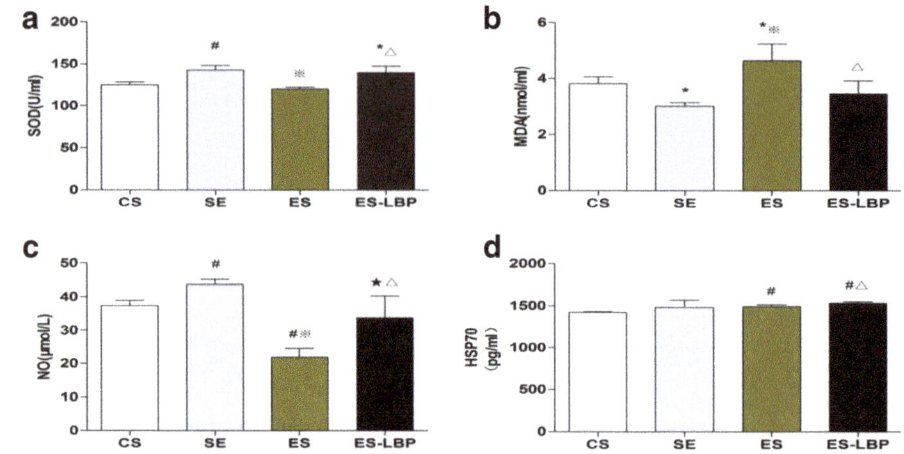

Figure 3 Effects of LBPs supplement and exhaustive exercise on SOD (a), MDA (b), NO (c) and HSP70 (d) expression in the rats. Values are expressed as mean ± SD (*n* = 10). **P* < 0.05 and #*P* < 0.01 *vs* CS; ★*P* < 0.05 and ※< 0.01 *vs* SE; △*P* < 0.01 vs ES.

compliance [30], which may interfere with NA-dependent vasoconstriction. The present study indicated that a bout of exhaustive swimming exercise caused a significant increase in oxidative stress, which decreased the serum antioxidant enzyme SOD and increased the lipid hydroperoxides MDA. LBPs were shown to be effective in avoiding oxidative stress and cleaning out the excess free radical and decreasing the level of lipid peroxidation [10,31,32]. These increases in super oxide levels were correlated with attenuated responsiveness to NA. Our previous study also showed that LBPs could enhance the immune function in exhausted swimming rat [33]. Combination with results of this study, LBPs is a useful protective agent in rats of exhaustive exercise, and whether LBPs are helpful for athletes needs a further research to confirm.

NO, derived from a biochemical reaction catalyzed by eNOS [34], plays an important role in the regulation of vascular tension [35]. The most important activity of NO may be vasodilation in the cardiovascular system, which is usually used as a surrogate index of endothelial function [35]. Studies have demonstrated that arterial stiffness was regulated by the endothelium through the release of NO [36]. Our data showed that LBPs could enhance the expression of eNOS, elevate NO levels and consequently inhibit the contractile response to NA. Previous studies have suggested that N-nitro-L-arginine methyl ester increased the contraction to phenylephrine in the aortic rings of LBPs-treated rats in vitro. LBPs reduced the phenylephrine-induced contraction which may be mediated by increasing the production of endothelium-derived relaxation factor (EDRF) [18]. In addition, aortic contractility of LBPs-treated rats reduced due to attenuated responsiveness to NA and probably to increase in plasmic level of NO. The up-regulation of SOD levels during exercise training might lead to improvement in endothelial function through an increase in NO production [37].

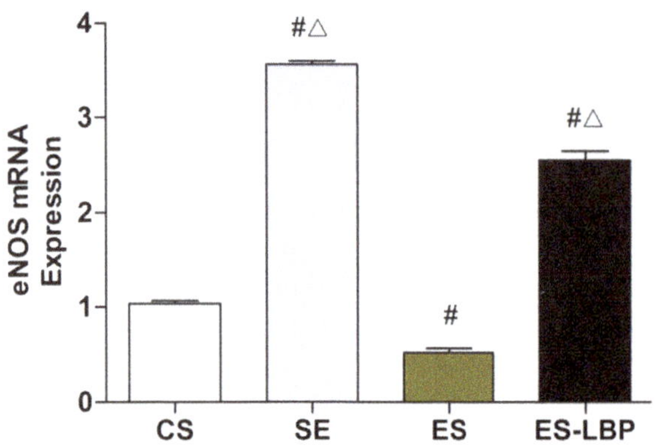

Figure 4 Effects of LBPs on eNOS mRNA expression in thoracic aorta separated from rats in different groups. Values are expressed as mean ± SD (*n* = 10). #*P*<0.01 *vs* CS; △*P*<0.01 vs ES.

Heat shock proteins (HSP) belong to the family of stress-responsive proteins that are induced by oxidative stress, which are essential for modulating cell function and maintaining protein homeostasis [38,39]. As a stress protein, the response of HSP70 is different according to the intensity and form of movement, which provides new ideas and methods to further understand the campaign laws and institute more scientific physical training and exercise training [40,41]. In ES-LBP, the HSP70 levels were significantly increased compared with that of ES. Meanwhile, the attenuation of the NA-induced aortic contraction was observed in ES-LBP rats. Thus, HSP70 may take part in this attenuation through protecting the cells from the deleterious effects of ROS and reducing oxidative stress.

Conclusion

In conclusion, this study clearly indicates that the contractile response to NA is attenuated by LBPs treatment in ES-LBP rats. The exhaustive swim time is also prolonged by LBPs supplement through activation of the antioxidant defense system. Meanwhile, LBPs can upregulate the expression of eNOS, NO and HSP70. However, the mechanism of blunted contractile response to NA in aorta of LBPs-treated rats is not fully investigated in this study, further research including molecular study is required to investigate this mechanism.

Competing interests

The authors declare that they have no competing interests.

Authors' contributions

GL: dissertation guidance, interpretation of the data and and drafted the manuscript; ZZ: randomization of the protocol training of animals, literature review; YL: molecular biology assays; LZ: ELISA assays assistance and biochemical assays; YW: paper revise; XZ: animal training assistance; All authors read and approved the final manuscript.

Acknowledgements

This study was supported by National Natural Science Foundation of China, No. 81060230, 81050352 and Ningxia Natural Science Foundation No. NZ10111, NZ13055. The authors also wish to thank Jason Zhang for English assistance.

Author details

[1]Department of Physiology, School of Basic Medical Science, Ningxia Medical University, Yinchuan 750004, China. [2]Department of Pediatrics, General Hospital of Ningxia Medical University, Yinchuan 750004, China.

References

1. Cavalcante JL, Lima JAC, Redheuil A, *et al*: **Aortic stiffness current understanding and future directions.** *J Am Coll Cardiol* 2011, **57**(14):1511–1522.
2. Heffernan K, Collier S, Kelly E, *et al*: **Arterial stiffness and baroreflex sensitivity following bouts of aerobic and resistance exercise.** *Int J Sports Med* 2007, **28**(3):197.
3. Song JK, Stebbins CL, Kim TK, *et al*: **Effects of 12 weeks of aerobic exercise on body composition and vascular compliance in obese boys.** *J Sports Med Phys Fitness* 2012, **52**(5):522–529.
4. Otsuki T, Maeda S, Iemitsu M, *et al*: **Vascular endothelium-derived factors and arterial stiffness in strength-and endurance-trained men.** *American J Physiol-Heart Circ Physiol* 2007, **292**(2):H786–H791.
5. Kawano H, Tanimoto M, Yamamoto K, *et al*: **Resistance training in men is associated with increased arterial stiffness and blood pressure but does not adversely affect endothelial function as measured by arterial reactivity to the cold pressor test.** *Exp Physiol* 2008, **93**(2):296–302.
6. Burr J, Bredin SS, Phillips A, *et al*: **Systemic arterial compliance following ultra-marathon.** *Int J Sports Med* 2012, **33**(03):224–229.
7. Vlachopoulos C, Kardara D, Anastasakis A, *et al*: **Arterial stiffness and wave reflections in marathon runners.** *Am J Hypertens* 2010, **23**(9):974–979.
8. Fujimoto N, Prasad A, Hastings JL, *et al*: **Cardiovascular effects of 1 year of progressive endurance exercise training in patients with heart failure with preserved ejection fraction.** *Am Heart J* 2012, **164**(6):869–877.
9. Deli MA, Yang D, Li S-Y, *et al*: **Lycium barbarum extracts protect the brain from blood–brain barrier disruption and cerebral edema in experimental stroke.** *Plos One* 2012, **7**(3):e33596.
10. Shan XZ, Zhou JL, Ma T, *et al*: **Lycium barbarum polysaccharides reduce exercise-induced oxidative stress.** *Int J Mol Sci* 2011, **12**(2):1081–1088.
11. Potterat OG: **(Lycium barbarumandL. chinense): phytochemistry, pharmacology and safety in the perspective of traditional uses and recent popularity.** *Planta Med* 2009, **76**(01):7–19.
12. Chang RC-C, So K-F: **Use of anti-aging herbal medicine, lycium barbarum, against aging-associated diseases. What do we know so far?** *Cell Mol Neurobiol* 2007, **28**(5):643–652.
13. Ho YS, Yu MS, Yik SY, *et al*: **Polysaccharides from wolfberry antagonizes glutamate excitotoxicity in rat cortical neurons.** *Cell Mol Neurobiol* 2009, **29**(8):1233–1244.
14. Wu HT, He XJ, Hong YK, *et al*: **Chemical characterization of Lycium barbarum polysaccharides and its inhibition against liver oxidative injury of high-fat mice.** *Int J Biol Macromol* 2010, **46**(5):540.
15. Tang W-M, Chan E, Kwok C-Y, *et al*: **A review of the anticancer and immunomodulatory effects of Lycium barbarum fruit.** *Inflammopharmacology* 2012, **20**(6):14–307.
16. Chang HM, But PPH, Yao SC: *Pharmacology and applications of Chinese materia medica*. Singapore: World Scientific Publishing Company Incorporated; 2001.
17. Potterat O: **Phytochemistry, pharmacology and safety in the perspective of traditional uses and recent popularity.** *Planta Med* 2010, **76**:7–19.
18. Jia YX, Dong JW, Wu XX, *et al*: **The effect of lycium barbarum polysaccharide on vascular tension in two-kidney, one clip model of hypertension.** *Sheng Li Xue Bao* 1998, **50**(3):309–314.
19. Sampaio-Barros M, Farias-Silva E, Grassi-Kassisse D, *et al*: **Effect of swimming session duration and repetition on metabolic markers in rats.** *Stress: Int J Biol Stress* 2003, **6**(2):127–132.
20. Thomas D, Marshall K: **Effects of repeated exhaustive exercise on myocardial subcellular membrane structures.** *Int J Sports Med* 1988, **9**(4):257–260.
21. Skarpańska-Stejnborn A, Basta P, Pilaczyńska-Szcześniak Ł, *et al*: **Black grape extract supplementation attenuates blood oxidative stress in response to acute exercise.** *Biol Sport* 2010, **27**(1):41–46.
22. Fehrenbach E, Northoff H: **Free radicals, exercise, apoptosis, and heat shock proteins.** *Exerc Immunol Rev* 2001, **7**:66–89.
23. Noble EG, Moraska A, Mazzeo RS, Roth DA, Olsson MC, Moore RL, Fleshner M: **Differential expression of stress proteins in rat myocardium after free wheel or treadmill run training.** *J Appl Physiol* 1999, **86**(5):1696–701.
24. Dunbar SL, Tamhidi L, Berkowitz DE, *et al*: **Hindlimb unweighting affects rat vascular capacitance function.** *American J Physiol-Heart Circ Physiol* 2001, **281**(3):H1170–H1177.
25. Kass DA, Saeki A, Tunin RS, *et al*: **Adverse influence of systemic vascular stiffening on cardiac dysfunction and adaptation to acute coronary occlusion.** *Circulation* 1996, **93**(8):1533–1541.
26. Belz GG: **Elastic properties and Windkessel function of the human aorta.** *Cardiovasc Drugs Ther* 1995, **9**(1):73–83.
27. Nickel KJ, Acree LS, Gardner AW: **Effects of a single bout of exercise on arterial compliance in older adults.** *Angiology* 2011, **62**(1):33–37.
28. Ahmadi N, Nabavi V, Hajsadeghi F, *et al*: **Impaired aortic distensibility measured by computed tomography is associated with the severity of coronary artery disease.** *Int J Cardiovasc Imaging (formerly Cardiac Imaging)* 2011, **27**(3):459–469.
29. Knez WL, Coombes JS, Jenkins DG: **Ultra-endurance exercise and oxidative damage: implications for cardiovascular health.** *Sports Med* 2006, **36**(5):429–441.
30. Wilkinson IB, MacCallum H, Cockcroft JR, *et al*: **Inhibition of basal nitric oxide synthesis increases aortic augmentation index and pulse wave velocity in vivo.** *Br J Clin Pharmacol* 2002, **53**(2):189–192.
31. Niu A-J, Wu J-M, Yu D-H, *et al*: **Protective effect of Lycium barbarum polysaccharides on oxidative damage in skeletal muscle of exhaustive exercise rats.** *Int J Biol Macromol* 2008, **42**(5):447–449.
32. Duan CB, Sun ZJ: **Supplementation of Lycium barbarum polysaccharides protection of skeletal muscle from exercise-induced oxidant stress in mice.** *African J Pharm Pharmacol* 2012, **6**(9):643–647.
33. Jing H, Hong-peng L, Zhou X, Guang-hua L: **The effect of LBP on immune function of exhausted swimming exercise in mice.** *J Liaoning University of TCM* 2009, **11**(8):234–236.
34. Li GH, Katakura M, Maruyama M, *et al*: **Changes of noradrenaline-induced contractility and gene expression in aorta of rats acclimated to heat in two different modes.** *Eur J Appl Physiol* 2008, **104**(1):29–40.
35. Maiorana A, O'Driscoll G, Taylor R, *et al*: **Exercise and the nitric oxide vasodilator system.** *Sports Med* 2003, **33**(14):1013–1035.
36. Bellien J, Favre J, Iacob M, *et al*: **Arterial stiffness is regulated by nitric oxide and endothelium-derived hyperpolarizing factor during changes in blood flow in humans.** *Hypertension* 2010, **55**(3):674–680.

37. Higashi Y, Yoshizumi M: **Exercise and endothelial function: role of endothelium-derived nitric oxide and oxidative stress in healthy subjects and hypertensive patients.** *Pharmacol Ther* 2004, **102**(1):87–96.
38. Asea A: **Hsp70: a chaperokine.** In *Novartis Foundation symposium; 2008*, Volume 1999. Chichester; New York: John Wiley; 2008:173.
39. Atalay M, Oksala N, Lappalainen J, *et al*: **Heat shock proteins in diabetes and wound healing.** *Curr Protein Pept Sci* 2009, **10**(1):85.
40. Banfi G, Dolci A, Verna R, *et al*: **Exercise raises serum heat-shock protein 70 (Hsp70) levels.** *Clin Chem Lab Med* 2004, **42**(12):1445–1446.
41. Guixia C, Junwei B: **Progress of the research on the effect of exercises on HSP70 expression in cardiac and skeletal muscles.** *J Jilin Institute of Phys Educ* 2010, **26**(5):83–85.

Does carbohydrate supplementation enhance tennis match play performance?

Rodrigo Vitasovic Gomes[1], Caroline Dario Capitani[2], Carlos Ugrinowitsch[1], Michael Christopher Zourdos[3], Jaime Fernandez-Fernandez[4], Alberto Mendez-Villanueva[5] and Marcelo Saldanha Aoki[6*]

Abstract

Background: Carbohydrate (CHO) ingestion may be an interesting approach to avoid significant decrement to the tennis match performance. The aim of the present investigation was to assess the effects of CHO supplementation on tennis match play performance.

Methods: Twelve young tennis players (18.0 ± 1.0 years; 176 ± 3.4 cm; 68.0 ± 2.3 kg; body fat: 13.7 ± 2.4%) with national rankings among the top 50 in Brazil agreed to participate in this study, which utilized a randomized, crossover, double blind research design. The experiment was conducted over a 5-day period in which each player completed two simulated tennis matches of a 3-hour duration. The players received either a CHO or a placebo (PLA) drinking solution during simulated tennis matches. Athlete's performance parameters were determined by filming each match with two video cameras. Each player was individually tracked for the entire duration of the match to measure the following variables: (1) games won; (2) rally duration; (3) strokes per rally; (4) effective playing time (%); (5) aces; (6) double faults; (7) first service in; (8) second service in; (9) first return in and (10) second return in.

Results: There were no differences between trials in any of the variables analyzed.

Conclusions: CHO supplementation did not improve tennis match play performance under the present experimental conditions.

Keywords: Match analysis, Glycemia, Performance

Background

There is strong evidence that appropriate selection of nutrients, timing of intake, and proper supplement choice are associated with optimal health and exercise performance [1]. During exercise, carbohydrate (CHO) supplementation is one of the most popular dietary recommendations to provide energy to skeletal muscles and the central nervous system [1-6]. Further, to ensure proper CHO delivery to the contracting skeletal muscles, the American College of Sports Medicine along with the Academy of Nutrition and Dietetics (AND) (formerly recognized as the American Dietetic Association) each recommend ingestion of a CHO solution during prolonged exercise [1,5]. This recommendation is supported by early empirical evidence regarding the positive effects of CHO supplementation to enhance endurance exercise performance [7,8].

However, even though a tennis match encompasses a long total period of time, the overall exercise requirements of a match differ from traditional endurance exercise. To illustrate, a tennis match involves intermittent bouts of high-intensity effort interspersed with periods of low-intensity activity, during which active recovery (between points) and passive periods (between changeover breaks in play) take place (20 s), over an extended period of time [9-11]. In the major international tournaments (e.g. Grand Slam events and Davis Cup), male players may play several matches within a relatively short period of time (i.e. <2 hours), however, some matches may extend to greater than 5 hours. Consequently, it is conceivable that such a long tennis match may deplete glycogen stores and produce a state of hypoglycemia [12]. Therefore, CHO ingestion may be an interesting approach to avoid significant decrements to a player's performance. Presently, only a

* Correspondence: aoki.ms@usp.br
[6]School of Arts, Sciences and Humanities, University of São Paulo, Av Arlindo Bettio, 1000, São Paulo 03828-000, Brazil
Full list of author information is available at the end of the article

few studies have investigated the effects of CHO supplementation on tennis performance [13-18].

Moreover, the available data regarding the benefits of CHO supplementation on tennis performance are equivocal. For example, hitting accuracy decreased in the PLA trial when compared to the CHO trial [16]. Similarly, CHO supplementation maintained ground stroke accuracy and increased muscle power after simulated tennis tournament [17]. Conversely, a previous study did not observe any significant positive effect of CHO ingestion on serve and ground stroke velocity as well as stroke accuracy during tennis match play [13]. Additional investigations observed similar results showing no significant effect in the CHO condition when compared to a PLA regarding serve velocity or unforced error [14], fan drill speed and percentage points won and lost [15] during tennis match play. In contrast, Ferrauti & Weber [18] reported that CHO supplementation improved tennis specific running speed test, but interestingly this improvement in speed had no effect on stroke accuracy and games won during a match simulation. Ultimately, there have been controversial results regarding the effects of CHO supplementation on tennis performance [13-18], however, the authors of the present investigation hypothesized that CHO supplementation would serve to avoid performance decrement during prolonged tennis match play. Therefore, the aim of the present investigation was to assess the effect of CHO supplementation on tennis match play performance among nationally ranked young players.

Methods

Participants

A total of 12 (mean and SD: 18.0 ± 1.0 years; 176 ± 3.4 cm; 68.0 ± 2.3 kg; body fat: 13.7 ± 2.4%), competitive male tennis, involved in regular tennis competitions at the national level, with a national ranking between 10 and 55, volunteered to participate in this study. The mean training background of the players was 15 hoursper week, for a minimum of 5 years. Prior to participation, the experimental procedures and potential risks were fully explained to the athletes and their parents. Additionally, written informed consent was obtained from both the players and their parents. Players with any pre-existing medical conditions (i.e. musculoskeletal injuries, metabolic disorders, severe illness) that could have influence in their hormonal responses or performance were excluded from the study. The study protocol was approved by the Human Subject Committee of the University of São Paulo, CAAE: 09860412.6.0000.5391.

Experimental design

This study was conducted over a 5-day period, in which each player completed 3 hours of simulated tennis match play, on 2 separate occasions (Figure 1). Subjects ingested either a CHO or PLA beverage in a double blind, randomized, placebo-controlled crossover design. A 48-hour recovery period was granted between each match. During the 2 weeks prior to commencing the study, all players decreased training volume (from 2 sessions to 1 session per day) to ensure each athlete was properly recovered at the study's onset. Additionally, this study was conducted during a training camp and researchers carefully controlled food and fluid ingestion, and exercise volume.

With the exception of the modified match structure, all games were played according the rules of the International Tennis Federation (ITF) [19] and conducted on an outdoor red clay court. Following the ITF rules, tennis balls (Fort Clay Court Dunlop©, Philippines) were

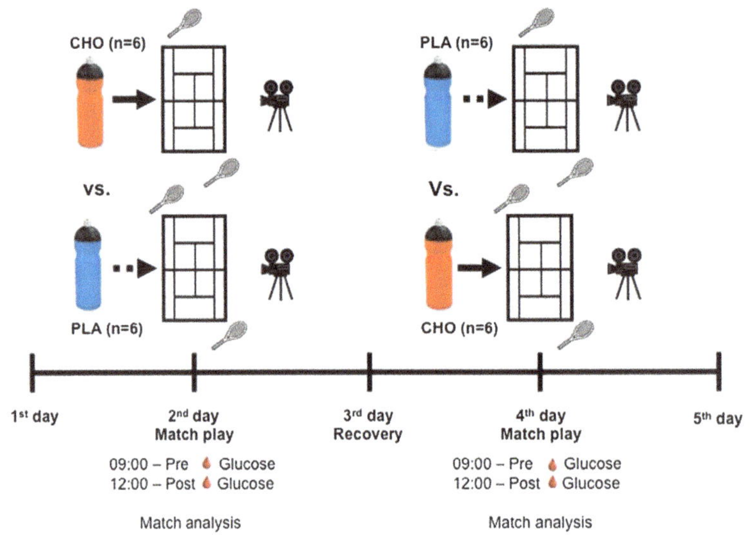

Figure 1 Experimental design.

replaced with new balls after the 7th game of each set and again every nine games afterward. Each match was structured so that each 'set' lasted 1 hour, regardless of the current score. Additionally, players competed against a different opponent each set to ensure a similar competition stimulus during each simulation. The athletes were divided into 3 groups of 4 players, and were allocated the same opponents in the same order (i.e. 1st hour: Player A vs. Player B; Player C x Player D, 2nd hour: Player A vs. Player C, Player B vs. Player D, and 3rd hour: Player A vs. Player D; Player C vs. Player B) for both conditions. The player who won the greatest number of points in each set was considered the winner. Each match was officiated by a qualified tennis referee, who also annotated points won by each player. Finally, the athletes were instructed to put maximal effort in both matches.

Finally, before each match, players performed a standardized warm-up, which consisted of 5-min of groundstrokes, volleys + overheads, and serves. The ambient temperature (day 1: 22.0 ± 1.8°C and day 2: 22.6 ± 1.5°C) and relative humidity (day 1: 77 ± 3% and day 2: 75 ± 2%) were similar between testing days.

CHO supplementation

The sequence of CHO or PLA conditions was randomized as part of the double-blind, crossover study design. At the start of each hour, all athletes ingested either a bottle of CHO solution (6%) containing maltodextrin or water artificially sweetened to comprise the PLA. Thus, players ingested three bottles during each 180-minute match (1 bottle per h - $0.5\,g \cdot kg^{-1} \cdot h^{-1}$) [1,4,20]. The solutions were similar in taste and served chilled in opaque containers. Once these solutions were consumed, players were allowed to drink water ad libitum from individually labelled bottles of known volumes. All of the subjects consumed the total volume of the experimental solution in both the CHO and PLA conditions. Therefore, the total volume of fluid consumption was similar between trials (CHO vs. PLA).

During the 24 hours prior both trials, players consumed an isoenergetic-diet prepared by a sports dietitian (CHO: $8.33 \pm 0.58\,g \cdot kg^{-1}$; Protein: $2.10 \pm 0.14\,g \cdot kg^{-1}$; Fat: $1.58 \pm 0.13\,g \cdot kg^{-1}$). Additionally, before each match (7:30), subjects received a standardized CHO solution (Maltodextrin solution; $1\,g \cdot kg^{-1}$; 10%). The daily energy expenditure of athletes was estimated from the following steps:

a) Basal energy expenditure (BEE) was estimated in accordance with the World Health Organization
b) Diet induced thermogenesis was calculated as 10% BEE, and
c) Energy expenditure for physical activity was estimated using metabolic equivalents (METs) [21].

Match analysis

The activity profile (specific measures of this profile are described later in this section) of each match was determined by filming the matches with two video cameras (DCR-HC17E, Sony©, Japan) positioned 2 meters away from the side of the court, at the level with the service line and approximately 6 meters above the court. Each player was individually 'tracked' to record for the activity profile measures for the entire duration of each match. The video recordings were replayed on a monitor to measure each player's activity profile in detail. The same researcher performed the video analysis of each player's activity profile. A modified match analysis protocol developed by Smekal *et al.* [22] was used to extract the following information as variables of a tennis match to comprise the activity profile: 1. games won; 2. rally duration (seconds); 3. strokes per rally; 4. effective playing time (%); 5. aces; 6. double faults; 7. first service in; 8. second service in; 9. first return in and 10. second return in. The validity and reliability of this protocol has been previously described in the literature [23].

Match analysis included (1) rally duration (s); (2) strokes per rally; (3) effective playing time (%). Rally duration was recorded from the time the service player served the first ball until the moment when one of the players won the point. Strokes per rally were quantified as the number of balls hit by the players from the first serve in to the end of the point. Therefore, for rally duration and strokes per rally, the time for first serve faults, as well as the stroke for the serve fault, and the time between first and second service were excluded from the analysis. Effective playing time was defined as the real playing time (sum of all the rally durations) divided by the total match duration multiplied by 100, as described by Fernandez-Fernandez *et al.* [9].

Blood glucose

Glycemia was determined from a blood sample drawn from the ear lobe and analyzed in the Accu-Chek© monitor (Accu-Chek Active, Roche©, Germany). This method of analysis is in accordance with a previous study, which categorized this monitor as "clinically accurate" [24]. Blood samples were drawn while the players were seated prior to and immediately after the matches. The glycemia test-retest had a coefficient of variation (CV) of 3.1%.

Statistical analyses

All variables were checked for normal distribution and extreme observations using standard procedures. Blood glucose level was analysed using linear mixed models having condition (i.e. CHO and PLA) and time (i.e. Pre and Post) as fixed factors and subjects as a random factor. Whenever a significant F-value was obtained a post-hoc test with a Tukey adjustment was performed for multiple comparison purposes. Match analysis variables were analysed using paired t-test with Bonferroni correction for multiple comparisons. Significance level was set at $p<0.05$.

Results

Blood glucose

There were no significant changes in blood glucose between conditions and from pre- to post-match. However, blood glucose in the CHO condition approached significance ($p = 0.06$) to being higher ($113.4\pm18.0\ mg \cdot dL^{-1}$), when compared to PLA ($93.6\pm9.0\ mg \cdot dL^{-1}$) (Figure 2), at the end of the tennis match play.

Match analysis

Match analysis of the activity profile revealed no significant differences in the number of games won between conditions (Figure 3). Similarly, there were no differences in rally duration (Figure 4) and number of strokes per rally (Figure 5) between the CHO supplementation and PLA conditions. Additionally, there were no differences in all parameters evaluated between conditions (first service in; second service in; first return in; second return in and baseline return in) (Table 1). Finally, effective playing time was (CHO: 19.1% and PLA: 19.3%), and the number of aces and double faults were similar between experimental conditions (Table 2).

Discussion

The purpose of this investigation was to assess the effects of CHO supplementation on variables related to match play performance in young tennis players. The main finding of the present study was that CHO supplementation did not affect match play performance variables or have a statistically significant effect on blood glucose level. However, blood glucose in the CHO condition showed a trend toward higher concentration as the statistical analysis approached significance ($p = 0.06$).

In agreement with the present results, CHO supplementation has been shown to have no effect on tennis match play performance [13-15]. However, previous research has also demonstrated that CHO supplementation is beneficial for improving elements of tennis match play such as stroke performance (accuracy and consistency) [16,17,25] as well as jumping and sprinting performance following a match [17,18]. It should be noted however, that the improvement of stroke accuracy or consistency in a well-controlled research setting may not represent the practical challenges during an actual tennis match play, which include serious tactical, technical and psychological challenges and components. Similarly, although improvements in jumping and sprinting are related to greater anaerobic power, it is not certain that these benefits in a research setting will directly translate to a better match play performance.

The effects of CHO supplementation on exercise performance are associated with the maintenance of blood glucose and the sparing of muscle glycogen stores through the exercise duration [2,3,6,20,26]. However, the results of the present study reveal no significant difference in blood glucose level between PLA and CHO conditions. A possible explanation for the lack of difference in blood glucose level may be that the present study design simulated match play performance, possibly causing the athletes to have a higher sympathetic activity compared with traditional laboratory settings [27]. The hepatic and pancreatic sympathetic activation causes an increased glucose output from the liver as well as a

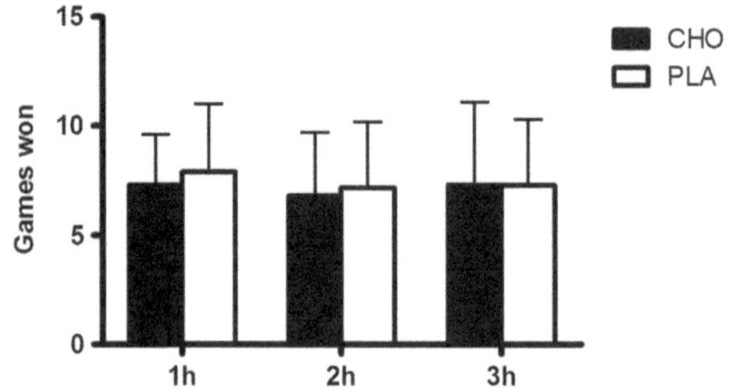

Figure 3 Sum of games won between PLA and CHO conditions.

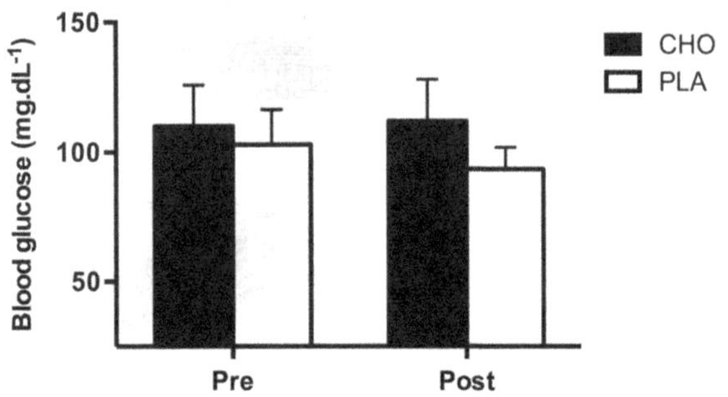

Figure 2 Blood glucose concentration (mean±SD) during PLA and CHO conditions.

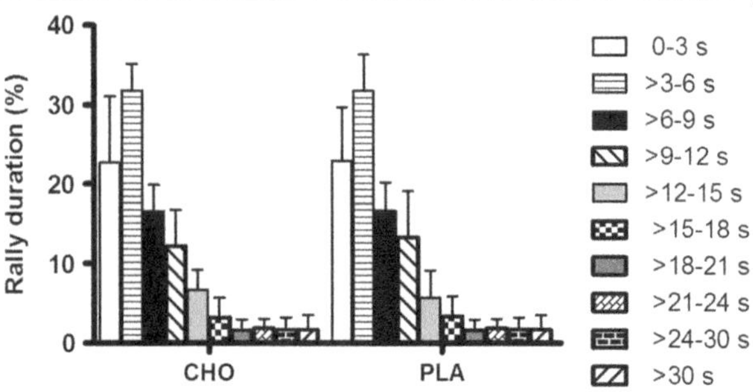

Figure 4 Distribution of rallies duration (%; mean±SD) during PLA and CHO conditions.

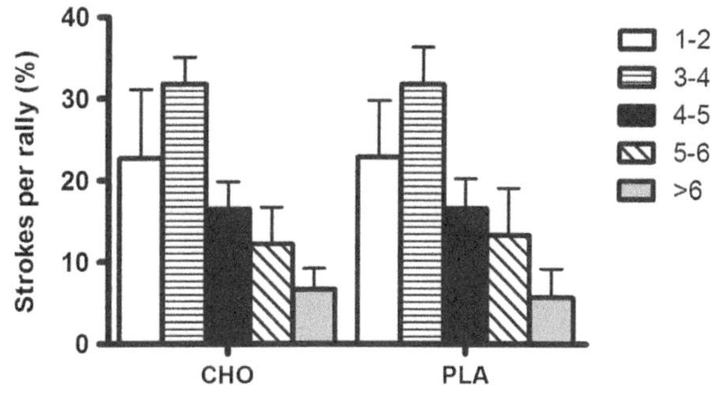

Figure 5 Distribution of strokes per rally (%; mean±SD) during PLA and CHO conditions.

Table 2 Number of aces and double faults during PLA and CHO conditions

	1st hour		2nd hour		3rd hour	
	CHO	PLA	CHO	PLA	CHO	PLA
Aces	4.0±1.4	3.8±1.5	3.5±1.2	2.9±1.2	3.7±1.2	3.2±1.1
Double faults	4.9±3.3	4.4±3.5	3.5±2.3	3.7±2.5	2.3±2.1	3.1±2.1

stimulation of glucagon secretion and an inhibition of insulin release from the pancreas [28,29]. Thus, it is reasonable to suggest that interplay of these factors could have prevented the fall of the blood glucose observed in the present study.

Further analysis unravels that the presented findings are consistent with the suggestion of Mitchell *et al.* [14] who note that blood glucose concentration in tennis players may remain stable for up to 180 min of match play. In additional corroboration to the results of the present study, Bergeron *et al.* [30] demonstrated that blood glucose was not significantly decreased following 85 minutes of match play.

Conversely, previous research does exist that prolonged strenuous exercise decreases blood glucose [6,20], and glycogen stores [26] suggesting the necessity of CHO supplementation for similar exercise activities and possibly sports with requirements of intermittent high intensity bouts. For instance, Curell *et al.* [31] reported that CHO supplementation improved performance in 90 minutes of soccer performance test and Winnick *et al.* [32] observed improvements in physical and central nervous system (CNS) functioning tests while mimicking intermittent sports. These studies, however, were in a laboratory setting and did not replicate an actual match or game, thus as suggested earlier it is possible that sympathetic activity was not elevated to same degree during the simulated match play in the present study.

To further explain the absence of difference in blood glucose between conditions, it has been reported that as exercise intensity increases CHO oxidation increases as well lowering blood glucose [33]. To illustrate, Gomes *et al.* [34] reported no significant change in blood glucose level following prolonged tennis match play (197 min), which was accompanied by an increase in blood cortisol. This maintenance of blood glucose with an increased cortisol concentration is quite possibly associated with the activation of gluconeogenesis and glycogenolysis [35]. These factors suggest the possibility that cortisol release might activate gluconeogenesis eliciting the maintenance of blood glucose. Ultimately, the lack of difference in blood glucose between conditions yielded similar patterns of performance during both trails (CHO vs. PLA). Therefore, it is possible that the metabolic demands of tennis are not sufficient to significantly alter blood glucose during tennis match play to warrant supplementation with CHO [14].

Even though CHO supplementation is often used to spare muscle glycogen stores during prolonged exercise, as performance seems to be impaired by low CHO availability [2,3,20,26,36] that did not seem to be the case in the present study. However, prolonged exercise (> 90 min

Table 1 Technical tennis match play analysis (%; mean±SD) during PLA and CHO conditions

	%					
	1st hour		2nd hour		3rd hour	
	CHO	PLA	CHO	PLA	CHO	PLA
First serves in	57±8	53±12	59±8	60±9	61±10	58±11
Second serves in	75±8	82±10	80±15	80±9	87±11	81±12
Return first serve in	70±19	79±12	74±14	73±12	73±18	75±18
Return second serve in	68±9	83±12	75±17	82±16	80±20	82±19
Return first serve in (Forehand)	69±17	76±13	76±17	71±20	74±17	75±13
Return first serve in (Backhand)	71±23	84±21	74±14	73±19	62±23	69±17
Return second serve in (Forehand)	72±9	85±6	74±12	82±12	78±8	74±10
Return second serve in (Backhand)	70±15	71±8	81±4	86±7	83±10	95±8
Baseline return in (Forehand)	75±8	78±4	76±8	76±8	67±10	71±12
Baseline return in (Backhand)	71±10	75±7	71±8	75±7	74±13	73±11

at 55–75% of maximum oxygen uptake - VO_{2max}) does seem to decrease blood glucose and muscle glycogen stores [20,26]. Therefore, it is worth noting that as the results of the present investigation demonstrated a trend toward higher blood glucose level in the CHO condition, one may speculate that decrement in blood glucose concentration could reach significance during a second match performed with less than 24 hours of rest interval, leading to deleterious performance effects. These data, make it is reasonable to presume that CHO supplementation may be beneficial to maintain blood glucose level and augment performance under tournament conditions (i.e. ATP, Challengers, Future and national tournaments), when matches are performed within 24 hours as a moderate impairment of glycogen stores during the initial match may cause a drop in blood glucose in the subsequent match [12].

CHO supplementation during exercise may have several benefits including an attenuation in central fatigue; a better maintenance of blood glucose and CHO oxidation rate an improved muscle glycogen sparing effect; a reduced exercise-induced strain; and a better maintenance of excitation-contraction coupling [36]. The maintenance of blood glucose might delay fatigue by attenuating the rise in free fatty acids. This process may convincingly limit the increase of precursors related to central fatigue (i.e. serotonin) [37,38]. Further, support is mounting to provide a link between reduced neural drive to skeletal muscle and fatigue throughout tennis matches [39-41]. Moreover it has been suggested that CHO supplementation may increase neural drive thus leading to an attenuation of fatigue and increased exercise performance [36].

A limitation of the present was that the protocol simulated tennis match play conditions, however, it did not simulate tournament conditions in which athletes would play multiple matches with short recovery periods. Thus, the presented findings cannot be extrapolated to tournament conditions that include multiple matches. A second limitation is that athletes received a high CHO diet (~60% daily energy expenditure; $8.33\ g \cdot kg^{-1} \cdot day^{-1}$) during the experiment, which may have diminished the need for exogenous ingestion of CHO during the tennis match play. It is likely, that the high CHO diet and the rest period between matches (48 hours) was an ample protocol to fill glycogen stores, explaining the maintenance of blood glucose observed in the PLA condition. However, it is important to mention that previous investigations have reported that athletes do not achieve the daily CHO intake recommended during training and competitions [2,42] and as a result liver and muscle glycogen stores might be compromised. In such scenario, CHO supplementation could be alternative to provide energy and spare glycogen stores, delaying fatigue and attenuating performance decrement. Finally, the results of the present study should be interpreted with caution considering that the study's sample consisted of well-trained athletes, who might have advanced physiological adaptations that could modulate the responses observed (e.g. more efficient counter-regulatory hormonal response, greater hepatic glucose production, lower reliance on carbohydrates and higher utilization of lipids as energy substrate [43]), which may not otherwise occur in a less-advance athletic population.

Conclusions

The main finding of the present study were: first, CHO supplementation does not augment measures of tennis match play performance and, second, no significant difference in blood glucose was detected after CHO trial compared to a PLA during 180 minutes of simulated match play, however there was a trend toward higher blood glucose in the CHO trial. It is possible that the metabolic demands of 180 minutes of tennis match play are not great enough to significantly lower blood glucose when players were fed a sufficient CHO diet (>$8\ g \cdot kg^{-1} \cdot day^{-1}$). However, during prolonged matches or tournaments that require multiple matches in a 24-hour time span an athlete may benefit from CHO supplementation. Therefore, coaches and athletes should carefully assess the timing and requirements of a single match or a tournament and determine if CHO supplementation is necessary. Further research is necessary to investigate the effects of CHO supplementation during longer matches and in tournament-style play of multiple matches in a 24-hour time span to clarify recommendations.

Competing interests

The authors declare that they have no competing interests.

Authors' contributions

RVG was responsible for data collection, data analysis and interpretation, and the writing of the draft. CDC helped with data collection and contributed to data analysis and interpretation. CU helped with statistical analysis and writing of the manuscript. MCZ participated in data analysis and the writing of the manuscript. JFF and AMV helped in data analysis and interpretation. MSA designed the study and supervised the data collection, analysis, and helped with the writing of the manuscript. All authors read and approved the final manuscript.

Author details

[1]School of Physical Education and Sport, University of São Paulo, Av Prof Mello Moraes 65, São Paulo, SP 05508-030, Brazil. [2]School of Applied Sciences, University of Campinas, Av Pedro Zacaria, 1300, Limeira, SP 13484-350, Brazil. [3]Department of Exercise Science and Health Promotion, Florida Atlantic University, 777 Glades Road, FH 11 Boca Raton, FL 33431, USA. [4]Sports Research Centre, Miguel Hernandez University, Avda. Universidad s/n, Elche, Alicante 03202, Spain. [5]ASPIRE Academy for Sports Excellence, Al Waab, Doha 22287, Qatar. [6]School of Arts, Sciences and Humanities, University of São Paulo, Av Arlindo Bettio, 1000, São Paulo 03828-000, Brazil.

References

1. American Dietetic Association, Dietitians of Canada, American College of Sports Medicine, Rodriguez NR, Di Marco NM, Langley S: **American College of Sports Medicine position stand. Nutrition and athletic performance.** *Med Sci Sports Exerc* 2009, **41**:709–731.
2. Burke LM, Cox GR, Culmmings NK, Desbrow B: **Guidelines for daily carbohydrate intake: do athletes achieve them?** *Sports Med* 2001, **31**:267–299.
3. Jeukendrup AE: **Carbohydrate intake during exercise and performance.** *Nutrition* 2004, **20**:669–677.
4. Kerksick C, Harvey T, Stout J, Campbell B, Wilborn C, Kreider R, Kalman D, Ziegenfuss T, Lopez H, Landis J, Ivy JL, Antonio J: **International Society of Sports Nutrition position stand: Nutrient timing.** *J Int Soc Sports Nutr* 2008, **3**:5–17.
5. American College of Sports Medicine, Sawka MN, Burke LM, Eichner ER, Maughan RJ, Montain SJ, Stachenfeld NS: **American College of Sports Medicine position stand. Exercise and fluid replacement.** *Med Sci Sports Exerc* 2007, **39**:377–390.
6. Coggan AR, Coyle EF: **Carbohydrate ingestion during prolonged exercise: effects on metabolism and performance.** *Exerc Sport Sci Rev* 1991, **19**:1–40.
7. Krogh A, Lindhard J: **The relative value of fat and carbohydrate as sources of muscular energy: with appendices on the correlation between standard metabolism and the respiratory quotient during rest and work.** *Biochem J* 1920, **14**:290–363.
8. Levine SA, Gordon B, Derick CL: **Some changes in chemical constituents of blood following a marathon race.** *JAMA* 1924, **82**:1778–1779.
9. Fernandez-Fernandez J, Mendez-Villanueva A, Fernandez-Garcia B, Terrados N: **Match activity and physiological responses during a junior female singles tennis tournament.** *Br J Sports Med* 2007, **41**:711–716.
10. Fernandez-Fernandez J, Sanz-Rivas D, Sanchez-Muñoz C, Pluim BM, Tiemessen I, Mendez-Villanueva A: **A comparison of the activity profile and physiological demands between advanced and recreational veteran tennis players.** *J Strength Cond Res* 2009, **23**:604–610.
11. Fernandez-Fernandez J, Kinner V, Ferrauti A: **The physiological demands of hitting and running in tennis on different surfaces.** *J Strength Cond Res* 2010, **24**:3255–3264.
12. Ferrauti A, Pluim BM, Busch T, Weber K: **Blood glucose responses and incidence of hypoglycaemia in elite tennis under practice and tournament conditions.** *J Sci Med Sport* 2003, **6**:28–39.
13. Hornery DJ, Farrow D, Mujika I, Young WB: **Caffeine, carbohydrate, and cooling use during prolonged simulated tennis.** *Int J Sports Physiol Perform* 2007, **2**:423–438.
14. Mitchell JB, Cole KJ, Grandjean PW, Sobczak RJ: **The effect of a carbohydrate beverage on tennis performance and fluid balance during prolonged tennis play.** *J Appl Sport Sci Res* 1992, **6**:174–180.
15. McCarthy PR, Thorpe RD, Williams C: **The influence of a carbohydrate-electrolyte beverage on tennis performance.** *Sports Med Sci* 1995, **22**:210–218.
16. McCarthy PR: *Influence of fatigue and dietary manipulation strategies on skilled tennis hitting performance*, PhD thesis. Department of Physical Education, Sports Science and Recreation Management: Loughborough University; 1997.
17. Burke ER, Ekblom B: **Influence of fluid ingestion and dehydration on precision and endurance in tennis.** *Athletic Trainer* 1982, **17**:275–277.
18. Ferrauti A, Weber K: **Metabolic and ergogenic effects of carbohydrate and caffeine beverages in tennis.** *J Sports Med Phys Fitness* 1997, **37**:258–266.
19. ITF: *Official Rules of Tennis*. Chicago IL: Triumph Books; 2002.
20. Coyle EF, Montain SJ: **Benefits of fluid replacement with carbohydrate during exercise.** *Med Sci Sports Exer* 1992, **24**:S324–S330.
21. Ainsworth BE, Haskell WL, Leon AS, Jacobs DR Jr, Montoye HJ, Sallis JF, Paffenbarger RS Jr: **Compendium of physical activities: classification of energy costs of human physical activities.** *Med Sci Sports Exer* 1993, **25**:71–80.
22. Smekal G, Von Duvillard SP, Rihacek C, Pokan R, Hofmann P, Baron R, Tschan H, Bachl N: **A physiological profile of tennis match play.** *Med Sci Sports Exerc* 2001, **33**:999–1005.
23. Mendez-Villanueva A, Fernandez-Fernandez J, Bishop D, Fernandez-Garcia B, Terrados N: **Activity patterns, blood lactate concentrations and ratings of perceived exertion during a professional singles tennis tournament.** *Br J Sports Med* 2007, **41**:296–300.
24. Freckman G, Baumstark A, Jendrike N, Zschornack E, Kocher S, Tshiananga J, Heister F, Haug C: **System accuracy evaluation of 27 blood glucose monitoring systems according to DIN EN ISO 15197.** *Diabetes Technol Ther* 2010, **12**:221–231.
25. Vergauwen L, Brouns F, Hespel P: **Carbohydrate supplementation improves stroke performance in tennis.** *Med Sci Sports Exerc* 1998, **30**:1289–1295.
26. Coyle EF, Hagberg JM, Hurley BF, Martin WH, Ehsani AA, Holloszy JO: **Carbohydrate feeding during prolonged strenuous exercise can delay fatigue.** *J Appl Physiol* 1983, **55**:230–235.
27. Kovacs MS: **Carbohydrate intake and tennis: are there benefits?** *Br J Sports Med* 2006, **40**:e13.
28. Järhult J, Falck B, Ingemansson S, Nobin A: **The functional importance of sympathetic nerves to the liver and endocrine pancreas.** *Ann Surg* 1979, **189**:96–100.
29. Yamaguchi N: **Sympathoadrenal system in neuroendocrine control of glucose: mechanisms involved in the liver, pancreas, and adrenal gland under hemorrhagic and hypoglycemic stress.** *Can J Physiol Pharmacol* 1992, **70**:167–206.
30. Bergeron MF, Maresh CM, Kraemer WJ, Abraham A, Conroy B, Gabaree C: **Tennis: a physiological profile during match play.** *Int J Sports Med* 1991, **12**:474–479.
31. Currell K, Conway S, Jeukendrup AE: **Carbohydrate ingestion improves performance of a new reliable test of soccer performance.** *Int J Sport Nutr Exerc Metab* 2009, **19**:34–46.
32. Winnick JJ, Davis JM, Welsh RS, Carmichael MD, Murphy EA, Blackmon JA: **Carbohydrate feedings during team sport exercise preserve physical and CNS function.** *Med Sci Sports Exerc* 2005, **37**:306–315.
33. Van Loon LJ, Greenhaff PL, Constantin-Teodosiu D, Saris WH, Wagenmakers AJ: **The effects of increasing exercise intensity on muscle fuel utilization in humans.** *J Physiol* 2001, **536**:295–304.
34. Gomes RV, Coutts AJ, Viveiros L, Aoki MS: **Physiological demands of match-play in elite tennis: A case study.** *Eur J Sport Sci* 2011, **11**:105–109.
35. Kjaer M: **Hepatic glucose production during exercise.** *Adv Exp Med Biol* 1998, **441**:117–127.
36. Karelis AD, Smith JW, Passe DH, Péronnet F: **Carbohydrate administration and exercise performance: what are the potential mechanisms involved?** *Sports Med* 2010, **40**:747–763.
37. Davis JM, Bailey SP, Woods JA, Galiano FJ, Hamilton MT, Bartoli WP: **Effects of carbohydrate feedings on plasma free tryptophan and branched-chain amino acids during prolonged cycling.** *Eur J Appl Physiol Occup Physiol* 1992, **65**:513–519.
38. Hornery DJ, Farrow D, Mujika I, Young W: **Fatigue in tennis: mechanisms of fatigue and effect on performance.** *Sports Med* 2007, **37**:199–212.
39. Girard O, Lattier G, Maffiuletti NA, Micallef JP, Millet GP: **Neuromuscular fatigue during a prolonged intermittent exercise: application to tennis.** *J Electromyogr Kinesiol* 2008, **18**:1038–1046.
40. Girard O, Lattier G, Micallef JP, Miller GP: **Changes in exercise characteristics, maximal voluntary contraction, and explosive strength during prolonged tennis playing.** *Br J Sports Med* 2006, **40**:521–526.
41. Girard O, Miller GP: **Neuromuscular fatigue in racquet sports.** *Phys Med Rehabil Clin N Am* 2009, **20**:161–173.
42. Gomes RV, Ribeiro SML, Veibig RF, Aoki MS: **Food intake and anthropometric profile of amateur and professionals tennis players.** *Rev Bras Med Esporte* 2009, **15**:436–440.
43. Brun JF, Dumortier M, Fedou C, Mercier J: **Exercise hypoglycemia in nondiabetic subjects.** *Diabetes Metab* 2001, **27**:92–106.

Creatine supplementation and oxidative stress in rat liver

Michel B Araújo[1*], Leandro P Moura[1], Roberto C Vieira Junior[2], Marcelo C Junior[1], Rodrigo A Dalia[1], Amanda C Sponton[1], Carla Ribeiro[1] and Maria Alice R Mello[1]

Abstract

Background: The objective of this study was to determine the effects of creatine supplementation on liver biomarkers of oxidative stress in exercise-trained rats.

Methods: Forty 90-day-old adult male Wistar rats were assigned to four groups for the eight-week experiment. Control group (C) rats received a balanced control diet; creatine control group (CCr) rats received a balanced diet supplemented with 2% creatine; trained group (T) rats received a balanced diet and intense exercise training equivalent to the maximal lactate steady state phase; and supplemented-trained (TCr) rats were given a balanced diet supplemented with 2% creatine and subjected to intense exercise training equivalent to the maximal lactate steady state phase. At the end of the experimental period, concentrations of creatine, hydrogen peroxide (H_2O_2) and thiobarbituric acid reactive substances (TBARS) were measured as well as the enzyme activity of superoxide dismutase (SOD), glutathione peroxidase (GSH-GPx) and catalase (CAT). Liver tissue levels of reduced glutathione (GSH), oxidized glutathione (GSSG) and the GSH/GSSG ratio were also determined.

Results: Hepatic creatine levels were highest in the CCr and TCr groups with increased concentration of H_2O_2 observed in the T and TCr animal groups. SOD activity was decreased in the TCr group. GSH-GPx activity was increased in the T and TCr groups while CAT was elevated in the CCr and TCr groups. GSH, GGS and the GSH/GSSG ratio did not differ between all animal subsets.

Conclusions: Our results demonstrate that creatine supplementation acts in an additive manner to physical training to raise antioxidant enzymes in rat liver. However, because markers of liver oxidative stress were unchanged, this finding may also indicate that training-induced oxidative stress cannot be ameliorated by creatine supplementation.

Keywords: Creatine supplementation, Oxidative stress, Enzymes, Treadmill exercise

Background

Physical activity modifies the balance between oxidative stress and antioxidant defense mechanisms. For both athletes and fitness enthusiasts, the combination of regular physical activity and antioxidant supplementation may have important restorative effects on the body's oxidation-reduction or redox balance.

Dietary supplementation with creatine (CrS) is popular in the sports and fitness industry, wherein CrS is believed to aid in the maintenance of high-energy phosphate reserves during exercise. While certain mechanisms of action involved in improved physical exercise performance with CrS have been established [1,2], recent research efforts have focused on other CrS benefits, specifically, the use of CrS in reducing the cellular oxidative stress associated with strenuous long-term exercise [3-5]. Creatine is an end-product of the metabolism of amino acids glycine and arginine, producing guanidinoacetate and participating in the urea cycle. Arginine also acts as a substrate in the nitric oxide synthase pathway and can stimulate the production of nitric oxide free radicals that modulate skeletal muscle and liver metabolism, contractility and glucose uptake [6-8].

Certain amino acids such as histidine, methionine and cysteine are particularly susceptible to oxidation by free radicals [9]. Sulfhydryl cysteine groups are known modulators

* Correspondence: mbujo@ig.com.br
[1]Laboratory of Nutrition, Metabolism and Exercise, Department of Physical Education, Universidade Estadual Paulista (UNESP), 24ª avenue nº 1515, P.O. Box 199, Bela Vista, Rio Claro, São Paulo, Brazil
Full list of author information is available at the end of the article

of the redox state across many protein functions that also appear to protect protein sulfhydryl groups and to improve liver function [10].

The antioxidant effects of creatine may derive from different mechanisms of action such as the indirect mechanisms involved in cell membrane stabilization and improved cellular energy capacity [11] and from its direct antioxidant properties [5]. Recently, creatine's potential to act directly to remove reactive oxygen species was investigated [12]. Lawler et al. [5] concluded that creatine has a significant role as a primary antioxidant. Using in vitro techniques, these authors found a dose-response relationship between creatine concentration and the ability to remove superoxide anions (O_2•-) and peroxynitrite (OONO). As creatine has not shown significant antioxidant activity against hydrogen peroxide (H_2O_2), these findings also demonstrate creatine's selective antioxidant capacity.

Sestili et al. [4] postulated a direct antioxidant role for creatine in cells exposed to various oxidative agents. These authors demonstrated that creatine in doses similar to those found in plasma after supplementation exerts cytoprotective antioxidant activity in three different cell lines against three different oxidative agents: H_2O_2, $OONO^-$ and t-butyl hydroperoxide (tB-OOH), an organic peroxide widely used in a variety of oxidation processes. Furthermore, cytoprotection was observed independent of the anti-oxidative state of the cell, as evaluated by the antioxidant enzymes catalase and glutathione peroxidase, which suggests a direct interaction between creatine and oxidizing agents and/or free radicals.

In humans, creatine synthesis appears to occur mainly in the liver [13], an organ that requires vast amounts of generated energy to perform its various functions. The high metabolic rate of the liver (200 kcal/kg of tissue per day) is directly associated with the high flow of electrons in the mitochondrial respiratory chain [14]. However, some of these electrons are diverted to produce reactive oxygen species (ROS). Several authors have demonstrated that the liver undergoes increased oxidative stress following exercise [14,15].

Thus, we sought to investigate the effects of CrS on oxidative balance, injury and liver antioxidant defense mechanisms during exercise in a laboratory model. The aims of this study were to: 1) determine whether creatine supplementation increased liver creatine stores and 2) determine whether creatine supplementation improved markers of liver oxidative stress following exercise training.

Methods

Animals and treatment

Forty 90-day-old male Wistar rats were given free access to water and food. The animals were housed in collective polyethylene cages measuring 37.0 × 31.0 × 16.0 cm with 5 animals per cage, all under controlled conditions of temperature (22°C) and light/dark cycle (12 h/12 h). The experiment was submitted to and approved by the Animal Experimentation Ethics Committee at the University of Taubaté - UNITAU, São Paulo State, Brazil (register CEEA / UNITAU nº 018/08).

Exercise training was performed and creatine supplementation given over eight weeks with animals allocated into four groups of ten animals in each group: control group (C), sedentary rats that received a balanced control diet; creatine control group (CCr), sedentary rats that received a balanced diet supplemented with 2% creatine; trained group (T), rats that were subjected to a training protocol and received a balanced diet; and supplemented trained group (TCr), rats that were subjected to a training protocol and received a balanced diet supplemented with 2% creatine.

Diet

The animals in the creatine-supplemented groups (CCr and TCr) received the balanced, isocaloric AIN-93 M diet [16] supplemented with 13% or 2% monohydrated creatine (All Chemistry, São Paulo, SP, Brazil) [17].

According to Hutman et al. [18] and Vandenbergue et al. [19] creatine supplementation must be provided in two phases, which aims to promote an overload state of this substrate. These phases were designated as a first peak phase and a subsequent maintenance phase. During the peak phase, rats received the 13% creatine diets for seven days followed by a maintenance phase for the remaining days of the experiment during which rats were fed a 2% creatine diet. We used the dosage of creatine based on dose for human but there was an adjustment for employment with the animals. The addition of 2% in diet creatine during the maintenance phase equals 20 g.kg-1 peak in the phase of 13% were used equivalent to 130 g.kg-1. Still, according to Altman and Dittmer [20], sets the speed rat metabolism is 5 times greater than the human being for this reason these present values of creatine supplementation. Thus, animals that received creatine-supplemented feed were supplemented seven days a week for eight weeks of the experiment.

The animals from groups C and T received the balanced isocaloric diet AIN-93 M [16] without addition of creatine. The detailed diet composition is provided in Table 1.

Training protocol

To determine the Maximum Lactate Steady State (MLSS), series of exercises was performed, rats bearing rectangular loads ran for 25 minutes on a treadmill at different fixed speeds for each series and a 48-hour interval between series. Blood sample was obtained every five minutes for lactate measurement and were taken from a small incision at the end of the tail that was made prior to the beginning

Table 1 Diets compositions

Components	AIN - 93M* (g_kg−1)	Addition of 2% creatine** (g_kg−1)	Addition of 13% creatine*** (g_kg−1)
Creatine	0.0	20.0	130.0
Cornstarch	465.7	444.7	335.7
Casein (85% protein)	140.0	140.0	140.0
Dextrin	155.0	155.0	155.0
Sucrose	100.0	100	100
Soybean oil	40.0	40.0	40.0
Fiber	50.0	50.0	50.0
Mineral mix	35.0	35.0	35.0
Vitamin min	10.0	10.0	10.0
L-cystine	1.8	1.8	1.8
Choline bitartrate	2.5	2.5	2.5
Kcal/Kg	3.802,77	3.802,77	3.802,77

*American Institute of Nutrition (AIN-93M) [16].
**Creatine maintenance diet according to Demenice et al. [17].
***Creatine peak diet addapted from Demenice et al. [17] and according to Hultman et al. [18] and Vandenbergue et al. [19].

of exercise and was sufficient for all specimen collections. The blood lactate concentration representative of the MLSS was considered that obtained from the highest speed where there was no variation in blood lactate between 10 and 25 min of exercise was no greater than 1.0 mmol/L [10,20]. The blood lactate concentration was determined by an enzymatic method [21].

The average MLSS for all rats was 26 m/min. Thus, all rats were trained at this intensity for 40 minutes/day, five days/week for the duration of the experiment.

Biochemical analysis

Animals were sacrificed after anesthesia with CO_2 at the conclusion of the experiment in the fed state and 48 hours after the last "in vivo" evaluation. Blood, liver and gastrocnemius muscle were removed for creatine measurement as described by Clark [22]. As biomarkers of oxidative stress, H_2O_2 was determined as hydrogen peroxide (Amplex UltraRed Reagent® kit, Life Technologies Corporation, Grand Island, New York, USA) and thiobarbituric acid reactive substances (TBARS) [23] were also evaluated.

As indicators of the antioxidant system, enzymatic activity was analyzed for superoxide dismutase (SOD) (Cayman Chemical commercial kit, Ann Arbor, Michigan, USA), glutathione peroxidase (GSH-GPx) (Cayman Chemical commercial kit, Ann Arbor, Michigan, USA) and catalase (CAT) [24]. Glutathione, both reduced (GSH) and oxidized (GSSG), were analyzed according to the method of Hissin and Hilf [25].

Statistical analysis

The normality of the data was confirmed by the Shapiro-Wilks test. The results are presented as the mean ± S.E. (standard error). Comparisons between groups were made through an analysis of variance (ANOVA *Two-Way*) and the Tukey HSD post-hoc test when necessary. A predetermined 5% significance level was used for all the analyses. The statistical program used was the STATISTICA®, version 7.0.

Results

Creatine concentration in the liver

Animals supplemented with creatine showed significant increase in hepatic creatine concentration when were compared to animals that received no supplementation (Figure 1).

Concentration of hydrogen peroxide (H_2O_2) and thiobarbituric acid reactive substances (TBARS) in the liver

Liver H_2O_2 levels obtained at the end of the experiment were significantly increased in the exercise-trained groups T and TCr in relation to control groups C and CCr (Figure 2A).

The values for hepatic TBARS at the end of experiment did not differ between groups (Figure 2B).

Activity of superoxide dismutase (SOD), glutathione peroxidase (GSH-GPx) and catalase (CAT) in the liver

Hepatic SOD activity at the end of the experiment showed decreased activity in rats from the TCr group when they were compared with rats from CCr group (Figure 3A). Hepatic GSH-GPx activity at the end of the experiment was elevated in groups T and TCr compared

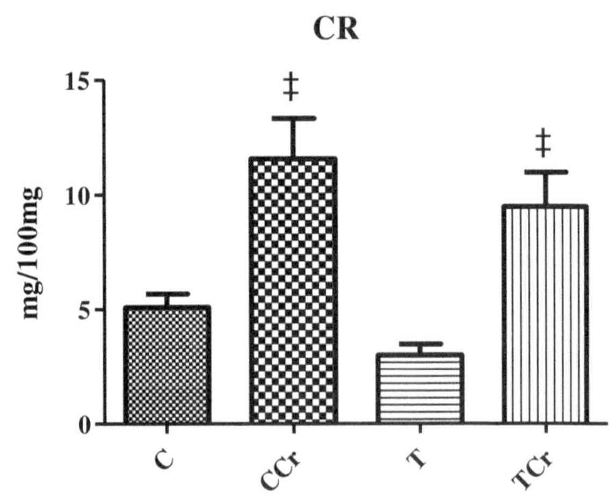

Figure 1 Creatine concentration (CR) in the liver the animals at the end of the experiment. The results are expressed as the mean + S.E. of 10 animals per group. TCr = Trained creatine; T = Trained; CCr = Control Creatine; C = Control not trained. ‡ different T/C.

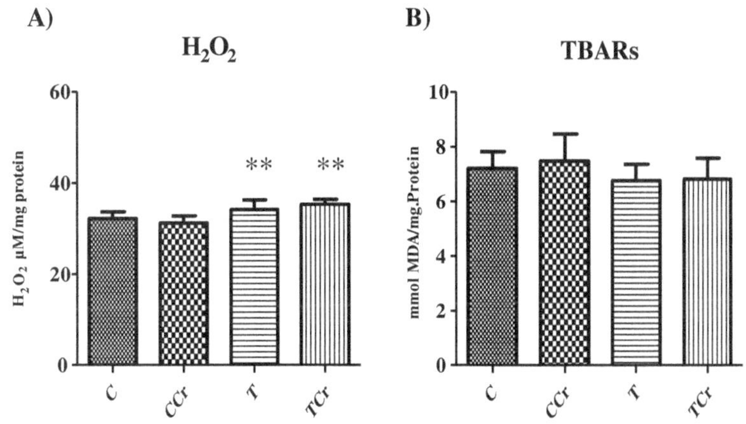

Figure 2 Analysis of pro-oxidants. A) Concentration of H_2O_2 **B)** Concentration of TBARs. The results are expressed as the mean + S.E. of 10 animals per group. TCr = Trained Creatine; T = Trained; CCr = Control Creatine; C = Control not trained ** different C e CCr.

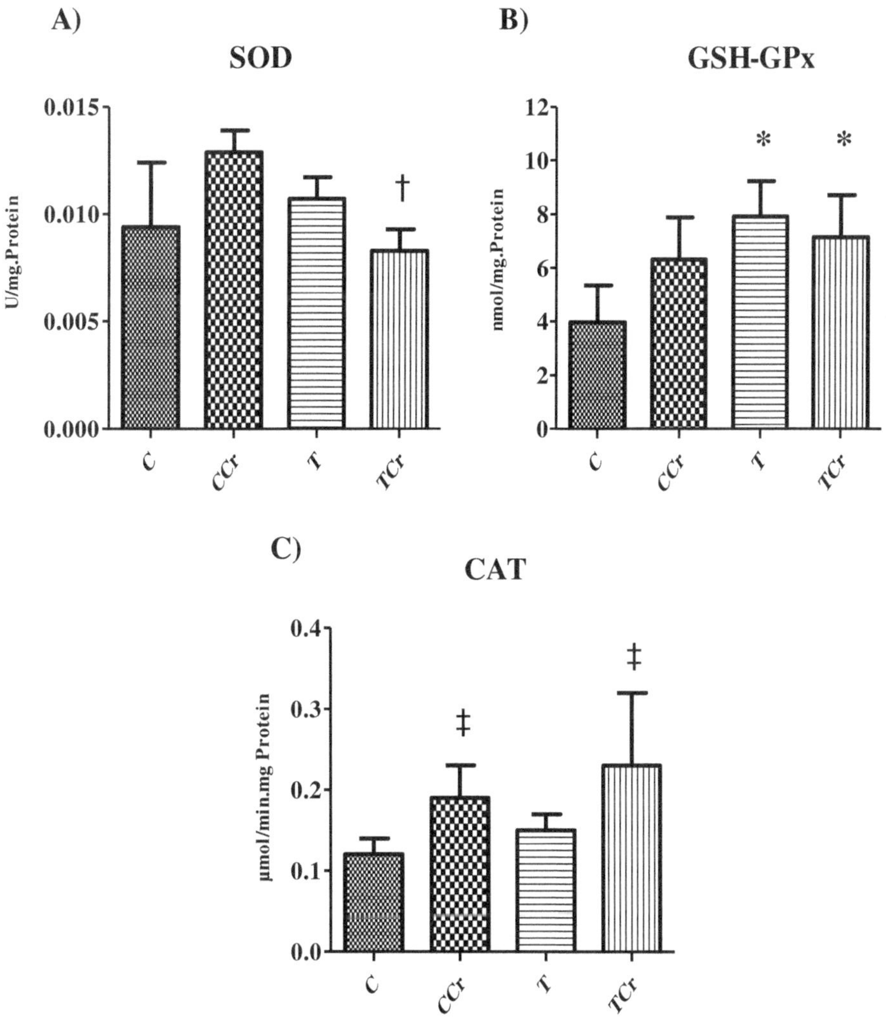

Figure 3 Analysis of antioxidants. A) Activity of SOD; **B)** GSH-GPx and **C)** CAT. The results are expressed as the mean + S.E. of 10 animals per group. TCr = Trained Creatine; T = Trained; CCr = Control Creatine; C = Control not trained. * different C; † different CCr; ‡ different T/C.

with group C rats (Figure 3B). Values obtained for hepatic CAT activity at the end of the experiment showed no differences between groups (Figure 3C). There was an increase in the activity of CAT in rats from the CCr and TCr groups in relation to those in control groups C and T (Figure 3C).

Concentration of reduced glutathione (GSH), oxidized glutathione (GSSG) and ratio between reduced glutathione and oxidized glutathione (GSH/GSSG) in liver

Rat liver values for GSH, GSSG and GSH/GSSG ratio at the end of the experiment showed no differences between groups (Figure 4).

Discussion

In recent years the use of creatine supplementation (CrS) whith antioxidant function has increased. Several studies have confirmed these effects and pointed to creatine as a new alternative in the prevention of oxidative stress in which creatine appears to play a crucial role in reducing the toxic effects of endogenous production of reactive oxygen species (ROS) [5,26-28].

The literature indicates that 2% CrS in animal feed is able to trigger a significant increase in phosphocreatine (PCr) and creatine levels in rat tissues [29,30]. Using this amount of creatine, McMillen et al. [30] observed a significant increase in the total creatine content of rat gastrocnemius muscle in two weeks of supplementation. In the present study, significant increase in the hepatic creatine concentrations were demonstrated in CCr and TCr rats compared to the non-supplemented control groups, which supports prior findings in the literature [30,31].

After confirming that dietary supplementation increased creatine concentration in rat liver, this study aimed to evaluate the possible antioxidant effects of CrS in vivo. The results demonstrate that creatine exerts indirect antioxidant activity in rat liver, i.e., creatine increased the activity of antioxidant enzymes GSH-GPx and CAT. However, CrS was not effective in normalizing the increased concentrations of H_2O_2 triggered by exercise. In addition, no significant differences were observed in the concentration of TBARS between groups.

H_2O_2 plays an important role in homeostasis. It participates in cellular induction of gene expression, among which are those genes responsible for antioxidant enzyme synthesis [32-34]. In the present study, we demonstrated

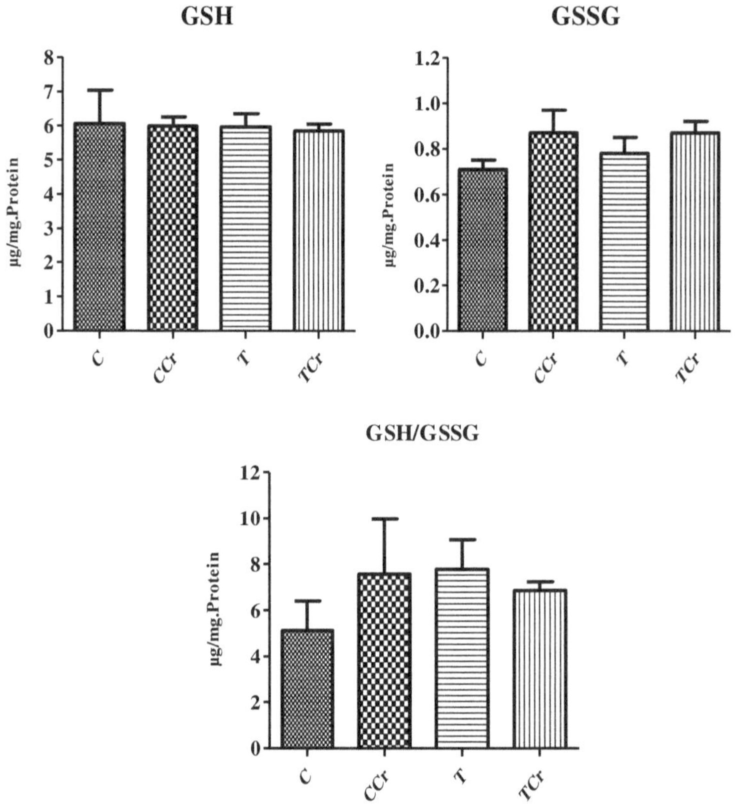

Figure 4 Concentration of reduced glutathione, oxidized glutathione and ratio reduced glutathione/oxidized glutathione in the liver the animals at the end of the experiment. The results are expressed as the mean + S.E. of 10 animals per group. TCr = Trained Creatine; T = Trained; CCr = Control Creatine; C = Control not trained.

that exercise-trained rats (T and TCr) had higher concentrations of H_2O_2 than sedentary rats (C and CCr). These data reinforce the observations of several authors that indicate that creatine appears to exert selective antioxidant effects [26,27]. Lawler et al. [5] have shown that creatine was able to remove $O_2\bullet$- and $OONO^-$ but had no effect on H_2O_2. Thus, the direct antioxidant actions of creatine appear to be limited to certain types of free radicals or reactive oxygen species. Sestili et al. [4] have found that creatine was not able to significantly counteract the concentrations of H_2O_2 and the compound tB-OOH that is derived from •OH and RO• radicals.

With regard to levels of TBARS, our results are consistent with previous findings [35] that showed no change in hepatic TBARS levels in treadmill exercise-trained rats. Taken in aggregate, these results for pro-oxidant markers underscore the findings of Sjodin et al. [36] and Souza et al. [37], that is, predominantly aerobic exercise causes increased oxygen flow in the mitochondria and approximately five percent of this oxygen is not completely reduced, thereby forming ROS.

As H_2O_2 levels rise, homeostasis requires increased production of antioxidant enzymes such as SOD, GSH-GPx and CAT to maintain the balance between oxidant production and the antioxidant system [8,38,39]. Our study results for SOD demonstrate decreased enzymatic activity in trained animals (T and TCR) when they were compared to group C rats. SOD is important in the metabolism of O2•- that results in the formation of H_2O_2 [34,40,41]. Thus, while SOD is an important combatant against oxidative stress, it also accelerates the formation of hydrogen peroxide, as occurs during physical exercise. In this situation, it has been suggested that reduced SOD activity is mainly explained by the inhibitory effect of increased H_2O_2 production [42].

In this study, a hypothesis may explain the decrease in SOD activity in response to CrS. Creatine may exert a sparing effect, i.e., creatine may act to neutralize ROS, resulting in down-regulation of the antioxidant system and specifically, the action of SOD. This hypothesis is based on research of antioxidant supplementation use that demonstrated inhibition of SOD, GSH-GPx and CAT activity [43,44]. However, a notable finding from these studies was that unlike SOD, the activity of GSH-GPx and CAT were increased in trained animals and CrS. Both GSH-GPx and CAT enzymes are present in most aerobic organisms and are responsible for conversion of intracellular H_2O_2 to water and oxygen [34,40].

Our study demonstrated increase in GSH-GPx levels in exercised-trained rat groups T and TCr compared to control group animals. This finding may be explained by the fact that regular physical training activates transcription factors such as NF-κB and Nrf2, which are responsible for triggering various genes, including mitochondrial GSH-GPx [45,46]. Moreover, the effect of training on the activity and expression of CAT is inconsistent and controversial [47]. However, increased activity of this enzyme has been observed in rat liver [48], mice liver [49] and trained rat heart [50].

The most striking finding we encountered was the increased CAT activity that occurred only in animals given CrS. This result appears to support an additive role for creatine on the actions of antioxidant enzymes. Physical training, as demonstrated by Halliwell and Gutteridge [51], activates transcription factors such as AMPK, which activate CAT mRNA, thereby stimulating protein synthesis and possibly increasing CAT activity. The ability of CrS to also exert this effect remains controversial. According to Sestile et al. [4], creatine has neutralizing effects on ROS production that do not interfere on the action of antioxidant enzymes. However, the increase in CAT activity observed in this study is attributed to the formation of H_2O_2 by SOD. According to Halliwel and Gutteridge [51], the chemical interaction of H_2O_2 at the catalase active site involves the transfer of a hydrogen ion between the two oxygen atoms, causing a heterolytic cleavage with water and oxygen end products. The findings in our study of increased H_2O_2 levels in trained and supplemented animals combined with the neutralizing action of creatine on this ROS may explain the reduced oxidative damage seen with increased CAT activity.

In contrast, the amounts of GSH and GSSG as well as the ratio between GSH/GSSG did not differ between the study groups. GSH has a central role in the biotransformation and elimination of xenobiotics, and protects cells against oxidative stress [52]. To maintain the protective activity of glutathione as expressed by the reduction of oxidizing species and consequent oxidation of GSH to GSSG, GSH must be regenerated through the catalytic cycle [52].

In summary, our study results demonstrate that creatine supplementation acts in an additive manner to physical training to increase antioxidant enzymes in rat liver. More studies are needed to expand our knowledge of the antioxidant effects of creatine and to investigate creatine's little-known effects on other body tissues.

Competing interests

The authors declare that they have no competing interests.

Authors' contributions

MBA (corresponding author) was responsible for the study design, execution of biochemical analysis, statistical analysis and writing of the manuscript. LPM held the writing of the manuscript. RCVJ, MCJ, RAD, ACS, CR and MARM participated in the realization of biochemical analysis. All authors read and approved the final manuscript.

Acknowledgements

The authors are grateful for the technical support of Clarice Y. Sibuya and José Roberto R. da Silva who contributed greatly to this Project.

Funding
This study was supported by "The State of São Paulo Foundation for Research Support" (FAPESP - Proc. 2009/52063-0).

Author details
[1]Laboratory of Nutrition, Metabolism and Exercise, Department of Physical Education, Universidade Estadual Paulista (UNESP), 24ª avenue n° 1515, P.O. Box 199, Bela Vista, Rio Claro, São Paulo, Brazil. [2]Post-Graduation Program – Graduation in Bioscience of Faculty of Nutrition from Federal University of Mato Grosso, UFMT, Cuiabá, Mato Grosso, Brazil.

References

1. Gama MS: **Efeitos da creatina sobre desempenho aeróbio: uma revisão sistemática.** *Revista Brasileira de Nutrição Esportiva* 2011, **5:**182–190.
2. Pereira Júnior M, Moraes AJP, Ornellas FH, Gonçalves MA, Liberalli R, Navarro F: **Eficiência da suplementação de creatina no desempenho físico humano.** *Revista Brasileira Prescrição e Fisiologia do Exercício* 2012, **6:**90–97.
3. Cruzat VF, Rogero MM, Borges MC, Tirapegui J: **Aspectos atuais sobre estresse oxidativo, exercícios físicos e suplementação.** *Rev Bras Med Esporte* 2007, **13:**336–342.
4. Sestili P, Martinelli C, Bravi G, Piccoli G, Curci R: **Creatine supplementation affords cytoprotection in oxidatively injured cultured mammalian cells via direct antioxidant activity.** *Free Radic Biol Med* 2006, **40:**837–849.
5. Lawler JM, Barnes WS, Wu G, Song W, Demaree S: **Direct antioxidant properties of creatine.** *Biochem Biophys Res Commun* 2009, **290:**47–52.
6. Reid MB: **Nitric oxide, reactive oxygen species, and skeletal muscle contraction.** *Med Sci Sports Exer* 2001, **33:**371–376.
7. Freire TO, Gualano B, Leme MD, Polacow VO, Lancha AH Jr: **Efeitos da Suplementação de Creatina na Captação de Glicose em Ratos Submetidos ao Exercício Físico.** *Rev Bras Med Esporte* 2008, **14:**431–435.
8. Araújo MB, Mello MAR: **Exercício, estresse oxidativo e suplementação com creatina.** *Revista Brasileira de Nutrição Esportiva* 2009, **3:**264–272.
9. Grune T, Reinheckel T, Davies KJA: **Degradation of oxidized proteins in mammalian cells.** *FASEB J* 1997, **11:**526–534.
10. Araújo MB, Moura LP, Ribeiro C, Dalia RA, Voltarelli FA, Mello MAR: **Oxidative stress in the liver of exercised rats supplemented with creatine.** *Int J Nutr Metab* 2011, **3:**58–64.
11. Wyss M, Schulze A: **Health implications of creatine: can oral creatine supplementation protect against neurological and atherosclerotic disease?** *Neuroscience* 2002, **112:**243–260.
12. Matthews RT, Yang L, Jenkins BG, Ferrante RJ, Rosen BR: **Neuroprotective effects of creatine and cyclocreatine in animal models of Huntington's disease.** *J Neurosci* 1998, **18:**156–163.
13. Williams MH, Kreider R, Branch JD: *Creatina.* São Paulo: Ed Manole; 2000.
14. Ogonovszky H, Sasvári M, Dosek A, Berkes I, Kaneko T, Tahara S: **The effects of moderate, strenuous, and overtraining on oxidative stress markers and DNA repair in rat liver.** *Can J Appl Physiol* 2005, **30:**186–195.
15. Navarro-Arevalo A, Sanchez-del-Pino MJ: **Age and exercise related changes in lipid peroxidation and superoxide dismutase activity in liver and soleus muscle tissues of rats.** *Mech Ageing Dev* 1998, **104:**91–102.
16. 0Reeves PG, Nielsen FH, Fahey GC Jr: **AIN-93 purified diets for laboratory rodents: final report of the American Institute of Nutrition ad hoc writing committee on the reformulation of the AIN-76A rodent diet.** *J Nutr* 1993, **123:**1939–195.
17. Deminice R, Portari GV, Vannucchi H, Jordao AA: **Effects of creatine supplementation on homocysteine levels and lipid peroxidation in rats.** *Br J Nutr* 2009, **102:**110–116.
18. Hultman E, Soderlund K, Timmons J, Cederblad G, Greenhaff P: **Muscle creatine loading in man.** *J Appl Physiol* 1996, **81:**232–237.
19. Vandenberghe K, Goris M, Van Hecke P, Van Leemputte M, Vangerven L, Hespel P: **Long-term creatine intake is beneficial to muscle performance during resistance training.** *J Appl Physiol* 1997, **83:**2055–2063.
20. Manchado FB, Gobatto CA, Contarteze RVL, Papoti M, Mello MAR: **Maximal lactate steady in running rats.** *J Exer Physiol Online* 2005, **8:**29–35.
21. Hill AV, Long CNH, Lupton H: **Muscular exercise, lactic acid, and the supply and utilization of oxygen: parts IV-VI.** *Proc R Soc B* 1924, **97:**84–138.
22. Clark LC, Thompson HL: **The determination of creatine and creatinine in urine.** *Anal Chem* 1949, **21:**1218–1221.
23. Mataix J, Quiles JL, Huertas JR, Battino M, Manas M: **Tissue specific interactions of exercise, dietary fatty acids, and vitamin E in lipid peroxidation.** *Free Radic Biol Med* 1998, **24:**511–521.
24. Aebi H: **Catalase in vitro.** *Methods Enzymol* 1984, **105:**121–126.
25. Hissin PJ, Hilf R: **A flurometric method for determination of oxidizid and reduced glutathione in tissues.** *Anal Biochem* 1976, **74:**214–226.
26. Souza Junior TP, Pereira B: **Creatina: auxílio ergogênico com potencial antioxidante?** *Rev Nutr* 2008, **21:**349–353.
27. Deminice R, Sicchieri T, Mialich MS, Milani F, Ovidio PP, Jordao AA: **Oxidative stress biomarker responses to an acute session of hypertrophy-resistance traditional interval training and circuit training.** *J Strength Cond Res* 2011, **25:**798–804.
28. Guimarães-Ferreira L, Hermano CJ, Gerlinger-Rom PF, Vitze KFL, Nachbar RT, Curi R, Nunes MT: **Short-term creatine supplementation decreases reactive oxygen species content with no changes in expression and activity of antioxidant enzymes in skeletal muscle.** *Eur J Appl Physiol* 2012, **2012**(112):801–1196.
29. Brannon TA, Adams GR, Gonniff CL, Baldwin KM: **Effects of creatine loading and training on running performance and biochemical properties of rat skeletal muscle.** *Med Sci Sports Exerc* 1997, **29:**489–495.
30. McMillen J, Donovan CM, Messer JI, Willis WT: **Energetic driving forces are maintained in resting rat skeletal muscle after dietary creatine supplementation.** *J Apply Physiol* 2001, **90:**62–66.
31. Rawson ES, Clarkson PM: **Scientifically debatable: Is creatine worth its weight?** *Sports Sci Exch* 2003, **16:**1–6.
32. Mandal BA, Chakraborty CD: **Oxidant, antioxidant and physical exercise.** *Mol Cell Biochem* 2003, **253:**307–312.
33. Ji LL, Gomez-Cabrera MC, Vina J: **Exercise and hormesis: activation of cellular antioxidant signaling pathway.** *Ann N Y Acad Sci* 2006, **1067:**425–435.
34. Ferreira F, Ferreira R, Duarte JÁ: **Stress oxidativo e dano oxidativo muscular esquelético: influência do exercício agudo inabitual e do treino físico.** *Revista Portuguesa de Ciência do Desporto* 2007, **7:**257–275.
35. Araújo MB, Voltarelli FA, Manchado-Gobatto FB, Moura LP, Mello MAR: **Treinamento em diferentes intensidades e biomarcadores de estresse oxidativo e do metabolismo glicídico musculoesquelético de ratos.** *Revista da Educação Física/UEM* 2010, **21:**695–707.
36. Sjodin B, Wesling HE, Apple S: **Biochemical mechanisms for oxygen free radical formation during exercise.** *Sports Med* 1990, **10:**236–254.
37. Souza RA, Santos RM, Osório RA, Cogo JC, Priati Júnior ACG: **Influência da suplementação aguda e crônica de creatina sobre as concentrações sanguíneas de glicose e lactato de ratos Wistar.** *Rev Bras Med Esporte* 2006, **12:**361–365.
38. Araújo MB, Prada FJA, Mello MAR: **Estresse oxidativo no exercício, modelos animais e intensidade do esforço.** *Motriz* 2006, **2006**(12):307–312.
39. Fisher-Wellman K, Bloomer RJ: **Acute exercise and oxidative stress: a 30 year history.** *Dyn Med* 2009, **8:**1–25.
40. Lee J, Koo N, Min DB: **Reactive oxygen species, aging, and antioxidative nutraceuticals.** *Compr Rev Food Sci Food Saf* 2004, **3:**21–33.
41. Mota MP, Figueiredo P, Duarte JÁ: **Teorias biológicas do envelhecimento.** *Revista Portuguesa de Ciências do Desporto* 2004, **4:**81–110.
42. Machefer G, Groussard C, Rannou-Bekono F, Zouhal H, Faure H: **Extreme Running Competition Decreases Blood Antioxidant Defense Capacity.** *J Am Coll Nutr* 2004, **23:**358–364.
43. Asha Devi S, Ravi Kiran T: **Regional responses in antioxidant system to exercise training and dietary Vitamin E in aging rat brain.** *Neurol Aging* 2004, **25:**501–508.
44. Hamid NAA, Hasrul MA, Ruzanna RJ, Ibrahim IA, Baruah PS: **Effect of vitamin E (Tri E®) on antioxidant enzymes and DNA damage in rats following eight weeks exercise.** *Nutr J* 2011, **10:**37.
45. Tromm CB, Rosa GL, Bom K, Mariano I, Pozzi B: **Efeito de diferentes frequências semanais de treinamento sobre parâmetros de estresse oxidativo.** *Revista Brasileira de Cineantropometria e Desempenho Humano* 2011, **14:**52–60.
46. Yu Z, Li D, Ling W, Jin T: **Role of nuclear factor (erythroid-derived 2)-like 2 in metabolic homeostasis and insulin action: A novel opportunity for diabetes treatment?** *World J Diabetes* 2012, **3:**19–28.
47. Pinho RA, Andrades ME, Oliveira MR, Pirola AC, Zago MS, Silveira PC: **Imbalance in SOD/CAT activities in rat skeletal muscles submitted to treadmill training exercise.** *Cell Biol Int* 2006, **30:**848–853.
48. Silva LA, Ronsanil MM, Souza PS, Severino BJ, Fraga DB: **Comparação do treinamento físico de quatro e oito semanas sobre atividade da cadeia**

transportadora de elétrons e marcadores de estresse oxidativo em fígado de camundongos. *Rev Bras Med Esporte* 2010, **16**:126–129.

49. Souza RA, Miranda H, Xavier M, Salles BF, Simão R: **Influência da suplementação aguda e crônica de creatina sobre marcadores enzimáticos de dano muscular de ratos sedentários e exercitados com natação.** *Revista Brasileira de Educação Física e Esporte* 2010, **24**:343–352.
50. Husain K, Somani SM: **Interaction of exercise and adenosine receptor agonist and antagonist on rat heart antioxidant defense system.** *Mol Cell Biochem* 2005, **270**:209–214.
51. Halliwell B, Gutteridge MC: *Free radicals in biology and medicine.* Oxford: University Press; 2007.
52. Huber PC, Almeida WP: **Glutationa e enzimas relacionadas: papel biológico e importância em processos patológicos.** *Quim Nova* 2008, **31**:S1–S4.

Effect of sodium bicarbonate and beta-alanine supplementation on maximal sprint swimming

Antti A Mero[1*], Petri Hirvonen[1], Janne Saarela[1], Juha J Hulmi[1], Jay R Hoffman[2] and Jeffrey R Stout[2]

Abstract

Background: This study examined the effect of simultaneous supplementation of extracellular buffer sodium bicarbonate (SB) and intracellular buffer beta-alanine (BA) on maximal sprint swimming.

Methods: Thirteen competitive male swimmers completed 4 different treatments (placebo [PL], SB, BA + PL, and BA + SB) in a crossover procedure. PL or SB supplementation (0.3 g/kg body weight) was ingested 60 min before two maximal 100-m freestyle swims that were performed with a passive recovery of 12-min between each swim. Because of the known long washout period for carnosine, four weeks of BA supplementation (4.8 g per day) was started after the first week of PL or SB supplementation and performance testing.

Results: The first maximal swims were similar, but the increase in time of the second versus the first 100-m swimming time was 1.5 s more ($p < 0.05$) in PL than in SB. Blood pH values were significantly ($p < 0.05$) greater in the SB and in the BA + SB groups compared to the PL and BA + PL values. There were no differences in peak blood lactate between the treatments.

Conclusion: Supplementing with SB prior to performing maximal sprint swimming with repetitions under 60 s improves performance. However, co-supplementation with SB and BA did not confer any added benefit on maximal swim performance.

Keywords: Alkalosis, Anaerobic exercise, Buffer, Ergogenic aid

Background

During intensive anaerobic exercise with a large glycolytic component, one major cause of fatigue is believed to be acidosis caused by high levels of hydrogen ions (H^+) in the muscle fibers. The increase in (H^+) corresponds to a decrease in muscle and blood pH [1], can slow glycolysis [2], interfere with calcium release from the endoplasmic reticulum and calcium ion binding [3,4], and increase the perception of fatigue after some types of exercises [5]. A number of buffers can be used by the body, but the primary method for buffering the H^+ is thought to be either bicarbonate or hemoglobin [6]. For the past 35 years, several studies have investigated the use of sodium bicarbonate (SB) as an ergogenic aid. The participants have typically been men, and efficacy (improved performance and a decrease in H^+ concentration after exercise) has generally been seen at doses of at least $0.3g \cdot kg^{-1}$ body mass [7-9].

A recent meta-analysis by Carr et al. [10] suggests that ingestion of SB at 0.3 - $0.5g \cdot kg^{-1}$ body mass improves mean power by 1.7 ± 2.0% during high-intensity races of short duration (1–10 min). Timing of ingestion ranging from 60 min - 180 min before exercise did not influence buffering capacity or the ergogenic potential of SB ($0.3g \cdot kg^{-1}$ body mass) as assessed by repeated sprint ability. However, visual analog scale scores indicated that at 180 minutes post-ingestion, an individual is less prone to experiencing significant gastrointestinal discomfort [11]. Gao et al. [3] and Siegler et al. [12] have demonstrated that swimmers ingesting $0.3g \cdot kg^{-1}$ body mass of SB can enhance blood buffering potential and positively influence interval swim performance. Lindh and colleagues [13] have also shown that SB supplementation ($0.3g \cdot kg^{-1}$ body mass) can improve a single 200 m freestyle performance time in elite male competitors, most likely by increasing extra-cellular buffering capacity.

* Correspondence: antti.a.mero@jyu.fi
[1]Department of Biology of Physical Activity, University of Jyväskylä, P.O. Box 35, Jyväskylä 40351, Finland
Full list of author information is available at the end of the article

Beta-alanine (BA) is a non-essential amino acid that combines with L-histidine, to form the dipeptide carnosine. BA is thought to be the rate-limiting step in the synthesis of carnosine [14]. Carnosine acts as an intracellular buffer during high-intensity exercise [15-18], and elevations in muscle carnosine concentration have been demonstrated to enhance cycling capacity [18], ventilatory threshold, and delay fatigue [19]. A recent meta-analysis [20] has shown a significant ergogenic effect of BA supplementation during high intensity exercise lasting 60–240 s in duration. However, the efficacy of BA supplementation during single exercise durations shorter than 60 s durations is not clear. Although the efficacy of BA on repeated sprint performance is not very well known, studies examining BA and resistance training performance have indicated significant increases in training volume [21,22], suggesting that BA ingestion would be beneficial for repetitive high intensity exercise activities.

There appears to be only a limited number of studies that have examined a combination of two supplemental buffers on exercise performance. Mero and colleagues [23] indicated that the combined ingestion of SB and creatine (Cr) enhanced performance in two consecutive maximal effort 100-m swims with a 10 min recovery to a greater extent than ingestion of the supplements separately. Hoffman et al. [22] were the first to examine the combination of both BA and Cr supplements. Results of their study demonstrated that this combination significantly improved the training volume more than creatine alone. Specifically, improvements in training volume were found to be associated with significantly greater gains in lean body mass and decreases in fat mass. Sale et al. [24] investigated the effects of the combination of SB and BA (4 weeks loading) on high intensity cycling endurance performance and found that BA alone improved cycling capacity. Despite a 6 s improvement in time to exhaustion with the addition of SB, it did not reach statistical significance. In another cycling study [25] acute SB supplementation significantly improved 4-min cycling performance, but there seemed to be only a minimal additive effect of combined BA and SB supplementation. In the study by Hobson et al. [26] it was shown that both chronic BA and acute SB supplementation alone had positive effects on 2000 m rowing endurance performance. The addition of acute SB to chronic BA supplementation may further enhance rowing performance. Chronic BA and SB supplementation alone equally enhanced high-intensity intermittent maximal upper-body performance (4 × 30 s with three minutes recovery) in well-trained athletes and combining BA and SB promoted a clear additive ergogenic effect [27]. Ducker et al. [28] investigated if combining BA and SB could lead to enhanced repeated-sprint performance (3 sets; 6 × 20 m departing every 25 s, 4 minutes recovery between sets). They concluded that supplementation with acute SB improved repeated-sprint performance more than either a combination of SB and BA or BA alone. In a recent study [29] the swimmers swam maximally at first 200 m and then 100 m with 30 minutes recovery. BA and SB supplementation improved both 200 m and 100 m swimming performance. The co-ingestion of BA and SB induced a further nonsignificant improvement in performance. The performance time in 100 m was a little bit over 60 s (60–64 s). This time limit 60 s [20] is interesting in races e.g. in swimming (100 m) and in running (400 m). Earlier Sostaric et al. [30] reported that SB supplementation lowered circulating potassium, enhanced muscle potassium uptake and sodium delivery with alkalosis, but there are no studies with BA supplementation. These physiological changes are all interesting with preservation of membrane excitability during exercise [30]. Therefore, the purpose of present study was to examine more the effect of SB (extracellular buffer), BA (intracellular buffer) and the combination of SB with BA on a maximal sprint performance under 60 s in swimmers in a simulated competition.

Methods

Participants

Thirteen national and international level male swimmers (mean ± SD: age 20.5 ±1.4 years, body mass 80.1 ± 8.1 kg, height 188 ± 8 cm, haemoglobin 150 ± 6 $g \cdot l^{-1}$ (average of the first and third test day), 100 m freestyle record 54.44 ± 2.41 s) were recruited from the local swimming team to serve as participants. All swimmers exercised in the same training group. Each participant provided a written informed consent, and was free to withdraw from the study at any time. This study was approved by Ethics Committee of the local University.

Experimental design and supplementation

Experimental design is shown in Figure 1. In the first part of the study the participants ingested gelatine covered capsules containing SB (1 g per capsule) or the placebo (calcium carbonate). Each participant was provided a dose equivalent to $0.3 g \cdot kg^{-1}$ body mass. The capsules were weighed to ensure the correct amount of substance in each capsule. Participants were provided with the SB supplement or with the placebo 60 minutes prior to performing the swimming protocol. This part of the experiments was randomized and double blinded. SB and calcium carbonate were acquired from the local pharmacy.

In addition to the acute SB or placebo ingestion, in the second part of the study the participants were provided a daily dose of BA for a 4-week period. Each participant was provided gelatine coated capsules, each containing 0.6 g of BA. Participants ingested eight capsules per day

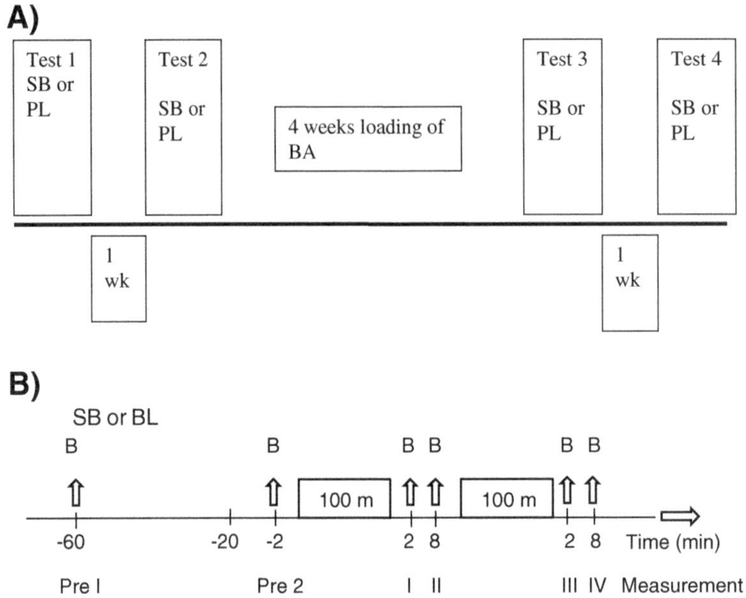

Figure 1 Experimental design. A) Swim test days 1–4, **B)** Timeline of each test day, SB = sodium bicarbonate, PL = placebo and BA = Beta-alanine supplementation, B = blood sample, 2 x 100 m swimming (swim 1 and 2).

in 1.5 - 2 h intervals throughout the 4 week period; therefore the total consumption of BA per day was 4.8 g [31]. Participants were instructed to consume the capsules at the same time every day which was controlled verbally by the researchers. The subjects and the researchers knew that every subject was consuming BA during a 4-week period (unblinded). After the period the participants were provided with the SB supplement or with the placebo supplement 60 minutes prior to performing the swimming protocol. Also this part of the experiments was randomized and double blinded. The subjects were told to keep a food diary for 24 hours prior to all tests, and to maintain similar eating habits and food prior to each test. All tests occurred at the beginning of the week (Monday & Tuesday), following a rest day. BA for the current study was provided by Manninen Nutraceuticals Ltd. (Oulu, Finland). Beta-alanine was not tested for contamination with stimulants or anabolic agents, however, the sponsoring company had certification on the quality of their beta-alanine product that it did not contain any banned substances.

Test day

The time line of the test day is shown in Figure 1B. On each test day participants consumed a self-prepared breakfast and arrived at the pool. Participants were grouped in pairs and were requested to arrive at 45 minute intervals to ensure a smooth flow of testing. Appointment times for each subject occurred at the same time of the day for both pre and post testing sessions. Actual performance testing took place in a 50-m pool during the afternoon. The water temperature during all tests was kept constant at 26.5° - 27.0°C and air temperature in the hall was 22° - 23°C. Participants provided their food diaries, and resting blood samples were obtained. They were then provided either with the SB supplement or the placebo 60 minutes prior to swimming. Following supplement ingestion the participants rested for 40 minutes by the pool. Easy walking and stretching was allowed during this time. After 40 minutes the subjects went to the pool to perform an 800-m standardized warm up. After the warm up, the actual test began. The test itself consisted of 2 × 100-m maximal freestyle sprints with a 12 min passive rest interval between each sprint. Just before the first swim, a blood sample was taken. The swimmers performed in pairs to create a competitive atmosphere and to motivate them to maximize their performance. The swimmers were paired according to their individual records in the 100-m freestyle. Every swim was timed with two experienced persons using stop-watches and their average value was used as the final swimming time. In all swimming times (n = 104) of the two timers, interclass correlation (ICC) was 0.99, standard error of measurement (SEM) was 0.16 seconds, and no significant difference was observed between the times of the two persons (57.2 ± 2.3 s and 57.2 ± 2.3 s). Subjects were also requested to report all any side effects to the investigators.

Blood collection and analysis

On the test day a total of six blood samples were obtained from every subject at six measurement points (Figure 1B). Whole blood samples were taken from a finger by using a sterile lancet, the first drop of blood was discarded, and free flow blood was collected in a balanced heparin 200-mL blood gas capillary tube. Two pre-exercise samples were obtained at 60 min (Pre 1) and 2 min (Pre 2) prior to commencing exercise, and post exercise blood samples were taken 2- and 8-min following each swim (I – IV, respectively). In addition, on the first and third measurement day a blood sample (2 ml) was obtained from a forearm vein using a needle and syringe. Blood samples were collected into an EDTA-vacuum tube to analyse haemoglobin.

All blood samples were analysed within six hours after collection. Blood lactate (B-Lactate), blood pH (B-pH), blood potassium (B-Potassium), blood sodium (B-Sodium), blood bicarbonate (B-Bicarbonate), blood base excess (B-Base excess) were analysed from all samples. The device used to measure lactate was an electro-chemical based EKF Biosen C-line Sport (EKF Diagnostic, Magdeburg, Germany). The reported coefficient of variation (CV) for the equipment is 1.5% according the manufacturer. Blood gases were analyzed instantly on site using a GEM Premier 3000 (Instrumentation Laboratory, Lexington, MA, USA) that uses a potentiometric system for analysis. The manufacturer reports following precision: in pH 7.15 level standard deviation (SD) is 0.009 and in pH level 7.46 SD is 0.005. In addition, blood bicarbonate and base excess were calculated. The coefficient of variation for sodium and potassium measures was 0.86% and 0.71% in our laboratory, respectively. Hemoglobin concentrations was analysed using Sysmex KX 21 N (Kobe, Japan) with a CV < 1.5% in our laboratory.

Nutrition

The participants were advised to maintain their normal dietary habits during the course of the study. Nutritional sports supplements (i.g. creatine, caffeine), except pure protein or carbohydrate, were forbidden during the study. All participants were instructed to keep a food diary 24 hours prior to each test. They were also instructed to eat as similarly (according to the first food diary) as possible before each test. The food diaries were analysed by using Micro Nutrica 3.0 software (Social Insurance Institution, Turku, Finland). The mean ± SD energy intake of four one day treatments was 3202 ± 478 kcal (carbohydrate 48 ± 4%, protein 24 ± 2%, and fat 28 ± 4%).

Training

The participants were allowed to train normally according to their training program. All participants had a minimum of four years of competitive swimming experience. The study occurred in the beginning of their training season, so that every participant would be in the similar preparation phase. The swimmers had six training days and one rest day per week. The average amount of training sessions was nine, but some swimmers trained 11 times per week (Table 1). Average length of each training session was two hours. In addition to swimming, all participants participated in three resistance training sessions per week for 60 minutes per session.

Statistical methods

All results were analysed with SPSS-statistics program (PASW statistics 17). Means ± SDs were calculated and the Wilcoxon Signed Rank Test was used to evaluate the differences between the means. A nonparametric test was chosen because the data was not normally distributed tested with the Shapiro-Wilk test. Statistical comparisons were considered significant when p values were < 0.05.

Results

Subjects reported no side effects related to SB intake, but symptoms of paraesthesia was experienced by all subjects consuming BA.

Swimming times

There were no significant differences in the time of the first 100-m sprint between the groups. In the second 100-m swim, the increase in time of the second versus the first 100-m swimming time was 1.5 s less ($p < 0.05$) in the SB group compared to the PL group (Figure 2). No significant differences were noted between the first or second sprint in either BA + SB or BA + PL.

Blood variables

Lactate, pH

There were no significant differences between the groups although lactates in measurements III and IV

Table 1 Average training week during the study

	Days						
Variable	1	2	3	4	5	6	7
Physical activity							
Morning	Aer	Aer/Anaer	Rest	Aer/Anaer	Drills	Strength	Rest
Evening	Speed	Strength	Speed	Strength	Speed	Aer/Anaer	
Load	Medium	High	Light	High	Light	High	

Aer = aerobic training, anaer = anaerobic training.

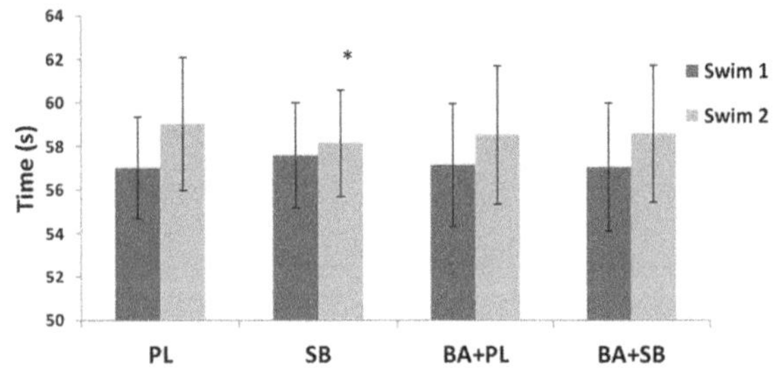

Figure 2 Swimming times (mean ± SD) in the supplemented groups. PL = placebo, SB = sodium bicarbonate, BA + PL = beta-alanine and placebo, BA + SB = beta-alanine and sodium bicarbonate, *Indicates a significant difference ($p < 0.05$) compared to PL.

tended ($p < 0.08$-0.09) to be greater in SB supplemented groups (Figure 3A). Blood pH values (Figure 3B) were significantly ($p < 0.05$) greater in the SB and in the BA + SB combination group 2 min before the first swim and in all measurement points following swimming compared to the PL measurement values.

Sodium, potassium

Significantly ($p < 0.05$) greater increases in plasma sodium concentrations were observed in SB and in BA + SB at every measurement point (except pre 1) compared to the PL values. A significant decrease in sodium concentrations was seen at BA + PL compared with PL during IV (Figure 4A). Significantly ($p < 0.05$) smaller plasma potassium concentrations were observed in SB and in the SB + BA groups at Pre 2, II and III compared to the PL values (Figure 4B).

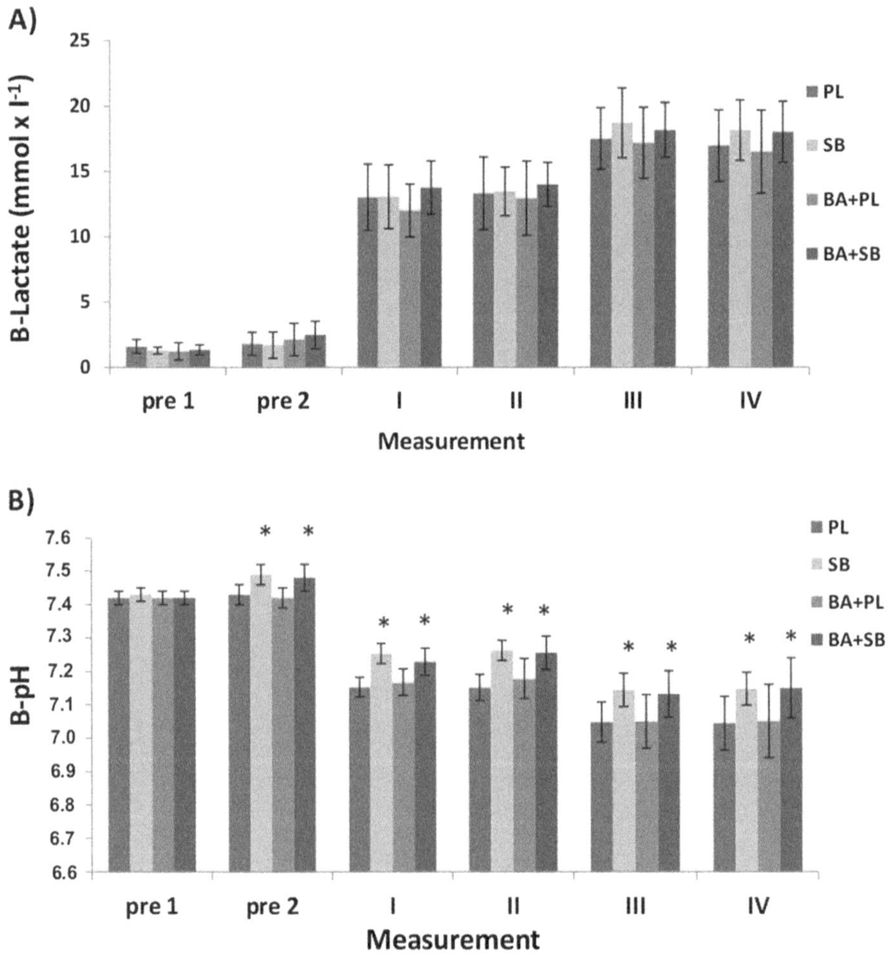

Figure 3 Blood lactate and pH values (mean ± SD) in the supplemented groups in different measurement time points. A) Blood lactate (B-Lactate), **B)** pH (B-pH), PL = placebo, SB = sodiumbicarbonate, BA + PL = beta-alanine and placebo, BA + SB = beta-alanine and sodium bicarbonate, pre 1 = 60 min before swimming, pre 2 = 2 min before swimming the first 100 m, I and III 2 min after both 100 m swimming, II and IV 8 min after both 100 m swimming, * Indicates a significant ($p < 0.05$) difference compared to PL.

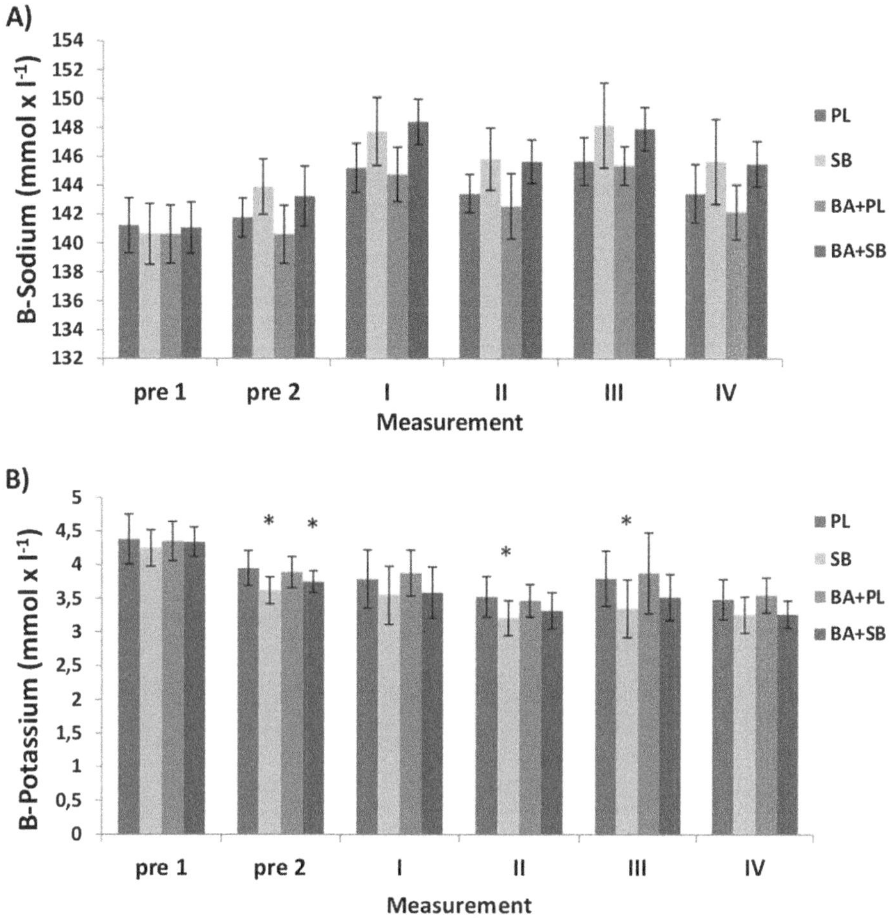

Figure 4 Blood sodium and potassium values (mean ± SD) in the supplemented groups in different measurement time points. **A)** Blood sodium (B-Sodium), **B)** potassium (B-Potassium), PL = placebo, SB = sodium bicarbonate, BA + PL = beta-alanine and placebo, BA + SB = beta-alanine and sodium bicarbonate. pre 1 = 60 min before swimming, pre 2 = 2 min before swimming the first 100 m, I and III 2 min after both 100 m swimming, II and IV 8 min after both 100 m swimming, * Indicates a significant ($p < 0.05$) difference compared to PL.

Bicarbonate, base excess

There were significantly greater values in blood bicarbonate and base excess values in SB and in BA + SB at every measurement point (except pre 1) compared to the PL values (Figures 5A and 5B).

Discussion

Main results

The primary findings from this investigation were that there was a significantly less attenuation in swim time for the second 100 m sprint following SB supplementation. However, co-supplementation of SB with BA did not add any further benefit.

Swim times

The subjects that ingested SB swam the second 100-m sprint 1.5 s (2.4%) faster compared to the PL trial. This improvement confirms the results previously reported by Mero et al. [23], who used a similar testing protocol and reported a 0.6 s ($p < 0.05$) improvement in subjects ingesting SB. Also in support of the present results, Gao et al. [4], demonstrated that pre - exercise supplementation with SB does not improve the first sprint but may be beneficial in later repetitions. In swimming races, an improvement of 1.5 s in performance may have a decisive effect on success in the final competition. During swimming competitions swimmers are often required to perform multiple heats during one day [32,33]. For example, in the 2012 London Olympics a female swimmer came in first in semifinals 200-m free style and then won the gold medal 15 min later in the 100-m backstroke. In our study the combined SB and BA supplementation did not improve swimming times. Recently Hobson et al. [26] showed that chronic BA and acute SB supplementation improved 2000 m rowing performance and they concluded that the addition of acute SB to chronic BA supplementation may further enhance rowing performance. They used a BA dose of 6.4 g per day during four weeks. In our study we used only 4.8 g per day for four weeks. Muscle carnosine is important in buffering and the muscle

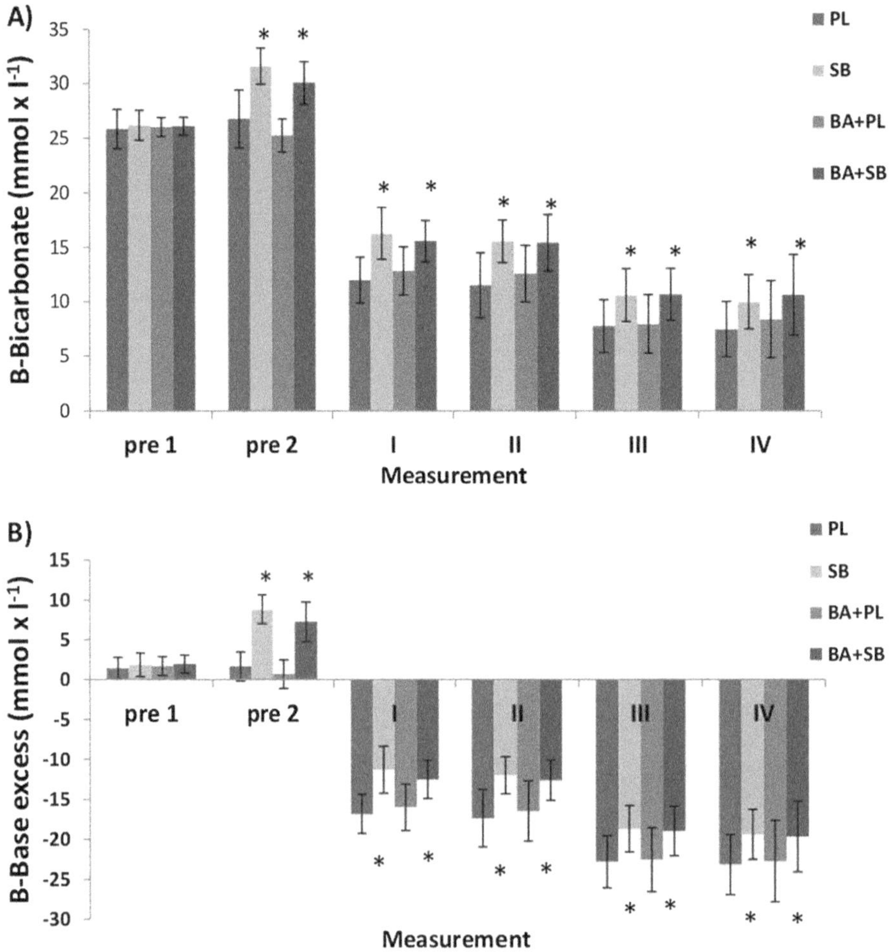

Figure 5 Blood bicarbonate and base excess values (mean ± SD) in the supplemented groups in different measurement time points. **A)** Blood bicarbonate (B-Bicarbonate) and **B)** base excess (B-Base excess) values (mean ± SD) in the supplemented groups in different measurement time points, PL = placebo, SB = sodium bicarbonate, BA + PL = beta-alanine and placebo, BA + SB = beta-alanine and sodium bicarbonate, pre 1 = 60 min before swimming, pre 2 = 2 min before swimming the first 100 m, I and III 2 min after both 100 m swimming, II and IV 8 min after both 100 m swimming, * Indicates a significant ($p < 0.05$) difference compared to PL.

content is dependent on BA ingestion [15] it would be interesting to use either bigger doses and/or longer supplementation periods in future studies.

Blood pH

Blood pH values were significantly greater when ingesting SB and with SB plus BA supplementation prior to the first swim compared to PL. The increase in blood pH was similar as in the earlier studies because the SB dose ($0.3 g \cdot kg^{-1}$ body mass) used was comparable. However, time for the first swim trial was not improved with SB or with SB + BA ingestion. In all four treatments following the swim trials, blood pH values were significantly lower compared to pre-values. Consequently, the second swim trial was performed in stronger acidosis than the first, and in this state the best performances were seen during SB treatment. These results in part confirm those by Gordon et al. [34], who observed that the alkalotic condition attenuates the increase in blood H^+ concentration. We hypothesized that the extracellular buffering action of SB and the intracellular pH-buffering action of carnosine through BA ingestion would be additive, resulting in an increased protection against the acidosis produced during anaerobic interval swimming. Our results appear to support the work of Hobson et al. [20] that suggested that benefits of BA supplementation may be dependent upon high intensity exercise durations lasting more than 60 s. However, it was a bit surprising that when SB and BA were combined the benefit observed with SB only was negated. This is difficult to explain but, although speculative, it may be related to muscle carnosine concentations. Although several studies have suggested that trained anaerobic athletes have higher muscle carnosine concentrations [35-37], the ability to enhance muscle carnosine concentration from training only has not been established. Therefore, the effect of supplementing for some individuals may be small.

It is possible that the effect of lowering intracellular acidity in this type of exercise is not the only factor for muscle fatigue [38]. The other possible factors for muscle fatigue may be phosphocreatine stores, maximal oxygen uptake and some neural factors.

Blood lactate

There were no significant differences in blood lactate concentrations between the treatment groups, although it seems to be higher with SB and SB + BA supplementation indicating increased buffering activity in muscle. The increase in peak blood lactate (change between PL and the SB groups) was about 1 $mmol \cdot l^{-1}$. This change was smaller than reported by Ibanez et al. [39] who demonstrated a difference in peak blood lactate between treatments of 2 $mmol \cdot l^{-1}$or more is needed to observe a strong and significant improvement in performance following SB supplementation. During intensive anaerobic work [40,41], it has been shown that lactate produced in fast-twitch muscle fibers can circulate to other fast-twitch or slow-twitch fibers for conversion to pyruvate. Pyruvate, in turn, converts to acetyl-CoA for entry into the citric acid cycle for aerobic energy metabolism. Lactate shuttling between cells enables glycogenolysis in one cell to supply other cells with fuel for oxidation [42]. Swimmers generally utilize both aerobic and combined aerobic-anaerobic training, and this may enhance the capacity of the lactate shuttling. In the present study, the effect of this lactate shuttling on peak blood lactate values remains an open question. However, the performance in the second 100 m swim following SB supplementation improved compared to PL, but co-supplementation with SB and BA did not confer any further significant benefit.

Blood bicarbonate, base excess, sodium and potassium

Blood analyses confirmed that SB and SB with BA were successful in increasing blood bicarbonate concentration and base excess consistent with previous studies of SB ingestion [43]. Both SB and SB with BA supplementations increased blood sodium as expected but blood potassium decreased. Earlier Sostaric et al. [30] reported that SB supplementation lowered circulating potassium and enhanced muscle potassium uptake, sodium delivery and chloride uptake with alkalosis. These physiological changes are all consistent with preservation of membrane excitability during exercise [30]. This suggests that lesser exercise-induced membrane depolarization may be an important mechanism underlying enhanced exercise performance with alkalosis. Thus alkalosis is associated with improved regulation of potassium, sodium, chloride and lactate. On the other hand, ingestion of BA significantly decreased blood sodium 8 min after the second swim compared with placebo, and tended to decrease at the other measurement points. Whereas potassium levels were very similar compared to placebo treatment. Consequently, ingestion of BA may affect membrane excitability differently during exercise compared with SB ingestion.

Conclusions

The results of this study indicate that there was a significant improvement in swimming time during the second 100 m swim trial following acute SB supplementation compared to PL, but the addition of chronic BA to acute SB did not provide any additional ergogenic benefit. Results indicate the efficacy of SB supplementation when performing maximal interval swimming lasting under 60 s but do not support any additional benefit of SB combined with BA.

Competing interests

The authors declare that they have no competing interests.

Authors' contributions

AAM (corresponding author) was responsible for the study design, the execution of the measurements, the statistical analysis and the writing of the manuscript. PH and JS participated in the study design, execution of the measurements, the statistical analysis and the writing of the manuscript. JRH and JRS participated in the study design and in the writing of the manuscript. All authors read and approved the final manuscript.

Acknowledgements

The authors would like to thank Mr. Risto Puurtinen for carrying out all the blood sampling and analysis.

Funding

This study project was funded by University of Jyväskylä, Department of Biology of Physical Activity.

Author details

[1]Department of Biology of Physical Activity, University of Jyväskylä, P.O. Box 35, Jyväskylä 40351, Finland. [2]Sport and Exercise Science, University of Central Florida, Orlando, Florida, USA.

References

1. Medbo JI, Sejersted OM: **Acid base and electrolyte balance after exhausting exercise in endurance and sprint trained subjects.** *Acta Physiol Scand* 1985, **125:**97–109.
2. Sutton JR, Jones NL, Toews CJ: **Effect of pH on muscle glucolysis during exercise.** *Clin Sci* 1981, **61**(3):331–338.
3. Fabiato A, Fabiato F: **Effects of pH on the myofilaments and the sarcoplasmic reticulum of skinned cells from cardiac and skeletal muscles.** *J Physiol* 1978, **75:**233–238.
4. Gao J, Costill DL, Horswill CA, Park SH: **Sodium bicarbonate ingestion improves performance in interval swimming.** *Eur J Appl Physiol* 1988, **78:**171–174.
5. Swank A, Robertson RJ: **Effect of induced alkalosis on perception during intermittent exercise.** *J Appl Physiol* 1989, **67:**1862–1867.
6. McNaughton LR, Ford S, Newbold C: **Effect of sodium bicarbonate ingestion on high intensity exercise in moderately trained women** *J Strength Cond Res* 1997, **11:**98–102.
7. Jones N, Sutton JR, Taylor R, Toews CJ: **Effects of pH on cardiorespiratory and metabolic responses to exercise.** *J Appl Physiol* 1977, **43:**959–964.
8. Siegler JC, Gleadall-Siddal DO: **Sodium bicarbonate ingestion and repeated swim sprint performance.** *J Strength Cond Res* 2010, **24**(11):105–111.
9. Wilkes D, Gledhill N, Smyth R: **Effect of acute induced metabolic alkalosis on 800-m racing time.** *Med Sci Sports Exerc* 1983, **15:**277–280.

10. Carr AJ, Hopkins WG, Gore CJ: **Effects of acute alkalosis and acidosis on performance: a meta-analysis.** *Sports Med* 2011, **41**(10):801–814.
11. Siegler JC, Marshall PWM, Bray J, Towlson C: **Sodium bicarbonate supplementation and ingestion timing: Does it matter?** *J Strength Cond Res* 2012, **26**(7):1953–1958.
12. Siegler JC, Midgley AW, Polman AWR, Remco CJ, Lever R: **Effects of various sodium bicarbonate loading protocols on the time-dependent extracellular buffering profile.** *J Strength Cond Res* 2010, **24**(9):2551–2557.
13. Lindh AM, Peyrebrune MC, Ingham SA, Bailey DM, Folland JP: **Sodium Bicarbonate Improves Swimming Performance.** *Int J Sports Med* 2008, **29**:519–523.
14. Artioli GG, Gualano B, Smith A, Stout J, Lancha AH Jr: **Role of beta-alanine supplementation on muscle carnosine and exercise performance.** *Med Sci Sports Exerc* 2010, **42**(6):1162–1173.
15. Baguet A, Reyngoudt H, Pottier A, Everaert I, Callens S, Achten E, Derave W: **Carnosine loading and washout in human skeletal muscles.** *J Appl Physiol* 2009, **106**:837–842.
16. Derave W, Özdemir MS, Harris RC, Pottier A, Reyngoudt H, Koppo K, Wise JA, Achten E: **Beta-alanine supplementation augments muscle carnosine content and attenuates fatigue during repeated isokinetic contraction bouts in trained sprinters.** *J Appl Physiol* 2007, **104**:1736–1743.
17. Harris RC, Marlin DJ, Dunnett M, Snow DH, Hultman E: **Muscle buffering capacity and dipeptide content in the thoroughbred horse, greyhound dog and man.** *Comp Biochem Physiol A Comp Physiol* 1990, **97**(2):249–251.
18. Hill CA, Harris RC, Kim HJ, Harris BD, Sale C, Boobis LH, Kim CK, Wise JA: **Influence of β-alanine supplementation on skeletal muscle carnosine concentrations and high intensity cycling capacity.** *Amino Acids* 2006, **32**:225–233.
19. Stout JR, Cramer JT, Zoeller RF, Torok D, Costa P, Hoffman JR, Harris RC, O'Kroy JO: **Effects of beta-alanine supplementation on the onset of neuromuscular fatigue and ventilatory thereshold in women.** *Amino Acids* 2007, **32**:381–386.
20. Hobson R, Saunders B, Ball G, Harris RC, Sale C: **Effects of β-alanine supplementation on exercise performance: a meta-analysis.** *Amino Acids* 2012, **43**:25–37.
21. Hoffman JR, Ratamess NA, Kang J, Mangine G, Faigenbaum AD, Stout JR: **Effect of creatine and β-alanine supplementation on performance and endocrine responses in strength/power athletes.** *Int J Sport Nutr Exer Metab* 2006, **16**:430–446.
22. Hoffman JR, Ratamess NA, Faigenbaum AD, Ross R, Kang J: **Short-duration β-alanine supplementation increases training volume and reduces subjective feelings of fatigue in college football players.** *Nutr Res* 2008, **28**:31–35.
23. Mero AA, Keskinen KL, Malvela MT, Sallinen JM: **Combined creatine and sodium bicarbonate supplementation enhances interval swimming.** *J Strength Cond Res* 2004, **18**(2):306–310.
24. Sale C, Saunders B, Hudson S, Wise JA, Harris RC, Sunderland CD: **Effect of β-alanine plus sodium bicarbonate on high-intensity cycling capacity.** *Med Sci Sports Exerc* 2011, **43**(10):1972–1978.
25. Bellinger PM, Howe ST, Shing CM, Fell JW: **Effect of combined β-alanine and sodium bicarbonate supplementation on cycling performance.** *Med Sci Sports Exerc* 2012, **44**(8):1545–1551.
26. Hobson RM, Harris RC, Martin D, Smith P, Macklin B, Gualano B, Sale C: **Effect of β-Alanine, With & Without Sodium Bicarbonate, on 2000m Rowing Performance.** *Int J Sport Nutr Exerc Metab* 2013 [Epub ahead of print].
27. Tobias G, Benatti FB, Painelli De Salles V, Roschel H, Gualano B, Sale C, Harris RC, Lancha AH Jr, Artioli GG: **Additive effects of beta-alanine and sodium bicarbonate on upper-body intermittent performance.** *Amino Acids* 2013, **45**:309–317.
28. Ducker KJ, Dawson B, Wallman KE: **Effect of beta-alanine and sodium bicarbonate supplementation on repeated-sprint performance.** *J Strength Cond Res* 2013. Epub ahead of print.
29. Painelli De Salles V, Roschel H, De Jesus F, Sale C, Harris RC, Solis MY, Benatti FB, Gualano B, Lancha AH Jr, Artioli GG: **The ergogenic effect of beta-alanine combined with sodium bicarbonate on high-intensity swimming performance.** *Appl Physiol Nutr Metab* 2013, **38**(5):525–532.
30. Sostaric SM, Skinner SL, Brown MJ, Sangkabutra T, Medved I, Medley T, Selig SE, Fairweather I, Rutar D, McKenna MJ: **Alkalosis increases muscle K+ release, but lowers plasma [K+] and delays fatigue during dynamic forearm exercise.** *J Physiol* 2006, **570**(1):185–205.
31. Campbell B, Wilborn C, Bounty PL, Taylor L, Nelson MT, Greenwood M, Ziegenfuss TN, Lopez HL, Hoffman JR, Stout JR, Stephen Schmitz S, Collin R, Kalman DS, Antonio J, Kreider RB: **International Society of Sports Nutrition position stand: energy drinks.** *J Int Soc Sports Nutr* 2013, **10**:1. http://www.jissn.com/content/10/1/1.
32. Capelli C, Pendergast DR, Termin B: **Energetics of swimming at maximal speeds in humans.** *Eur J Appl Physiol* 1998, **78**:385–393.
33. Gledhill N: **Haemoglobin, blood volume and endurance.** In *Endurance in Sport.* 1st edition. Edited by Shephard RJ, Astrand P-OA. Oxford: Blackwell Scientific Publications; 1992:208–214.
34. Gordon SE, Kraemer WJ, Vos NH, Lynch JM, Knuttgen HG: **Effect of acid–base balance on the growth hormone response to acute high-intensity cycle exercise.** *J Appl Physiol* 1994, **76**:821–829.
35. Harris RC, Tallon MJ, Dunnet M, Boobis L, Coakley J, Kim HJ, Fallowfield JL, Hill CA, Sale C, Wise JA: **The absorption of supplied beta-alanine and its effect on muscle carnosine synthesis in human vastus lateralis.** *Amino Acids* 2006, **30**:279–289.
36. Suzuki Y, Ito O, Takahashi H, Takamatsu K: **The effect of sprint training on skeletal muscle carnosine in humans.** *Int J Sport Health Sci* 2004, **2**:105–110.
37. Tallon MJ, Harris RC, Boobis LH, Fallowfield JL, Wise JA: **The carnosine content of vastus lateralis is elevated in resistance trained bodybuilders.** *J Strength Cond Res* 2005, **19**(4):725–729.
38. Allen DG, Lamb GD, Westerblad H: **Skeletal muscle fatigue: cellular mechanisms.** *Physiol Rev* 2008, **88**(1):287–332.
39. Ibanez J, Pullinen T, Gorostiaga E, Postigo A, Mero A: **Blood lactate and ammonia in short-term anaerobic work following induced alkalosis.** *J Sports Med Phys Fitness* 1995, **35**(3):187–193.
40. Kinderman W, Keul J: *Anaerobe Energiebereitstellung im Hochleistungssport.* Schorndorf: Verlag Karl Hofmann; 1977.
41. Newsholme EA, Blomstrand E, McAndrew N, Parry-Billings M: **Biochemical causes of fatigue and overtraining.** In *Endurance in Sport.* 1st edition. Edited by Shephard RJ, Astrand P-O. Oxford: Blackwell Scientific Publications; 1992:351–364.
42. Brooks GA: **Lactate: Glycolytic end product and oxidative substrate during sustained exercise in mammals -The "Lactate Shuttle'.** In *Circulation, Respiration and Metabolism: Current Comparative Approaches.* Edited by Gillis R. Berlin: SpringerVerlag; 1985:208–218.
43. Robergs RA, Ghiasvand F, Parker D: **Biochemistry of exercise-induced metabolic acidosis.** *Am J Physiol Regul Integ Comp Physiol* 2004, **287**:R502–R516.

11

Effects of betaine on body composition, performance, and homocysteine thiolactone

Jason M Cholewa[1*], Monika Wyszczelska-Rokiel[2], Rafal Glowacki[2], Hieronim Jakubowski[3,4], Tracey Matthews[5], Richard Wood[5], Stuart AS Craig[6] and Vincent Paolone[5]

Abstract

Background: This study investigated the effects of long term betaine supplementation on body composition, performance, and homocysteine thiolactone (HCTL) in experienced strength trained men.

Methods: Twenty-three subjects were matched for training experience (4.8 ± 2.3 years) and body fat percentage (BF%: 16.9 ± 8.0%), randomly assigned to either a placebo (PL; $n = 12$) or betaine group (BET; $n = 11$; 2.5 g/day), and completed a 6 week periodized training program consisting of 3 two-week micro-cycles. Bench press and back squat training volumes were recorded and changes in training volume were assessed at each micro-cycle. Fasting urine was collected at baseline (BL), weeks 2, 4 and 6, and assayed for HCTL. Subjects were tested prior to and following 6 weeks of treatment. Arm and thigh cross sectional area (CSA) was estimated via girth and skin fold measurements. Body density was estimated via skin fold calipers and used to estimate BF%, fat mass (FM), and lean body mass (LBM). Performance was assessed via vertical jump (VJ), bench press 1 RM (BP), and back squat 1 RM (BS).

Results: Arm CSA increased significantly ($p < .05$) in BET but not PL. No differences existed between group and time for changes in thigh CSA. Back squat training volume increased significantly ($p < .05$) for both groups throughout training. Bench press training volume was significantly ($p < .05$) improved for BET compared to PL at microcycles one and three. Body composition (BF%, FM, LBM) improved significantly ($p < .05$) in BET but not PL. No differences were found in performance variables (BP, BS, VJ) between groups, except there was a trend ($p = .07$) for increased VJ power in BET versus PL. A significant interaction ($p < .05$) existed for HCTL, with increases from BL to week 2 in PL, but not BET. Additionally, HCTL remained elevated at week 4 in PL, but not BET.

Conclusion: Six-weeks of betaine supplementation improved body composition, arm size, bench press work capacity, attenuated the rise in urinary HCTL, and tended to improve power ($p = .07$) but not strength.

Keywords: Hypertrophy, Strength, Power, Supplementation, Trimethylglycine

Background

Betaine (trimethylglycine) is an organic osmolyte found in many foods, including spinach, beets, and whole grains [1]. Administration of supplemental betaine for 10–15 days has enhanced performance in several studies but with varying results: Lee et al. [2] reported increased power output and force production, whereas others [3,4] reported improvements in muscular endurance but not power. On the other hand, Del Favero et al. [5] reported no improvements in power output, strength, or body composition with 10 days of betaine treatment; however, subjects were instructed to avoid training and supplementation was ceased 5 days prior to performance testing.

To the author's knowledge, only two studies have examined the effects of betaine on body composition and hypertrophy in humans. Betaine did not improve body composition in obese, sedentary subjects on a 500 kcal/day caloric deficit following 12 weeks of supplementation [6]. Similarly, 10 days of betaine supplementation did not improve body composition in sedentary young male subjects [5]. Though research is limited in humans, chronic

* Correspondence: jcholewa@coastal.edu
[1]Department of Kinesiology, Recreation, and Sport Studies, Coastal Carolina University, Conway, SC, USA
Full list of author information is available at the end of the article

betaine supplementation has been shown to reduce adipose mass and increase muscle mass in animals [7-9]. Greater improvements in body composition with betaine supplementation were observed when pigs were given extra pen space to move and exercise [9], suggesting that betaine may exert the most influential effects on growth under conditions of metabolic or nutritional stress. Because the subjects in Schwab et al. [6] and Del Favero et al. [5] were instructed not to exercise, the absence of a metabolic stressor may have compromised the effects of betaine. Given the enhanced effects of movement in pigs and the ineffectiveness reported in sedentary, non-exercising humans, we hypothesize that the effects of betaine on body composition, strength and power may be most apparent when supplementation occurs over several weeks accompanied by a resistance training program.

By donating a methyl group to transmethylate Hcy back to methionine (Met), betaine increases Hcy metabolism and the availability of the universal methyl donor, *S*-adenosylmethionine (SAM) [10]. We hypothesize betaine supplementation may enhance protein synthesis and thus improve body composition by reducing Hcy and homocysteine thiolactone (HCTL). Hcy directly impairs insulin signaling by reducing insulin receptor stubstrate-1 (IRS-1) activation and thus inhibiting Akt-phosphorylation [11]. Moreover, excess dietary Met is metabolized to form Hcy and both high dietary Met consumption and the resultant increase in plasma Hcy contributes to elevated HCTL [12]. A short (10 min) HCTL treatment inhibits insulin signaling, including insulin-mediated mRNA expression and protein synthesis [13]. This suggests that HCTL is more effective than Hcy in promoting insulin resistance. Additionally, HCTL has been shown to modify protein lysine residues, which causes protein aggregation, and inactivates enzymes associated with protein synthesis [14].

Concentrations of plasma Hcy or HCTL levels in strength athletes have yet to be reported. Given that transmethylation capacity is dependent upon plasma folate and betaine [15] and because weight trainers regularly consume excess Met and inadequate folate and betaine [16], Hcy transmethylation may be impaired resulting in excess HCTL generation. Thus, by decreasing insulin receptor signaling [11], elevated HCTL in weight lifters may compromise body composition directly by inhibiting mRNA expression and protein synthesis.

In healthy adults the ingestion of 500 mg of betaine decreased fasting plasma Hcy and attenuated Hcy rise for 24 hr following a Met load [11], and betaine treatment lowers HCTL in patients with genetically compromised transmethylation capacities [12]; however, to date there are no published reports investigating the effects of betaine ingestion on HCTL in healthy subjects. We hypothesize that by increasing transmethylation capacity betaine supplementation reduces plasma Hcy and may thus decrease HCTL generation, resulting in improved insulin signaling and myofibril protein synthesis, and ultimately enhancing muscle and strength gains. Therefore, the purpose of this study was to investigate the sub-chronic effects of betaine on strength, power, and body composition during resistance training in experienced strength trained males. Additionally, urine HCTL was measured to determine if betaine affects performance by reducing plasma HCTL. We hypothesized that betaine supplementation would improve strength, vertical jump, limb CSA, and body composition between the 1st week and 6th week over placebo. We also hypothesized that betaine supplementation would reduce urinary HCTL over the course of 6 weeks.

Methods

Experimental design

To investigate the effects of betaine supplementation, subjects were matched, and randomly assigned to a treatment or placebo group in a double-blinded study. Subjects underwent 6 weeks of supplementation with either betaine or placebo administered in identical gelatin capsules. Before and after the treatment period skin fold and girth measurements were taken, and subjects completed a strength testing protocol. Additionally, urine was collected prior to treatment and at 2 week intervals thereafter.

Subjects

Twenty three experienced recreationally strength trained males (weight: 86.8 ± 9.1 kg; training experience: 4.8 ± 2.3 months; BF%: 16.9 ± 8%) between the ages of 18 and 35 were recruited divided into two groups based on training experience (6 month intervals) and body fat percentage (2 percentage point intervals starting at 6%), and randomly assigned to receive either the treatment ($n = 11$) or placebo ($n = 12$). Medical histories were obtained to exclude medical, musculoskeletal, and endocrine disorders, concurrent nutritional supplementation, and anabolic drugs. Additionally, subjects must have met the inclusion criteria to be classified as experienced in resistance training [17]: previous consecutive resistance training equal to or greater than 24 months; a frequency of at least 3 resistance training sessions per week; at least 24 months experience in the back squat and bench press; and the ability to bench press a load equal to body weight and back squat at least 1.25 fold that of body weight. All subjects signed an informed consent form following verbal and written explanation of benefits and potential risks associated with participating in the study.

Experimental controls

Subjects were required to complete a 3-day food diary, and were instructed to consume a similar quantity/

quality of foods throughout the study in order avoid changes in nutritional status. Subjects were also required to perform all prescribed resistance training sessions, complete and submit training logs to the primary investigator on a weekly basis, and abstain from performing other structured exercise programs throughout the duration of the study. Subjects were required to render urine upon waking following an overnight fast. Limb girth, skin fold, strength, and power testing was carried out at the same time of day within 2 days prior to and immediately following the 6 week trial period. Prior to all exercise tests, subjects were familiarized with the assessment protocols. All methods and procedures were approved by the Institutional Review Board of Springfield College prior to data collection.

Procedures

All testing was conducted at the Springfield College Human Performance Laboratory (HPL). Subjects were required to report to the HPL on two separate occasions (pre-treatment and post treatment) where height, nude body mass, skin fold, anthropometric measurements, and maximal strength testing was performed.

Body fat

Lange skin fold calipers (Cambridge Scientific Industries Inc: Cambridge, MD) were calibrated before testing each subject, and measurements were performed by the primary investigator to eliminate inter-rater variability. Skin folds (mm) were measured on the right side of the body in the following rotation: sub-scapular (X_1), abdominal (X_2), triceps brachii (X_3), and chest at the mix-auxiliary line (X_4). Body density (BD) was estimated via the following equation [18]: $BD = 1.03316 - .00164X_1 + .0041H - .00144X_2 - .00069X_3 + .00062X_4$, and then used to estimate BF % [19]: BF % = [(4.57 / BD) – 4.142] × 100. Lean body mass (LBM) and fat mass (FM) were then calculated from the BF % and body weight.

Cross sectional area

A 6-week trial period was chosen to allow for detectable changes in muscle CSA to occur. Changes in limb muscle mass have been demonstrated to be detectable via CSA measurements after four weeks of training and continue to increase week to week [20]. Limb muscle volume was assessed by evaluating differences in CSA via the Moritani and DeVries (MD) method [21]. The MD method is both sensitive ($SEE = 3.25\ cm^2$) and highly correlated ($r = .98$) to computed tomography, the gold standard of CSA measurement [22].

Girth and skin fold measurements were performed on the right limbs to determine CSA via the MD method. Cross sectional area of the arm was determined at the midpoint between the humeral greater tuberosity and lateral epicondyle, whereas CSA of the thigh was determined at the midpoint of the distance between the greater trochanter and lateral epicondyle of the femur. Skin fold measurements were performed three times at the four quadrants of the limb at the location where the circumference was measured. Cross sectional area was calculated via the following equation [21]: $CSA = \pi \left[\frac{C}{2\pi} - \frac{\sum_{i=1}^{4} fi}{4}\right]$, where C = limb circumference and $\sum_{i=1}^{4} fi$ = sum of skin folds. All measurements were performed by the primary investigator to eliminate inter-rater variability. Distances from the proximal boney land mark (humeral greater tuberosity and greater trochanter) where measurements were performed were recorded and used again for post treatment measuring to minimize intra-rater variability.

Strength and power testing

All strength and power testing was conducted under the supervision of a National Strength and Conditioning Association (NSCA) Certified Strength and Conditioning Specialist. Power was assessed via vertical jump using the Just Jump! Mat (Probotics Inc.: Huntsville, AL). Maximal strength was assessed with the free weight bench press and back squat. The heaviest resistance lifted in each exercise was considered the 1 RM. The bench press and back squat were chosen for strength assessment because: they are common exercises performed by weight lifters and the standardized strength training program in this study utilized the two exercises. Additionally, 1 RM testing has been shown to be a reliable (ICC = .96) [17] measure to assess changes in muscle strength following an exercise intervention.

All subjects completed a standardized dynamic warm up prior to performance testing. Following a 5-min rest subjects performed 3 trials of counter-movement vertical jumps separated by a 3-min rest. Vertical jumps were measured in inches on the Just Jump! mat. Subjects were instructed to perform a rapid lower body eccentric contraction followed immediately by a maximal intensity concentric contraction. Subjects were instructed to jump straight up and minimize any in-air hip flexion. The best of the three trials was recorded as vertical jump height.

Subjects were then given a 3-min rest prior to the strength specific warm ups. Subjects performed three sets of four repetitions with a progressively heavier load, three sets of one repetition with a progressively heavier load, and then a 3 min rest prior to attempting the first 1 RM. The first load used was 90% of the subject's most recent 1 RM or predicted from the subject's most recent RM [23]: 1-RM = 100 * rep wt / (101.3 – 2.67123 * reps). Loads were increased by 5 – 10% and 10 – 20% for bench press and squat, respectively, and then the 1 RM was determined in fewer than 5 sets with a rest interval of 3–5 min between sets. There were no significant differences in attempts between pre- and post-testing (3.4 ± .82, $p = .71$). The bench press 1 RM was tested first, and then a rest interval of at least 10 min was provided prior to determining the back squat 1 RM.

Homocysteine thiolactone

HCTL is a toxic metabolite in humans and renal excretion serves as the primary method of HCTL elimination [14]. Urinary concentrations of HCTL are 100 fold greater than those found in the plasma [24]. Urine was rendered upon waking following an overnight fast prior to treatment administration (baseline) and at the end of week 2, 4 and 6 throughout the study. The urine samples were collected by the primary investigator on the same day that urine was rendered and stored in 1-mL aliquots at −80°C prior to being sent for analysis. Urine was analyzed for HCTL via the cation-exchange high pressure liquid chromatography (HPLC) at the Institute of Bioorganic Chemistry, Polish Academy of Sciences, Poznan, Dept. of Biochemistry and Biotechnology, Life Sciences University, Poznan, Poland, as described Jakubowski et al. [24-26]. The cation-exchange HPLC is highly sensitive with a 0.36 nmol/L detection limit [24].

Treatments

Treatments were administered double blind and consisted of either a placebo (flour) or betaine (DuPont Nutrition & Health: Tarrytown, NY). The blind was not removed until all data had been collected. The primary investigator filled identical, unmarked gelatin capsules with either 0.42 g white flour or 0.42 g betaine. Subjects consumed three capsules (1.25 g) twice per day yielding an absolute total of 2.5 g betaine. This dosage was chosen because: betaine is safe at a dietary intake of 9 – 12 g/day [1]; 2.5 - 5 g betaine has been shown to significantly elevate plasma betaine [6]; 2.5 g positively affects strength

Table 1 Non-linear 6 week resistance training program

Monday	Micro cycle 1	Micro cycle 2	Micro cycle 3
Exercise	**Week 1 - 2**	**Week 3 - 4**	**Week 5 - 6**
Barbell Bench Press	3 × (12–15) / 90 sec	4 × (4–6) / 3 min	3 × (8–10) / 2 min
Barbell Incline Press	3 × (12–15) / 90 sec	4 × (4–6) / 3 min	3 × (8–10) / 2 min
Bent Over Barbell Row	3 × (12–15) / 90 sec	4 × (4–6) / 3 min	3 × (8–10) / 2 min
Seated Cable Row	3 × (12–15) / 90 sec	4 × (4–6) / 3 min	3 × (8–10) / 2 min
Biceps Barbell Curl	3 × (12–15) / 90 sec	4 × (4–6) / 3 min	3 × (8–10) / 2 min
Lying Triceps Extension	3 × (12–15) / 90 sec	4 × (4–6) / 3 min	3 × (8–10) / 2 min
Tuesday	**Micro cycle 1**	**Micro cycle 2**	**Micro cycle 3**
Exercise	**Week 1 - 2**	**Week 3 - 4**	**Week 5 - 6**
Free Weight Back Squat	3 × (8–10) / 2 min	3 × (12–15) / 90 sec	4 × (4–6) / 3 min
Barbell Rumanian Dead Lift	3 × (8–10) / 2 min	3 × (12–15) / 90 sec	4 × (4–6) / 3 min
Leg Extension Machine	3 × (8–10) / 2 min	3 × (12–15) / 90 sec	4 × (4–6) / 3 min
Abdominal Crunches	3 × (20–30) / 1 min	3 × (20–30) / 1 min	3 × (20–30) / 1 min
Thursday	**Micro cycle 1**	**Micro cycle 2**	**Micro cycle 3**
Exercise	**Week 1 - 2**	**Week 3 - 4**	**Week 5 - 6**
Barbell Military Press	3 × (12–15) / 90 sec	4 × (4–6) / 3 min	3 × (8–10) / 2 min
Wide Grip Front Lat Pull Down	3 × (12–15) / 90 sec	4 × (4–6) / 3 min	3 × (8–10) / 2 min
Dumbbell Row	3 × (12–15) / 90 sec	4 × (4–6) / 3 min	3 × (8–10) / 2 min
Dumbbell Lateral Shoulder Raise	3 × (12–15) / 90 sec	4 × (4–6) / 3 min	3 × (8–10) / 2 min
Alternating Curls with Dumbbells	3 × (12–15) / 90 sec	4 × (4–6) / 3 min	3 × (8–10) / 2 min
Triceps Extension with Cables	3 × (12–15) / 90 sec	4 × (4–6) / 3 min	3 × (8–10) / 2 min
Friday	**Micro cycle 1**	**Micro cycle 2**	**Micro cycle 3**
Exercise	**Week 1 - 2**	**Week 3 - 4**	**Week 5 - 6**
Standard Dead Lift	3 × (8–10) / 2 min	3 × (12–15) / 90 sec	4 × (4–6) / 3 min
Barbell Split Squat	3 × (8–10) / 2 min	3 × (12–15) / 90 sec	4 × (4–6) / 3 min
Prone Leg Curl Machine	3 × (8–10) / 2 min	3 × (12–15) / 90 sec	4 × (4–6) / 3 min
Hanging Leg Raises	3 × (20–30) / 1 min	3 × (20–30) / 1 min	3 × (20–30) / 1 min

Note: Volume is prescribed as: Sets × (Rep Range) / Rest Periods.

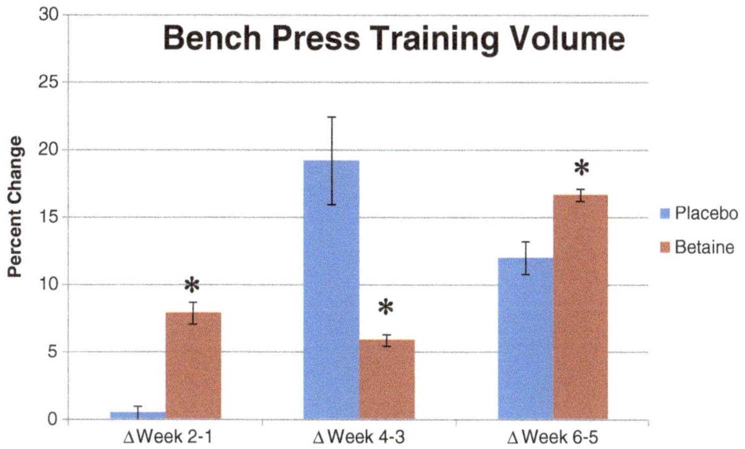

Figure 1 Percent change in bench press volume for placebo (n = 12) and betaine (n = 11) for 3 training micro-cycles. Note: * = Significantly (p < .05) different than placebo.

performance [2,4]; and the average relative dosage (34.8 mg/kg-LBM) in the present study is similar to the average relative dosage (36.3 mg/kg-LBM) reported previously to improve performance [3]. Subjects were provided with 42 capsules per week and were required to log and submit consumption times in accordance with the treatment protocol.

Training program

Subjects assigned to the betaine and placebo groups performed the same exercises, sets and repetitions during the six week investigation. A non-linear periodization (NLP) training program consisting of three 2-week micro-cycles was prescribed because NLP has been shown to produce larger increases in strength [27] and muscle volume [28] compared to linear or non-periodized programs. Upper body training was performed on Monday and Thursday, whereas lower body training took place on Tuesday and Friday. The prescription for exercises, training days, loads, rest period, warm ups, and resistance progression can be found in Table 1.

The training sessions were not monitored; however, subjects were required to submit training logs to the primary investigator on a biweekly basis (at the conclusion of each micro-cycle). Training volume was calculated as the sum of the load lifted multiplied by the number of repetitions performed during each week for the bench press and back squat, respectively. Work capacity for bench press and back squat was assessed by comparing percent improvement in training volume for each micro-cycle (week 1 vs. week 2; week 3 vs. week 4; week 5 vs. week 6).

Statistical analysis

An independent samples *t*-test was used to examine differences between groups for pre-trial BF % and training experience. A 2 × 5 Mixed Factorial ANOVA with Repeated Measures was used to determine the difference between groups (placebo and betaine) and time for changes in urinary HCTL from baseline and week to week. Two 2 × 6 Mixed Factorial ANOVA with Repeated Measures were used to determine differences between groups and time for bench press and back squat work capacity at each training micro-cycle. If significant interactions were found, percent improvements at each micro-cycle was calculated and compared between groups with an independent samples *t*-test. Eight 2 × 2 Mixed Factorial ANOVAs with Repeated Measures were used to determine differences in arm CSA, thigh CSA, BF %, LBM, FM, vertical jump, bench press 1 RM, and back squat 1 RM between groups and time (pre- vs. post-trial). All statistical analyses were analyzed using Statistical Package for the Social Sciences (SPSS v. 19, IBM) and the alpha level was set at .05.

Table 2 Changes in bench press training volume (kg) for placebo (n = 12) and betaine (n = 11) between three micro-cycles

	Pre	Post	Δ	*P*
Micro Cycle 1				
Betaine	2736 ± 463	2953 ± 500	216 ± 39	.01
Placebo	3154 ± 553	3170 ± 555	15 ± 70	.44
Micro Cycle 2				
Betaine	1755 ± 296	1858 ± 315	103 ± 25	.30
Placebo	2320 ± 406	2903 ± 672	583 ± 288	.01
Micro Cycle 3				
Betaine	2160 ± 365	2520 ± 427	360 ± 101	.01
Placebo	2481 ± 435	2779 ± 487	298 ± 62	.01

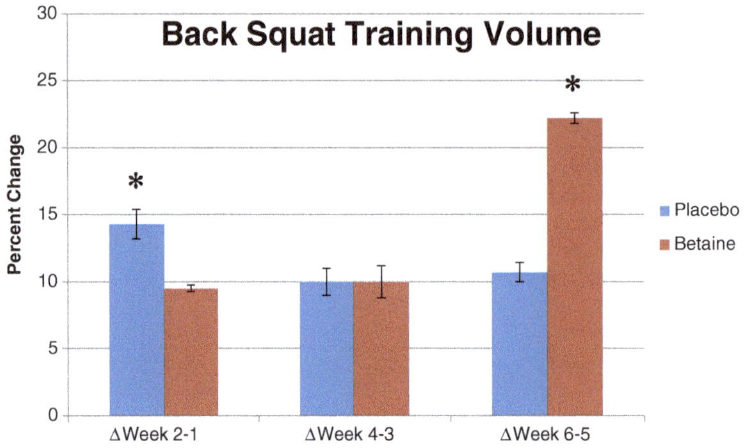

Figure 2 Percent change in back squat volume for placebo (n = 12) and betaine (n = 11) for 3 training micro-cycles. Note: * = Significantly ($p < .05$) different than placebo.

Results

All values are presented as means ± standard deviations. A significant interaction ($p = .001$) between group and time existed for bench press work capacity (Figure 1). Bench press training volume increased with placebo at micro-cycles 2 and 3, and for betaine at micro-cycles 1 and 3 (Table 2). *Post hoc* analysis revealed the betaine group improved significantly more than placebo at micro-cycle one (7.89 ± 2.65% vs. 0.49 ± 1.69%, $p = .001$) and three (16.67 ± 1.51% vs. 12.00 ± 4.21%, $p = .05$); however, the percent improvement for placebo was significantly greater than betaine at micro-cycle two (19.2 ± 11.2% vs. 5.9 ± 1.4%, $p = .001$).

A significant main effect ($p = .001$) of time existed for squat work capacity. Both groups increased squat volume at the second week of each training micro-cycle (Figure 2 & Table 3); however, *post-hoc* analysis revealed the percent improvement in squat training volume was significantly greater with placebo than betaine at micro-cycle one (14.3 ± 3.8% vs. 9.5 ± 0.8%, $p = .001$), and significantly greater with betaine than placebo at micro-cycle three (22.2 ± 1.3% vs. 10.7 ± 2.5%, $p = .001$). There were no differences ($p = .68$) between groups for percent improvement at micro-cycle two.

Table 3 Changes in back squat training volume (kg) for placebo (n = 12) and betaine (n = 11) between three micro-cycles

	Pre	Post	Δ	P
Micro Cycle 1				
Betaine	2760 ± 482	3022 ± 527	262 ± 43	.01
Placebo	3003 ± 695	3364 ± 779	360 ± 84	.01
Micro Cycle 2				
Betaine	3736 ± 652	4084 ± 712	347 ± 76	.01
Placebo	4015 ± 930	4444 ± 1030	428 ± 159	.01
Micro Cycle 3				
Betaine	2056 ± 357	2541 ± 444	484 ± 91	.01
Placebo	2350 ± 545	2655 ± 633	305 ± 85	.01

No significant ($p = .70$) main effect or interaction existed between group and time for thigh CSA (Table 4). A significant ($p = .03$) interaction was found between groups and time for arm CSA (Figure 3). Arm CSA increased significantly post-trial vs. pre-trial with betaine but not placebo (Table 4).

All body composition data can be found in Table 5. Significant interactions between group and time were found for BF% ($p = .007$), LBM ($p = .03$), and FM ($p = .01$). BF% and FM both decreased significantly post-trial vs. pre-trial with betaine but not placebo (Figures 4, 5). Post-trial LBM increased significantly over pre-trial with betaine but not placebo.

Vertical jump, bench press 1RM and back squat 1Rm data can be found in Table 6. An interaction trend ($p = .07$) was found for vertical jump. Vertical jump decreased with placebo and increased in betaine. No significant ($p = .99$) interaction or main effect ($p = .12$) existed between group and time for bench press. A significant ($p = .001$) main effect for time was found for back squat 1 RM. Mean post-trial back squat 1 RM was significantly greater than pre-trial squat 1 RM; however, no significant interaction ($p = .18$) existed between group and time.

There was a trend ($p = .06$) for greater baseline HCTL concentrations in betaine. A significant ($p = .002$) interaction between group and time was found for urinary HCTL. The change in urinary HCTL with placebo was significantly greater than that of betaine between baseline and week 2, and baseline and week 4, respectively (Figure 6 & Table 7). No significant changes in HCTL were found for either group when comparing the change between week 2 and 4 or week 4 and week 6; however,

Table 4 Changes in thigh and arm cross sectional area (cm³) for placebo (n = 12) and betaine (n = 11) between pre- and post-treatment

	Pre	Post	Δ	P
Thigh CSA				
Betaine	85.0 ± 12.2	87.7 ± 12.2	2.7 ± 4.2	.254
Placebo	87.6 ± 17.7	89.0 ± 13.9	2.3 ± 10	.254
Arm CSA				
Betaine	49.5 ± 8.7	54.1 ± 6.6	4.6 ± 4.3	.01
Placebo	53.4 ± 10.2	53.5 ± 11.2	-.1 ± 5	.98

a main effect of time was found when comparing week 6 to week 4.

Discussion

We hypothesized body composition would improve with 6 weeks of betaine supplementation. This hypothesis was supported by significant increases in lean mass, and decreases in fat mass and body fat percentage with betaine compared to placebo. Increases in arm CSA were found to be greater with betaine than placebo; however, thigh CSA did not increase in either group. We also expected strength and power performance to improve with betaine supplementation. While back squat 1 RM increased for both groups, there were no differences in improvement between betaine and placebo. There was a trend ($p = .07$) for greater vertical jump power with betaine versus placebo, however there were no increases in bench press 1 RM.

The improvements in lean mass, fat mass and body fat percentage with betaine supplementation contrast previous investigations [5,6]. Differences in methodology may explain these discrepancies: subjects in the previous studies were both sedentary and instructed not to exercise, whereas the subjects in the present study were currently training and given a structured exercise program. Betaine has been suggested to act as a nutrient partitioner and thereby accelerate lean mass gains in pigs. By increasing Hcy transmethylation, betaine spares Met, allows for more efficient use of dietary protein, and increases nitrogen retention [7]. Due to the inclusion of resistance training in this study but not previous studies [5,6], the demand for Met in the initiation of translation in protein synthesis was likely elevated, thereby leading to a greater utilization of elevated Met, and thus improvements in lean mass. Therefore, the results from the present study lend support to the hypothesis that the action of betaine to improve body composition in humans may be most effective when accompanied by exercise.

The increase in arm CSA in the betaine group compared to placebo was accompanied by an improvement in bench press work capacity. The greatest improvements in volume over placebo occurred during the first and third training micro-cycles, where subjects were instructed to perform 3 sets of 12–15 repetitions with 90 sec rest periods and 3 sets of 8–10 repetitions with 120 sec rest periods, respectively. Given the relationship between training volume and hypertrophy [29], betaine may have positively impacted muscle growth by promoting a greater training load over a series of subsequent workouts.

The improvements in bench press work capacity differ from previous studies where betaine did not improve single-set repetitions to fatigue at 75% [3] or 3 sets of repetitions to fatigue at 85% 1 RM [2]. In contrast, betaine improved work capacity for 10 sets of repetitions to fatigue at 50% 1 RM [4]. Given improved work capacity with higher volume resistance training prescriptions, and the lack of improvement during micro-cycle 2 which imposed less of a metabolic demand (4 sets of 4–6

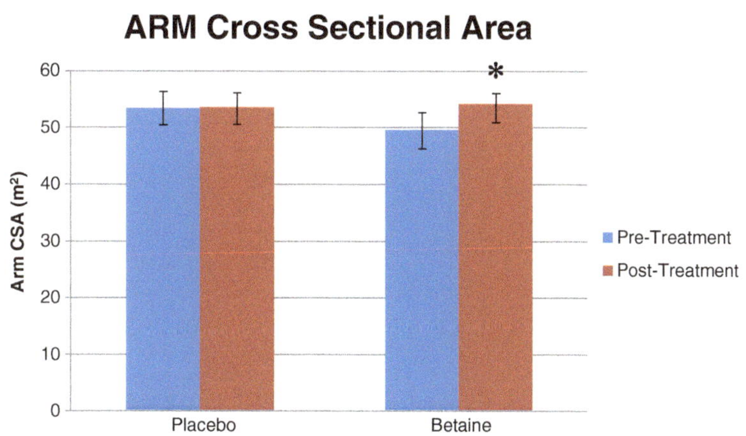

Figure 3 Bar graph for arm cross sectional area (cm²) for placebo (n = 12) and betaine (n = 11) for pre- and post-treatment.
Note: * = Significantly (p < .05) different than pre-treatment.

Table 5 Changes in body composition for placebo (n = 12) and betaine (n = 11) for pre- and post-treatment

	Pre	Post	Δ	*P*
Body Fat (%)				
Betaine	17.5 ± 8.3	14.3 ± 5.7	−3.2 ± 2.5	.01
Placebo	16.4 ± 8.1	16.6 ± 8.2	0.2 ± 2.7	.82
Lean Body Mass (kg)				
Betaine	69.5 ± 8.8	71.2 ± 7.9	2.4 ± 2.6	.01
Placebo	74.2 ± 9.1	74.5 ± 9.4	0.3 ± 2.6	.68
Fat Mass (kg)				
Betaine	15.0 ± 7.9	12.1 ± 5.4	−2.9 ± 2.0	.01
Placebo	14.8 ± 8.0	15.1 ± 8.5	0.3 ± 2.3	.68

repetitions with 3 min rest), it is likely that betaine poses the most ergogenic potential in resistance training exercise protocols that impose higher metabolic demands. Betaine is actively taken up by skeletal muscle during periods of stress, and may be ergogenic as an osmolyte by protecting sensitive metabolic pathways against cellular hypertonicity such as protein turnover, amino acid and ammonia metabolism, pH regulation, and gene expression [30]. Specifically, betaine maintains cellular hydration to protect myosin ATPase and myosin heavy chain proteins against denaturation by urea [31]. Moreover, the affinity of troponin for Ca^{2+} and thus force production, is negatively affected by reductions in protein hydration [32].

Contrary to the changes in arm CSA, no differences in leg CSA were found between groups. Similar results have been reported in animal studies investigating the effects of betaine supplementation on carcass cuts where betaine supplementation improved shoulder and butt, but not ham meat yield [9]. Additionally, changes in upper body muscle thickness occur at a greater magnitude and earlier than do the lower extremities [33]. Therefore, it is possible that changes in thigh CSA may have occurred with a longer study period.

Although the back squat requires recruitment of the quadriceps femoris, it also has a high gluteal/hip requirement. Increases in muscle mass may have occurred predominantly in the gluteals as seen in animal studies, or the adaptations leading to greater back squat volume and 1 RM occurred separately from increased muscle CSA. Back squat work capacity increased for each group at each training micro-cycle; however, the betaine group improved nearly two-fold compared to placebo during micro-cycle three (4 sets of 4–6 repetitions with 3 min rest) which posed a higher neural and lower metabolic demand than the previous micro-cycles. These improvements in back squat work capacity contrasts previous results [34] whereby betaine did not improve mean or peak isokinetic power during 5 sets of 6 repetitions at 80% peak force. The improvements in work capacity at micro-cycle three but not micro-cycle one or two also contradict our hypothesis that betaine may be most ergogenic when combined with exercise protocols producing higher levels of metabolic stress. Given the improvement in bench press work capacity that also occurred at micro-cycle three but not two, and the lack of improvement with only 2 weeks of supplementation [2,4], it may also be that the effects of increased intramuscular betaine manifest over a longer period of time, and therefore require at least a 4–6 week ingestion period.

There were no differences between groups for back squat 1 RM improvements, and despite increases in bench press training volume with betaine, bench press 1 RM did not improve. This contrasts previous reports [2], and may be partially explained by difference in subject training status. Lee et al. employed recreationally trained

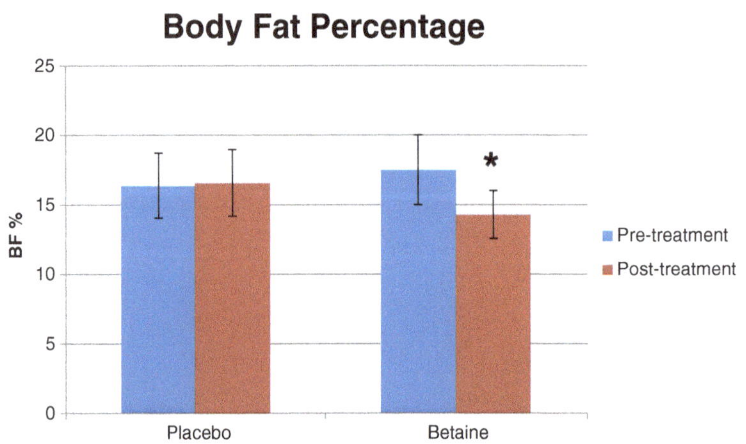

Figure 4 Bar graph for body fat percentage for placebo (n = 12) and betaine (n = 11) for pre- and post-treatment. Note: Significantly ($p < .05$) different than pre-treatment.

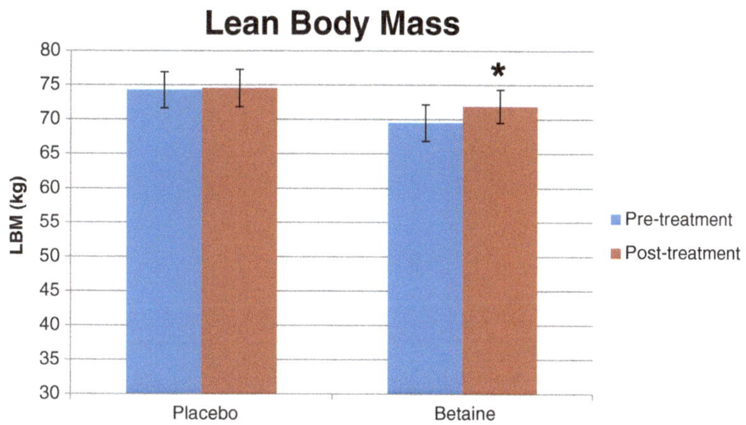

Figure 5 Bar graph for lean body mass (kg) for placebo (n = 12) and betaine (n = 11) for pre- and post-treatment. Note: Significantly ($p < .05$) different than pre-treatment.

subjects, whereas subjects in the present study averaged 4.8 years of training experience. The ability to make large performance gains, termed the "window of adaptation" [35], decreases with training experience. The "window of adaptation" was likely smaller for the subjects in the present study, thus reducing the ability to detect changes in strength. Finally, the primary aim of this study was to evaluate the effects of betaine on muscle growth; thus, the training program utilized was selected because it provided the greatest stimulation for hypertrophy. Given the high training status of the subjects, a strength concentrated program (i.e.: 4–6 sets of 1–3 repetitions) may have been needed to induce further improvements in bench press and back squat 1 RM with betaine supplementation.

There was a trend ($p = .07$) toward an increased vertical jump with betaine supplementation. The positive trend in the present study and improvements reported by Lee et al. [2] differs from the results reported by other researchers where vertical jump did not increase with betaine [3,4]. Variances in training prescription may account for these

Table 6 Changes in vertical jump (cm), Back squat 1RM (kg), and Bench press 1RM (kg) for Placebo (n = 12) and Betaine (n = 11) for pre- and post-treatment

	Pre	Post	Δ	P
Vertical Jump				
Betaine	68.1 ± 8.4	68.8 ± 8.4	0.8 ± 3.3	.45
Placebo	65.5 ± 10.4	63.0 ± 9.9	−2.5 ± 4.0	.09
Bench Press				
Betaine	118.2 ± 19.3	120.0 ± 20.3	1.8 ± 4.3	.20
Placebo	137.7 ± 25.0	140.0 ± 24.5	2.3 ± 6.0	.31
Back Squat				
Betaine	148.6 ± 26.7	151.4 ± 26.4	2.7 ± 4.5*	.09
Placebo	159.1 ± 38.8	164.5 ± 38.1	5.5 ± 4.0	.01

* Non Significant Time × Treatment Interaction: $p = .18$.

discrepancies. In Lee et al. and the present study subjects were assigned standardized training between testing sessions, whereas subjects in Hoffman et al. [4] and Trepanowski et al. [3] were not. Because detections in power improvements are compromised when power movements are not a regular part of training [34], future researchers should include exercises that train muscular contractile velocity when investigating the effects of betaine supplementation on power output.

We hypothesized that subjects would have high urinary HCTL values due to reduced Hcy transmethylational capacity; however, the results did not support this hypothesis. The normal range for urinary HCTL is .011-.473 nmol/mL [24]. Mean pretreatment HCTL was .028 nmol/mL (± .02 nnmol/mL), which suggests that the subjects began the study with low HCTL levels. Betaine supplementation attenuated the rise in HCTL observed in placebo at weeks 2 and 4, but did not appear to reduce HCTL values. Many subjects moved from the campus dormitories to live with their parents for the summer. It is possible that subjects had access to foods higher in protein quality and richer in fats and cholesterol than when living on campus, and this led to the increase in HCTL. Increases in dietary fat and cholesterol have been shown to increase plasma Hcy [36] as 3 Hcy are produced during the methylation of phosphatidylethanolamine in very low density lipoprotein synthesis. Thus, higher methionine and fat intakes may have increased Hcy generation, leading to higher levels of HCTL. Given the ability of betaine to increase Hcy transmethylation, it is possible that betaine supplementation attenuated the dietary induced rise in HCTL.

HCTL decreased in both groups between week 4 and week 6, although there was a trend for a reduction in HCTL when comparing week 6 to baseline with betaine and not placebo. While subjects were instructed to maintain the same diet throughout the study, many

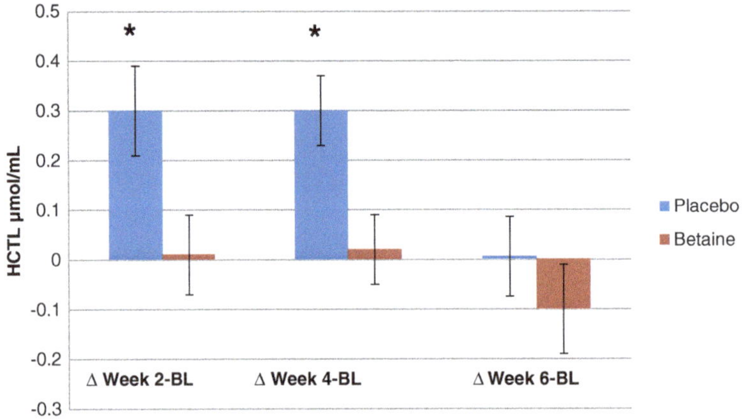

Figure 6 Changes in urinary homocysteine thiolactone values for placebo (n = 12) and Betaine (n = 11) between baseline and three time intervals. Note: * = Significantly (p < .05) different than betaine.

foods rich in betaine and folate come into season in June including spinach (0.3 mg/cup folate) and collard greens (0.2 mg/cup folate), and the consumption of two-three servings of folate rich food per day will reduce Hcy by 20% [37]. Because the start of June corresponded with week 4 of the study, it is possible that the consumption of local greens and the resultant increase in folate consumption may have reduced HCTL values in week 6.

Based on the small differences in HCTL changes, betaine supplementation may have impacted body composition via other mechanisms. Betaine has been shown to elevate plasma GH and IGF-1, and increase Akt phosphorylation in human skeletal muscle [38]. In mice betaine improves insulin sensitivity by restoring activation of IRS1 and the subsequent phosphorylation of PI3K/Akt by 50-100% in a concentration-dependent manner [39]. Thus, it is possible that by elevating anabolic hormones and enhancing downstream cellular signaling, betaine may have improved muscle protein synthesis, thus leading to an increase in lean mass. Finally, because betaine is a powerful osomylte, the increases in lean mass may have been due to cellular swelling without an appreciable increase in myofibril protein accretion.

Table 7 Changes in urinary homocysteine thiolactone (nmol/mL) for Placebo (n = 12) and Betaine (n = 11) between baseline and three time intervals

	Concentration	Δ From baseline	*P*
	Baseline		
Betaine	.037 ± .024*	NA	NA
Placebo	.019 ± .018	NA	NA
	Week 2		
Betaine	.038 ± .02	.001 ± .02	.95
Placebo	.049 ± .03	.029 ± .01	.01
	Week 4		
Betaine	.039 ± .01	.002 ± .01	.74
Placebo	.048 ± .02	.029 ± .01	.01
	Week 6		
Betaine	.027 ± .03	-.024 ± .03	.29
Placebo	.026 ± .02	.011 ± .03	.48

* Not significantly different than placebo at baseline: $p = .06$.

Limitations

The MD method for estimating muscle CSA presents a potential limitation when interpreting the limb CSA results of the present study. The *SEE* for the MD method is 3.25 cm^2. In the present study, the betaine group increased arm CSA by 4.6 cm^2 compared to a 0.1 cm^2 decrease with placebo. The difference in change for thigh CSA between betaine and placebo was 2.7 and 1.4 cm^2, respectively. It is possible that a non-significant difference in arm CSA change or a significant difference in thigh CSA change may have been observed if CSA was measured differently. Future studies examining the effects of betaine on muscle CSA change should utilize an analysis with a lower *SEE*.

Caution should also be taken when interpreting the HCTL results. The primary aim in the present study was to determine the effectiveness of betaine supplementation to improve strength and body composition in weight trained males. A secondary aim was investigate if a relationship between changes in HCTL values and body composition or performance existed. Because improvements in strength were reported in previous studies without controlling for micronutrients [2,4], subjects were instructed to consume a similar quantity and quality of foods throughout the study to control for energy and protein intake. Because subject diets were not analyzed for micronutrients, it is possible that dietary fluctuations in folate, betaine, or other B-vitamin consumption occurred and influenced urinary HCTL. Future studies should provide standard control meals and/or analyze micronutrient intake to investigate clinical relationships between betaine supplementation and HCTL.

Conclusions

In summary, the major findings of the present study are that 6 weeks of betaine supplementation improved body composition, muscle size, work capacity, attenuated a rise in HCTL, tended to improve power, but not strength in resistance trained men. Further work is warranted to confirm any role of HCTL on body composition compared to other mechanisms like lipogenic enzymatic activity, growth hormones, cellular signaling, or gene expression. Betaine attenuated an increase in urinary HCTL; however, because strength trained men in this study had low baseline HCTL betaine likely affected body composition via another mechanism. HCTL has been implicated in vascular disease [40], insulin resistance [13], diabetic retinopathy [41], seizures, and Alzheimer's disease [42]. Thus, future investigations are needed to evaluate the clinical ability of betaine to reduce HCTL in at risk populations with elevated Hcy.

Competing interests

DuPont Nutrition & Health (Tarrytown, NY) provided funding for this project. SASC is employed by DuPont Nutrition & Health. All other authors declare they have no competing interests. All authors involved collected, analyzed, or interpreted results from this study. Publication of these findings should not be viewed as endorsement by the editorial board of the Journal of International Society of Sports Nutrition.

Authors' contributions

JMC was the primary investigator, designed the study, obtained grant funds, supervised subject recruitment, data acquisition, data specimen collection, and manuscript preparation. MWR, RG, and HJ performed data specimen analysis. JMC was primarily responsible for writing the manuscript. TM, RW, SASC, and VP made substantial contributions to manuscript writing and preparation. All authors read and approved the final manuscript.

Author details

[1]Department of Kinesiology, Recreation, and Sport Studies, Coastal Carolina University, Conway, SC, USA. [2]Department of Environmental Chemistry, University of Lodz, Pomorska 163, 90-236, Lodz, Poland, USA. [3]Institute of Bioorganic Chemistry, Polish Academy of Sciences, Poznan, Department of Biochemistry and Biotechnology, Life Sciences University, Poznan, NJ, Poland. [4]UNDMJ-New Jersey Medical School, Newark, NJ, USA. [5]Department of Exercise Science and Sport Studies, Springfield College, Springfield, MA, USA. [6]DuPont Nutrition & Health, Tarrytown, NY, USA.

References

1. Craig SAS: **Betaine in human nutrition.** *Am J Clin Nutr* 2004, **80:**539–549.
2. Lee EC, Maresh CM, Kraemer WJ, Yamamoto LM, Hatfield DL, Bailey BL, Armstrong LE, Volek JS, McDermott BP, Craig SA: **Ergogenic effects of betaine supplementation on strength and power performance.** *J Int Soc Sports Nutr* 2010, **7:**27.
3. Hoffman JR, Ratamess NA, Kang J, Rashti SL, Faigenbaum AD: **Effect of betaine supplementation on power performance and fatigue.** *J Int Soc Sports Nutr* 2009, **6:**7.
4. Trepanowski JF, Farney TM, McCarthy CG, Schilling BK, Craig SA, Bloomer RJ: **The effects of chronic betaine supplementation on exercise performance, skeletal muscle oxygen saturation and associated biochemical parameters in resistance trained men.** *J Strength Cond Res* 2011, **25:**3461–3471.
5. Del Favero S, Roschel H, Artioli G, Ugrinowitsch C, Tricoli V, Costa A, Barroso R, Negrelli AL, Otaduy MC, da Costa Leite C, Lancha-Junior AH, Gualano B: **Creatine but not betaine supplementation increases muscle phosphorylcreatine content and strength performance.** *Amino Acids* 2011.
6. Schwab U, Törrönen A, Toppinen L, Alfthan G, Saarinen M, Aro A, Uusitupa M: **Betaine supplementation decreases plasma homocysteine concentrations but does not affect body weight, body composition, or resting energy expenditure in human subjects.** *Am J Clin Nutr* 2002, **76:**961–967.
7. Huang QC, Xu ZR, Han XY, Li WF: **Effect of betaine on growth hormone pulsatile secretion and serum metabolites in finishing pigs.** *J Anim Physiol Anim Nutr* 2007, **91:**85–90.
8. Huang Q, Xu Z, Han X, Li W: **Effect of dietary betaine supplementation on lipogenic enzyme activities and fatty acid synthase mRNA expression in finishing pigs.** *Anim Feed Sci Technol* 2008, **140:**365–375.
9. Matthews JO, Southern LL, Higbie AD, Persica MA, Bidner TD: **Effects of betaine on growth, carcass characteristics, pork quality, and plasma metabolites of finishing pigs.** *J Anim Sci* 2001, **79:**722–728.
10. Garcia MM, Guéant-Rodriguez R-M, Pooya S, Brachet P, Alberto J-M, Jeannesson E, Maskali F, Gueguen N, Marie P-Y, Lacolley P, Herrmann M, Juillière Y, Malthiery Y, Guéant J-L: **Methyl donor deficiency induces cardiomyopathy through altered methylation/acetylation of PGC-1α by PRMT1 and SIRT1.** *J Pathol* 2011, **225:**324–335.
11. Li Y, Jiang C, Xu G, Wang N, Zhu Y, Tang C, Wang X: **Homocysteine upregulates resistin production from adipocytes in vivo and in vitro.** *Diabetes* 2008, **57:**817–827.
12. Chwatko G, Boers GHJ, Strauss KA, Shih DM, Jakubowski H: **Mutations in methylenetetrahydrofolate reductase or cystathionine beta-synthase gene, or a high-methionine diet, increase homocysteine thiolactone levels in humans and mice.** *Journal Fed Am Soc Exp Biol* 2007, **21:**1707–1713.
13. Najib S, Sánchez-Margalet V: **Homocysteine thiolactone inhibits insulin-stimulated DNA and protein synthesis: possible role of mitogen-activated protein kinase (MAPK), glycogen synthase kinase-3 (GSK-3) and p70 S6K phosphorylation.** *J Mol Endocrinol* 2005, **34:**119–126.
14. Jakubowski H: **Pathophysiological consequences of homocysteine excess.** *J Nutr* 2006, **136:**1741–1749.
15. Williams KT, Schalinske KL: **New insights into the regulation of methyl group and homocysteine metabolism.** *J Nutr* 2007, **137:**311–314.
16. Kleiner SM, Bazzarre TL, Litchford MD: **Metabolic profiles, diet, and health practices of championship male and female bodybuilders.** *J Am Diet Assoc* 1990, **90:**962–967.
17. Ritti-Dias RM, Avelar A, Salvador EP, Cyrino ES: **Influence of previous experience on resistance training on reliability of one-repetition maximum test.** *J Strength Cond Res* 2011, **25:**1418–1422.
18. Forsyth HL, Sinning WE: **The anthropometric estimation of body density and lean body weight of male athletes.** *Med Sci Sports Exerc* 1973, **5:**174–180.
19. Brozek J, Grande F, Anderson JT, Keys A: **Densitometric analysis of body composition: revision of some quantitative assumptions.** *Ann NY Acad Sci* 1963, **110:**113–140.
20. DeFreitas JM, Beck TW, Stock MS, Dillon MA, Kasishke PR: **An examination of the time course of training-induced skeletal muscle hypertrophy.** *Eur J Appl Physiol* 2011, **111:**2785–2790.
21. Moritani T, DeVries HA: **Neural factors versus hypertrophy in the time course of muscle strength gain.** *Am J Phys Med* 1979, **58:**115–130.
22. DeFreitas JM, Beck TW, Stock MS, Dillon MA, Sherk VD, Stout JR, Cramer JT: **A comparison of techniques for estimating training-induced changes in muscle cross-sectional area.** *J Strength Cond Res* 2010, **24:**2383–2389.
23. Lander J: **Maximum based on reps.** *J Strength Cond Res* 1985, **6:**60–61.
24. Chwatko G, Jakubowski H: **The determination of homocysteine-thiolactone in human plasma.** *Anal Biochem* 2005, **337:**271–277.
25. Głowacki R, Bald E, Jakubowski H: **An on-column derivatization method for the determination of homocysteine-thiolactone and protein N-linked homocysteine.** *Amino Acids* 2011, **41:**187–194.
26. Jakubowski H: **The determination of homocysteine-thiolactone in biological samples.** *Anal Biochem* 2002, **308:**112–119.
27. Monteiro AG, Aoki MS, Evangelista AL, Alveno DA, Monteiro GA, Piçarro I da C, Ugrinowitsch C: **Nonlinear periodization maximizes strength gains in split resistance training routines.** *J Strength Cond Res* 2009, **23:**1321–1326.

28. Spineti J, de Salles BF, Rhea MR, Lavigne D, Matta T, Miranda F, Fernandes L, Simão R: **Influence of exercise order on maximum strength and muscle volume in nonlinear periodized resistance training.** *J Strength Cond Res* 2010, **24:**2962–2969.
29. Schoenfeld BJ: **The mechanisms of muscle hypertrophy and their application to resistance training.** *J Strength Cond Res* 2010, **24:**2857–2872.
30. Häussinger D: **The role of cellular hydration in the regulation of cell function.** *Biochem J* 1996, **313**(3):697–710.
31. Ortiz-Costa S, Sorenson MM, Sola-Penna M: **Betaine protects urea-induced denaturation of myosin subfragment-1.** *FEBS J* 2008, **275:**3388–3396.
32. Suarez MC, Machado CJV, Lima LMTR, Smillie LB, Pearlstone JR, Silva JL, Sorenson MM, Foguel D: **Role of hydration in the closed-to-open transition involved in Ca2+ binding by troponin C.** *Biochemistry* 2003, **42:**5522–5530.
33. Abe T, DeHoyos DV, Pollock ML, Garzarella L: **Time course for strength and muscle thickness changes following upper and lower body resistance training in men and women.** *Eur J Appl Physiol* 2000, **81:**174–180.
34. Hoffman JR, Ratamess NA, Kang J, Gonzalez AM, Beller NA, Craig SAS: **Effect of 15 days of betaine ingestion on concentric and eccentric force outputs during isokinetic exercise.** *J Strength Cond Res* 2011, **25:**2235–2241.
35. Newton RU, Kraemer WJ: **Developing explosive muscular power: implications for a mixed methods training strategy.** *J Strength Cond Res* 1994, **16:**20–31.
36. Verhoef P: **Homocysteine–an indicator of a healthy diet?** *Am J Clin Nutr* 2007, **85:**1446–1447.
37. Olthof MR, Verhoef P: **Effects of betaine intake on plasma homocysteine concentrations and consequences for health.** *Curr Drug Metab* 2005, **6:**15–22.
38. Apicella JM, Lee EC, Bailey BL, Saenz C, Anderson JM, Craig SAS, Kraemer WJ, Volek JS, Maresh CM: **Betaine supplementation enhances anabolic endocrine and Akt signaling in response to acute bouts of exercise.** *Eur J Appl Physiol* 2012. In Press.
39. Jakubowski H: **The pathophysiological hypothesis of homocysteine thiolactone-mediated vascular disease.** *J Physiol Pharmacol* 2008, **59**(Suppl 9):155–167.
40. Kathirvel E, Morgan K, Nandgiri G, Sandoval BC, Caudill MA, Bottiglieri T, French SW, Morgan TR: **Betaine improves nonalcoholic fatty liver and associated hepatic insulin resistance: a potential mechanism for hepatoprotection by betaine.** *Am J Gastrointestinal Liver Physiol* 2010, **299:**1068–1077.
41. Barathi S, Angayarkanni N, Pasupathi A, Natarajan SK, Pukraj R, Dhupper M, Velpandian T, Muralidharan C, Sivashanmugham M: **Homocysteinethiolactone and paraoxonase: novel markers of diabetic retinopathy.** *Diabetes care* 2010, **33:**2031–2037.
42. Borowczyk K, Shih DM, Jakubowski H: **Metabolism and neurotoxicity of homocysteine thiolactone in mice: evidence for a protective role of paraoxonase 1.** *J Alzheimers Dis* 2012, **30:**225–231.

The effect of an acute antioxidant supplementation compared with placebo on performance and hormonal response during a high volume resistance training session

James Ackerman[1], Tom Clifford[2], Lars R McNaughton[3] and David J Bentley[4*]

Abstract

Antioxidant supplementation is known to increase human endogenous antioxidant (AOX) capacity providing a means of blunting exercise induced reactive oxygen species (ROS). The purpose of this study was to compare the effects of a single acute dose of an AOX (vs blinded placebo) on muscle contractile performance and hormonal responses to a single bout of lower limb 'hypertrophic' resistance training (RT). Fifteen resistance trained subjects (age 23 ± 4 years: body mass 86 ± 6 kg) volunteered to participate in the study. Each subject attended the laboratory on three occasions, firstly to determine three repetition maximum (3-RM) isotonic strength in the back squat and perform a familiarisation of the experimental task. On the second/third visits subjects completed the hypertrophic training session (HTS) which consisted of six sets of 10 repetitions of 70% of a predicted 1 RM load (kg). Four hours prior to the HTS the subjects consumed 2 $ml \cdot kg^{-1}$ total body mass of either the placebo mixture or AOX supplement in a randomised order. Work completed during the strength training session was completed with equipment that had an integrated linear force transducer (Gymaware system, Kinetic Performance Technology, Canberra, Australia). During the placebo trials concentric mean power significantly ($p < 0.05$) decreased from sets 1–6. Accumulated power output during the AOX HTS was 6746 ± 5.9 W which was significantly greater compared to the placebo HTS of 6493 ± 17.1 W ($p < 0.05$, ES'r = 0.99). Plasma growth hormone (GH) concentration was significantly less immediately following AOX supplementation (6.65 ± 1.84 vs 16.08 ± 2.78 $ng \cdot ml^{-1}$; $p < 0.05$, ES'r = 0.89). This study demonstrates ingestion of an AOX cocktail prior to a single bout of resistance training improved muscle contractile performance and modulated the GH response following completion of the resistance exercise. Future studies should explore the mechanisms associated with the performance modification and specific muscle adaptations to AOX supplementation in conjunction with heavy RT.

Keywords: Fatigue, Ergogenic, Response, Anabolic, Exercise

Background

Reactive oxygen species (ROS) have been implicated as one of the causes of skeletal muscle fatigue during both aerobic and anaerobic exercise [1]. Although small increases in exercise induced ROS are important for stimulating cellular growth and maximising muscular force production [2,3], excessive accumulation leads to a pro-oxidant environment which can damage DNA, lipid and protein membranes [4,5]. Cellular damage may also impair cross-bridge cycling during skeletal muscle contraction and accelerate the onset of fatigue [2,6,7]. This is supported by previous work suggesting that a bout of resistance training induces an excessive increase in ROS production which could be implicated in the reduction in skeletal muscle force generating capacity observed during exercise [4,8,9].

To maximise gains in muscular hypertrophy an RT session would typically involve exercising at a moderate intensity, defined as lifting a load between 65-85% of an individual's one repetition maximum (RM), and using a

* Correspondence: david.bentley@adelaide.edu.au
[4]Human Exercise Performance Laboratory, School of Medical Sciences, University of Adelaide, Adelaide 5005, South Australia
Full list of author information is available at the end of the article

high volume, typically 3–6 sets of 6–15 repetitions of the exercise [10]. Goldfarb and colleagues [8] found significant increases in the plasma ROS markers malondialdehyde (MDH) and protein carbonyls (PC) following arm flexor exercise involving four sets of a 12 repetition maximum (RM) load. Similar results have also been found for lower body resistance exercise where plasma measures of oxidised gluthanione (GSSG) and protein oxidation were elevated following 30 min of sub-maximal squatting exercise [4]. The primary cause of RT induced oxidative damage appears to result from increased xanthine and nicotinamide adenine dinucleotide phosphate (NADPH) oxidase production, together with ischemia–reperfusion which results in an increase in xanthine oxidase (XO) and peroxynitrite [9,11,12]. Xanthine oxidase production appears to be a primary cause of oxidative stress during vigorous exercise [13], and plasma concentrations have been shown to increase dramatically after performing an RT session [14]. Other sources such as a decrease in intracellular pH, lactate accumulation and sarcomere disruption can also contribute to RT induced ROS production [4,2].

It has been suggested that a supplementation regime of antioxidants could reinforce the body's endogenous antioxidant system providing a means of blunting exercise induced ROS molecules [15,16]. Several studies have demonstrated that AOX supplementation can minimise damage to cellular structures caused by RT [8,17] and also help maintain muscular force [18] during isometric maximal contractions. However, there are also a number of studies that have found no benefit of AOX supplementation on markers of oxidative stress or performance [19-21]. Differing exercise protocols, subjects and types/amounts of AOX supplements used, have been suggested as the cause of the inconsistency between findings [21]. It appears that RT protocols employing a higher volume and intensity invokes the greatest oxidative stress response, while there is some support for the effectiveness of Vitamins C and E and flavonoid supplements at attenuating acute muscle injury in untrained individuals [21].

Most AOX studies have focused on the effects of vitamin C and/or E supplementation to attenuate the oxidative stress caused by RT [8,18-20]. There has been little focus on plant polyphenols, which have potent antioxidants qualities [22,23]. Pycnogenol (PYC) is a particularly effective antioxidant polyphenol, comprised of several proanthocyanidins and phenolic acids and has been shown to blunt elevated ROS [24,25], increase growth hormone (GH) secretion [26] and stimulate muscle blood flow [27]. It has also previously been shown that the supplement Lactaway©, containing PYC, acutely improves endurance cycle performance without improving AOX capacity [28,29]. There are no studies that have yet assessed the effects of Lactaway© containing PYC on RT performance and the associated bio-molecular responses. Hence, this study aimed to assess the effect of a PYC mixture, on performance during lower limb 'hypertrophic' RT (HRT) and the resulting acute endocrine, physiological and oxidative stress response.

Methods

Subjects

Fifteen healthy subjects volunteered to participate in the study (age 23 ± 4 yr: body mass 86 ± 6 kg: height 179.4 ± 6.1 cm). Each subject had been resistance training for a minimum of 2 yr prior to recruitment for the study. All the subjects were familiar with the back squat exercise (BS) and could perform the activity satisfactorily from a technique perspective. Assessment was carried out by the primary researcher who was a certified strength and conditioning coach. Each subject completed a consent form and pre activity screening questionnaire to identify any musculoskeletal and orthopaedic problems that could affect performance of the exercise. The study gained approval from the University of New South Wales, Human Research Ethics Committee.

Study design

A double blind repeated measures design was employed where the subjects ingested either the AOX treatment or a placebo version prior to completing the training session. In the 48 h leading up to these sessions the subjects were instructed to refrain from intense physical exercise in order to eliminate residual fatigue. The supplements were provided using a randomized and counterbalanced design. The subjects visited the laboratory on three occasions, firstly to record their physical characteristics and determine their 3 RM BS which was used to predict 1RM strength [1.06 × 3RM (kg) [30]]. On their second and third visits subjects completed the hypertrophic training session (HTS) which consisted of six sets of 70% of 1RM. The BS was performed with an Olympic barbell using a power rack (Body Maker, Nantong, China). The depth of the squat was controlled by placing the safety spot inserts of the squat rack device just below of the level the barbell when subject's thighs were parallel to the ground. This acted as a feedback mechanism for the participant and researcher but participants were asked to refrain from "bouncing" on the parallel bars. The subjects were instructed to refrain from alcohol, foods with high AOX capacity and caffeine for 24 h prior to HTS. This information was in a document which was read to each subject prior to commencement of participation in the study. Subjects recorded their diet and were asked to replicate the same dietary intake 24 hrs prior to each session.

Preliminary measures and familiarisation

On the subjects' first visit, their body mass (kg) was measured using a balance beam (Weylux, England) and height (cm) with a stadiometer (Holtain Ltd). Subjects then undertook a warm on up on a cycle ergometer (Schroberer Rad MeBtechnik (SRM), Weldorf, Germany), cycling at 1 watt·kg^{-1} for five min. The determination of the 3RM was followed according to methods previously described [31]. Briefly, it required approximately four to six sets to determine the 3RM with progressively heavier loads per set. Three min rest was allowed between each set and the 3RM was determined as the load lifted three times and when no extra weight could be added. The 3RM was used to predict 1RM for each participant. After a five min break a squat session of 10 repetitions at 70% 1RM load for five sets was performed.

Experimental procedures and supplements

Four hours prior to the HTS the subjects consumed 2 ml·kg^{-1} body mass of either the placebo mixture or AOX supplement [Lactaway©, Away Australia Pty Ltd, Sydney, Australia] containing 2.4 g·L of PYC in a randomised order. The placebo and AOX mixtures tasted and appeared the same. The participants and researchers were not aware of which substance was supplement or placebo until after the completion of the study when details were released by an independent person. The placebo mixture contained the exact energy content (315 KJ) and constituents (pineapple pulp, molasses, sodium chloride, flavour, steviol glycosides, sodium benzoate, potassium sorbate) as the Lactaway© mixture (315 KJ) but it did not include any of the active AOX ingredient PYC.

After a brief cycling warm up, the subjects completed a warm up set consisting of 10 repetitions at 50% of the actual load to be used during the work sets. After a two min rest period the subjects performed the second warm up set at 80% of the load to be used during the work sets. After a three min rest period, subjects completed six sets, separated by 2 min rest periods. The subjects were instructed to lower the barbell under control (eccentric) and then verbally encouraged to "drive" the barbell upwards in as short as time possible (concentric). The squat training session lasted ~18 min. After the completion of each set the subjects were also asked their rate of perceived exertion (RPE) using the Borg scale [32]. Five microliter (μL) finger tip capillary blood samples were collected under standard aseptic procedures before, immediately after and twenty min post-exercise to analyse blood lactate (LT 1710 Lactate Pro, KDK Corporation, Shiga, Japan).

An integrated linear force transducer (Gymaware system, Kinetic Performance Technology, Canberra, Australia) was used to determine barbell displacement for each repetition and set completed. This system allows for the determination of concentric mean power (W), and concentric velocity (m·s) to be determined. The system was set up according to the manufacturer's guidelines and has been shown to provide a reliable (Coefficients of variation (CV) = 3.3%) and valid estimate of power during resistance training [33].

Blood collection and analysis

Venous blood was withdrawn via venepuncture before, immediately after and twenty min after the HTS. Blood was collected from a vein in the cubital fossa in ethylenediaminetetraacetic acid (EDTA) (10 ml tube) vacutainers (BD367863, NJ, USA). The samples were then centrifuged at 3000 rpm for 10 min, at 4°C. The plasma top layer was placed into Eppendorf tubes (Oldenburg, Germany) and snapped frozen and stored at −80°C until analysis.

Plasma GH, an indicator of the anabolic hormonal milieu during RT [34] was determined pre-exercise, immediately post-exercise and 20 min post-exercise. Plasma GH was assayed by a radio-immunoassay using a commercially available kit (human growth hormone ELISA DSL-10-1900, Diagnostic Systems Laboratories, Webster, USA). The assay was performed in duplicate as per the instructions from DSL and determined the levels of the 22 kDa GH isoform. The CV was less than 7% for the assays and the limit detection was 0.03 ng/ml.

Plasma cortisol (CORT) was measured as an indicator of the catabolic hormonal environment during RT [34], and was determined by a radio-immunoassay using a commercially available kit (cortisol ELISA DSL-10-2000, Diagnostic Systems Laboratories, Webster, USA). Plasma CORT was assayed pre-exercise, immediately post-exercise and 20 min post-exercise. The assay was performed in duplicate as per the instructions from DSL and the CV was less than 10%.

Xanthine oxidase (XO) was measured because it is involved in free radical production and its elevation contributes to oxidative stress [12,13]. The XO was assayed in duplicate using a commercially available kit (Invitrogen, Carlsbad, California, USA). Plasma was assayed pre-exercise and immediately post-exercise. The XO stock solution was used to construct a standard curve. The standards and serum were pipetted into a high binding enzyme immunoassay (Caymen Chemical Co. Ann Arbor, MI USA) 96 well plate. The plasma samples were diluted 1 fold by the placement of a buffer solution, and the XO reaction was started when a composition of amplex red, horseradish peroxidase, hypoxanthine and buffer solution was added to each well. The plate was incubated at 37°C for 30 min and the absorbance was read at 550 nm using a PolarStar Galaxy plate reader (BMG Laboratory Technologies, Offenburg, Germany).

Statistical analysis

A two way repeated measures analysis of variance (ANOVA) was used to evaluate changes over time and condition for power and velocity along with lactate, RPE, GH, CORT and XO. If a significant F value was achieved the Bonferroni post hoc test was performed. The level of significance was set at $p \leq 0.05$. All data was analysed using SPSS for Windows version 16. Data are presented as mean ± standard error of the mean (SEM). Where relevant effect size ratios (ES'r) were calculated using Cohens *d* [35]. An ES'r of ≥0.5 was considered to display a moderate effect and ≥0.8 a large effect.

Results

The pre to post HTS, blood lactate concentrations (B_{lac}) increased significantly after both AOX supplementation; 1.23 ± 0.08 to 7.68 ± 3.01 $mmol \cdot l^{-1}$ ($p < 0.05$) and placebo supplementation; 1.79 ± 0.30 $mmol \cdot l^{-1}$ to 8.11 ± 2.98 $mmol \cdot l^{-1}$ ($p < 0.05$). Blood lactate continued to be significantly elevated twenty min post-exercise for both groups, but there was no significant difference in B_{lac} levels between the two conditions at any time point ($p > 0.05$). The RPE was significantly increased in both groups for sets three to six compared to set one. There were however no significant differences in RPE between the AOX and placebo conditions at any point during the HTS ($p < 0.05$).

The concentric mean power and velocity are presented in Figures 1 and 2 respectively. Following AOX supplementation concentric mean power remained consistent across all six sets of the HTS. However, during the placebo trials concentric mean power significantly decreased from sets 1–6. During the placebo trial concentric mean power was significantly lower in comparison to each set in the AOX condition, with sets five and six having the greatest decrease ($p < 0.05$, ES'r = 0.52). Similarly average velocity during the AOX was higher compared to placebo. Accumulated power output during the AOX HTS was 6746 ± 5.9 W which was significantly greater compared to the placebo HTS of 6493 ± 17.1 W ($p < 0.05$, ES'r = 0.99).

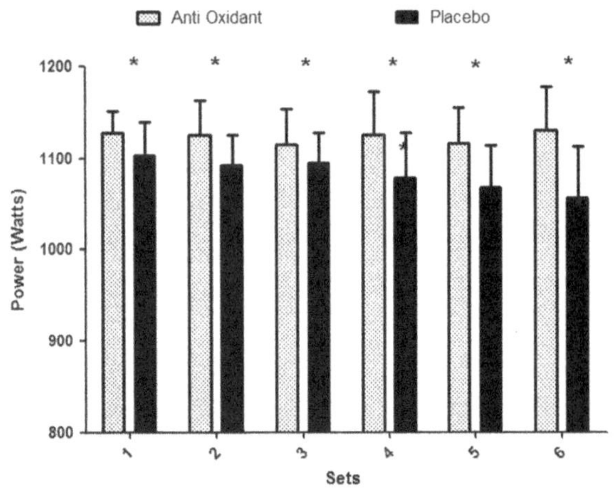

Figure 1 Concentric power output for each set during the resistance training session (HTS) when AOX or placebo was ingested (mean ± SEM). Statistically significant difference (*$p < 0.05$ and **$p < .001$) between the AOX and placebo trials.

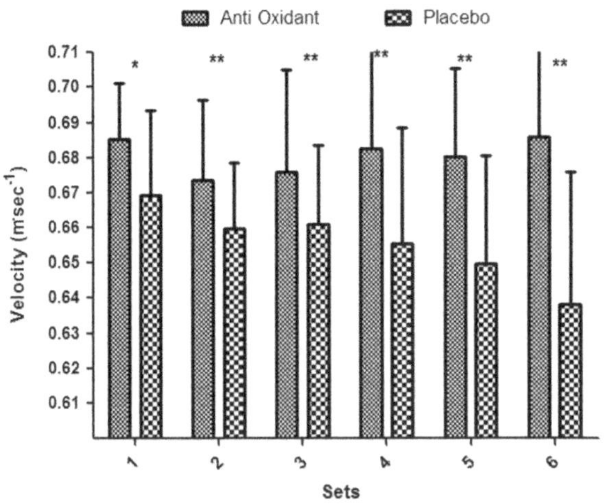

Figure 2 Velocity (m.s) during each set of the resistance training session (HTS) when AOX or placebo was ingested (mean ± SEM). Statistically significant difference (*$p < 0.05$ and **$p < .001$) between the AOX and placebo trials.

The HTS resulted in a significantly elevated XO in both the placebo (pre: 11.05 ± 0.94 to immediately post: 15.47 ± 1.11 $mU \cdot ml^{-1}$) and AOX condition's (pre: 9.16 ± 0.93 to immediately post: 11.2 ± 2.48 $mU \cdot ml^{-1}$, $p < 0.05$). The difference between the two conditions was not statistically significant ($p > 0.05$). Circulating GH levels increased significantly after both trials, however the increase was significantly less immediately following AOX supplementation; 6.65 ± 1.84 $ng \cdot ml^{-1}$ compared to the placebo trials;16.08 ± 2.78 $ng \cdot ml^{-1}$ ($p < 0.05$, ES'r = 0.89). GH continued to be significantly elevated 20 min after the HTS for both treatments, and was still significantly greater following the placebo trial in comparison to the AOX trial ($p < 0.05$) (Figure 3). Cortisol increased significantly immediately after the HTS following AOX and placebo supplementation to 567.25 ± 20.12 $nmol \cdot l^{-1}$ and 571.43 ± 18.77 $nmol \cdot l^{-1}$, respectively ($p < 0.05$). Cortisol was still significantly elevated 20 min post exercise for both treatments ($p < 0.05$) however there was no significant difference between the AOX and placebo HTS at any time point ($p < 0.05$).

Discussion

The primary aim of the present research was to assess the effect of a PYC mixture on performance during lower limb 'hypertrophic' RT and the resulting acute endocrine, physiological and oxidative stress response. It was found that in comparison to a placebo mixture, subjects were able to perform 3.75% more work (W), and

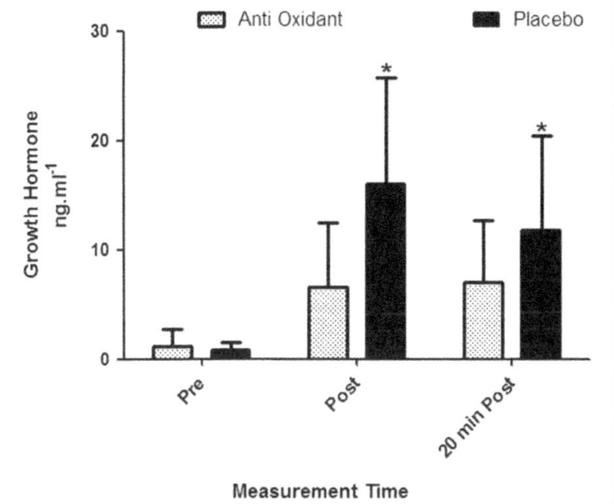

Figure 3 Growth hormone (GH) in response to the AOX and placebo HTS (mean ± SEM). Statistically significant difference (*$p < 0.05$) between the AOX and placebo trials.

generate greater mean concentric power and velocity throughout the HTS after consuming the AOX mixture. An additional aim was to establish the physiological, endocrine and oxidative stress response to a HTS. There were no significant differences between RPE, B_{lac}, CORT and XO between the two trials, however circulating GH levels was significantly reduced in the AOX trial compared to the placebo trial. This is the first study to demonstrate that an AOX mixture containing PYC can improve RT performance. There was a significant increase in B_{lac} levels immediately after both trials and 20 min post HTS from pre exercise values. The observed increase was similar to other RT protocols using high volume moderate loading intensity [36,37].

The attenuation of power decrement during the AOX trial agrees with previous studies that have shown that PYC AOX supplementation improves high intensity cycling and running performance [28,29]. This study was unique in that performance was monitored for each repetition and did not rely solely on the total volume for the session. Instead, concentric performance was measured by mean power output. The key finding from the performance data was that AOX supplementation was effective in attenuating the decrease in mean power which occurred in the placebo trial, meaning concentric power output was greater during the AOX trial (see Figure 1). During the placebo trial the mean power decrements per set ranged from 5% to 10% (specific data not shown). These observations are similar to the decrements observed by Baker and Newton [38], however their study employed a series of jump squats to elucidate a ROS response, and therefore comparisons between the two studies should be approached with caution.

The present study also found the oxidative stress response as measured by the marker XO was significantly increased after the HTS following both the placebo and AOX trials. This is similar to other studies which also observed an elevated XO response following strenuous exercise [13,39]. The significant rise in XO would suggest that the HTS in the present study invoked a substantial ROS response, which can lead to skeletal muscle injury and fatigue [1,39,40]. Indeed, reduced XO activity during RT has been linked to less oxidative damage and enhanced recovery from RT sessions [13]. It was therefore hypothesised that the AOX treatment would blunt the oxidative stress response, preserving skeletal muscle integrity and force production when performing strenuous RT such as BS exercise.

Yet, there was no significant difference in XO levels between the placebo and AOX trials, although a slight trend towards a reduction in XO following the AOX trials was observed ($p = 0.069$). There was also no difference in blood lactate concentration between the two conditions suggesting that differences in anaerobic fatigue were not the cause for the disparity in performance. This data suggests other mechanisms of muscular fatigue may have been involved in the performance changes observed. One possible mechanism is a decrease in Na+/K + ATPase pump activity [41]. A previous study found AOX supplementation in the form of N-acetylcysteine is effective in preserving Na+/K + ATPase activity during strenuous exercise, acting as a reduced thiol donor and promoting the regeneration of the endogenous AOX glutathione (GSH) [1,42]. Similarly, PYC supplementation has been shown to enhance GSH activity and decrease the levels of GSSG [43]. It is therefore possible that in the present study, the PYC based AOX supplement supported GSH levels which then lead to decreased thiol oxidation thus maintaining Na+/K + ATPase activity and attenuating muscular fatigue. Another possibility for the attenuation of muscular fatigue during the AOX trial may be a result of nitric oxide (NO) stimulated increased blood flow during exercise [44]. It has been repeatedly shown that PYC can enhance blood flow [23,25] and decrease platelet aggregation [45] which can decrease peripheral blood flow to contracting muscles during high intensity exercise [45]. At present it can only be speculated that these mechanisms were involved as GSH or muscular blood flow were not measured in this study. Further research with additional measures of oxidative stress is required to help determine the precise mechanisms involved in the performance improvements observed.

Cortisol increased significantly in both groups after the HTS and remained significantly elevated twenty min post exercise. However, there was no significant difference between the two groups at any time. Previous studies also found that similar RT protocols consisting of multiple set sessions with moderately high repetitions increases CORT secretion [34,46]. The catabolic activity of CORT may affect nitrogen balance after RT which in turn may hinder strength and/or MH development [47]. It would therefore be beneficial to attenuate CORT secretion during and after RT to avoid the deleterious effects that may interfere with training adaptations. At present, the effects of AOX supplementation on attenuating CORT and the underlying biochemical mechanisms involved is not well understood. Previous investigations with a similar design to the present study have produced mixed results. One study found positive results, where Vitamin C and E supplementation for 28 days significantly reduced post exercise increases in CORT following a lower body RT session. However, others agree with the present study, finding that an AOX treatment failed to mitigate the increase in CORT after a 90 min basketball training session [48] and a 90 min intermittent shuttle running protocol [49]. The discrepancy in results between the studies could be due to the type and duration of exercise sessions, and in particular the AOX supplementation type and dosage. Additional research should focus on using a greater dosage of PYC to further understand this compounds effects on CORT.

The GH response to the HTS was significantly affected by the AOX supplement. Immediately after the HTS the AOX group had a significantly lower GH response compared to the placebo group. This decreased circulating GH was also evident in the AOX group 20 min post exercise. This finding was unexpected as previous research showed PYC to be a potent secretagogue of GH in genetically engineered cells [26]. That the opposite occurred in this study is possibly related to the differing protocols and test subjects between the two, considering their findings were not observed in human subjects undertaking RT as in the present study. Another possible explanation is that GH secretion appears to be influenced by the degree of skeletal muscular fatigue induced by an exercise protocol. It has been demonstrated how increasing local muscular fatigue in the thigh by using forced exercise repetitions significantly increased GH response [50]. It's therefore possible that during the placebo trials participants' experienced greater levels of muscular fatigue, as evidenced by the reduced mean power output compared to the AOX trials, and thus leading to a greater GH response. Further research is needed to help determine this possibility and the potential role AOX supplementation has on GH secretion. Furthermore, as GH is an anabolic hormone its elevation during RT coupled with appropriate mechanical strain may be important for the process of muscular hypertrophy [51,52]. This would suggest that the GH results from this study indicate they may be undesirable in regards to promoting muscular hypertrophy. It is therefore of interest for future studies to examine whether this decreased circulating GH would affect muscular hypertrophy after a prolonged period of use or whether it acutely affects IGF-1 levels. Moreover, recent research suggests excessive AOX supplementation may hinder important physiological training adaptations [3,53]. This has prompted the suggestion that optimal oxidant content for maximal force production exists within the muscle [53]. These recent findings and the GH results in this study, highlight the need to further our understanding of the effect of AOX supplementation on training adaptations.

Conclusions

In conclusion, an acute dose of a PYC based AOX supplement enhanced lower body RT performance in trained males by improving mean concentric power, velocity and total work output. The mechanisms involved are still unclear considering oxidative stress response (measured as plasma XO) was not significantly reduced in the AOX treatment, as hypothesised. Future studies should incorporate further measures of oxidative stress, particularly GSH, and muscle blood flow which may help determine the biochemical and physiological mechanisms that led to the results in this study. Furthermore, GH secretion was significantly attenuated in the AOX trial compared to the placebo. The mechanisms that led to these results are not fully understood, but further research is required as GH secretion is involved in MH and strength development and its attenuation may negatively impact training adaptations.

Competing interests

The authors declare they have no competing interests.

Authors' contributions

DB and LRM conceived the concept for the investigation and contributed significantly to the drafting of the manuscript. JA was primary investigator in this study conducted the majority of testing and biochemical analysis. TC and DB assisted in data collection and provided a significant contribution to composition and review of the manuscript. All authors read and approved the final manuscript.

Author details

[1]Health and Exercise, School of Medical Sciences, University of New South Wales, Sydney, Australia. [2]Department of Exercise Science, University of Portsmouth, Portsmouth, UK. [3]Department of Sport and Physical Activity, Edge Hill University, Ormskirk, UK. [4]Human Exercise Performance Laboratory, School of Medical Sciences, University of Adelaide, Adelaide 5005, South Australia.

References

1. Ferreira LF, Reid MB: **Muscle-derived ROS and thiol regulation in muscle fatigue.** *J Appl Phys* 2008, **104:**853–860.
2. Finaud J, Lac G, Filaire E: **Oxidative stress relationship with exercise and training.** *Sports Med* 2006, **36:**327–358.
3. Peternelj TT, Coombes JS: **Antioxidant supplementation during exercise training beneficial or detrimental?** *Sports Med* 2011, **41:**1043–1069.

4. Bloomer RJ, Goldfarb AH, Wideman L, McKenzie MJ, Consitt LA: **Effects of acute aerobic and anaerobic exercise on blood markers of oxidative stress.** *J Strength Con Res* 2005, **19**:276–285.
5. Hoffman JR IMJ, Kang J, Maresh CM, Kraemer WJ, French D, Nioka S, Kime R, Rundell KW, Ratamess NA, Faigenbaum AD, Chance B: **Comparison of low- and high-intensity resistance exercise on lipid peroxidation: role of muscle oxygenation.** *J Strength Cond Res* 2007, **21**:118–122.
6. Powers SK, Nelson BW, Hudson MB: **Exercise-induced oxidative stress in humans: cause and consequences.** *Free Rad Bio Med* 2011, **51**:942–950.
7. Oh J, Shin Y, Yoon J, Kim SH, Shin H, Hwang HJ: **Effect of supplementation with *Ecklonia cava* polyphenol on endurance performance of college students.** *Int J of Sport Nutr Exerc Metab* 2010, **20**:72–79.
8. Goldfarb AH, Bloomer RJ, McKenzie MJ: **Combined antioxidant treatment effects on blood oxidative stress after eccentric exercise.** *Med Sci Sports Exerc* 2005, **37**:234–239.
9. Cross AR, Jones OT: **Enzymic mechanisms of superoxide production.** *Biochim Biophys Acta* 1991, **1057**:281–298.
10. Baechle TR, Earle RW, Wathen D: *Essentials of strength training and conditioning.* 3rd edition. Champaign, IL: Human Kinetics; 2008.
11. Koyama K, Kaya M, Ishigaki T, Tsujita J, Hori S, Seino T, Kasugai A: **Role of xanthine oxidase in delayed lipid peroxidation in rat liver induced by acute exhausting exercise.** *Eur J Appl Physiol Occup Physiol* 1999, **80**:28–33.
12. Pattwell D, Ashton T, Mcardle A, Griffiths RD, Jackson MJ: **Ischemia and reperfusion of skeletal muscle lead to the appearance of a stable lipid free radical in the circulation.** *Am J Physiol Heart Circ Physiol* 2003, **284**:2400–2404.
13. Vina J, Gimeno A, Sastre J, Desco C, Asensi M, Pallardo FV, Cuesta A, Ferrero JA, Terada LS, Repine JE: **Mechanism of free radical production in exhaustive exercise in humans and rats; role of xanthine oxidase and protection by allopurinol.** *IUBMB Life* 2009, **49**:539–44.
14. Volek JS, Kraemer WJ, Rubin MR, Gomez AL, Ratamess NA, Gaynor P: **L-Carnitine L-tartrate supplementation favourably affects markers of recovery from exercise stress.** *Am J Physiol Endocrinol Metab* 2002, **282**:474–482.
15. Powers SK, DeRuisseau KC, Quindry J, Hamilton KL: **Dietary antioxidants and exercise.** *J Sports Sci* 2004, **22**:81–94.
16. Powers SK, Smuder AJ, Kavazis AN, Hudson MB: **Experimental guidelines for studies designed to investigate the impact of antioxidant supplementation on exercise performance.** *Int J of Sport Nutr and Exerc Metab* 2010, **20**:2–14.
17. Bloomer RJ, Goldfarb AH: **Anaerobic exercise and oxidative stress: a review.** *Can J Appl Physiol* 2004, **29**:245–263.
18. Shafat A, Butler P, Jensen RL, Donnelly AE: **Effects of dietary supplementation with vitamins C and E on muscle function during and after eccentric performance in humans.** *Eur J Appl Physiol* 2004, **93**:196–202.
19. Childs A, Jacobs C, Kaminski T, Haliwell B, Leeuwenburgh C: **Supplementation with vitamin C and N-acetyl-cysteine increases oxidative stress in humans after an acute muscle injury induced by eccentric exercise.** *Free Radic Biol Med* 2001, **31**:745–753.
20. Viitalal PE, Newhouse IJ, Lavoie N, Gottardo C: **The effects of antioxidant vitamin supplementation on resistance exercise induced lipid peroxidation in trained and untrained subjects.** *Lipids Health Dis* 2004, **3**:14–22.
21. Bloomer RJ, Falvo MJ, Schilling BK, Smith WA: **Prior exercise and antioxidant supplementation: effect on oxidative stress and muscle injury.** *Jour Int Soc of Sports Nutr* 2007, **4**(9):9–19.
22. Scalbert A, Williamson G: **Dietary intake and bioavailability of polyphenols.** *J Nutr* 2000, **130**(8):2073–2085.
23. Chang AS, Yeong BY, Koh WP: **Symposium on Plant Polyphenols: Nutrition, Health and Innovations.** *Nutr Rev* 2009, **68**:246–252.
24. Slayback DL, Watson RR: **Bioflavonoids and Cardiovascular health: tea, red wine, cocoa and Pycnogenol.** *JANA* 2006, **9**:16–21.
25. D'Andrea G: **Pycnogenol: A blend of procyanidins with multifaceted therapeutic applications.** *Fitoterapia* 2010, **81**(7).724–736.
26. Buz'Zard AR, Peng Q, Lau BH: **Kyolic and Pycnogenol increase human growth hormone secretion in genetically-engineered keratinocytes.** *Growth Horm IGF Res* 2002, **12**:34–40.
27. Nishioka K, Hidaka T, Nakamura A, Umemura A, Jitsuiki D, Soga J, Chayama K, Yoshizumi M, Higashi Y: **Pycnogenol french maritime pine bark extract, augments endothelium-dependent vasodilation in humans.** *Hypertens Res* 2007, **30**:775–780.
28. Mach J, Midgley AW, Dank S, Grant RS, Bentley DJ: **The Effect of Antioxidant Supplementation on Fatigue during Exercise: Potential Role for NAD$^+$ (H).** *Nutrients* 2010, **2**:319–329.
29. Bentley DJ, Dank S, Coupland R, Midgley A, Spence I: **Acute antioxidant supplementation improves endurance performance in trained athletes.** *Res in Sports Med: An Int Jour* 2012, **20**:1–12.
30. Baker D: **The use of submaximal repetitions to predict maximal squat and bench press strength in trained athletes.** *Strength Cond. Coach* 1996, **3**:17–19.
31. Astorino TA, Rohmann RL, Firth K: **Effect of caffeine ingestion on one-repetition maximum muscular strength.** *Eur J Appl Physiol* 2008, **102**:127–132.
32. Borg G, Hassmen P, Lagerstrom M: **Perceived exertion related to heart rate and blood lactate during arm and leg exercise.** *Eur Jour Appl Phys Occ Phys* 1987, **56**:679–685.
33. Crewther BT, Kilduff LP, Cunningham DJ, Cook C, Owen N, Yang G-Z: **Validating two systems for estimating force and power.** *Int J Sports Med* 2011, **32**:254–258.
34. Kraemer WJ, Ratamess NA: **Hormonal responses and adaptations to resistance exercise and training.** *Sports Med* 2005, **35**:339–361.
35. Cohen J: *Statistical power analysis for the behavioral sciences.* 2nd edition. Hillsdale, NJ: Lawrence Earlbaum Associates; 1988.
36. Williams AG, Ismail AN, Sharma A, Jones DA: **Effects of resistance exercise volume and nutritional supplementation on anabolic and catabolic hormones.** *Eur J Appl Physiol* 2002, **86**:315–321.
37. Smilios I, Pilianidis T, Karamouzis M, Tokmakdis SP: **Hormonal responses after various resistance exercise protocols.** *Med Sci Sports Exerc* 2003, **35**:644–654.
38. Baker DG, Newton RU: **Change in power output across a high-repetition set of bench throws and jump squats in highly trained athletes.** *J Strength Cond Res* 2007, **21**:1007–1111.
39. Bloomer RJ, Smith WA: **Oxidative stress in response to aerobic and anaerobic power testing: influence of exercise training and carnitine supplementation.** *Res Sports Med* 2009, **17**:1–16.
40. Friedl HP, Smith DJ, Till GO, Thomson PD, Louis DS, Ward PA: **Ischemia-reperfusion in humans: appearance of xanthine oxidase activity.** *Am J Pathol* 1990, **136**:491–495.
41. Allen DG, Lamb GD, Westerblad H: **Impaired calcium release during fatigue.** *J Appl Physiol* 2008, **104**:296–305.
42. Sen CK: **Glutathione homeostasis in response to exercise training and nutritional supplements.** *Mol Cell Biochem* 1999, **196**:31–42.
43. Dvorakova M, Sivonova M, Trebaticka J, Skodacek I, Waczulikova I, Muchova J, Durackova Z: **The effect of polyphenolic extract from pine bark, Pycnogenol on the level of glutathione in children suffering from attention deficit hyperactivity disorder (ADHD).** *Redox Report* 2006, **11**:163–172.
44. Watson RR: **Pycnogenol and cardiovascular health.** *Ev-Based Integ Med*, **1**(1):27–32.
45. Li N, He S, Blomback M, Hjemdahl P: **Platelet activity, coagulation, and fibrinolysis during exercise in healthy males: effects of thrombin inhibition by argatroban and enoxaparin.** *Arterioscler Thromb Vasc Biol* 2007, **27**:407–413.
46. Hakkinen K, Pakarinen A: **Acute hormonal responses to two different fatiguing heavy-resistance protocols in male athletes.** *J Appl Physiol* 1993, **74**:882–887.
47. Bird SP, Tarpenning KM, Marino FE: **Independent and combined effects of liquid carbohydrate/essential amino acid ingestion on hormonal and muscular adaptations following resistance training in untrained men.** *Eur J Appl Physiol* 2006, **97**(2):225–238.
48. Galiano D, Tramullas A, Mora J, Navarro E, Schroder H: **Effects of alpha-tocopherol, beta-carotene and ascorbic acid on oxidative, hormonal and enzymatic exercise stress markers in habitual training activity of professional basketball players.** *Eur J Nutr* 2001, **40**:178–184.
49. Thomson D, Williams C, McGregor SJ, Nicholas CW, Mcardle F, Jackson MJ, Powell JR: **Prolonged vitamin C supplementation and recovery from demanding exercise.** *Int J Sport Nutr Exerc Metab* 2001, **11**:466–481.
50. Ahtiainen JP, Pakarinen A, Kraemer WJ, Hakkinen K: **Acute hormonal and neuromuscular responses and recovery to forced vs maximum repetitions multiple resistance exercises.** *Int J Sports Med* 2003, **24**:410–418.

51. McCall GE, Byrnes WC, Fleck SJ, Dickinson A, Kraemer WJ: **Acute and chronic hormonal responses to resistance training designed to promote muscle hypertrophy.** *Can J Appl Physiol* 1999, **24**:96–107.
52. Kraemer WJ, Gordon SE, Fleck SJ, Marchitelli LJ, Mello R, Dziados JE, Friedl K, Harman E, Maresh C, Fry AC: **Endogenous anabolic hormonal and growth factor responses to heavy resistance exercise in males and females.** *Int J Sports Med* 1991, **12**:228–235.
53. Reid MB: **Invited Review: redox modulation of skeletal muscle contraction: what we know and what we don't.** *J Appl Phys* 2001, **90**:724–731.

Metabolic adaptation to weight loss: implications for the athlete

Eric T Trexler[1], Abbie E Smith-Ryan[1*] and Layne E Norton[2]

Abstract

Optimized body composition provides a competitive advantage in a variety of sports. Weight reduction is common among athletes aiming to improve their strength-to-mass ratio, locomotive efficiency, or aesthetic appearance. Energy restriction is accompanied by changes in circulating hormones, mitochondrial efficiency, and energy expenditure that serve to minimize the energy deficit, attenuate weight loss, and promote weight regain. The current article reviews the metabolic adaptations observed with weight reduction and provides recommendations for successful weight reduction and long term reduced-weight maintenance in athletes.

Keywords: Weight loss, Energy restriction, Body composition, Energy expenditure, Metabolic rate, Energy deficit, Weight maintenance, Uncoupling proteins, Mitochondrial efficiency

Introduction

In a variety of competitive sports, it is considered advantageous to achieve low levels of body fat while retaining lean body mass. The metabolic effects of this process have been given little context within athletics, such as physique sports (i.e. bodybuilding, figure), combat sports (i.e. judo, wrestling), aesthetic sports (i.e. gymnastics, figure skating), and endurance sports. Previous literature has documented cases of male bodybuilders reducing body fat to less than 5% of total body mass [1,2], and studies documenting physiological profiles of male wrestlers [3] and judo athletes [4] present body fat ranges that extend below 5%. A study on elite female gymnasts and runners reported an average body fat percentage (BF%) of 13.72% for the entire sample, with subgroups of middle-distance runners and artistic gymnasts averaging 12.18% and 12.36%, respectively [5]. Elite female runners have also reported percent body fat levels below 10% [6]. Energy deficits and extremely low levels of body fat present the body with a significant physiological challenge. It has been well documented that weight loss and energy restriction result in a number of homeostatic metabolic adaptations aimed at decreasing energy expenditure, improving metabolic efficiency, and increasing cues for energy intake [7-9]. While the unfavorable endocrine effects of contest preparation have been documented in male bodybuilders [1,2,10], anecdotal reports from physique athletes also describe a state in which metabolic rate has slowed to an extent that exceeds the predicted magnitude, making weight loss increasingly difficult despite low caloric intakes and high training volumes. Although such reports could potentially be related to inaccurate dietary reporting [11,12], these claims may be substantiated by a number of metabolic adaptations to weight loss, including adaptive thermogenesis [13-15], increased mitochondrial efficiency [16-19], and hormonal alterations that favor decreased energy expenditure, decreased satiety, and increased hunger [1,2,10]. As a dieting phase progresses, such adaptations may threaten dietary adherence, make further weight loss increasingly difficult, and predispose the individual to rapid weight regain following the cessation of the diet. Although data documenting the attainment and recovery from extreme changes in body composition is limited, the present article aims to investigate the condition of metabolic adaptation described by competitors and identify potential mechanisms to explain such a phenomenon.

* Correspondence: abbsmith@email.unc.edu
[1]Department of Exercise and Sport Science, University of North Carolina at Chapel Hill, 209 Fetzer Hall, CB# 8700, Chapel Hill, NC 27599-8700, USA
Full list of author information is available at the end of the article

The endocrine response to an energy deficit

A number of hormones play prominent roles in the regulation of body composition, energy intake, and energy expenditure. The hormones of the thyroid gland, particularly triiodothyronine (T3), are known to play an important and direct role in regulating metabolic rate. Increases in circulating thyroid hormones are associated with an increase in the metabolic rate, whereas lowered thyroid levels result in decreased thermogenesis and overall metabolic rate [20]. Leptin, synthesized primarily in adipocytes, functions as an indicator of both short and long-term energy availability; short-term energy restriction and lower body fat levels are associated with decreases in circulating leptin. Additionally, higher concentrations of leptin are associated with increased satiety and energy expenditure [21]. Insulin, which plays a crucial role in inhibiting muscle protein breakdown [22] and regulating macronutrient metabolism, is considered another "adiposity signal" [23]. Similar to leptin, high levels of insulin convey a message of energy availability and are associated with an anorexigenic effect. Conversely, the orexigenic hormone ghrelin functions to stimulate appetite and food intake, and has been shown to increase with fasting, and decrease after feeding [24]. Testosterone, known primarily for its role in increasing muscle protein synthesis and muscle mass [22], may also play a role in regulating adiposity [25]. Changes in fat mass have been inversely correlated with testosterone levels, and it has been suggested that testosterone may repress adipogenesis [25]. More research is needed to delineate the exact mechanism (s) by which testosterone affects adiposity. Cortisol, a glucocorticoid that influences macronutrient metabolism, has been shown to induce muscle protein breakdown [22], and increased plasma cortisol within the physiologic range has increased proteolysis in healthy subjects [26]. Evidence also suggests that glucocorticoids may inhibit the action of leptin [27].

Results from a number of studies indicate a general endocrine response to hypocaloric diets that promotes increased hunger, reduces metabolic rate, and threatens the maintenance of lean mass. Studies involving energy restriction, or very low adiposity, report decreases in leptin [1,10,28], insulin [1,2], testosterone [1,2,28], and thyroid hormones [1,29]. Subsequently, increases in ghrelin [1,10] and cortisol [1,30,31] have been reported with energy restriction. Further, there is evidence to suggest that unfavorable changes in circulating hormone levels persist as subjects attempt to maintain a reduced body weight, even after the cessation of active weight loss [32,33].

Low energy intake and minimal body fat are perceived as indicators of energy unavailability, resulting in a homeostatic endocrine response aimed at conserving energy and promoting energy intake. It should be noted that despite alterations in plasma levels of anabolic and catabolic hormones, losses of lean body mass (LBM) often fail to reach statistical significance in studies on bodybuilding preparation [1,2]. Although the lack of significance may relate to insufficient statistical power, these findings may indicate that unfavorable, hormone-mediated changes in LBM can potentially be attenuated by sound training and nutritional practices. Previous research has indicated that structured resistance training [34] and sufficient protein intake [35-37], both commonly employed in bodybuilding contest preparation, preserve LBM during energy restriction. Further, Maestu et al. speculate that losses in LBM are dependent on the magnitude of weight loss and degree of adiposity, as the subjects who lost the greatest amount of weight and achieved the lowest final body fat percentage in the study saw the greatest losses of LBM [2]. The hormonal environment created by low adiposity and energy restriction appears to promote weight regain and threaten lean mass retention, but more research is needed to determine the chronic impact of these observed alterations in circulating anabolic and catabolic hormones.

Weight loss and metabolic rate

An individual's total daily energy expenditure (TDEE) is comprised of a number of distinct components (Figure 1). The largest component, resting energy expenditure (REE), refers to the basal metabolic rate (BMR) [8]. The other component, known as non-resting energy expenditure (NREE), can be further divided into exercise activity thermogenesis (EAT), non-exercise activity thermogenesis (NEAT), and the thermic effect of food (TEF) [8].

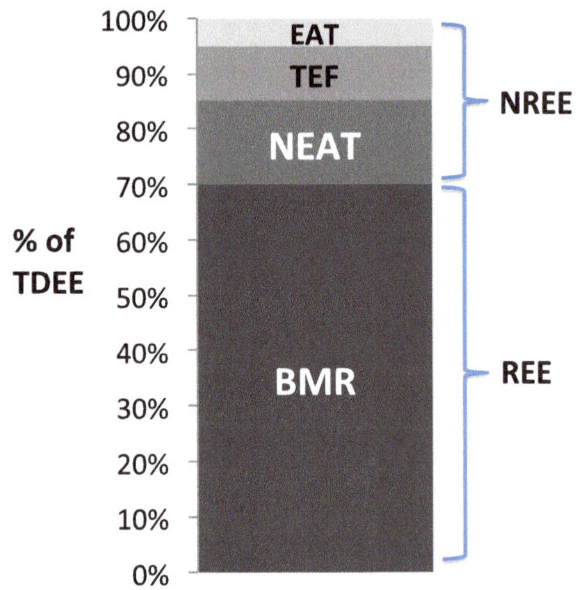

Figure 1 Components of total daily energy expenditure (TDEE). BMR = basal metabolic rate; NEAT = non-exercise activity thermogenesis; TEF = thermic effect of food; EAT = exercise activity thermogenesis; REE = resting energy expenditure; NREE = non-resting energy expenditure. Adapted from Maclean et al., 2011.

Metabolic rate is dynamic in nature, and previous literature has shown that energy restriction and weight loss affect numerous components of energy expenditure. In weight loss, TDEE has been consistently shown to decrease [38,39]. Weight loss results in a loss of metabolically active tissue, and therefore decreases BMR [38,39]. Interestingly, the decline in TDEE often exceeds the magnitude predicted by the loss of body mass. Previous literature refers to this excessive drop in TDEE as adaptive thermogenesis, and suggests that it functions to promote the restoration of baseline body weight [13-15]. Adaptive thermogenesis may help to partially explain the increasing difficulty experienced when weight loss plateaus despite low caloric intake, and the common propensity to regain weight after weight loss.

Exercise activity thermogenesis also drops in response to weight loss [40-42]. In activity that involves locomotion, it is clear that reduced body mass will reduce the energy needed to complete a given amount of activity. Interestingly, when external weight is added to match the subject's baseline weight, energy expenditure to complete a given workload remains below baseline [41]. It has been speculated that this increase in skeletal muscle efficiency may be related to the persistent hypothyroidism and hypoleptinemia that accompany weight loss, resulting in a lower respiratory quotient and greater reliance on lipid metabolism [43].

The TEF encompasses the energy expended in the process of ingesting, absorbing, metabolizing, and storing nutrients from food [8]. Roughly 10% of TDEE is attributed to TEF [44,45], with values varying based on the macronutrient composition of the diet. While the relative magnitude of TEF does not appear to change with energy restriction [46], such dietary restriction involves the consumption of fewer total calories, and therefore decreases the absolute magnitude of TEF [41,46]. NEAT, or energy expended during "non-exercise" movement such as fidgeting or normal daily activities, also decreases with an energy deficit [47]. There is evidence to suggest that spontaneous physical activity, a component of NEAT, is decreased in energy restricted subjects, and may remain suppressed for some time after subjects return to *ad libitum* feeding [29]. Persistent suppression of NEAT may contribute to weight regain in the post-diet period.

In order to manipulate an individual's body mass, energy intake must be adjusted based on the individual's energy expenditure. In the context of weight loss or maintaining a reduced body weight, this process is complicated by the dynamic nature of energy expenditure. In response to weight loss, reductions in TDEE, BMR, EAT, NEAT, and TEF are observed. Due to adaptive thermogenesis, TDEE is lowered to an extent that exceeds the magnitude predicted by losses in body mass. Further, research indicates that adaptive thermogenesis and decreased energy expenditure persist after the active weight loss period, even in subjects who have maintained a reduced body weight for over a year [14,48]. These changes serve to minimize the energy deficit, attenuate further loss of body mass, and promote weight regain in weight-reduced subjects.

Adaptations in mitochondrial efficiency

A series of chemical reactions must take place to derive ATP from stored and ingested energy substrates. In aerobic metabolism, this process involves the movement of protons across the inner mitochondrial membrane. When protons are transported by ATP synthase, ATP is produced. Protons may also leak across the inner membrane by way of uncoupling proteins (UCPs) [49]. In this "uncoupled respiration", energy substrate oxidation and oxygen consumption occur, but the process does not yield ATP. Proton leak is a significant contributor to energy expenditure, accounting for roughly 20-30% of BMR in rats [50-52].

In the condition of calorie restriction, proton leak is reduced [16-19]. Uncoupling protein-1 and UCP-3, the primary UCPs of brown adipose tissue (BAT) and skeletal muscle [53], are of particular interest due to their potentially significant roles in energy expenditure and uncoupled thermogenesis. Skeletal muscle's large contribution to energy expenditure [54] has directed attention toward literature reporting decreases in UCP-3 expression in response to energy restriction [55,56]. Decreased UCP-3 expression could potentially play a role in decreasing energy expenditure, and UCP-3 expression has been negatively correlated with body mass index and positively correlated with metabolic rate during sleep [57]. Despite these correlations, more research is needed to determine the function and physiological relevance of UCP-3 [58], as contradictory findings regarding UCP-3 and weight loss have been reported [18].

Uncoupling Protein-1 appears to play a pivotal role in the uncoupled thermogenic activity of BAT [59]. Energy restriction has been shown to decrease BAT activation [60] and UCP-1 expression [61], indicating an increase in metabolic efficiency. Along with UCP-1 expression, thyroid hormone and leptin affect the magnitude of uncoupled respiration in BAT. Thyroid hormone (TH) and leptin are associated with increased BAT activation, whereas glucocorticoids oppose the BAT-activating function of leptin [59]. Evidence indicates that TH plays a prominent role in modulating the magnitude of proton leak [53], with low TH levels associated with decreased proton leak [62]. The endocrine response to energy restriction, including increased cortisol and decreased TH and leptin [1,10,28-31], could potentially play a regulatory role in uncoupled respiration in BAT. It is not clear if decreases in proton leak and UCP expression persist until weight reverts to baseline, but there is evidence to suggest a persistent adaptation [19,55,56], which mirrors the persistent downregulation of TH and leptin [32,33].

Changes observed in proton leak, UCP expression, and circulating hormones appear to influence metabolic efficiency and energy expenditure. In the context of energy restriction, the observed changes are likely to make weight loss increasingly challenging and promote weight regain. It has been reported that females have more BAT than males [63], and that energy-restricted female rats see greater decreases in BAT mass and UCP-1 than males [64], indicating a potential sex-related difference in uncoupled respiration during weight loss. Subjects identified as "diet-resistant" show decreased proton leak and UCP-3 expression compared to "diet-responsive" subjects during maintenance of a reduced bodyweight [65]. More research is needed to determine if these differential responses to hypocaloric diets make sustained weight loss more difficult for females and certain predisposed "diet-resistant" individuals. While future research may improve our understanding of the magnitude and relative importance of mitochondrial adaptations to energy restriction, current evidence suggests that increased mitochondrial efficiency, and a decline in uncoupled respiration, might serve to decrease the energy deficit in hypocaloric conditions, making weight maintenance and further weight reduction more challenging.

Practical applications for weight loss in athletes

Hypocaloric diets induce a number of adaptations that serve to prevent further weight loss and conserve energy. It is likely that the magnitude of these adaptations are proportional to the size of the energy deficit, so it is recommended to utilize the smallest possible deficit that yields appreciable weight loss. This may decrease the rate of weight loss, but attenuate unfavorable adaptations that challenge successful reduction of fat mass. Weight reduction should be viewed as a stepwise process in this context; as weight loss begins to plateau, energy intake or expenditure should be adjusted to "re-open" the energy deficit. Large caloric deficits are also likely to induce greater losses of LBM [66,67] and compromise athletic performance and recovery [68,69], which are of critical importance to athletes. Participation in a structured resistance training program [34] and sufficient protein intake [35-37] are also likely to attenuate losses in LBM. Additionally, high protein diets (≥25% PRO) are associated with increased satiety and thermogenesis, making them a better option for the calorie-restricted athlete [70].

In the world of physique sports, periodic "refeeding" has become common in periods of extended dieting. A refeed consists of a brief overfeeding period in which caloric intake is raised slightly above maintenance levels, and the increase in caloric intake is predominantly achieved by increasing carbohydrate consumption. While studies have utilized refeeding protocols that last three days [71,72], physique athletes such as bodybuilders and figure competitors often incorporate 24-hour refeeds, once or twice per week. The proposed goal of periodic refeeding is to temporarily increase circulating leptin and stimulate the metabolic rate. There is evidence indicating that leptin is acutely responsive to short-term overfeeding [72], is highly correlated with carbohydrate intake [71,73], and that pharmacological administration of leptin reverses many unfavorable adaptations to energy restriction [33]. While interventions have shown acute increases in leptin from short-term carbohydrate overfeeding, the reported effect on metabolic rate has been modest [71]. Dirlewanger et al. reported a 7% increase in TDEE; this increase amounts to approximately 138 kilocalories of additional energy expenditure, of which 36 kilocalories can be attributed to the thermic effect of carbohydrate intake [71]. More research is needed to determine if acute bouts of refeeding are an efficacious strategy for improving weight loss success during prolonged hypocaloric states. A theoretical model of metabolic adaptation and potential strategies to attenuate adaptations is presented in Figure 2.

In the period shortly after cessation of a restrictive diet, body mass often reverts toward pre-diet values [29,74,75]. This body mass is preferentially gained as fat mass, in a phenomenon known as post-starvation obesity [29]. While many of the metabolic adaptations to weight loss persist, a dramatic increase in energy intake results in rapid accumulation of fat mass. It is common for individuals to "overshoot" their baseline level of body fat, and leaner individuals (including many athletes) may be more susceptible to overshooting than obese individuals [74,75]. In such a situation, the individual may increase body fat beyond baseline levels, yet retain a metabolic rate that has yet to fully recover. There is evidence to suggest that adipocyte hyperplasia may occur early in the weight-regain process [76], and that repeated cycles of weight loss and regain by athletes in sports with weight classes are associated with long-term weight gain [77]. Therefore, athletes who aggressively diet for a competitive season and rapidly regain weight may find it more challenging to achieve optimal body composition in subsequent seasons.

To avoid rapid fat gain following the cessation of a diet, "reverse dieting" has also become popular among physique athletes. Such a process involves slowly increasing caloric intake in a stepwise fashion. In theory, providing a small caloric surplus might help to restore circulating hormone levels and energy expenditure toward pre-diet values, while closely matching energy

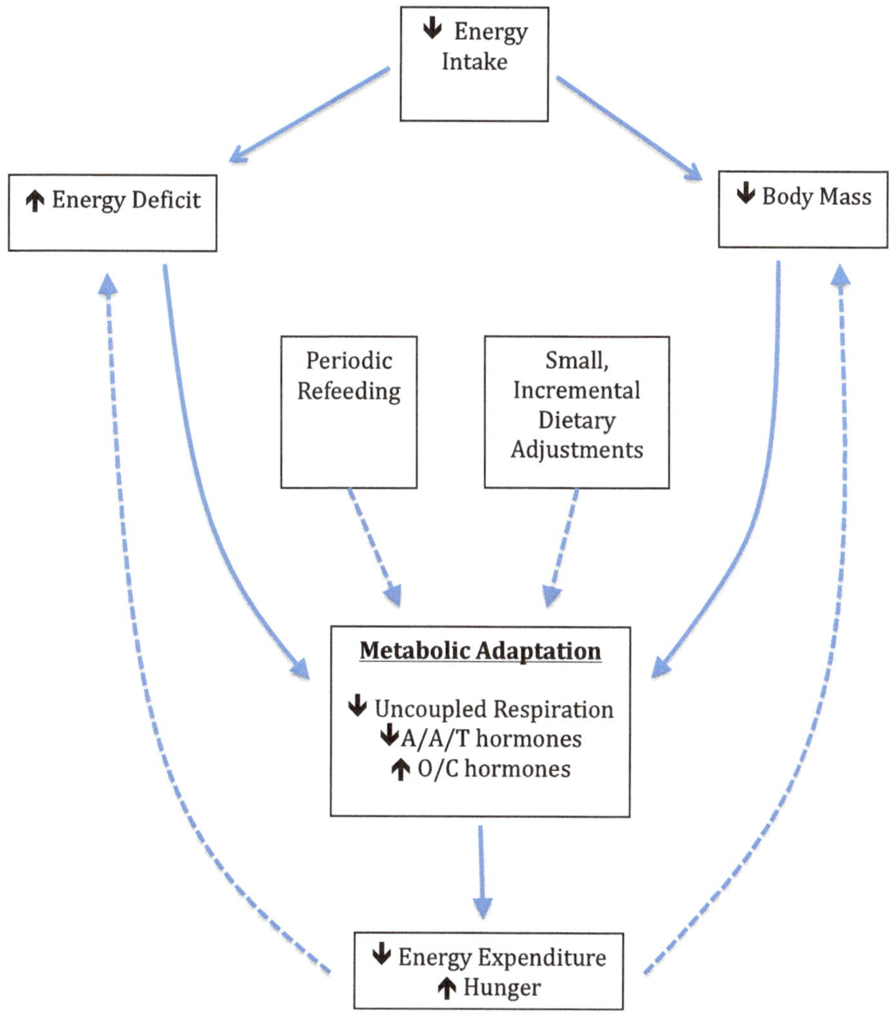

Figure 2 A theoretical model of metabolic adaptation and potential strategies to attenuate adaptations. A/A/T hormones = Anabolic, Anorexigenic, and Thermogenic hormones; O/C hormones = Orexigenic and Catabolic hormones. Dotted lines represent inhibition.

intake to the recovering metabolic rate in an effort to reduce fat accretion. Ideally, such a process would eventually restore circulating hormones and metabolic rate to baseline levels while avoiding rapid fat gain. While anecdotal reports of successful reverse dieting have led to an increase in its popularity, research is needed to evaluate its efficacy.

Limitations

Although there is a substantial body of research on metabolic adaptations to weight loss, the majority of the research has utilized animal models or subjects that are sedentary and overweight/obese. Accordingly, the current article is limited by the need to apply this data to an athletic population. If the adaptations described in obese populations serve to conserve energy and attenuate weight loss as a survival mechanism, one might speculate that the adaptations may be further augmented in a leaner, more highly active population. Another limitation is the lack of research on the efficacy of periodic refeeding or reverse dieting in prolonged weight reduction, or in the maintenance of a reduced bodyweight. Until such research is available, these anecdotal methods can only be evaluated from a mechanistic and theoretical viewpoint.

Conclusion

Weight loss is a common practice in a number of sports. Whether the goal is a higher strength-to-mass ratio, improved aesthetic presentation, or more efficient locomotion, optimizing body composition is advantageous to a wide variety of athletes. As these athletes create an energy deficit and achieve lower body fat levels, their weight loss efforts will be counteracted by a number of metabolic adaptations that may persist throughout weight maintenance. Changes in energy expenditure, mitochondrial efficiency, and circulating hormone concentrations work in concert to attenuate further weight loss and promote the restoration of baseline body mass. Athletes must aim to minimize the magnitude of these adaptations, preserve LBM, and adequately fuel performance and recovery during weight reduction. To accomplish these goals, it is recommended to approach weight loss in a stepwise, incremental fashion, utilizing small energy deficits to ensure a slow rate of weight loss. Participation in a structured resistance training program and adequate protein intake are also imperative. More research is needed to verify the efficacy of periodic refeeding and reverse dieting in supporting prolonged weight reduction and attenuating post-diet fat accretion.

Abbreviations

BAT: Brown adipose tissue; BF%: Body fat percentage; BMR: Basal metabolic rate; EAT: Exercise activity thermogenesis; LBM: Lean body mass; NEAT: Non-exercise activity thermogenesis; NREE: Non-resting energy expenditure; REE: Resting energy expenditure; TDEE: Total daily energy expenditure; TEF: Thermic effect of food; TH: Thyroid Hormone; T3: Triiodothyronine; UCP: Uncoupling protein.

Competing interests

The authors declare that they have no competing interests.

Authors' contributions

ETT conceived of the review topic and drafted the manuscript. AES conceived, drafted and revised the manuscript. LEN helped to draft and revise the manuscript. All authors read and approved the final manuscript.

Author details

[1]Department of Exercise and Sport Science, University of North Carolina at Chapel Hill, 209 Fetzer Hall, CB# 8700, Chapel Hill, NC 27599-8700, USA.
[2]BioLayne LLC, Tampa, FL, USA.

References

1. Rossow LM, Fukuda DH, Fahs CA, Loenneke JP, Stout JR: **Natural bodybuilding competition preparation and recovery: a 12-month case study.** *Int J Sports Physiol Perform* 2013, **8:**582–592.
2. Maestu J, Eliakim A, Jurimae J, Valter I, Jurimae T: **Anabolic and catabolic hormones and energy balance of the male bodybuilders during the preparation for the competition.** *J Strength Cond Res* 2010, **24:**1074–1081.
3. Yoon J: **Physiological profiles of elite senior wrestlers.** *Sports Med* 2002, **32:**225–233.
4. Franchini E, Del Vecchio FB, Matsushigue KA, Artioli GG: **Physiological profiles of elite judo athletes.** *Sports Med* 2011, **41:**147–166.
5. Deutz RC, Benardot D, Martin DE, Cody MM: **Relationship between energy deficits and body composition in elite female gymnasts and runners.** *Med Sci Sports Exerc* 2000, **32:**659–668.
6. Wilmore JH, Brown CH, Davis JA: **Body physique and composition of the female distance runner.** *Ann N Y Acad Sci* 1977, **301:**764–776.
7. Dulloo AG, Jacquet J: **Adaptive reduction in basal metabolic rate in response to food deprivation in humans: a role for feedback signals from fat stores.** *Am J Clin Nutr* 1998, **68:**599–606.
8. Maclean PS, Bergouignan A, Cornier MA, Jackman MR: **Biology's response to dieting: the impetus for weight regain.** *Am J Physiol Regul Integr Comp Physiol* 2011, **301:**R581–R600.
9. MacLean PS, Higgins JA, Jackman MR, Johnson GC, Fleming-Elder BK, Wyatt HR, Melanson EL, Hill JO: **Peripheral metabolic responses to prolonged weight reduction that promote rapid, efficient regain in obesity-prone rats.** *Am J Physiol Regul Integr Comp Physiol* 2006, **290:**R1577–R1588.
10. Maestu J, Jurimae J, Valter I, Jurimae T: **Increases in ghrelin and decreases in leptin without altering adiponectin during extreme weight loss in male competitive bodybuilders.** *Metabolism* 2008, **57:**221–225.
11. Lichtman SW, Pisarska K, Berman ER, Pestone M, Dowling H, Offenbacher E, Weisel H, Heshka S, Matthews DE, Heymsfield SB: **Discrepancy between self-reported and actual caloric intake and exercise in obese subjects.** *N Engl J Med* 1992, **327:**1893–1898.
12. Garriguet D: **Under-reporting of energy intake in the Canadian community health survey.** *Health Rep* 2008, **19:**37–45.
13. Doucet E, St-Pierre S, Almeras N, Despres JP, Bouchard C, Tremblay A: **Evidence for the existence of adaptive thermogenesis during weight loss.** *Br J Nutr* 2001, **85:**715–723.
14. Rosenbaum M, Hirsch J, Gallagher DA, Leibel RL: **Long-term persistence of adaptive thermogenesis in subjects who have maintained a reduced body weight.** *Am J Clin Nutr* 2008, **88:**906–912.
15. Rosenbaum M, Leibel RL: **Adaptive thermogenesis in humans.** *Int J Obes* 2010, **34**(Suppl 1):S47–S55.
16. Asami DK, McDonald RB, Hagopian K, Horwitz BA, Warman D, Hsiao A, Warden C, Ramsey JJ: **Effect of aging, caloric restriction, and uncoupling protein 3 (UCP3) on mitochondrial proton leak in mice.** *Exp Gerontol* 2008, **43:**1069–1076.
17. Bevilacqua L, Ramsey JJ, Hagopian K, Weindruch R, Harper ME: **Effects of short- and medium-term calorie restriction on muscle mitochondrial proton leak and reactive oxygen species production.** *Am J Physiol Regul Integr Comp Physiol* 2004, **286:**E852–E861.
18. Bevilacqua L, Ramsey JJ, Hagopian K, Weindruch R, Harper ME: **Long-term caloric restriction increases UCP3 content but decreases proton leak and reactive oxygen species production in rat skeletal muscle mitochondria.** *Am J Physiol Endocrinol Metab* 2005, **289:**E429–E438.
19. Hagopian K, Harper ME, Ram JJ, Humble SJ, Weindruch R, Ramsey JJ: **Long-term calorie restriction reduces proton leak and hydrogen peroxide production in liver mitochondria.** *Am J Physiol Endocrinol Metab* 2005, **288:**E674–E684.
20. Kim B: **Thyroid hormone as a determinant of energy expenditure and the basal metabolic rate.** *Thyroid* 2008, **18:**141–144.
21. Margetic S, Gazzola C, Pegg GG, Hill RA: **Leptin: a review of its peripheral actions and interactions.** *Int J Obes Relat Metab Disord* 2002, **26:**1407–1433.
22. Rooyackers OE, Nair KS: **Hormonal regulation of human muscle protein metabolism.** *Annu Rev Nutr* 1997, **17:**457–485.
23. Strohacker K, McCaffery JM, Maclean PS, Wing RR: **Adaptations of leptin, ghrelin or insulin during weight loss as predictors of weight regain: a review of current literature.** *Int J Obes* 2013:1–9. http://www.nature.com/ijo/journal/vaop/ncurrent/full/ijo2013118a.html.
24. Ariyasu H, Takaya K, Tagami T, Ogawa Y, Hosoda K, Akamizu T, Suda M, Koh T, Natsui K, Toyooka S, Shirakami G, Usui T, Shimatsu A, Doi K, Hosoda H, Kojima M, Kangawa K, Nakao K: **Stomach is a major source of circulating ghrelin, and feeding state determines plasma ghrelin-like immunoreactivity levels in humans.** *J Clin Endocrinol Metab* 2001, **86:**4753–4758.
25. De Maddalena C, Vodo S, Petroni A, Aloisi AM: **Impact of testosterone on body fat composition.** *J Cell Physiol* 2012, **227:**3744–3748.
26. Simmons PS, Miles JM, Gerich JE, Haymond MW: **Increased proteolysis. An effect of increases in plasma cortisol within the physiologic range.** *J Clin Invest* 1984, **73:**412–420.
27. Zakrzewska KE, Cusin I, Sainsbury A, Rohner-Jeanrenaud F, Jeanrenaud B: **Glucocorticoids as counterregulatory hormones of leptin: toward an understanding of leptin resistance.** *Diabetes* 1997, **46:**717–719.
28. Hagmar M, Berglund B, Brismar K, Hirschberg AL: **Body composition and endocrine profile of male Olympic athletes striving for leanness.** *Clin J Sport Med* 2013, **23:**197–201.
29. Weyer C, Walford RL, Harper IT, Milner M, MacCallum T, Tataranni PA, Ravussin E: **Energy metabolism after 2 y of energy restriction: the biosphere 2 experiment.** *Am J Clin Nutr* 2000, **72:**946–953.
30. Witbracht MG, Laugero KD, Van Loan MD, Adams SH, Keim NL: **Performance on the Iowa gambling task is related to magnitude of weight loss and salivary cortisol in a diet-induced weight loss intervention in overweight women.** *Physiol Behav* 2012, **106:**291–297.
31. Tomiyama AJ, Mann T, Vinas D, Hunger JM, Dejager J, Taylor SE: **Low calorie dieting increases cortisol.** *Psychosom Med* 2010, **72:**357–364.
32. Sumithran P, Prendergast LA, Delbridge E, Purcell K, Shulkes A, Kriketos A, Proietto J: **Long-term persistence of hormonal adaptations to weight loss.** *N Engl J Med* 2011, **365:**1597–1604.

33. Rosenbaum M, Goldsmith R, Bloomfield D, Magnano A, Weimer L, Heymsfield S, Gallagher D, Mayer L, Murphy E, Leibel RL: **Low-dose leptin reverses skeletal muscle, autonomic, and neuroendocrine adaptations to maintenance of reduced weight.** *J Clin Invest* 2005, **115:**3579–3586.
34. Bryner RW, Ullrich IH, Sauers J, Donley D, Hornsby G, Kolar M, Yeater R: **Effects of resistance vs. aerobic training combined with an 800 calorie liquid diet on lean body mass and resting metabolic rate.** *J Am Coll Nutr* 1999, **18:**115–121.
35. Mettler S, Mitchell N, Tipton KD: **Increased protein intake reduces lean body mass loss during weight loss in athletes.** *Med Sci Sports Exerc* 2010, **42:**326–337.
36. Layman DK, Boileau RA, Erickson DJ, Painter JE, Shiue H, Sather C, Christou DD: **A reduced ratio of dietary carbohydrate to protein improves body composition and blood lipid profiles during weight loss in adult women.** *J Nutr* 2003, **133:**411–417.
37. Bopp MJ, Houston DK, Lenchik L, Easter L, Kritchevsky SB, Nicklas BJ: **Lean mass loss is associated with low protein intake during dietary-induced weight loss in postmenopausal women.** *J Am Diet Assoc* 2008, **108:**1216–1220.
38. Ravussin E, Burnand B, Schutz Y, Jequier E: **Energy expenditure before and during energy restriction in obese patients.** *Am J Clin Nutr* 1985, **41:**753–759.
39. Leibel RL, Rosenbaum M, Hirsch J: **Changes in energy expenditure resulting from altered body weight.** *N Engl J Med* 1995, **332:**621–628.
40. Weigle DS: **Contribution of decreased body mass to diminished thermic effect of exercise in reduced-obese men.** *Int J Obes* 1988, **12:**567–578.
41. Weigle DS, Brunzell JD: **Assessment of energy expenditure in ambulatory reduced-obese subjects by the techniques of weight stabilization and exogenous weight replacement.** *Int J Obes* 1990, **14**(Suppl 1):69–77. discussion 77–81.
42. Doucet E, Imbeault P, St-Pierre S, Almeras N, Mauriege P, Despres JP, Bouchard C, Tremblay A: **Greater than predicted decrease in energy expenditure during exercise after body weight loss in obese men.** *Clin Sci* 2003, **105:**89–95.
43. Rosenbaum M, Vandenborne K, Goldsmith R, Simoneau JA, Heymsfield S, Joanisse DR, Hirsch J, Murphy E, Matthews D, Segal KR, Leibel RL: **Effects of experimental weight perturbation on skeletal muscle work efficiency in human subjects.** *Am J Physiol Regul Integr Comp Physiol* 2003, **285:**R183–192.
44. Tappy L: **Thermic effect of food and sympathetic nervous system activity in humans.** *Reprod Nutr Dev* 1996, **36:**391–397.
45. Ravussin E, Lillioja S, Anderson TE, Christin L, Bogardus C: **Determinants of 24-hour energy expenditure in man. Methods and results using a respiratory chamber.** *J Clin Invest* 1986, **78:**1568–1578.
46. Miles CW, Wong NP, Rumpler WV, Conway J: **Effect of circadian variation in energy expenditure, within-subject variation and weight reduction on thermic effect of food.** *Eur J Clin Nutr* 1993, **47:**274–284.
47. Levine JA: **Non-exercise activity thermogenesis (NEAT).** *Best Pract Res Clin Endocrinol Metab* 2002, **16:**679–702.
48. Leibel RL, Hirsch J: **Diminished energy requirements in reduced-obese patients.** *Metabolism* 1984, **33.**164–170.
49. Jastroch M, Divakaruni AS, Mookerjee S, Treberg JR, Brand MD: **Mitochondrial proton and electron leaks.** *Essays Biochem* 2010, **47:**53–67.
50. Rolfe DF, Brand MD: **Contribution of mitochondrial proton leak to skeletal muscle respiration and to standard metabolic rate.** *Am J Physiol* 1996, **271:**C1380–1389.
51. Rolfe DF, Brown GC: **Cellular energy utilization and molecular origin of standard metabolic rate in mammals.** *Physiol Rev* 1997, **77:**731–758.
52. Rolfe DF, Newman JM, Buckingham JA, Clark MG, Brand MD: **Contribution of mitochondrial proton leak to respiration rate in working skeletal muscle and liver and to SMR.** *Am J Physiol* 1999, **276:**C692–699.
53. Thrush AB, Dent R, McPherson R, Harper ME: **Implications of mitochondrial uncoupling in skeletal muscle in the development and treatment of obesity.** *FEBS J* 2013, **280:**5015–5029.
54. Zurlo F, Larson K, Bogardus C, Ravussin E: **Skeletal muscle metabolism is a major determinant of resting energy expenditure.** *J Clin Invest* 1990, **86:**1423–1427.
55. Esterbauer H, Oberkofler H, Dallinger G, Breban D, Hell E, Krempler F, Patsch W: **Uncoupling protein-3 gene expression: reduced skeletal muscle mRNA in obese humans during pronounced weight loss.** *Diabetologia* 1999, **42:**302–309.
56. Vidal-Puig A, Rosenbaum M, Considine RC, Leibel RL, Dohm GL, Lowell BB: **Effects of obesity and stable weight reduction on UCP2 and UCP3 gene expression in humans.** *Obes Res* 1999, **7:**133–140.
57. Schrauwen P, Xia J, Bogardus C, Pratley RE, Ravussin E: **Skeletal muscle uncoupling protein 3 expression is a determinant of energy expenditure in Pima Indians.** *Diabetes* 1999, **48:**146–149.
58. Harper ME, Dent RM, Bezaire V, Antoniou A, Gauthier A, Monemdjou S, McPherson R: **UCP3 and its putative function: consistencies and controversies.** *Biochem Soc Trans* 2001, **29:**768–773.
59. Cannon B, Nedergaard J: **Brown adipose tissue: function and physiological significance.** *Physiol Rev* 2004, **84:**277–359.
60. Rothwell NJ, Stock MJ: **Effect of chronic food restriction on energy balance, thermogenic capacity, and brown-adipose-tissue activity in the rat.** *Biosci Rep* 1982, **2:**543–549.
61. Young JB, Saville E, Rothwell NJ, Stock MJ, Landsberg L: **Effect of diet and cold exposure on norepinephrine turnover in brown adipose tissue of the rat.** *J Clin Invest* 1982, **69:**1061–1071.
62. Harper ME, Brand MD: **The quantitative contributions of mitochondrial proton leak and ATP turnover reactions to the changed respiration rates of hepatocytes from rats of different thyroid status.** *J Biol Chem* 1993, **268:**14850–14860.
63. Cypess AM, Lehman S, Williams G, Tal I, Rodman D, Goldfine AB, Kuo FC, Palmer EL, Tseng YH, Doria A, Kolodny GM, Kahn CR: **Identification and importance of brown adipose tissue in adult humans.** *N Engl J Med* 2009, **360:**1509–1517.
64. Valle A, Catala-Niell A, Colom B, Garcia-Palmer FJ, Oliver J, Roca P: **Sex-related differences in energy balance in response to caloric restriction.** *Am J Physiol Endocrinol Metab* 2005, **289:**E15–22.
65. Harper ME, Dent R, Monemdjou S, Bezaire V, Van Wyck L, Wells G, Kavaslar GN, Gauthier A, Tesson F, McPherson R: **Decreased mitochondrial proton leak and reduced expression of uncoupling protein 3 in skeletal muscle of obese diet-resistant women.** *Diabetes* 2002, **51:**2459–2466.
66. Chaston TB, Dixon JB, O'Brien PE: **Changes in fat-free mass during significant weight loss: a systematic review.** *Int J Obes* 2007, **31:**743–750.
67. Garthe I, Raastad T, Refsnes PE, Koivisto A, Sundgot-Borgen J: **Effect of two different weight-loss rates on body composition and strength and power-related performance in elite athletes.** *Int J Sport Nutr Exerc Metab* 2011, **21:**97–104.
68. American Dietetic A, Dietitians of C, American College of Sports M, Rodriguez NR, Di Marco NM, Langley S: **American College of Sports Medicine position stand. Nutrition and athletic performance.** *Med Sci Sports Exerc* 2009, **41:**709–731.
69. Burke LM, Loucks AB, Broad N: **Energy and carbohydrate for training and recovery.** *J Sports Sci* 2006, **24:**675–685.
70. Paddon-Jones D, Westman E, Mattes RD, Wolfe RR, Astrup A, Westerterp-Plantenga M: **Protein, weight management, and satiety.** *Am J Clin Nutr* 2008, **87:**1558S–1561S.
71. Dirlewanger M, di Vetta V, Guenat E, Battilana P, Seematter G, Schneiter P, Jequier E, Tappy L: **Effects of short-term carbohydrate or fat overfeeding on energy expenditure and plasma leptin concentrations in healthy female subjects.** *Int J Obes Relat Metab Disord* 2000, **24:**1413–1418.
72. Chin-Chance C, Polonsky KS, Schoeller DA: **Twenty-four-hour leptin levels respond to cumulative short-term energy imbalance and predict subsequent intake.** *J Clin Endocrinol Metab* 2000, **85:**2685–2691.
73. Jenkins AB, Markovic TP, Fleury A, Campbell LV: **Carbohydrate intake and short-term regulation of leptin in humans.** *Diabetologia* 1997, **40:**348–351.
74. Dulloo AG, Jacquet J, Girardier L: **Poststarvation hyperphagia and body fat overshooting in humans: a role for feedback signals from lean and fat tissues.** *Am J Clin Nutr* 1997, **65:**717–723.
75. Dulloo AG, Jacquet J, Montani JP: **How dieting makes some fatter: from a perspective of human body composition autoregulation.** *Proc Nutr Soc* 2012, **71:**379–389.
76. Jackman MR, Steig A, Higgins JA, Johnson GC, Fleming-Elder BK, Bessesen DH, MacLean PS: **Weight regain after sustained weight reduction is accompanied by suppressed oxidation of dietary fat and adipocyte hyperplasia.** *Am J Physiol Regul Integr Comp Physiol* 2008, **294:**R1117–1129.
77. Saarni SE, Rissanen A, Sarna S, Koskenvuo M, Kaprio J: **Weight cycling of athletes and subsequent weight gain in middleage.** *Int J Obes* 2006, **30:**1639–1644.

14

Controversies of antioxidant vitamins supplementation in exercise: ergogenic or ergolytic effects in humans?

Cainara Lins Draeger, Andréia Naves, Natália Marques, Ana Beatriz Baptistella, Renata Alves Carnauba, Valéria Paschoal and Humberto Nicastro*

Abstract

The aim of this commentary was to discuss the last studies regarding the effect of antioxidant vitamins supplementation on oxidative stress in exercise in humans. The inclusion criteria encompassed published studies done in adult males and females between 2006 and 2013. The keywords used in the search engine were: endurance athlete, diet, oxidative stress, physical activity, diet, nutrition, antioxidant, antioxidant status, vitamin C, vitamin A, vitamin E, β-carotene and combinations. Twelve studies were identified and organized according to the methodology and results of supplementation: ergogenic, ergolytic, partial or no difference between groups. The results of these studies showed no effect on physiological parameters and activity of antioxidant enzymes (n = 07), better response of the placebo treatment (ergolytic effect; n = 02), partial results (n = 01) and ergogenic results of antioxidant supplementation (n = 02). It is concluded that supplementation with antioxidant vitamins has controversial effects to oxidative damage induced by endurance exercise. The discordances among the studies are presented and discussed.

Keywords: Endurance, Oxidative stress, Antioxidant, Athlete, Diet, Physical activity, Vitamin A, Vitamin C, Vitamin E and β-caroten

Background

Oxidative stress occurs when there is an imbalance in the human body homeostasis, i.e. the production of pro-oxidants becomes excessive and the cellular antioxidant mechanisms cannot neutralize these radicals. Excessive production of free radicals can be triggered by several endogenous and exogenous factors and, among these, exposure to radiation, excessive heat, inflammation, infection, trauma and exhaustive physical exercise can be considered strong exogenous triggers [1].

The regular practice of exercise induces several adaptations in cardiovascular, skeletal muscle and respiratory systems providing positive results for the prevention and treatment of metabolic diseases [2]. However, despite the undeniable health benefits, exercise may increase mitochondrial formation of reactive oxygen species which may cause cellular damage [3]. When produced in excess, free radicals may promote cellular oxidation, damage in the DNA structure, aging and a variety of diseases [4], impair skeletal muscle function and pain and, thereby affecting exercise performance [5]. In an attempt to minimize the effects of oxidative stress during physical activity, many athletes and sports professionals are performing supplementation with antioxidant vitamins.

However, recent studies raise the assumption that exercise alone could increase the oxidative capacity of skeletal muscle and potentiate the action of endogenous antioxidants, which is sufficient to counteract the negative effects of oxidative stress induced by the mechanical stimuli [3,6-8]. In view of this background, the aim of this commentary was to systematize the results of the last studies published regarding the effects of antioxidant vitamins intake on oxidative stress in exercise in humans.

* Correspondence: nicastroh@yahoo.com.br
VP Research Institute, Rua Pedro Morganti, 103 – Vila Mariana, PO Box 04020-070, São Paulo, SP, Brazil

Table 1 Results of the studies with endurance trained volunteers supplemented with vitamins A, C, and E

Study	Experimental design	Sample	Duration	Suplementation protocol			Result	
				Vitamin A	Vitamin C	Vitamin E	Ergogenic	Ergolytic
Tauler et al. [6]	Randomized, double-blind	15 athletes	90 d*	30 mg (β-caroten)	1000 mg	500 mg	↔	↔
Gauche et al. [9]	Randomized, double-blind	22 athletes	21 d (pre-exercise) + 2 dias (post-exercise)	6 mg (β-caroten)	200 mg	32 mg	↑	N/R
Nielsen et al. [10]	Randomized, double-blind, cross-over	15 athletes	28 d	-	400 mg	180 mg	↔	↔
Patil et al. [11]	Randomized, double-blind	37 athletes	21 d	-	-	200 mg	↔	↔
Louis et al. [12]	Randomized, double-blind	16 athletes	21 d	17.1 mg (β-caroten)	319.2 mg	48 mg	↑	N/R

* Vitamin C supplementation occurred only in the last 15 days of the study; ↑ Improved exercise performance; ↔ No results on exercise performance; N/R – not reported.

Results and discussion

We included 12 studies published in the last years that addressed the supplementation of antioxidant vitamins in trained volunteers (n = 05; Table 1) and in volunteers submitted to endurance exercise (n = 07; Table 2).

In general, it was observed that there are controversial results about antioxidant supplementation during high-intensity exercise. According to two studies evaluated [3,7], the placebo group presented significant better physical performance, fatigue resistance and antioxidant protection when compared to the supplemented groups. In contrast, Gauche et al. [9] and Louis et al. [12] evaluated the effects of vitamin and mineral supplementation on muscle activity of athletes and observed that dietary supplementation provided a slight advantage over the placebo group in maximum voluntary muscle contraction after high-intensity exercise. This small advantage in the supplemented group compared to the placebo group was sufficient for the authors to consider the antioxidant supplementation as an ergogenic aid. Regarding the other studies, no differences were found between the groups.

Sample characteristics

The subjects included in the studies presented different metabolic and body composition patterns. It is known that untrained subjects are more responsive to an exercise bout and, consequently, much more susceptible to suffer cellular damage from oxidative stress than trained individuals. For example, muscle damage caused by

Table 2 Results of the studies with untrained volunteers submitted to endurance exercise and supplemented with vitamins C e E

Study	Experimental design	Sample	Duration	Supplementation protocol		Result	
				Vitamin C	Vitamin E	Ergogenic	Ergolytic
Bloomer et al. [13]	Randomized, double-blind	15 trained and e 15 untrained subjects	14 d (pre-exercise) + 2 d (post-exercise)	2000 mg	835 mg	↔	↔
Gomez-Cabrera et al. [7]	Randomized, double-blind	14 untrained subjects e 36 rats	8 weeks	1 g (humans) and 0.24 $mg \cdot cm^{-2}$ (rodents)	-	N/R	↓
Ristow et al. [3]	Randomized, double-blind	20 trained and e 20 untrained subjects	4 weeks	1000 mg	440 mg	N/R	↓
Yfanti et al. [14]	Randomized, double-blind	21 untrained subjects	16 weeks	500 mg	400 IU	↔	↔
Yfanti et al. [5]	Randomized, double-blind	21 untrained subjects	16 weeks	500 mg	400 IU	↔	↔
Nalbant et al. [8]	Randomized	57 elderly	6 months		900 IU	↔	↔
Nakhostin et al. [15]	Randomized	16 untrained subjects	N/R	1000 mg	-	↑↓	N/R

↑ Improved exercise performance; ↓ Impaired exercise performance; ↑↓ Partial result; ↔ No results on exercise performance; IU – International Units; N/R – not reported.

oxidative stress, in general, is more pronounced in untrained individuals [16].

Another point to be considered is the sample size of the studies. It was observed that the number of individuals that comprise the groups used in the studies listed in Table 1 is smaller than those in Table 2. This can be partially justified by the difficulty of recruiting athletes to be volunteers. Consequently, the statistical power and the effect size of such data can be compromised and should be carefully interpreted.

Dietary control

Parallel to vitamin supplementation, it was observed that several studies did not perform dietary control of the subjects [3] or performed an inadequate control [9-12] to assess the possible interference of diet on the outcome. The dietary control is quite important since some vitamins and minerals may compete in terms of absorption in the gastrointestinal tract. Thus, the absence or inadequate dietary control can be considered a bias of the published studies.

Tauler et al. [6] and Yfanti et al. [5,14] performed dietary control through food records before and after the intervention. Gomez-Cabrera et al. [7] instructed the subjects to repeat the diet in the day before the exercise test in the pre- and post-supplementation periods. Only in the study of Bloomer et al. [13] dietary control was performed through food records. The variables analyzed were: total caloric value of the meals, amount of proteins, carbohydrates and lipids and of vitamins A, C and E. Even using a better dietary control than the other studies, the authors did not identify differences in the diet that could justify the results obtained.

Controversies

The differences between the results in the studies described can also be mainly attributed to the different methodologies, conveyed vitamin dosage, study length, sample size, differences in gender, age, and subjects characteristics (athletes and non-athletes). These differences make it difficult to draw conclusion about the advantages and disadvantages of antioxidant vitamins supplementation.

So far, the results of the studies presented confirm that exercise is capable of increasing the oxidative capacity of skeletal muscle and potentiate the action of endogenous antioxidants [6]. Exercise increases the expression of reduced glutathione (GSH) and antioxidant enzymes (superoxide dismutase [SOD], and glutathione peroxidase [GSH-Px]), which appear to be sufficient to counteract the negative effects of exercise-induced oxidative stress [3,7,8]. In this context, the real need to use antioxidant vitamins supplements as ergogenic aids is questionable. The safest and effective alternative in attenuating exercise-induced oxidative stress could be a balanced diet based on foods with the recommended amounts of antioxidants in order to improve exercise performance.

Conclusions

The results obtained in the considered studies with antioxidant vitamins supplementation are contradictory. Some studies show that supplementation does not improve exercise performance but can impair it. Others show that supplementation provides a slight advantage over the placebo. Thus, although many athletes use antioxidant supplementation to improve their physical performance, there is no consistent evidence suggesting that supplementation reduces oxidative stress and ensures better results in exercise.

Abbreviations

DNA: Deoxyribonucleic acid; GSH: Reduced glutathione; GSH-Px: Glutathione peroxidase; SOD: Superoxide dismutase.

Competing interests

The authors declare that they have no competing interests.

Authors' contributions

CLD participate in the manuscript design and wrote the first draft of the manuscript. AN, NM, ANB, RAC, and VP participated in the interpretation and preparation of the manuscript. HN participated in the manuscript design, interpretation and preparation of the manuscript. All the authors read and approved the final manuscript.

References

1. Halliwell B: **The wanderings of a free radical.** *Free Radic Biol Med* 2009, **46**:531–542.
2. Chaput JP, Klingenberg L, Rosenkilde M, Gilbert JA, Tremblay A, Sjodin A: **Physical activity plays an important role in body weight regulation.** *J Obes* 2011, **2011**:11.
3. Ristow M, Zarse K, Oberbach A, Kloting N, Birringer M, Kiehntopf M, Stumvoll M, Kahn CR, Bluher M: **Antioxidants prevent health-promoting effects of physical exercise in humans.** *Proc Natl Acad Sci USA* 2009, **106**:8665–8670.
4. Sahlin K, Shabalina IG, Mattsson CM, Bakkman L, Fernstrom M, Rozhdestvenskaya Z, Enqvist JK, Nedergaard J, Ekblom B, Tonkonogi M: **Ultraendurance exercise increases the production of reactive oxygen species in isolated mitochondria from human skeletal muscle.** *J Appl Physiol (1985)* 2010, **108**:780–787.
5. Yfanti C, Fischer CP, Nielsen S, Akerstrom T, Nielsen AR, Veskoukis AS, Kouretas D, Lykkesfeldt J, Pilegaard H, Pedersen BK: **Role of vitamin C and E supplementation on IL-6 in response to training.** *J Appl Physiol (1985)* 2012, **112**:990–1000.
6. Tauler P, Aguilo A, Gimeno I, Fuentespina E, Tur JA, Pons A: **Response of blood cell antioxidant enzyme defences to antioxidant diet supplementation and to intense exercise.** *Eur J Nutr* 2006, **45**:187–195.
7. Gomez-Cabrera MC, Domenech E, Romagnoli M, Arduini A, Borras C, Pallardo FV, Sastre J, Vina J: **Oral administration of vitamin C decreases muscle mitochondrial biogenesis and hampers training-induced adaptations in endurance performance.** *Am J Clin Nutr* 2008, **87**:142–149.
8. Nalbant O, Toktas N, Toraman NF, Ogus C, Aydin H, Kacar C, Ozkaya YG: **Vitamin E and aerobic exercise: effects on physical performance in older adults.** *Aging Clin Exp Res* 2009, **21**:111–121.
9. Gauche E, Lepers R, Rabita G, Leveque JM, Bishop D, Brisswalter J, Hausswirth C: **Vitamin and mineral supplementation and neuromuscular recovery after a running race.** *Med Sci Sports Exerc* 2006, **38**:2110–2117.

10. Nielsen HG, Skjonsberg OH, Lyberg T: **Effect of antioxidant supplementation on leucocyte expression of reactive oxygen species in athletes.** *Scand J Clin Lab Invest* 2008, **68:**526–533.
11. Patil SM, Chaudhuri D, Dhanakshirur GB: **Role of alpha-tocopherol in cardiopulmonary fitness in endurance athletes, cyclists.** *Indian J Physiol Pharmacol* 2009, **53:**375–379.
12. Louis J, Hausswirth C, Bieuzen F, Brisswalter J: **Vitamin and mineral supplementation effect on muscular activity and cycling efficiency in master athletes.** *Appl Physiol Nutr Metab* 2010, **35:**251–260.
13. Bloomer RJ, Falvo MJ, Schilling BK, Smith WA: **Prior exercise and antioxidant supplementation: effect on oxidative stress and muscle injury.** *J Int Soc Sports Nutr* 2007, **4:**9.
14. Yfanti C, Akerstrom T, Nielsen S, Nielsen AR, Mounier R, Mortensen OH, Lykkesfeldt J, Rose AJ, Fischer CP, Pedersen BK: **Antioxidant supplementation does not alter endurance training adaptation.** *Med Sci Sports Exerc* 2010, **42:**1388–1395.
15. Nakhostin-Roohi B, Babaei P, Rahmani-Nia F, Bohlooli S: **Effect of vitamin C supplementation on lipid peroxidation, muscle damage and inflammation after 30-min exercise at 75% VO2max.** *J Sports Med Phys Fitness* 2008, **48:**217–224.
16. Lamprecht M, Greilberger J, Oettl K: **Analytical aspects of oxidatively modified substances in sports and exercises.** *Nutrition* 2004, **20:**728–730.

Antioxidant and anti-nociceptive effects of *Phyllanthus amarus* on improving exercise recovery in sedentary men: a randomized crossover (double-blind) design

Thapanee Roengrit[1,5], Panakaporn Wannanon[1,5], Piyapong Prasertsri[2,5], Yupaporn Kanpetta[3,5], Bung-orn Sripanidkulchai[4,6] and Naruemon Leelayuwat[1,5*]

Abstract

Background: *Phyllanthus amarus* (PA) is a herbal plant containing antioxidant compounds that scavenge free radicals. The reduced oxidative stress may decrease muscle damage leading to early recovery from muscle soreness. This study aimed to evaluate the effects of PA powder on oxidative stress, muscle damage, leukocyte counts, inflammation, and muscle soreness after a single bout of high-intensity exercise.

Methods: Twelve men participated in two 3-day phases separated by a 1-week washout in a randomized double-blinded, crossover design. On day 1, randomly divided participants ingested two capsules of either PA (PA group) or placebo (PLA group) 20 min before a single bout of cycling at high intensity for 20 min followed by four capsules (two capsules after lunch and dinner), and six capsules/day for the next 2 days. Blood samples were collected before, immediately after, and 24 and 48 h after the exercise. Pain threshold was measured at the mid-thigh on both legs.

Results: Malondialdehyde concentration in the PA group was lower than that in the PLA group ($p < 0.05$) 48 h after high-intensity exercise. Vitamin C concentration was greater in the PA than in the PLA group ($p < 0.05$) immediately after high-intensity exercise. Pain threshold in both legs in the PA group was higher than in the PLA group 24 and 48 h after high-intensity exercise. There were no significant differences in creatine kinase, leukocyte counts or inflammation between groups.

Conclusion: Acute PA supplementation reduced oxidative stress and muscle soreness induced by high-intensity exercise.

Keywords: Herbal plant, Pain threshold, Malondialdehyde, Vitamin C, Muscle damage, Leukocytes, Inflammation

Introduction

Physical inactivity is the fourth-greatest risk factor for global mortality [1] (World Health Organization [WHO]), because it is an important cause of noncommunicable diseases (NCDs) [2]. To prevent NCDs, WHO introduced the *Global Recommendations on Physical Activity for Health* [3], which encourage people of all ages to begin moderately and gradually progress to higher levels of physical activity. Athletes often perform exercise at high intensity, aiming to win a competition. At the start of an exercise program, muscle damage both in sedentary participants [4] and athletes has often occurred [5]. Exercise-induced muscle damage is attributed to an exercise intensity-dependent increase in oxidative stress [6] produced by mitochondrial process (6). The oxidant damages the plasma membrane, which leads to leakage of creatine kinase (CK) into the blood [7]. This damage generates the inflammatory C-reactive protein (CRP), which facilitates the influx of inflammatory cells to

* Correspondence: naruemon@kku.ac.th
[1]Department of Physiology, Faculty of Medicine, Khon Kaen University, Khon Kaen 40002, Thailand
[5]The Exercise and Sport Sciences Research and Development Group, Khon Kaen University, Khon Kaen 40002, Thailand
Full list of author information is available at the end of the article

repair the damage [8]. Neutrophils and monocytes then repair the muscle via the oxidative or proteolytic modification to remove tissue debris in the injured muscle [9]. This process, known as the acute inflammatory response, causes muscle soreness after exercise [8]. Alternatively, the muscle soreness may be induced by increased hydrogen ion concentration or decreased pH of the muscle [10]. Rapid recovery from the prior exercise is important for both beginners performing regular exercise to improve their health and athletes preparing for competition. Thus, antioxidant supplementation to attenuate exercise-induced muscle injury, inflammation, and pain may facilitate success in both health promotion and sport competition.

Phyllanthus amarus (PA) is a herbal plant widely spread throughout tropical and subtropical areas, including in Thailand. PA extracts contain alkaloids, lignins, flavonoids, and polyphenol compounds [11]. These substances are known to have anti-carcinogenic and anti-inflammatory properties [12], anti-nociceptive effects [13], and hematological and immunological properties [14].

Although eccentric exercise was shown to damage active muscle, concentric exercise was also reported to cause muscular damage [6]. The previous study demonstrated that the high intensity concentric exercise (75% maximal oxygen consumption) increased CK activity immediately after the exercise. Moreover, the high-intensity exercise also increased neutrophil counts 24 h and monocyte counts 2 h after the exercise. These findings showed that the concentric exercise at high intensity causes the damage of active muscles and induces inflammation. Importantly, the reason for applying concentric exercise in this study is that we wanted to imitate real situation in daily life.

Thus far, no research investigating these effects of PA in exercise conditions in humans has been done; thus, we are interested in investigating its antioxidant, anti-inflammatory, and anti-nociceptive effects on improving exercise recovery. To test the hypothesis that acute PA supplementation reduces pain during recovery from high-intensity exercise, we examined the acute effects of PA on oxidative stress, muscle damage, leukocyte counts, inflammation, and muscle soreness after high-intensity exercise.

Materials and methods

Participants

Twelve sedentary men aged 22 ± 2.90 years participated in the study. They did not perform regular vigorous exercise and had never taken antioxidant supplements or medications. Prior to enrollment in the study, each subject's physical examination and electrocardiogram (ECG) were taken. Blood samples were collected after a 12-h overnight fast to measure glucose, creatinine, lipid profiles, and alanine aminotransferase (ALT), to check subjects' health status prior to the study. None of the subjects was a smoker or had cardiovascular, renal, neuromuscular, orthopedic, or liver disease. This study was approved by the Khon Kaen University Ethical Committee and conformed to the standards set by the Declaration of Helsinki in 2010 (HE531029). All participants provided informed consent to participate in the study after receiving both verbal and written explanations.

Power calculation

The sample size of this study was calculated by the WINPEPI program by using the study of Fenercioglu et al. [15] which reported that the antioxidant supplement prevent the increased MDA after the exercise. It was decided to require 80% power at a significance level of 0.05. Thus, the proposed size was 12 subjects per group.

Study design

This study was of a randomized crossover (double-blind) design. Subjects were blinded as to the composition of the PA and PLA or which supplement they were on at which times.

Supplement preparation

The supplements consisted of PA and placebo (PLA). The aerial parts of PA were collected from Khon Kaen Province. After washing with distilled water and drying at 50°C, the plant was ground and tested for microbial contamination. The plant powder was then placed into capsules containing excipients. One PA capsule contained 100 mg of dried PA powder and one placebo capsule contained Avicel® PH101 (microcrystalline cellulose; FMC BioPolymer, Philadelphia, PA, USA), Aerosil® (desiccant; Evonik Industries, China), and artificial colors. Both supplements were manufactured and controlled the contents by the Center for Research and Development of Herbal Health Products, Khon Kaen University. They were produced in the same lot of manufacture. The dosage of the PA was based on recommendations for the product in Thailand (Khaolaor Laboratories Co. Ltd, G 357/42). The PA contents in each capsule consisted of total polyphenol (33 mg/g) and vitamin C (1.60 mg/100 g) as measured by the Central Laboratory (Thailand) Co. Ltd., Thailand.

Baseline measurements

Before the experiment, anthropometric and body composition assessments were performed. Body composition was directly measured by Dual emission X-ray absorptiometry (DEXA) in the supine position. Fat distribution was indirectly measured by the ratio of waist and hip circumferences. A 3-day dietary and physical activity records were completed.

Peak oxygen consumption test

Each participant underwent an incremental exercise test on the cycle ergometer (Corival, Lode, The Netherlands). Oxygen consumption and carbon dioxide production were measured throughout the test using a gas analysis system (AD instrument, ML206, Australia). The test was started with a 12 min 4-stage incremental test in which workload was increased every 3 min for 4 workloads [16]. The workload was determined from an estimate of the participants' physical fitness status. The peak oxygen uptake value ($\dot{V}O_{2,peak}$) of the participant was determined when any of the following was achieved; the participant's $\dot{V}O_2$ reached a plateau with an increased workload, or a respiratory gas exchange ratio exceeded 1.15, or the heart rate (HR) reached a maximum HR (calculated by the equation: 220 − age), or maximal symptoms of dyspnea and fatigue by using the rating of perceived dyspnea (RPD) and the rating of perceived exertion (RPE) scales, or were unable to maintain cycling at a speed of 60 rpm. HR and ECG were continuously monitored during the test. After the participants reached the criteria, they rested, drank water, and measured their HR until it returned to normal. This test was done at least 1 wk before the initial exercise session.

Procedure

Participants participated randomly in two 3-day visits 2 weeks apart to prevent carryover effect. At the start of all visits they randomly ingested two capsules of either PA or PLA 20 min before performing exercise on the cycle ergometer. They then exercised without a workload for a 3-min warm-up. They then exercised for 20 min at high intensity (85% of peak oxygen consumption). On the same day and for the next 2 days, participants received the same supplement they had taken initially (two capsules three times per day after meals). Blood samples were collected immediately before ingestion of the supplement, immediately before exercise, and 24 and 48 h after exercise.

Blood chemistry

At each visit, a 12-mL blood sample was taken from an antecubital vein. After placing 6 mL into EDTA, 2 mL into lithium heparin, and 4 mL into clotting tubes, all samples were placed immediately on ice. One EDTA tube (2 mL) was then added to 1 mol/L of $HClO_4$ to precipitate the protein to measure vitamin C. All tubes were centrifuged at 4°C and 3,000 g for 15 min. The upper layer was transferred to a microcentrifuge tube and stored at −80°C until assay. CK, high-sensitivity CRP (hs-CRP), and complete blood count were analyzed in the clinical laboratory of the Srinagarind Hospital, Faculty of Medicine, Khon Kaen University, Thailand.

Malondialdehyde (MDA) assay

Plasma MDA, a marker of lipid peroxidation, was measured using the thiobarbituric acid (TBA) test according to the method of Draper [17]. The basis of the TBA method is the reaction of MDA with 0.6% of TBA at low pH and 95°C (boiled for 30 min) to form a colored complex. Acid hydrolysis and heat are necessary for the release of MDA bound to the amino groups of proteins and other amino compounds. The MDA-TBA complex, with an absorption at 532 nm, was measured using a spectrophotometer (Genesys 20, SN:35 gk 130009; Thermo Fisher Scientific, Waltham, MA, USA).

Vitamin C assay

Plasma vitamin C concentration was measured by using Zhang's method [18]. In this assay, Fe(III) is deoxidized to Fe(II) by ascorbate at pH 4.0 and Fe(II) reacts with potassium ferricyanide to form a blue product, soluble Prussian blue ($KFe^{III}[Fe^{II}(CN)_6]$). The absorbance of this product was monitored over time using a spectrophotometer at 735 nm and the amount of ascorbate was calculated based on absorbance.

Nitric oxide ($NO^{\cdot}$) assay

Plasma $NO^{\cdot}$ concentration was measured indirectly using inNO Nitric Oxide Measuring System and Sensors (Innovative Instruments, Inc., Brooks Court, FL, USA). The generation of $NO^{\cdot}$ is achieved by the addition of standard nitrite solution to an acidified solution in the presence of a reducing agent such as iodide ion according to the following equation:

$$2\,NO_2^- + 2I^- + 4H^+ \rightarrow 2\,NO^{\cdot} + I_2 + 2H_2O$$

As shown in the chemical equation, the molar ratio of nitrite to nitric oxide is 1:1. Thus, the amount of nitric oxide generated equals the amount of nitrite added.

Muscle damage

To determine the degree of muscle damage, serum CK activity was assessed. It is proportional to the rate of NADPH formation and was measured with a Roche/Hitachi cobas®c 502 analyzer (Roche, Basel, Switzerland) using standard automated laboratory methods.

Inflammation

CK activity and hsCRP concentration were determined using a Roche/Hitachi cobas c system (Cobas c 501, Roche Diagnostics, Indianapolis, IN, USA). The principle of CK activity measurement was the rate of the NADPH formation, which is directly proportional to the catalytic CK activity. It is determined by measuring the increase in absorbance. Equimolar quantities of NADPH and ATP are formed at the same rate. The photometrically measured rate of formation of NADPH is directly proportional to the CK activity. HsCRP level was determined using a particle enhanced immuno-turbidimetric assay method, in that agglutinates formation of human CRP with latex particles coated with monoclonal anti-CRP antibody was determined turbidimetrically.

Muscle soreness

Muscle soreness was measured by the pressure pain threshold of the quadriceps muscle at the mid-thigh using an algometer. Participants were asked to indicate verbally when they felt pain from the pressure.

Statistics

Data are presented as mean ± SD except when stated otherwise. Dependent variables were analyzed using repeated measure analysis of variance (ANOVA). Statistical analysis was performed using SPSS statistical software, version 18 (SPSS, Chicago, IL, USA). For all statistical tests, differences were considered significant when the p value was less than 0.05.

Results

Participant characteristics

The participants in this study were 12 healthy sedentary men. Anthropometry and physical fitness are summarized in Table 1. Baseline blood parameters are shown in Table 2. Regarding percentage of peak oxygen consumption, all participants performed exercise at high intensity (80.62 ± 3.3% and 82.39 ± 7.0 %$\dot{V}O_{2,peak}$ for PLA and PA groups, respectively). In addition, participants' dietary composition, energy intake, and energy expenditure are presented in Table 3. Physiological parameters, dietary composition (including vitamin C), energy intake, and energy expenditure were not different between groups.

Muscle soreness

The pain thresholds of both legs were lower at 24 h and 48 h ($p < 0.05$) after the high-intensity exercise in the PLA group than in the PA group (Figure 1A and 1B). In addition, the pain threshold of the right leg was lower 48 h after high-intensity exercise than pre-exercise in the PLA group (Figure 1A).

Oxidative stress, damage and inflammation

Plasma MDA concentration in the PA group was significantly lower than that of the PLA group 48 h after high-intensity exercise (1.92 ± 0.53 vs. 3.44 ± 1.27 nM; $p < 0.01$) (Figure 2). Vitamin C concentration was significantly

Table 1 Anthropometry, body composition and physical fitness of participants

	Mean ± SD
Age (yr)	22 ± 2.9
Height (m)	1.69 ± 0.06
BM (kg)	63.6 ± 10.7
BMI (kg/m^2)	22.8 ± 3.3
%BF	19.5 ± 9.0
FM (kg)	12.5 ± 7.3
FFM (kg)	48.4 ± 6.6
Waist circumference (cm)	76.7 ± 7.5
Hip circumference (cm)	94.8 ± 6.1
Waist: hip circumference ratio	0.81 ± 0.04
Physical fitness	
$\dot{V}O_{2,peak}$ (ml/kgBM/min)	36.9 ± 5.2
Work load$_{max}$ (watts)	136.0 ± 32.4

Values are presented as mean ± SD; n = 12.
BM, body mass; BMI, body mass index; %BF, percentage of body fat; FM, fat mass; FFM, fat free mass; $\dot{V}O_{2,peak}$, peak oxygen consumption.

Table 2 Baseline blood parameters of participants

	Mean ± SD
Blood glucose (mM)	4.6 ± 0.3
Creatinine (µmol/L)	0.01 ± 0.001
ALT (IU/L)	23.08 ± 24.91
TG (mM)	1.1 ± 0.3
TC (mM)	2.6 ± 1.4
LDL (mM)	2.8 ± 0.9
HDL (mM)	1.6 ± 0.4

Values are presented as mean ± SD; n = 12.
TG, triglycerides; TC, total cholesterol; LDL, low density lipoprotein; HDL, high density lipoprotein; ALT, alanine aminotransferase.

Table 3 Dietary composition, energy intake and energy expenditure of participants

	PLA	PA
Dietary composition (/day)		
- Protein (g)	122.9 ± 30.6	125.4 ± 35.6
- Fat (g)	89.3 ± 30.2	78.0 ± 17.4
- Carbohydrate (g)	254.3 ± 71.7	239.2 ± 62.9
- Fiber (g)	5.6 ± 2.0	7.1 ± 2.1
- Vitamin C (mg)	23.2 ± 18.4	27.1 ± 12.2
- Vitamin A (RE)	746.1 ± 1388.8	710.4 ± 1382.4
- Thiamine (mg)	1.3 ± 0.4	1.2 ± 0.5
- Riboflavin (mg)	1.9 ± 1.0	1.4 ± 0.5
- Niacin (mg)	20.7 ± 6.6	18.6 ± 6.5
Energy intake (kcal/day)	2289.2 ± 475.8	2112.0 ± 423.2
Energy expenditure (kcal/day)	2292.1 ± 388.1	2127.9 ± 654.6

Values are presented as mean ± SD; n = 12.
Vitamin A 1 RE = 12 µg alpha-carotene.
PLA, placebo group; PA, *Phyllanthus amarus* group; RE, retinol equivalent; kcal, kilocalories; g, grams; mg, milligrams; kg, kilograms.

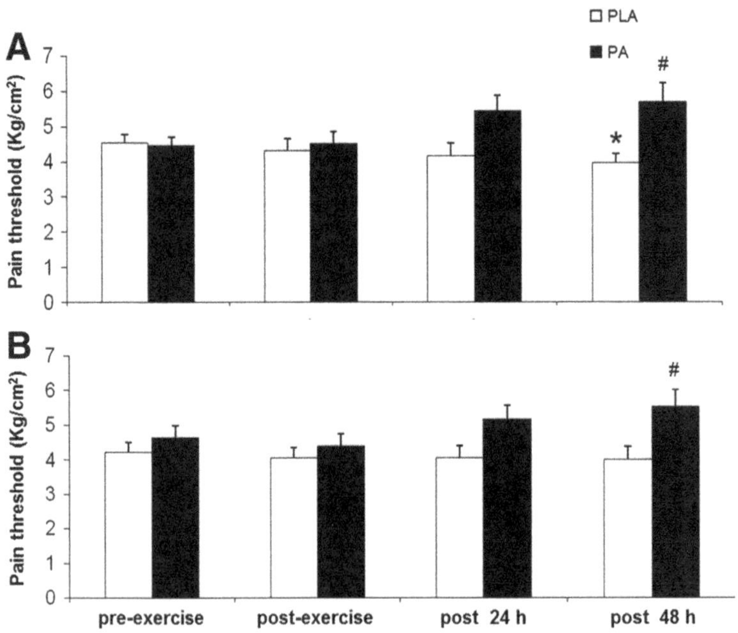

Figure 1 Levels of pain threshold on the right leg (A) and left leg (B) before exercise (pre-exercise), immediately after (post-exercise), and 24 h (post 24 h) and 48 h (post 48 h) after high-intensity exercise. Values are presented as mean ± SE (n = 12). PLA, placebo. *Significantly different from before exercise ($p < 0.05$), #significantly different from the PLA group at the same time point ($p < 0.05$).

higher in the PA group than in the PLA group immediately after high-intensity exercise (9.68 ± 2.21 vs. 5.91 ± 1.45 μg/mL; $p < 0.05$) (Figure 3). It then fell to baseline at 24 h after exercise. Plasma CK concentration were significantly higher immediately after exercise than before exercise (Table 4). However, CK, NO˙ and hs-CRP concentrations were not significantly different between groups at any time point (Table 4).

Leukocyte counts

Neutrophil count was significantly higher immediately after exercise than before exercise in both groups (Table 4). Neutrophil count at 24 h was significantly lower than immediately after exercise in the PA group ($p < 0.05$) (Table 4). Lymphocyte count significantly increased immediately after exercise when compared with pre-exercise ($p < 0.05$) (Table 4). Moreover lymphocyte counts at 48 h

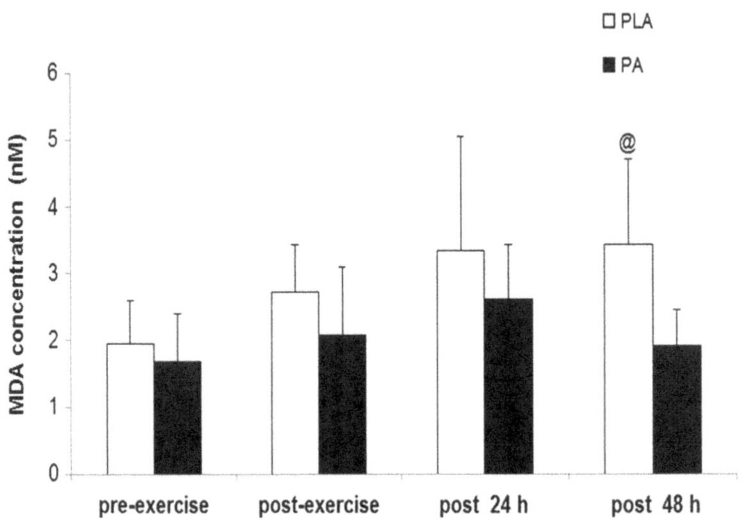

Figure 2 MDA concentration before exercise (pre-exercise), immediately after (post-exercise), and 24 h (post 24 h) and 48 h (post 48 h) after high-intensity exercise. Values are presented as mean ± SE (n = 12). MDA, malondialdehyde; PLA, placebo [@]Significantly different from the PLA group at the same time point ($p < 0.01$).

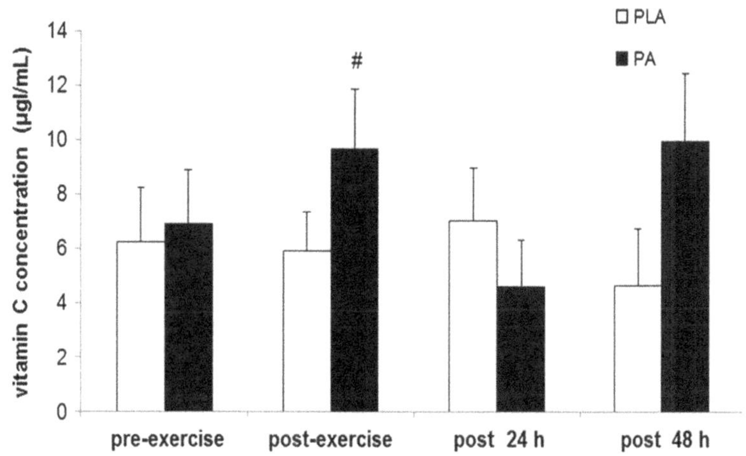

Figure 3 Vitamin C concentration before exercise (pre-exercise), immediately after (post-exercise), and 24 h (post 24 h) and 48 h (post 48 h) after high-intensity exercise. Values are presented as mean ± SE (n = 12). PLA, placebo. #Significantly different from the PLA group at the same time point ($p < 0.05$).

in the PA group and 24 h in the PLA group significantly lower than immediately after the exercise ($p < 0.05$) (Table 4). Monocyte count was significantly increased 24 h after the exercise when compared with pre-exercise ($p < 0.05$) (Table 4). There were no significant between-group differences in leukocyte count at any time point.

Discussion

Our results demonstrate that acute PA supplementation may reduce the muscle soreness of both legs during recovery from high-intensity exercise in healthy participants.

The results partially support our hypothesis that acute PA supplementation reduces pain during recovery from high-intensity exercise. Previous studies on PA supplementation have demonstrated the antioxidant and anti-nociceptive effects of PA in animals under non-exercise conditions [19-21]. Thus, the present study is the first to demonstrate a reduction in muscle pain after the ingestion of PA immediately before and a few days after the exercise with improved oxidative stress during recovery. A review of the literature suggests that muscle soreness is strongest 24–72 h after exercise [22]. Our finding of decreased muscle soreness at 24 h may demonstrate a potential effect of PA on recovery from muscle soreness and may enable beginners in sports activity to return to a competition or an exercise session the next day.

PA has been shown by this study to contain a wide variety of antioxidant compounds, such as vitamin C and total polyphenol compounds. The lack of difference in dietary vitamin C intake before the experiment between

Table 4 CK, NO˙, hs-CRP concentrations and leukocyte counts before the exercise (pre-exercise), immediately (post-exercise), 24 h (post 24 h) and 48 h (post 48 h) after the high–intensity exercise

		Pre-exercise	Post-exercise	Post-24 h	Post-48 h
CK (U/L)	PLA	151.8 ± 22.4	166.0 ± 24.9*	164.8 ± 25.2	163.7 ± 30.1
	PA	132.3 ± 19.0	194.5 ± 21.5*	182.6 ± 41.5	145.6 ± 65.6
hs-CRP (mg/L)	PLA	1.24 ± 0.37	1.36 ± 0.43	1.58 ± 0.74	2.28 ± 1.11
	PA	1.24 ± 0.33	1.15 ± 0.33	1.57 ± 0.57	1.26 ± 0.42
Neutrophils (10^3/μL)	PLA	3.68 ± 0.33	4.80 ± 0.61*	4.05 ± 0.53	3.66 ± 0.19
	PA	3.53 ± 0.35	4.39 ± 0.45*	3.09 ± 0.25∞	3.37 ± 0.26
Lymphocytes (10^3/μL)	PLA	2.08 ± 0.19	2.57 ± 0.39	1.77 ± 0.08∞	1.75 ± 0.10
	PA	1.88 ± 0.16	2.61 ± 0.28*	2.13 ± 0.15	1.91 ± 0.09∞
Monocytes (10^3/μL)	PLA	0.41 ± 0.02	0.45 ± 0.05	0.44 ± 0.06	0.43 ± 0.03
	PA	0.31 ± 0.44	0.36 ± 0.41	0.48 ± 0.33∞	0.44 ± 0.06

Values are presented as mean ± SE; n = 12.
NO˙, nitric oxide; hs-CRP, high sensitive C-reactive protein.
*Significantly different from before the high-intensity exercise ($p < 0.05$).
∞Significantly different from immediately after the exercise (post-exercise) ($p < 0.05$).

the groups confirmed that the greater plasma vitamin C concentration was induced by the PA supplementation. The amount of vitamin C in the PA intake per day in this study seemed to be too small to increase plasma vitamin C concentration. In a previous study, vitamin C intake of less than 200 mg (9.60 mg in this study) increased the absorption rate to 98% [23]. This may contribute to the higher vitamin C concentration immediately after the exercise in the PA than the placebo group. Apart from vitamin C, the PA in each capsule contains 33 mg/g of total polyphenol. Although polyphenol compounds in participants' blood were not measured in this study, it may play antioxidant role during and immediately after the exercise. Polyphenol may spare the antioxidant activity of vitamin C at this period. Then the decreased vitamin C concentration at the following 24 h after the exercise may imply that vitamin C was greatly consumed in scavenging free radicals resulting in the decrease of lipid peroxidation indicated by MDA at 48 h after the exercise.

In addition, three possible mechanisms explaining important anti-nociceptive role of vitamin C and total polyphenol compounds induced by PA supplementation are: 1) stimulation of the secretion of beta-endorphin by vitamin C, which is effective at reducing neuropathic pain [24], 2) scavenging reactive oxygen species [25], which play an important role in reducing neuropathic pain [26]. The reduction in free radicals resulted in decreased prostaglandins [27], which are sympathetic nervous system pain mediators [28], as well as by central inhibitory pain mechanisms [29]. Unfortunately, beta-endorphin secretion and the pain mediators are not examined by this study. Therefore, the effects of acute PA supplementation on either beta-endorphin secretion or the liberation of pain mediators should be further investigated. 3) Reduction in hydrogen ion produced by high-intensity exercise may be one of the mechanisms that explain the effect of these antioxidants on pain reduction. Proton normally produced by high-intensity exercise was shown to increase pain and fatigue [30]. Recently polyphenol including flavonoid was demonstrated to scavenge free radicals by hydrogen ion transfer. This may thus reduce noxious effects due to oxidative stress [31].

The anti-nociceptive effect of antioxidants mentioned above was shown in non-exercise condition. This effect on exercise recovery in humans is still unclear. Some authors have reported reductions in muscle pain [32], but others did not demonstrate this effect [33,34]. The discrepancy may be due to the duration and timing of supplementation. The anti-nociceptive effect seems to be present if PA is ingested long before the exercise (>2 wk) [32,35,36] because this finding is not reported in previous studies with shorter durations of pre-exercise (2 h to 3 d) and post-exercise supplementation [33,34,37-39].

The significant increase in plasma CK concentration indicated increased muscle damage, as determined by both supplement groups immediately after the high-intensity exercise. This indicates that the single bout of high-intensity exercise for 20 min in this study was sufficient to cause muscle damage. However, we did not find any difference in CK concentration between groups, which, combined with the lack of differences in immune cell counts and inflammatory responses to the exercise between groups suggests that the development of cell damage and inflammation in this exercise was not attenuated by PA supplementation.

Improved oxidative stress after exercise by PA supplementation might be useful for some medical conditions generating high oxidative stress, such as type 2 diabetes mellitus [40] or for individuals with pre-hypertension who got benefit effect from the reduced oxidative stress [41] but further study would be required to prove this possibility. It is likely that acute supplementation during exercise may provide protection until patients can adapt to oxidative stress by modifying their own antioxidant status, which require a bit of time. Moreover, prolonged supplementation before exercise may provide protective effects against oxidative stress and exercise recovery in the patients who are not trained person.

We performed our research according to the guidelines proposed by a recent review article on studies investigating the impact of antioxidant supplementation on exercise performance [42] by carefully preparing and storing the antioxidant compounds; i.e., PA in this study, to prevent oxidation and degradation. Also, to ensure that the results in this study were really due to the PA ingested, we compared the dietary status of both groups and confirmed no difference between them. Moreover, the subjects had no other antioxidant supplementation at any time before or during the experiment.

A limitation of this study is that the dose of PA powder was the dose for resting conditions. This was intended to avoid adverse effects on participants. A longer duration of PA supplementation before exercise, or a higher dose of PA, might be required to yield muscle damage and inflammation and greater and earlier beneficial effects on muscle soreness after high-intensity exercise, which in turn may contribute to rapid recovery after high-intensity exercise.

Conclusions

The present study shows that PA supplementation improved oxidative stress and muscle soreness induced by high-intensity exercise. This may encourage beginners or novices in sports activity or fitness to return to a competition or an exercise session the next day, with early recovery from muscle soreness. The present results add a treatment value of PA, a herb generally found in Thailand, in aspects of both health and sport.

Abbreviations
ALT: Alanine aminotransferase; ANOVA: Analysis of variance; CK: Creatine kinase; ECG: Electrocardiogram; DEXA: Dual emission x-ray absorptiometry; EDTA: Ethylene diamine tetra acetic acid; HDL: High-density lipoprotein; hs CRP: high sensitive C reactive protein; MDA: Malondialdehyde; NO˙: Nitric oxide; NCDs: noncommunicable diseases; PA: *Phyllanthus amarus*; PLA: Placebo; RE: retinol equivalent; TBA: Thiobarbituric acid; $\dot{V}O_{2,peak}$: Peak oxygen consumption; WHO: World Health Organization.

Competing interests
The authors declare that they have no competing of interest.

Authors' contributions
NL conceived and designed the study and prepared the manuscript. PW provided medical coverage throughout the experiment. TR carried out all the experimental work and statistical analysis and helped to draft the manuscript. PP and YK assisted the experimental work. BS provided PA and PLA supplements. All authors read and approved the final manuscript.

Acknowledgments
This study was supported by the Graduate Research Fund Academic Year 2010 (53212102) Khon Kaen University, National Research University (MIH-2554-Ph.D-10), and Invitation research (I 55145). It was partially supported by the Exercise and Sport Sciences Research and Development Group and Back, Neck and Other Joint Pain Research Group, Khon Kaen University. We thank the Center for Research and Development of Herbal Health Products, Khon Kaen University, for the supplement manufacture. We thank Professor Yukifumi Nawa for his excellent proofreading of this manuscript. Finally, we thank the volunteers for their enthusiastic participation in this study.

Author details
[1]Department of Physiology, Faculty of Medicine, Khon Kaen University, Khon Kaen 40002, Thailand. [2]Faculty of Allied Health Sciences, Burapha University, Chonburi 20130, Thailand. [3]Exercise and Sport Sciences Program, Graduate School, Khon Kaen University, Khon Kaen 40002, Thailand. [4]Faculty of Pharmaceutical Sciences, Khon Kaen University, Khon Kaen 40002, Thailand. [5]The Exercise and Sport Sciences Research and Development Group, Khon Kaen University, Khon Kaen 40002, Thailand. [6]The Center for Research and Development of Herbal Health Products, Khon Kaen University, Khon Kaen 40002, Thailand.

References
1. World Health Organization: *Global health risks: mortality and burden of disease attributable to selected major risks.* Geneva: World Health Organization Press; 2009.
2. World Health Organization: *The global burden of disease: 2004 update.* Geneva: World Health Organization Press; 2008.
3. World Health Organization: *Global recommendations on physical activity for health.* Geneva. ISBN 9789241599979. 2010.
4. Moflehi D, Kok LY, Tengku-Kamalden TF, Amri S: **Effect of single-session aerobic exercise with varying intensities on lipid peroxidation and muscle-damage markers in sedentary males.** *Glob J Health Sci* 2012, **4**:48–54. doi:10.5539/gjhs.v4n4p48.
5. Teixeira VH, Valente HF, Casal SI, Marques FP, Moreira PA: **Blood antioxidant and oxidative stress biomarkers acute responses to a 1000-m kayak sprint in elite male kayakers.** *J Sports Med Phys Fitness* 2013, **53**:71–79.
6. Seifi-Skishahr F, Siahkohian M, Nakhostin-Roohi B: **Influence of aerobic exercise at high and moderate intensities on lipid peroxidation in untrained men.** *J Sports Med Phys Fitness* 2008, **48**:515–521.
7. Brancaccio P, Maffulli N, Limongelli FM: **Creatine kinase monitoring in sport medicine.** *Br Med Bull* 2007, **81–82**:209–230.
8. Semple SJ, Smith LL, McKune AJ, Neveling N, Wadee A: **Alterations in acute-phase reactants (CRP, rheumatoid factor, complement, Factor B, and immune complexes) following an ultramarathon.** *SA Sports Medicine* 2004, **16**:17–21.
9. Nieman DC: **Immune response to heavy exertion.** *J Appl Physiol* 1997, **82**:1385–1394.
10. Issberner U, Reeh PW, Steen KH: **Pain due to tissue acidosis: a mechanism for inflammatory and ischemic myalgia?** *Neurosci Lett* 1996, **208**:191–194.
11. Kumaran A, Karunakaran RJ: **In vitro antioxidant activities of methanol extracts of five Phyllanthus species from India.** *LWT. Food Sci Technol* 2007, **40**:344–352. DOI:10.1016/j.lwt.2005.09.011
12. Kiemer AK, Hartung T, Huber C, Vollmar AM: **Phyllanthusamarus has anti-inflammatory potential by inhibition of iNOS, COX-2, and cytokines via the NF-kappaB pathway.** *J Hepatol* 2003, **38**:289–297.
13. Santos AR, Filho VC, Yunes RA, Calixto JB: **Analysis of the mechanisms underlying the antinociceptive effect of the extracts of plants from the genus Phyllanthus.** *Gen Pharmacol* 1995, **26**:1499–1506.
14. Taiwo IA, Oboh BO, Francis-Garuba PN: **Haematological properties of aqueous extracts of Phyllantus amarus (Schum and Thonn.) and Xylopia aethiopica (Dunal) A. Rich in albino rats.** *Ethno-Med* 2009, **3**:99–103.
15. Fenercioglu AK, Saler T, Genc E, Sabuncu H, Altuntas Y: **The effects of polyphenol-containing antioxidants on oxidative stress and lipid peroxidation in Type 2 diabetes mellitus without complications.** *J Endocrinol Invest* 2010, **33**:118–124. doi:10.3275/6564. Epub 2009 Oct 15.
16. Prasertsri P, Roengrit T, Kanpetta Y, Tong-un T, Muchimapura S, Wattanathorn J, Leelayuwat N: **Cashew apple juice supplementation enhanced fat utilization during high-intensity exercise in trained and untrained men.** *J Int Soc Sports Nutr* 2013, **10**:13. doi:10.1186/1550-2783-10-13.
17. Draper HH, Squires EJ, Mahmoodi H, Wu J, Agarwal S, Hadley M: **A comparative evaluation of thiobarbituric acid methods for the determination of malondialdehyde in biological materials.** *Free Radic Biol Med* 1993, **15**:353–363.
18. Zhang H, Li J, Wang K, Du X, Li Q: **A simple and sensitive assay for ascorbate using potassium ferricyanide as spectroscopic probe reagent.** *Anal Biochem* 2009, **388**:40–46.
19. Karuna R, Reddy SS, Baskar R, Saralakumari D: **Antioxidant potential of aqueous extract of Phyllanthusamarus in rats.** *Indian J Pharmacol* 2009, **41**:64–67. doi:10.4103/0253-7613.51342.
20. Maity S, Chatterjee S, Variyar PS, Sharma A, Adhikari S, Mazumder S: **Evaluation of antioxidant activity and characterization of phenolic constituents of Phyllanthusamarus root.** *J Agric Food Chem* 2013, **61**:3443–3450.
21. Obidike IC, Salawu OA, Ndukuba M, Okoli CO, Osunkwo UA: **The anti-inflammatory and antinociceptive properties of the chloroform fraction from Phyllanthusniruri plant is mediated via the peripheral nervous system.** *J Diet Suppl* 2010, **7**:341–350. doi:10.3109/19390211.2010.522553.
22. Nosaka K: **Muscle soreness and damage and the repeated-bout effect.** In *Skeletal muscle damage and repair 2008 (pp. 63).* Edited by Tiidus PM. Champaign, IL: Human Kinetics. ISBN 978-0-7360-5867-4.
23. Levine M, Conry-Cantilena C, Wang Y, Welch RW, Washko PW, Dhariwal KR, Park JB, Lazarev A, Graumlich JF, King J, Cantilena LR: **"Vitamin C pharmacokinetics in healthy volunteers: evidence for a recommended dietary allowance".** *Proc Natl Acad Sci USA* 1996, **93**:3704–3709. Bibcode:1996PNAS…93.3704L. doi:10.1073/pnas.93.8.3704.
24. Yang Z, Copolov DL, Lim AT: **Ascorbic acid augments the adenylyl cyclase-cAMP system mediated POMC mRNA expression and beta-endorphin secretion from hypothalamic neurons in culture.** *Br Res* 1996, **706**:243–248.
25. Rice ME: **Ascorbate regulation and its neuroprotective role in the brain.** *Trends Neurosci* 2000, **23**:209–216.
26. Kim HK, Park SK, Zhou JL, Taglialatela G, Chung K, Coggeshall RE, Chung JM: **Reactive oxygen species (ROS) play an important role in a rat model of neuropathic pain.** *Pain* 2004, **111**:116–124.
27. Ye Y, Guo Y, Luo YT: **Anti-inflammatory and analgesic activities of a novel biflavonoid from shells of Camellia oleifera.** *Int J Mol Sci* 2012, **13**:12401-12411. doi:10.3390/ijms131012401.
28. Duarte JDG, Nakamura M, Ferreira SH: **Participation of the sympathetic system in acetic acid induced writhing in mice.** *Braz J Med Biol Res* 1988, **21**:341–343.
29. Ren W, Kiritoshi T, Gregoire S, Ji G, Guerrini R, Calo G, Neugebauer V: **Neuropeptide S: a novel regulator of pain-related amygdala plasticity and behaviors.** *J Neurophysiol* 2013, **110**:1765–1781. doi:10.1152/jn.00874.2012. Epub 2013 Jul 24.
30. Pollak KA, Swenson JD, Vanhaitsma TA, Hughen RW, Jo D, Light KC, Schweinhardt P, Amann M, Light AR: **Exogenously applied muscle metabolites synergistically evoke sensations of muscle fatigue and pain in human subjects.** *Exp Physiol* 2014, **99**:368–380. doi:10.1113/expphysiol.2013.075812. Epub 2013 Oct 18.

31. Di Meo F, Lemaur V, Cornil J, Lazzaroni R, Duroux JL, Olivier Y, Trouillas P: **Free radical scavenging by natural polyphenols: atom versus electron transfer.** *J Phys Chem A* 2013, **117**:2082–2092. doi:10.1021/jp3116319. Epub 2013 Mar 5.
32. Bloomer RJ, Goldfarb AH, McKenzie MJ, You T, Nguyen L: **Effects of antioxidant therapy in women exposed to eccentric exercise.** *Int J Sport Nutr Exerc Metab* 2004, **14**:377–388.
33. Close GL, Ashton T, Cable T, Doran D, Holloway C, McArdle F, MacLaren DP: **Ascorbic acid supplementation does not attenuate post-exercise muscle soreness following muscle-damaging exercise but may delay the recovery process.** *Br J Nutr* 2006, **95**:976–981.
34. Thompson D, Williams C, Garcia-Roves P, McGregor SJ, McArdle F, Jackson MJ: **Post-exercise vitamin C supplementation and recovery from demanding exercise.** *Eur J Appl Physiol*, **89**:393–400. Epub 2003 Apr 1.
35. Bryer SC, Goldfarb AH: **Effect of high dose vitamin C supplementation on muscle soreness, damage, function, and oxidative stress to eccentric exercise.** *Int J Sport Nutr Exerc Metab* 2006, **16**:270–280.
36. Thompson D, Williams C, McGregor SJ, Nicholas CW, McArdle F, Jackson MJ, Powell JR: **Prolonged vitamin C supplementation and recovery from demanding exercise.** *Int J Sport Nutr Exerc Metab* 2001, **11**:466–481.
37. Thompson D, Williams C, Kingsley M, Nicholas CW, Lakomy HK, McArdle F, Jackson MJ: **Muscle soreness and damage parameters after prolonged intermittent shuttle-running following acute vitamin C supplementation.** *Int J Sports Med* 2001, **22**:68–75.
38. Childs A, Jacobs C, Kaminski T, Halliwell B, Leeuwenburgh C: **Supplementation with vitamin C and N-acetyl-cysteine increases oxidative stress in humans after an acute muscle injury induced by eccentric exercise.** *Free Radic Biol Med* 2001, **31**:745–753.
39. Connolly DA, Lauzon C, Agnew J, Dunn M, Reed B: **The effects of vitamin C supplementation on symptoms of delayed onset muscle soreness.** *J Sports Med Phys Fitness* 2006, **46**:462–467.
40. Leelayuwat N, Tunkumnerdthai O, Donsom M, Punyaek N, Manimanakorn A, Kukongviriyapan U, Kukongviriyapan V: **An alternative exercise and its beneficial effects on glycaemic control and oxidative stress in participants with type 2 diabetes.** *Diabetes Res Clin Pract* 2008, **82**:e5–e8.
41. Wichitsranoi J, Weerapreeyakul N, Boonsiri P, Settasatian C, Settasatian N, Komanasin N, Sirijaichingkul S, Teerajetkul Y, Jungtrakul D, Leelayuwat N: **Antihypertensive and antioxidant effects of dietary black sesame meal in pre-hypertensive humans.** *Nutr J* 2011, **9**:10–82.
42. Powers SK, Smuder AJ, Kavazis AN, Hudson MB: **Experimental guidelines for studies designed to investigate the impact of antioxidant supplementation on exercise performance.** *Int J Sport Nutr Exerc Metab* 2010, **20**:2–14.

16

The effects of pre versus post workout supplementation of creatine monohydrate on body composition and strength

Jose Antonio* and Victoria Ciccone

Abstract

Background: Chronic supplementation with creatine monohydrate has been shown to promote increases in total intramuscular creatine, phosphocreatine, skeletal muscle mass, lean body mass and muscle fiber size. Furthermore, there is robust evidence that muscular strength and power will also increase after supplementing with creatine. However, it is not known if the timing of creatine supplementation will affect the adaptive response to exercise. Thus, the purpose of this investigation was to determine the difference between pre versus post exercise supplementation of creatine on measures of body composition and strength.

Methods: Nineteen healthy recreational male bodybuilders (mean ± SD; age: 23.1 ± 2.9; height: 166.0 ± 23.2 cm; weight: 80.18 ± 10.43 kg) participated in this study. Subjects were randomly assigned to one of the following groups: PRE-SUPP or POST-SUPP workout supplementation of creatine (5 grams). The PRE-SUPP group consumed 5 grams of creatine immediately before exercise. On the other hand, the POST-SUPP group consumed 5 grams immediately after exercise. Subjects trained on average five days per week for four weeks. Subjects consumed the supplement on the two non-training days at their convenience. Subjects performed a periodized, split-routine, bodybuilding workout five days per week (Chest-shoulders-triceps; Back-biceps, Legs, etc.). Body composition (Bod Pod®) and 1-RM bench press (BP) were determined. Diet logs were collected and analyzed (one random day per week; four total days analyzed).

Results: 2x2 ANOVA results - There was a significant time effect for fat-free mass (FFM) ($F = 19.9$; $p = 0.001$) and BP ($F = 18.9$; $p < 0.001$), however, fat mass (FM) and body weight did not reach significance. While there were trends, no significant interactions were found. However, using magnitude-based inference, supplementation with creatine post workout is possibly more beneficial in comparison to pre workout supplementation with regards to FFM, FM and 1-RM BP. The mean change in the PRE-SUPP and POST-SUPP groups for body weight (BW kg), FFM (kg), FM (kg) and 1-RM bench press (kg) were as follows, respectively: Mean ± SD; BW: 0.4 ± 2.2 vs. 0.8 ± 0.9; FFM: 0.9 ± 1.8 vs. 2.0 ± 1.2; FM: -0.1 ± 2.0 vs. −1.2 ± 1.6; Bench Press 1-RM: 6.6 ± 8.2 vs. 7.6 ± 6.1.
Qualitative inference represents the likelihood that the true value will have the observed magnitude. Furthermore, there were no differences in caloric or macronutrient intake between the groups.

Conclusions: Creatine supplementation plus resistance exercise increases fat-free mass and strength. Based on the magnitude inferences it appears that consuming creatine immediately post-workout is superior to pre-workout vis a vis body composition and strength.

Keywords: Creatine, Supplement timing, Body composition, Fat free mass, Dietary supplement

* Correspondence: ja839@nova.edu
Exercise and Sports Sciences, Nova Southeastern University, 3532 S. University Drive, University Park Plaza Suite 3532, Davie, FL 33314, USA

Introduction

Chronic supplementation with creatine has been shown to increase lean body mass and enhance exercise performance [1-10]. Creatine supplementation for as brief a period as 3 days has been shown to produce a significant increase in skeletal muscle volume and exercise performance according to Ziegenfuss et al. [9]. One week of supplementation has been shown to increase body weight 1.4 kg (range 0.00 to 2.7 kg) [11]. Furthermore, creatine supplementation combined with resistance training resulted in a 6.3% increase in body weight and fat-free mass after a 12 week treatment period [12]. Subjects with initially low levels of intramuscular creatine (e.g. vegetarians) are more responsive to supplementation than those who regularly consume meat [13]. However, not all investigations demonstrate a positive effect of creatine supplementation vis a vis body composition [14-18].

It has not yet been fully elucidated what effect nutrient timing (i.e. consuming nutrients pre, during and/or post workout) has on the adaptive response to exercise [19-24]. However, based on the preponderance of evidence, it is apparent that consuming the proper nutrients during the periworkout time period may enhance lean body mass and expedite skeletal muscle recovery [25-29]. For instance, Tipton et al. demonstrated that consuming an essential amino acid solution pre workout resulted in a greater net muscle protein synthesis than that when the solution is consumed after exercise; this increase in muscle protein synthesis is believed to be the result of an increased delivery of amino acids to the leg [29]. Cribb and Hayes discovered that consuming a protein-carbohydrate-creatine supplement immediately pre and post workout resulted in greater gains in lean body mass, muscle fiber size and muscular strength in comparison to morning and evening consumption [25]. It is apparent that the timing of nutrient intake does indeed affect the adaptive response to exercise but it is not known if there is a difference between pre versus post workout consumption of a supplement or nutrient combination. Therefore, the purpose of this investigation was to determine if there was a difference in pre versus post workout supplementation of creatine on body composition and muscular strength.

Methods

Subjects

Nineteen male recreational bodybuilders (mean ± SD: age, 23.1 ± 2.9 years; height, 166.0 ± 23.2 cm; body weight, 80.2 ± 10.4 kg) completed this study. Participants were otherwise healthy college-age students who had been resistance training regularly for over a year. Individuals who were currently consuming other workout supplements or ergogenic aids were instructed to immediately stop consumption and complete at least a four-week washout period before entering the study. All procedures involving human subjects were approved by Nova Southeastern University's Human Subjects Institutional Review Board in accordance with the Helsinki Declaration, and written informed consent was obtained prior to participation.

Experimental design

Subjects were randomly assigned to one of two groups: a PRE-SUPP or POST-SUPP group. The PRE-SUPP group consumed 5 grams of creatine monohydrate immediately prior to training. The POST-SUPP group consumed the same amount of creatine immediately after training. Following pre-testing data collection, participants began a periodized four-week resistance training program that was self-administered. On off-training days, subjects consumed creatine at their convenience. The total treatment duration was four weeks.

Resistance training protocol

All subjects followed a periodized, split-routine bodybuilding training regimen geared primarily for skeletal muscle hypertrophy. The participants trained 5 days a week for 4 weeks for a total of 20 training sessions. Each training session lasted approximately 60 minutes. The program was as follows:

Week 1
Mon – Chest, Shoulder, Triceps (3 × 15, sets × reps; does not include 2 warm up sets)
Tues – Hips, Legs (3 × 15)
Wed – Back, Biceps (3 × 15)
Thurs – Chest, Shoulders, Triceps (3 × 10)
Fri – Hips, Legs (3 × 10)
Sat – REST
Sun - REST
Week 2
Mon – Back, Biceps (3 × 10)
Tues – Chest, Shoulder, Triceps (3 × 5)
Wed – Hips, Legs (3 × 5)
Thurs – Back, Biceps (3 × 5)
Fri – Chest, Shoulder, Triceps (3 × 15)
Sat – REST
Sun – REST
Week 3
Mon – Hips, Legs (3 × 15)
Tues – Back, Biceps (3 × 15)
Wed – Chest, Shoulders, Triceps (3 × 10)
Thurs – Hips, Legs (3 × 10)
Fri – Back, Biceps (3 × 10)
Sat – REST
Sun – REST

Week 4
Mon – Chest, Shoulders, Triceps (3 × 5)
Tues – Hips, Legs (3 × 5)
Wed – Back, Biceps (3 × 5)
Thurs – Chest, Shoulder, Triceps (3 × 15)
Fri – Hip, Legs (3 × 15)
Sat – REST
Sun – REST

Choice of exercises for each body part split

Chest – (subject performed 3 of these) flat bench press, incline bench press, cable cross-overs, pec deck, flat bench flies, decline bench press; Shoulders (subject performed 3 of these) – upright row, machine military press, dumbbell overhead presses, lateral dumbbell raises, shoulder shrugs; Triceps (subject performed two of these) – triceps pushdowns, dips, French press; Back (subject performed four of these) – Wide grip lat pulldown, narrow grip lat pulldown, chin ups, cable rows, dumbbell rows, dumbbell flies; Biceps (subject performed three of these) – standing barbell curls, standing EZ bar curl, concentration curls, preacher curls, hammer curls; Legs/Hips (subject performed five of these) – Back squats, Smith machine squats, Leg Press, Lunges, Leg curls, Leg extensions, calf raise (seated or standing), Stiff-legged deadlift. On test days, participants reported to NSU's Exercise and Sports Science lab after a 3 hour fast and refrained from participating in vigorous activity or exercise in the 24-hour period prior to testing. Subjects were asked to maintain their normal dietary intake for the duration of the study and to refrain from ingesting any other dietary supplement that may enhance body composition (e.g. protein, amino acids, etc.).

Food diary, workout log, body composition

Subjects provided a 24-hour diet recall on one random day on week 1, 2, 3, and 4 (as determined by the investigators). Dietary intake was measured using the Nutribase® program. Height was measured using standard anthropometry and total body weight was measured using a calibrated scale. Body composition was assessed by whole body densitometry using air displacement via the Bod Pod® (COSMED USA, Concord, CA). All testing was performed in accordance with the manufacturer's instructions. Briefly, subjects were tested while wearing only tight fitting clothing (swimsuit or undergarments) and an acrylic swim cap. The subjects wore the exact same clothing for all testing. Thoracic gas volume was estimated for all subjects using a predictive equation integral to the Bod Pod® software. The calculated value for body density used the Siri equation to estimate body composition. Data from the Bod Pod® included body weight, % body fat, fat free mass and fat mass. All testing was done with each subject at the same time of day (plus or minus 1 hour). Also, all subjects were required to keep a workout log showing the exercises with reps and sets performed.

Exercise performance assessment

Subjects performed a 1 repetition maximum lifts (1-RM) on the bench press. Subjects warmed up (2 sets of 8–10 repetitions at approximately 50% of anticipated maximum) on the bench press. Subjects performed successive 1-RM lifts starting at about 70% of anticipated 1-RM and increased it by 5–10 lbs until the reaching a 1-RM. There was a two minute rest interval between sets. Each subject was allowed a maximum of three attempts.

Statistical analysis

Data were analyzed utilizing five separate 2-way [group (Pre-Treatment [aka PRE-SUPP] vs. Post-Treatment [aka POST-SUPP]) × time (pre vs. post)] Analysis of Variance (ANOVA). When appropriate, follow-up analysis included paired sample *t*-test. An alpha level was set at $p \leq 0.05$, and all analyses were performed using PASW version 18.0 (SPSS, Inc., Chicago, IL). The effects of nutrient timing plus resistance exercise were calculated as the changes from pretraining to post-training body composition and performance measurements among Pre-Treatment vs. Post-Treatment groups. Magnitude-based inferences were used to identify clinical differences in the measurement changes between the Pre-Treatment and Post-Treatment. Several studies have supported the use of magnitude-based inference statistics as a complementary tool for null hypothesis testing to reduce errors in interpretation and to provide more clinically meaningful results [30,31]. The precision of the magnitude inference was set at 90% confidence limits, using a p value derived from an independent *t*-test. Threshold values for positive and negative effect were calculated by multiplying standard deviations of baseline values by 20% [30]. Inferences on true differences between the exercise and control group were determined as positive, trivial, or negative according to methods previously described by Batterham and Hopkins [31]. Inferences were based on the confidence interval range relative to the smallest clinically meaningful effect to be positive, trivial, or negative. Unclear results are reported if the observed confidence interval overlaps both positive and negative values. The probability of the effect was evaluated according to the following scale: : <0.5%, most unlikely; 0.5-5%, very unlikely; 5-25%, unlikely; 25-75%, possibly; 75-95%, likely; 95–99.5%, very likely; >99.5%, most likely (Hopkins, 2010).

Results

Twenty-two subjects were initially recruited for this investigation. Three subjects dropped out for no given reason. Nineteen healthy recreational male bodybuilders (age: 23.1 ± 2.9; height: 166.0 ± 23.2 cm; weight: 80.2 ± 10.4 kg) completed the study. There were no differences between groups for any of the baseline measures. 2×2 ANOVA results - There was a significant time effect for FFW ($F = 19.9$; $p = 0.001$) and BP ($F = 18.9$; $p < 0.001$), however FM and BW did not reach significance. While there were trends, no significant interactions were found (Table 1).

Thus, using magnitude-based inference, supplementation with creatine post-workout is possibly more beneficial in comparison to pre-workout supplementation with regards to FFM, FM (Table 2, Figure 1, Figure 2) and 1-RM BP. It is apparent that everyone in the POST-SUPP group improved vis a vis FFM; however, this was not the case with the PRE-SUPP group (Figures 1 and 2).

Dietary variables

The macronutrient intake for the PRE-SUPP and POST-SUPP groups are summarized in Table 3. There were no significant differences between the groups. On average, both groups consumed a diet of 39-40% carbohydrate, 26% protein, and 35% fat. Both groups consumed 1.9 grams of protein per kg body weight.

Discussion

The results from this study suggest that consuming creatine monohydrate post exercise may be superior to consuming it pre exercise with regards to improving body composition (i.e. gains in FFM, loss of FM). This is the first investigation to demonstrate that the timing of creatine intake affects the adaptive response to exercise. When subjects were pooled together, the gains in fat-free mass and muscular strength in the current investigation were similar to others. Rugby union football players who supplemented daily with creatine monohydrate over an 8-week period decreased fat mass (−1.9 kg) and increased lean tissue (+1.2 kg). They also performed better in bench and leg press tests [15]. Older men (71 yrs) who consumed creatine increased lean tissue mass (+3.3 kg) and improved lower body strength as measured using a 1-RM [32]. Using a single-limb training model, men and women who supplemented with creatine after training of the arms increased their muscle thickness. Interestingly, males had a greater increase in lean tissue mass with creatine supplementation than females [4]. In elite male handball players, creatine supplementation for 32 days resulted in an increase in 1-RM bench press (8.30 vs. 5.29 kg; creatine versus control) [33]. These and other investigations indeed show that creatine supplementation in general has a significant anabolic and performance-enhancing effect [34,35] which is in agreement with the current investigation. Mechanistically, creatine supplementation has been shown to increase muscle fiber size, enhance myosin heavy chain protein synthesis, activate satellite cells as well as increase the concentrations of intramuscular ATP and PCr [6,7,12,36,37].

However, whether supplement timing has a role in the adaptive response vis a vis creatine has not been previously investigated. Certainly, the most important aspect of the current investigation is that post workout supplementation of creatine may indeed be superior to pre workout supplementation. Data on protein and amino acid supplementation indicate that indeed the pre, during and post workout window are important times to consume nutrients though some studies demonstrate a neutral effect [20-24,38]. One study examined the effects of a solution of whey protein consumed either immediately before exercise or immediately following exercise. They found no difference in amino acid uptake between the groups [18]. In six subjects (3 men, 3 women) that randomly consumed a treatment drink (6 g essential amino acids, 35 g sucrose) or a flavored placebo drink 1 hour or 3 hours after a bout of resistance exercise,

Table 1 Body composition and strength

		Baseline	Post-test	Mean change
PRE-SUPP N = 9	BW (kg)	82.5 ± 10.5	82.9 ± 10.6	0.4 ± 2.5
POST-SUPP N = 10		78.1 ± 10.4	78.9 ± 10.0	0.8 ± 0.9
PRE-SUPP	FFM (kg)	66.7 ± 6.9	67.6 ± 7.6	0.9 ± 1.8
POST-SUPP		65.9 ± 8.0	67.9 ± 8.6	2.0 ± 1.2
PRE-SUPP	FM (kg)	15.4 ± 4.9	15.3 ± 5.5	−0.1 ± 2.0
POST-SUPP		13.00 ± 4.0	11.8 ± 3.6	−1.2 ± 1.6
PRE-SUPP	% Body Fat	18.4 ± 4.1	18.2 ± 5.1	−0.2 ± 2.2
POST-SUPP		16.9 ± 4.8	15.0 ± 4.7	−1.9 ± 2.3
PRE-SUPP	1-RM BP	96.7 ± 21.9	103.3 ± 19.5	6.6 ± 8.2
POST-SUPP		103.2 ± 24.0	110.9 ± 25.4	7.7 ± 6.2

Values are mean ± SD. *1-RM* one repetition maximum, *BP* Bench Press, *BW* body weight, *FFM* fat-free mass, *FM* fat mass.

Table 2 Magnitude-based inference results

	POST-SUPP	PRE-SUPP		
Measures	**Mean ± SD**	**Mean ± SD**	**Difference ± 90CI[a]**	**Qualitative Inference**
BW (kg)	0.8 ± 0.9	0.4 ± 2.2	0.4 ± 1.3	Trivial
FFM (kg)	2.0 ± 1.2	0.9 ± 1.8	1.1 ± 1.2	Possibly beneficial
FM (kg)	−1.2 ± 1.6	−0.1 ± 2.0	1.1 ± 1.5	Possibly beneficial
1-RM BP (kg)	7.6 ± 6.2	6.6 ± 8.2	1.2 ± 1.7	Likely beneficial

Changes in body composition and performance in PRE-SUPP vs. POST-SUPP groups, and qualitative inferences about the effects on body composition and bench press strength.
Values reported as mean ± standard deviation (SD); *BW* body weight, *FFM* fat-free mass, *FM* fat mass. [a] ± 90% CI: add and subtract this number to the mean difference to obtain the 90% confidence intervals for the true difference. Qualitative inference represents the likelihood that the true value will have the observed magnitude.

investigators found no difference in the anabolic response whether the drink was consumed 1 hour or 3 hours post exercise [39]. Indeed, others have found that timed protein supplementation immediately before and after exercise does not further enhance muscle mass or strength in healthy elderly men who habitually consume adequate amounts of dietary protein [40]. Also, timed protein-supplement ingestion in resistance-trained athletes during a 10-week training program does not further enhance strength, power, or body-composition changes [41].

On the other hand, consuming an essential amino acid solution immediately before resistance exercise elevates muscle protein synthesis to a greater extent than when the solution is consumed after exercise. The investigators postulated that this may be due to an increased delivery of amino acids to the leg [29]. Clearly, issues related to blood flow would not be advantageous to the POST-SUPP group in the current study.

Another study investigated the importance of immediate (P0) or delayed (P2: 2 hours post exercise) intake of an oral protein supplement upon muscle hypertrophy and strength over a period of resistance training in elderly males. In response to training, the cross-sectional area of the quadriceps femoris muscle and mean fiber area increased in the P0 group, whereas no significant increase was observed in P2. These investigators found no difference in the glucose or insulin response at P0 or P2, thus, it is not likely that differences in the hormonal environment contributed to the difference in muscle mass gain. Thus, the early intake of an oral protein supplement after resistance training is important for skeletal muscle hypertrophy [42].

Perhaps the seminal study vis a vis nutrient timing compared taking a protein-carbohydrate-creatine supplement either immediately pre and post exercise (PRE-POST) or in the morning and evening (MOR-EVE). Indeed the PRE-POST group demonstrated a greater increase in lean body mass and 1-RM strength in two of three assessments. Furthermore, type II muscle fiber cross-sectional area was larger in the PRE-POST group

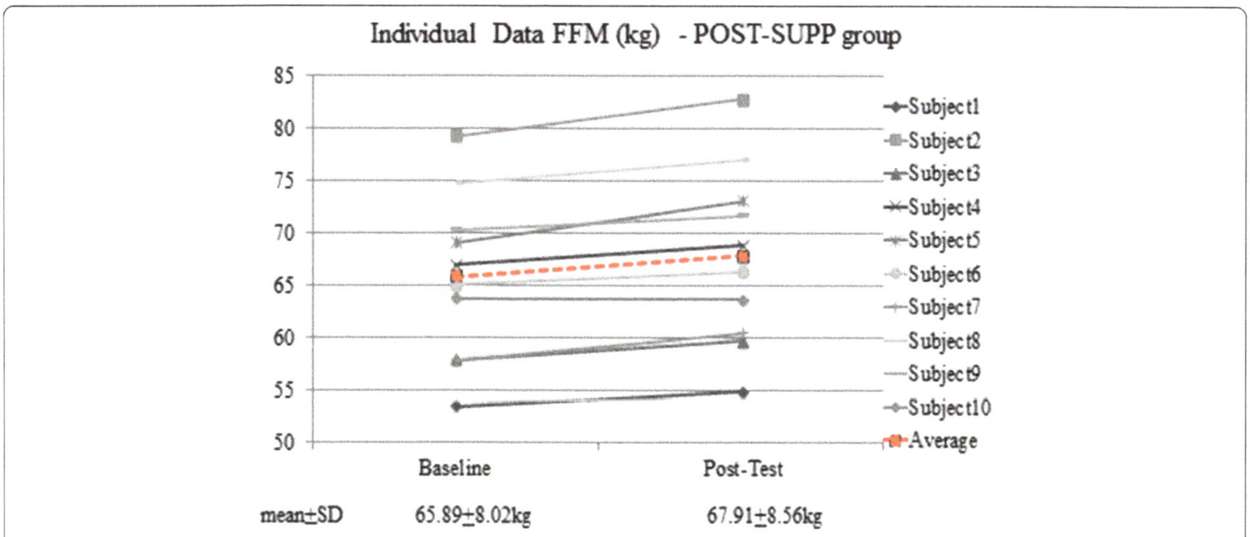

Figure 1 Individual data for FFM in the POST-SUPP group.

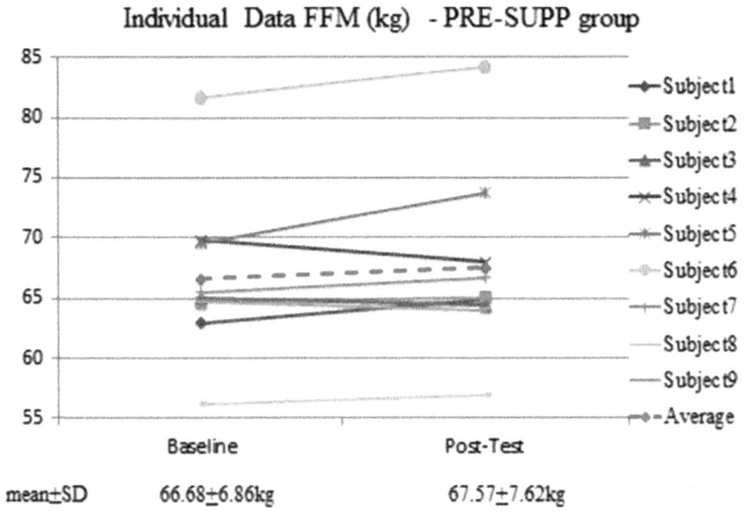

Figure 2 Individual data for FFM in the PRE-SUPP group.

as well as intramuscular concentrations of creatine and glycogen [25]. Data from this investigation showed the intramuscular creatine and glycogen concentrations were greater in the PRE-POST versus MOR-EVE groups. Thus, taking the exact same supplement (but timed pre and post exercise) is significantly better than consuming it in the morning and evening.

Our investigation did not involve the use of protein, carbohydrate or amino acids. Whether creatine uptake is truly sensitive to timed intake is not entirely known despite the superior gains in the POST-SUPP group. Moreover, it is entirely possible that the difference in body composition and muscular strength between the two groups was the result of a small sample size. One individual in the POST-SUPP and three individuals in the PRE-SUPP group experienced a minor reduction in FFM. With regards to 1-RM bench press performance, two subjects in the PRE-SUPP group showed either no change or a decline in strength; on the other hand, only one subject in the POST-SUPP group showed no change in strength. All other subjects experienced an increase in strength.

The use of recreational bodybuilders in the current investigation is advantageous because it is difficult for highly trained individuals to experience an increase in FFM or muscular strength in the time frame allotted for this study. Nonetheless, of the 19 subjects that completed the study, 16-21% were non-responders regarding muscular strength and FFM. It should be noted that the nutrient intake (kcals, carbohydrate, fat and protein) was similar between the groups. In fact, each group consumed a high protein diet (1.9 grams of protein per kg bw daily); thus, it is not likely that dietary factors caused the discrepancy in the adaptive response to creatine supplementation and resistance training. Nevertheless, another consideration to take into account would be that because these recreational bodybuilders were already consuming large quantities of protein, this could have affected the results (i.e. they could already have a high amount of creatine stored intramuscularly and this may have blunted the results).

In conclusion, post workout supplementation with creatine for a period of 4 weeks in recreational bodybuilders may produce superior gains in FFM and strength in comparison to pre workout supplementation. The major limitations of this study include the small sample size as well as the brief treatment duration. Future studies should investigate creatine supplementation using resistance trained individuals for a longer duration.

Table 3 Dietary intake

	PRE-SUPP	POST-SUPP
Total kcals	2416 ± 438	2575 ± 842
CHO g	229 ± 53	261 ± 120
CHO kcal	915 ± 213	1046 ± 479
CHO %	39 ± 11	40 ± 10
PRO g	159 ± 41	147 ± 41
PRO kcal	637 ± 165	590 ± 163
PRO %	26 ± 4	25 ± 7
FAT g	96 ± 39	104 ± 48
FAT kcal	863 ± 359	939 ± 433
FAT %	35 ± 10	35 ± 8

Values are mean ± SD; no significant differences for any of the variables.
CHO carbohydrate, *PRO* protein.

Competing interests
Jose Antonio PhD was a former sports science consultant to VPX® Sports.

Authors' contributions
VC and JA contributed significantly to all aspects of this study. Both authors read and approved the final manuscript.

Acknowledgements
The creatine monohydrate (Creatine Plasma™) was provided by VPX® Sports, Davie FL. Many thanks to Jeff Stout PhD for running the stats on this project.

References
1. Aguiar AF, Januario RS, Junior RP, Gerage AM, Pina FL, do Nascimento MA, Padovani CR, Cyrino ES: **Long-term creatine supplementation improves muscular performance during resistance training in older women.** *Eur J Appl Physiol* 2013, **113**:987–996.
2. Rawson ES, Stec MJ, Frederickson SJ, Miles MP: **Low-dose creatine supplementation enhances fatigue resistance in the absence of weight gain.** *Nutrition* 2011, **27**:451–455.
3. Gotshalk LA, Kraemer WJ, Mendonca MA, Vingren JL, Kenny AM, Spiering BA, Hatfield DL, Fragala MS, Volek JS: **Creatine supplementation improves muscular performance in older women.** *Eur J Appl Physiol* 2008, **102**:223–231.
4. Chilibeck PD, Stride D, Farthing JP, Burke DG: **Effect of creatine ingestion after exercise on muscle thickness in males and females.** *Med Sci Sports Exerc* 2004, **36**:1781–1788.
5. Cooke MB, Rybalka E, Williams AD, Cribb PJ, Hayes A: **Creatine supplementation enhances muscle force recovery after eccentrically-induced muscle damage in healthy individuals.** *J Int Soc Sports Nutr* 2009, **6**:13.
6. Spillane M, Schoch R, Cooke M, Harvey T, Greenwood M, Kreider R, Willoughby DS: **The effects of creatine ethyl ester supplementation combined with heavy resistance training on body composition, muscle performance, and serum and muscle creatine levels.** *J Int Soc Sports Nutr* 2009, **6**:6.
7. Buford TW, Kreider RB, Stout JR, Greenwood M, Campbell B, Spano M, Ziegenfuss T, Lopez H, Landis J, Antonio J: **International Society of Sports Nutrition position stand: creatine supplementation and exercise.** *J Int Soc Sports Nutr* 2007, **4**:6.
8. Mendel RW, Blegen M, Cheatham C, Antonio J, Ziegenfuss T: **Effects of creatine on thermoregulatory responses while exercising in the heat.** *Nutrition* 2005, **21**:301–307.
9. Ziegenfuss TN, Rogers M, Lowery L, Mullins N, Mendel R, Antonio J, Lemon P: **Effect of creatine loading on anaerobic performance and skeletal muscle volume in NCAA Division I athletes.** *Nutrition* 2002, **18**:397–402.
10. Mihic S, MacDonald JR, McKenzie S, Tarnopolsky MA: **Acute creatine loading increases fatfree mass, but does not affect blood pressure, plasma creatinine, or CK activity in men and women.** *Med Sci Sports Exerc* 2000, **32**:291–296.
11. Volek JS, Kraemer WJ, Bush JA, Boetes M, Incledon T, Clark KL, Lynch JM: **Creatine supplementation enhances muscular performance during high-intensity resistance exercise.** *J Am Diet Assoc* 1997, **97**:765–770.
12. Volek JS, Duncan ND, Mazzetti SA, Staron RS, Putukian M, Gomez AL, Pearson DR, Fink WJ, Kraemer WJ: **Performance and muscle fiber adaptations to creatine supplementation and heavy resistance training.** *Med Sci Sports Exerc* 1999, **31**:1147–1156.
13. Burke DG, Chilibeck PD, Parise G, Candow DG, Mahoney D, Tarnopolsky M: **Effect of creatine and weight training on muscle creatine and performance in vegetarians.** *Med Sci Sports Exerc* 2003, **35**:1946–1955.
14. Sakkas GK, Mulligan K, Dasilva M, Doyle JW, Khatami H, Schleich T, Kent-Braun JA, Schambelan M: **Creatine fails to augment the benefits from resistance training in patients with HIV infection: a randomized, double-blind, placebo-controlled study.** *PLoS One* 2009, **4**:e4605.
15. Chilibeck PD, Magnus C, Anderson M: **Effect of in-season creatine supplementation on body composition and performance in rugby union football players.** *Appl Physiol Nutr Metab* 2007, **32**:1052–1057.
16. Bemben MG, Witten MS, Carter JM, Eliot KA, Knehans AW, Bemben DA: **The effects of supplementation with creatine and protein on muscle strength following a traditional resistance training program in middle-aged and older men.** *J Nutr Health Aging* 2010, **14**:155–159.
17. Tipton KD, Wolfe RR: **Protein and amino acids for athletes.** *J Sports Sci* 2004, **22**:65–79.
18. Tipton KD, Elliott TA, Cree MG, Aarsland AA, Sanford AP, Wolfe RR: **Stimulation of net muscle protein synthesis by whey protein ingestion before and after exercise.** *Am J Physiol Endocrinol Metab* 2007, **292**:E71–E76.
19. Candow DG, Chilibeck PD: **Timing of creatine or protein supplementation and resistance training in the elderly.** *Appl Physiol Nutr Metab* 2008, **33**:184–190.
20. Aragon AA, Schoenfeld BJ: **Nutrient timing revisited: is there a post-exercise anabolic window?** *J Int Soc Sports Nutr* 2013, **10**:5.
21. Stark M, Lukaszuk J, Prawitz A, Salacinski A: **Protein timing and its effects on muscular hypertrophy and strength in individuals engaged in weight-training.** *J Int Soc Sports Nutr* 2012, **9**:54.
22. Kerksick C, Harvey T, Stout J, Campbell B, Wilborn C, Kreider R, Kalman D, Ziegenfuss T, Lopez H, Landis J, *et al*: **International Society of Sports Nutrition position stand: nutrient timing.** *J Int Soc Sports Nutr* 2008, **5**:17.
23. Wilson J, Wilson GJ: **Contemporary issues in protein requirements and consumption for resistance trained athletes.** *J Int Soc Sports Nutr* 2006, **3**:7–27.
24. White JP, Wilson JM, Austin KG, Greer BK, St John N, Panton LB: **Effect of carbohydrateproteinsupplement timing on acute exercise-induced muscle damage.** *J Int Soc Sports Nutr* 2008, **5**:5.
25. Cribb PJ, Hayes A: **Effects of supplement timing and resistance exercise on skeletal muscle hypertrophy.** *Med Sci Sports Exerc* 2006, **38**:1918–1925.
26. Levenhagen DK, Gresham JD, Carlson MG, Maron DJ, Borel MJ, Flakoll PJ: **Postexercise nutrient intake timing in humans is critical to recovery of leg glucose and protein homeostasis.** *Am J Physiol Endocrinol Metab* 2001, **280**:E982–E993.
27. Tipton KD, Ferrando AA, Phillips SM, Doyle D Jr, Wolfe RR: **Postexercise net protein synthesis in human muscle from orally administered amino acids.** *Am J Physiol* 1999, **276**:E628–E634.
28. Tipton KD, Ferrando AA: **Improving muscle mass: response of muscle metabolism to exercise, nutrition and anabolic agents.** *Essays Biochem* 2008, **44**:85–98.
29. Tipton KD, Rasmussen BB, Miller SL, Wolf SE, Owens-Stovall SK, Petrini BE, Wolfe RR: **Timing of amino acid-carbohydrate ingestion alters anabolic response of muscle to resistance exercise.** *Am J Physiol Endocrinol Metab* 2001, **281**:E197–E206.
30. Hopkins WG, Marshall SW, Batterham AM, Hanin J: **Progressive statistics for studies in sports medicine and exercise science.** *Med Sci Sports Exerc* 2009, **41**:3–13.
31. Batterham AM, Hopkins WG: **Making meaningful inferences about magnitudes.** *Int J Sports Physiol Perform* 2006, **1**:50–57.
32. Chrusch MJ, Chilibeck PD, Chad KE, Davison KS, Burke DG: **Creatine supplementation combined with resistance training in older men.** *Med Sci Sports Exerc* 2001, **33**:2111–2117.
33. Percario S, Domingues SP, Teixeira LF, Vieira JL, de Vasconcelos F, Ciarrocchi DM, Almeida ED, Conte M: **Effects of creatine supplementation on oxidative stress profile of athletes.** *J Int Soc Sports Nutr* 2012, **9**:56.
34. Jagim AR, Oliver JM, Sanchez A, Galvan E, Fluckey J, Riechman S, Greenwood M, Kelly K, Meininger C, Rasmussen C, Kreider RB: **A buffered form of creatine does not promote greater changes in muscle creatine content, body composition, or training adaptations than creatine monohydrate.** *J Int Soc Sports Nutr* 2012, **9**:43.
35. Souza-Junior TP, Willardson JM, Bloomer R, Leite RD, Fleck SJ, Oliveira PR, Simao R: **Strength and hypertrophy responses to constant and decreasing rest intervals in trained men using creatine supplementation.** *J Int Soc Sports Nutr* 2011, **8**:17.
36. Willoughby DS, Rosene J: **Effects of oral creatine and resistance training on myosin heavy chain expression.** *Med Sci Sports Exerc* 2001, **33**:1674–1681.
37. Olsen S, Aagaard P, Kadi F, Tufekovic G, Verney J, Olesen JL, Suetta C, Kjaer M: **Creatine supplementation augments the increase in satellite cell and myonuclei number in human skeletal muscle induced by strength training.** *J Physiol* 2006, **573**:525–534.
38. Lemon PW, Berardi JM, Noreen EE: **The role of protein and amino acid supplements in the athlete's diet: does type or timing of ingestion matter?** *Curr Sports Med Rep* 2002, **1**:214–221.

39. Rasmussen BB, Tipton KD, Miller SL, Wolf SE, Wolfe RR: **An oral essential amino acidcarbohydrate supplement enhances muscle protein anabolism after resistance exercise.** *J Appl Physiol* 2000, **88:**386–392.
40. Verdijk LB, Jonkers RA, Gleeson BG, Beelen M, Meijer K, Savelberg HH, Wodzig WK, Dendale P, van Loon LJ: **Protein supplementation before and after exercise does not further augment skeletal muscle hypertrophy after resistance training in elderly men.** *Am J Clin Nutr* 2009, **89:**608–616.
41. Hoffman JR, Ratamess NA, Tranchina CP, Rashti SL, Kang J, Faigenbaum AD: **Effect of protein-supplement timing on strength, power, and body-composition changes in resistancetrained men.** *Int J Sport Nutr Exerc Metab* 2009, **19:**172–185.
42. Esmarck B, Andersen JL, Olsen S, Richter EA, Mizuno M, Kjaer M: **Timing of postexercise protein intake is important for muscle hypertrophy with resistance training in elderly humans.** *J Physiol* 2001, **535:**301–311.

Effects of creatine supplementation associated with resistance training on oxidative stress in different tissues of rats

Giuseppe Potrick Stefani[1], Ramiro Barcos Nunes[1*], André Zuanazzi Dornelles[1], Jadson Pereira Alves[1], Marcella Ody Piva[2], Marlise Di Domenico[2], Cláudia Ramos Rhoden[2] and Pedro Dal Lago[1,3]

Abstract

Background: Creatine supplementation is known to exert an effect by increasing strength in high intensity and short duration exercises. There is a hypothesis which suggests that creatine supplementation may provide antioxidant activity by scavenging Reactive Oxygen Species. However, the antioxidant effect of creatine supplementation associated with resistance training has not yet been described in the literature. Therefore, we investigated the effect of creatine monohydrate supplementation associated with resistance training over maximum strength gain and oxidative stress in rats.

Methods: Forty male Wistar rats (250-300 g, 90 days old) were randomly allocated into 4 groups: Sedentary (SED, n = 10), Sedentary + Creatine (SED-Cr, n = 10), Resistance Training (RT, n = 10) and Resistance Training + Creatine (RT-Cr, n = 10). Trained animals were submitted to the RT protocol (4 series of 10–12 repetitions, 90 second interval, 4 times per week, 65% to 75% of 1MR, for 8 weeks).

Results: In this study, greater strength gain was observed in the SED-Cr, RT and RT-Cr groups compared to the SED group ($P < 0.001$). The RT-Cr group showed a higher maximum strength gain when compared to other groups ($P < 0.001$). Creatine supplementation associated with resistance training was able to reduce lipoperoxidation in the plasma ($P < 0.05$), the heart ($P < 0.05$), the liver ($P < 0.05$) and the gastrocnemius ($P < 0.05$) when compared to control groups. However, the supplementation had no influence on catalase activity (CAT) in the analyzed organs. Only in the heart was the CAT activity higher in the RT-Cr group ($P < 0.05$). The activity of superoxide dismutase (SOD) was lower in all of the analyzed organs in the SED-Cr group ($P < 0.05$), while SOD activity was lower in the trained group and sedentary supplemented group ($P < 0.05$).

Conclusions: Creatine was shown to be an effective non-enzymatic antioxidant with supplementation alone and also when it was associated with resistance training in rats.

Keywords: Creatine, Supplementation, Resistance training, Oxidative stress, Lipoperoxidation, Antioxidant, Maximum strength, Rats

Background

Creatine supplementation has been extensively studied since the 1990s and several studies [1-3] have analyzed its effects on maximum strength and body mass increase, which are well understood. The muscular storages of free creatine (Cr) and phosphorylated creatine (PCr) can be increased with creatine supplementation, leading to improvements in energy production by anaerobic systems in the first instances of physical exercises. Furthermore, this PCr increase can contribute to elevated protein synthesis and proteolysis prevention in muscular tissue [4].

From a different perspective, other studies have in investigated the antioxidant effect of creatine supplementation. In a cell-free experiment, the ability of creatine to quench reactive oxygen and nitrogen species, such as H_2O_2 and $ONOO^-$, in muscle homogenates was observed

* Correspondence: ramiro.barcos@gmail.com
[1]Laboratório de Fisiologia – UFCSPA/Porto Alegre, Rua Sarmento Leite, 245, 900050-170 Porto Alegre, RS, Brazil
Full list of author information is available at the end of the article

[5]. On the other hand, the first study reporting antioxidant activity related to creatine supplementation in living cells was performed by Sestili and colleagues in 2006 [6]. However, few studies have assessed the antioxidant effect of creatine supplementation in biological systems, such as in humans or animals. A recent study pointed out the pleiotropic effects of creatine and its possible direct antioxidant effect in scavenging Reactive Oxygen Species (ROS) and Reactive Nitrogen Species (RNS) [7].

Oxidative stress and the subsequent damage to lipids, proteins and nucleic acids in acute response to aerobic exercise is well established in the literature [8-10]. In the same way, some studies have demonstrated an oxidative response when resistance exercises are performed [11-13]. Since systematic training can lead to increases in the activity of antioxidant enzymes (modulated by exercise adaptations) [14], it is still not clear whether Resistance Training (RT) can attenuate the acute oxidative damage experienced after exercise. Moreover, until now, there have been few studies that have evaluated the effect of creatine supplementation on resistance training maximum strength gain and oxidative stress.

Considering this, it is not clear whether creatine supplementation exerts intra and/or extracellular antioxidant effects and it plays a synergistic role in the adaptation of antioxidant enzymes associated with RT. Thus, the aim of this study was to evaluate the effects of monohydrate creatine supplementation associated, or not, with RT on oxidative stress and antioxidant enzymatic activity in the plasma, the heart, the liver and the gastrocnemius of rats.

Materials and methods

Animals

Forty male Wistar rats (250 to 300 g; 90 days old) from the UFCSPA Breeding Unit were divided into four groups: Sedentary (SED, n = 10), Sedentary + Creatine (SED-Cr, n = 10), Resistance Training (RT, n = 10) and Resistance Training + Creatine (RT-Cr, n = 10). The animals were housed under standard conditions (food and water *ad libitum*, temperature between 22 and 24°C, light–dark cycle of 12 hours).

The handling of the animals obeyed Law nº 11,794 of 10/08/2008, Law nº 6,899 of 07/15/2009, and Resolution nº 879 of 02/15/2008 (CFMV), as well as other provisions applicable to the use of animals for teaching and research, in particular the resolutions of the National Council on Animal Experimentation. This study was approved by CEUA/UFCSPA, under the protocol number 060/11.

Resistance training protocol

Before the beginning of the experiment, the animals from the training groups were submitted to a familiarization period in the adapted squat apparatus designed by Krisan et al. [15]. The animals were placed in the apparatus and performed between 5 and 10 repetitions with 40% to 60% of their body weight, three times per week for one week. This load was considered low intensity as it has already been demonstrated that non-trained rats can lift up to three times their body weight upon first contact with the referred apparatus [16].

The rats were placed in a neoprene vest leaving them in bipedal position of the lower limbs. An electrical stimulus (4–5 mA, 0.3 seconds long, with a 3 second interval between each repetition) was applied in the rat's tail using a surface electrode, in order to provoke the extension movement of the lower limbs of the rat, thus raising the load imposed in the squat apparatus. As this stimulus is considered low intensity, it is not expected to cause any physical injury to the animals [17]. All training sessions were performed in a dark room.

To determine the maximum lifted load in one repetition, the One Maximum Repetition (1MR) was utilized. From the obtained value, the load percentages required to perform the training protocol were determined. In response to training, strength gains were reported, making the realization of retests every two weeks necessary, in order to adjust the training load.

The training protocol lasted for a total eight weeks, at a frequency of four times per week. Each training session consisted of four series of 10–12 repetitions with a load of 65-75% of 1MR with a 90 second interval between each series [18]. The training program followed the guidelines of the American Physiological Society (2006) [19].

Creatine supplementation protocol

The groups that were administered creatine monohydrate (presentation form: powder, purity: 99.9%, Delaware Laboratory, RS, Brazil) were given this by gavage solutions, as this resembles human oral consumption and ensures that the desired dose is achieved. The dosage of supplement administered followed the recommendations of the International Society of Sports Nutrition (2007) [20]. During the saturation period, which was the first seven days prior to the initiation of training, the dosage of 0.3 g/kg/day of creatine, diluted with 1.5 ml distilled water, was established. In the maintenance period, which comprised the last seven weeks, the dosage was set at 0.05 g/kg/day of creatine, which was diluted with 1.5 ml of distilled water. The animals received the supplement every day before training for the entire period of the protocol (including the days on which they did not train).

Blood and tissues collection

The blood collection was performed through the decapitation method. The blood was stored in 2 ml Eppendorf microtubes containing EDTA and subsequently centrifuged (3,000 rpm for 10 minutes at 4°C) to separate the supernatant plasma. After blood collection, the collection of tissues (heart, liver and gastrocnemius) was performed, and samples were frozen at -80°C.

Oxidative stress evaluation

Tissues homogenization

The heart, liver and gastrocnemius were defrosted, weighed in an analytical balance and homogenized in KPi buffer (KCl 1.15%), pH 7.4, with proportion of 9 ml/1 g of tissue. The proteases were inactivated with the addition of 0.5 mM phenylmethanesulfonyl fluoride (Sigma-Aldrich®, SP, Brazil) in anhydrous ethanol (1 µl of PMSF/1 ml of KPi buffer). The homogenization was performed manually in a glass macerator, with a Teflon pistil, counting 30 rotation movements and structure compression [21]. The homogenized samples were then centrifuged (3,000 rpm for 10 minutes at 6°C) and the supernatants utilized to determine the malondialdehyde (MDA), catalase (CAT) and superoxide dismutase (SOD) activities.

Determination of total protein by the Bradford method

This technique is based in the interaction between the *coomassie brilliant blue* pigment BG 250 (Sigma-Aldrich®, SP, Brazil) and the protein macromolecules that contain aromatic or basic lateral amino acids. The interaction between the high molecular weight protein and the pigment provokes a shift of this in the equilibrium to the anionic form, which absorbs strongly at 595 nm [22]. To assess the dosage of protein in the tissue, 10 µl of homogenized sample was diluted in 190 µl of distilled water. Twenty microliters of this solution was placed in plastic cuvettes (optical path: 10 mm), containing 1 ml of Bradford reagent. The sample absorbances were determined at 595 nm, in a Lambda 35 spectrophotometer (Perkin-Elmer of Brazil, SP, Brazil). The protein standard curve was obtained from known concentrations of standard solutions of bovine albumin (1 mg/ml).

Determination of malondialdehyde (MDA) through the thiobarbituric acid reactive substances test

To determine the MDA concentration, the technique according to JA Buege and SD Aust [23]. To promote the precipitation of proteins, 125 µl of tissue homogenate or plasmatic supernatant was added to 375 µl of 10% trichloroacetic acid solution. Next, the samples were centrifuged (3,000 rpm for 10 minutes at 6°C) and 250 µl of 0.670% thiobarbituric acid was added to 250 µl of supernatant. The solution was agitated and heated at 100°C in a water-bath for 15 minutes. After cooling, 750 µl of n-butanol was added. Then, following the second agitation, the samples were centrifuged (3,000 rpm for 5 minutes at 6°C). The stained supernatant was placed in glass microcuvettes to determine the absorbance at 535 nm in a Lambda 35 spectrophotometer (Perkin-Elmer of Brazil, SP, Brazil). The MDA concentration in each cuvette was expressed in nmol per mg of total proteins. To calculate the MDA concentration, the standard curve generated from the known concentrations of 1, 1, 3, 3-Tetrametoxypropane 100 nmol/ml in 1% H_2SO_4 solution was utilized.

Determination of superoxide dismutase activity (SOD)

SOD activity was determined according to the technique of [24] at 420 nm. This reaction consisted of the inhibition of pyrogallol auto-oxidation by SOD activity. One unit of SOD is defined as the enzyme quantity capable of inhibiting 50% of the reaction. A total of 930 µl of TRIS buffer (TRIS 50 mM/EDTA 1 mM; pH 8.2), 4 µl of 30 µM catalase and 50 µl of homogenized tissue or plasmatic supernatant was placed into cuvettes. Then, 16 µl of 24 mM pyrogallol in 10 mM HCl was added to the solution. The sample absorbances were determined in a Lambda 35 spectrophotometer (Perkin-Elmer of Brazil, SP, Brazil), at 420 nm after 60 and 120 s. The results were expressed in SOD units/mg of total protein.

Determination of catalase activity (CAT)

The CAT activity was determined through the decomposition of hydrogen peroxide at 25°C. In a quartz cuvette, 2865 µl of phosphate buffer 50 mM (pH 7.0) and 30 µl of homogenized tissue or plasmatic supernatant were added. Then, 35 µl of 0.02 M hydrogen peroxide was added to the solution. The sample absorbances were determined in a Lambda 35 spectrophotometer (Perkin-Elmer of Brazil, SP, Brazil), at 240 nm, and the results are expressed in pmol/mg of total protein [25].

Statistical analysis

The data were evaluated using the software SigmaPlot version 12.0 for *Windows*. To detect a minimal difference of 18.91%, with an alpha error of 5% and a power of 80%, the minimal number of animals calculated to be required for each group was ten. This difference was based on a previous study in our laboratory, which utilized an outcome of maximum strength gain (Alves JP, personal communication, 2011). The results were expressed as the mean ± SD. Here, the two-way ANOVA test followed by the Student-Newman-Keuls' *Post Hoc* test was used to make comparisons among groups. For associations among variables, the Pearson Correlation Test was performed. The accepted significance level was 5% ($P < 0.05$). For sample size calculations, the software SigmaPlot version 12.0 for *Windows* was utilized. To perform correlations and graphics, the software GraphPad 5.0 for *Windows* was used.

Results

The body weight of the animals at the beginning of the study was similar ($P > 0.05$), but was different by the end. The trained groups demonstrated lower body weight gain when compared to the SED-Cr group ($P < 0.01$), while the RT group presented lower body weight gain compared to the SED and RT-Cr groups ($P < 0.05$).

Maximum strength gain

In relation to absolute maximal strength gain (Figure 1a), a higher strength gain was observed in the creatine supplemented groups and in the group only submitted to RT, compared to the SED group ($P < 0.001$). The RT-Cr group presented higher maximum strength gain when compared to other groups ($P < 0.001$).

When the analysis related to body weight and maximal strength gain was performed (Figure 1b), a higher strength gain was only observed in the trained groups when compared to the sedentary groups ($P < 0.001$).

Oxidative stress and antioxidant enzymes activity

With regard to the plasma concentration of MDA (Figure 2a), a lower concentration was observed in the creatine supplemented groups, when compared to the SED and RT groups ($P < 0.01$). The activity of plasmatic SOD (Figure 2b) was lower in the SED-Cr group, compared to the SED group ($P < 0.05$), but there were no differences between trained groups. The activity of plasmatic CAT (Figure 2c) was only higher in the RT group in relation to other groups (P < 0.05). No correlation was observed between SOD activity and MDA concentration in plasma ($r = 0.0321$; $P > 0.05$).

Likewise, in relation to the heart concentration of MDA (Figure 3a), a lower concentration was observed in the creatine supplemented groups compared to the SED and RT groups ($P < 0.01$). The activity of SOD in the heart (Figure 3b) was lower in the SED-Cr group compared to the SED and RT-Cr groups ($P < 0.05$), but there were no differences seen with the RT group. The CAT activity in the heart (Figure 3c) was only higher in the RT-Cr group, in relation to sedentary groups ($P < 0.05$). Also, a positive correlation was observed between SOD activity with MDA concentration in the heart ($r = 0.4172$; $P < 0.05$).

In the liver, only the SED-Cr group demonstrated a lower MDA concentration (Figure 4a) in relation to the SED group ($P < 0.05$), without any differences reported between the trained groups. The SOD activity in the liver (Figure 4b) was lower in the SED-Cr group when compared to the SED and RT-Cr groups ($P < 0.01$). CAT activity in the liver (Figure 4c) was higher in the SED and trained groups in comparison with SED-Cr group ($P < 0.01$). A positive correlation was observed between SOD activity and MDA concentration in the liver ($r = 0.3722$; $P < 0.05$).

Considering the MDA concentration in the gastrocnemius (Figure 5a), only the RT-Cr group presented a lower concentration when compared to the SED group ($P < 0.05$). SOD activity in the gastrocnemius (Figure 5b) was lower in the trained and SED-Cr groups compared to SED group ($P < 0.01$). No differences were observed among groups in relation to CAT activity in the gastrocnemius ($P > 0.05$) (Figure 5c). Also, no correlation was observed between SOD activity and MDA concentration in the gastrocnemius ($r = 0.0283$; $P > 0.05$).

Discussion

This is one of the first studies to demonstrate a possible antioxidant effect of creatine supplementation either in association or not with an RT protocol. It is also one of the few studies to elucidate the antioxidant effect paradigm of creatine *in vivo*.

In our study, after 8 weeks of RT in squat apparatus adapted for rats, a significant increase in the maximum strength was observed in all groups. However, the strength was higher in the trained group supplemented with creatine. Similar results were observed in other studies that evaluated the gain of maximum strength in humans [26-28]. Although it has not been evaluated in the present study, the

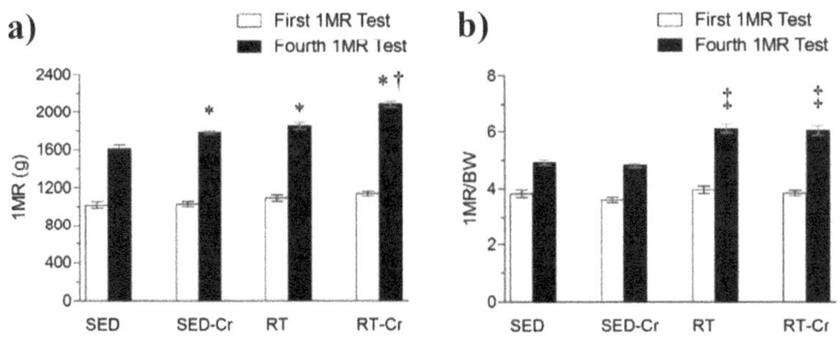

Figure 1 Maximum strength gain after 8 weeks of intervention. a) Absolute maximum strength gain related to the first to fourth tests of One Maximum Repetition (1MR); **b)** Relative maximum strength gain related to the first to fourth tests of One Maximum Repetition (1MR). Values in mean ± SD; n = 10 for all groups. SED, sedentary rats; SED-Cr, sedentary supplemented with creatine rats; RT, resistance training rats; RT-Cr, resistance training supplemented with creatine rats. Two way ANOVA, followed by the *post hoc* test of Student Newman-Keuls. *$P < 0.001$ vs. SED; †$P < 0.001$ vs. SED-Cr, RT; ‡$P < 0.05$ vs. SED, SED-Cr.

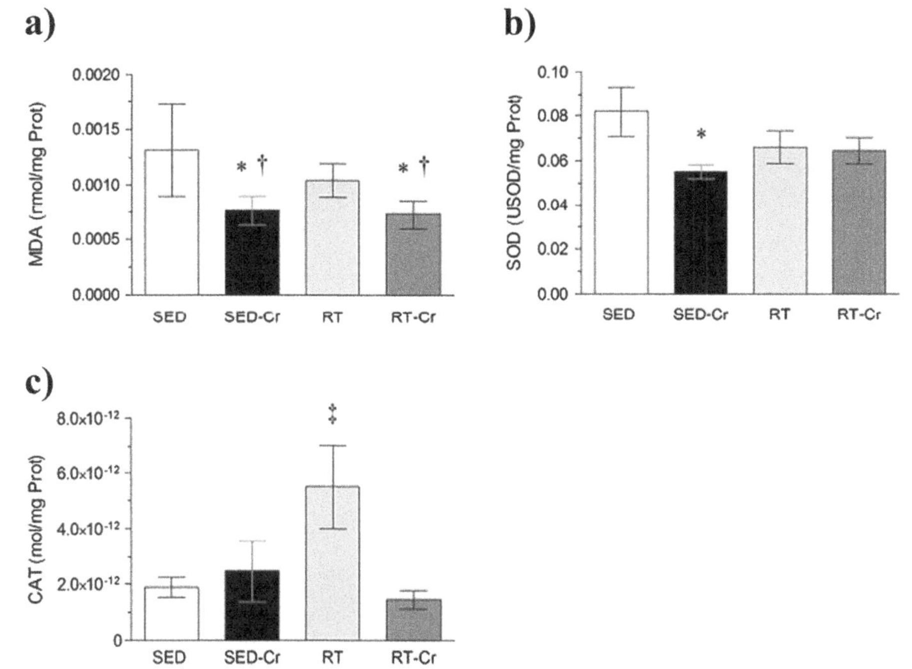

Figure 2 Oxidative stress in plasma after 8 weeks of intervention. Concentrations of **a)** MDA in plasma; **b)** SOD activity in plasma; and **c)** CAT activity in plasma. Values in mean ± SD; n = 10 for all groups. SED, sedentary rats; SED-Cr, sedentary supplemented with creatine rats; RT, resistance training rats; RT-Cr, resistance training supplemented with creatine rats. Two way ANOVA, followed by the *post hoc* test of Student Newman-Keuls. *$P < 0.05$ vs. SED; †$P < 0.05$ vs. RT; ‡$P < 0.05$ vs. all groups.

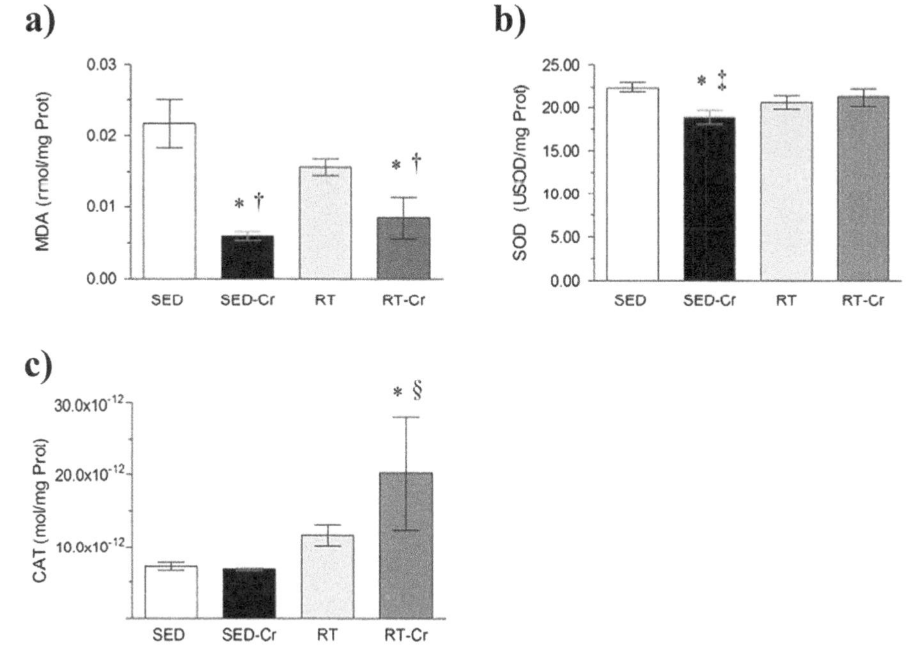

Figure 3 Oxidative stress in heart after 8 weeks of intervention. Concentrations of **a)** MDA in heart; **b)** SOD activity in heart; and **c)** CAT activity in heart. Values are mean ± SD; n = 10 for all groups. SED, sedentary rats; SED-Cr, sedentary supplemented with creatine rats; RT, resistance training rats; RT-Cr, resistance training supplemented with creatine rats. Two way ANOVA, followed by the *post hoc* test of Student Newman-Keuls. *$P < 0.05$ vs. SED; †$P < 0.05$ vs. RT; ‡$P < 0.05$ vs. RT-Cr; §$P < 0.05$ vs. SED-Cr.

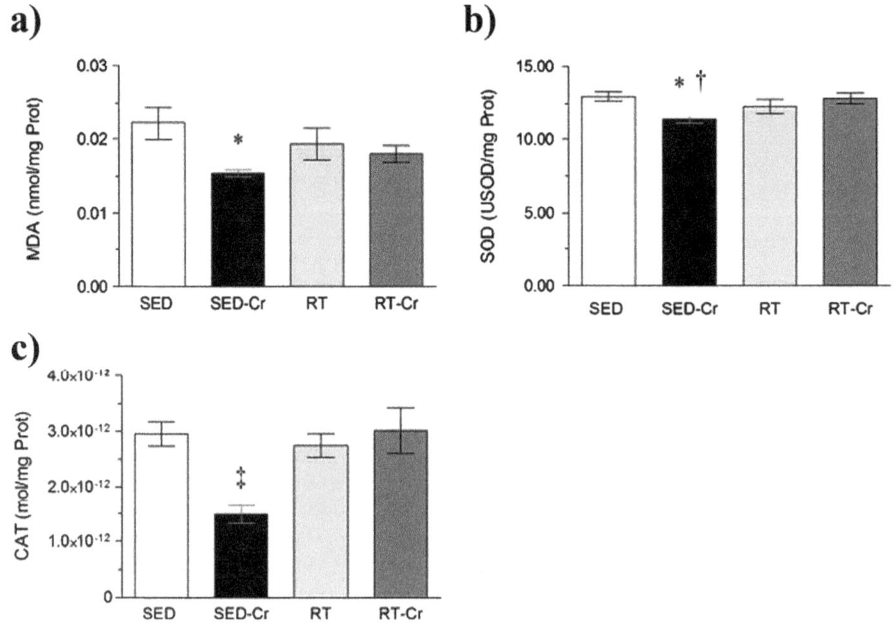

Figure 4 Oxidative stress in liver after 8 weeks of intervention. Concentrations of **a)** MDA in liver; **b)** SOD activity in liver; and **c)** CAT activity in liver. Values in mean ± SD; n = 10 for all groups. SED, sedentary rats; SED-Cr, sedentary supplemented with creatine rats; RT, resistance training rats; RT-Cr, resistance training supplemented with creatine rats. Two way ANOVA, followed by the *post hoc* test of Student Newman-Keuls. *$P < 0.05$ vs. SED; †$P < 0.05$ vs. RT-Cr; ‡$P < 0.001$ vs. all groups.

muscular content of free creatine and creatine-phosphate storage appear to contribute to an increase in the maximum strength of creatine supplemented individuals submitted to the RT protocol, as demonstrated by Buford and colleagues in 2007 [20].

In the present work, a lower plasmatic lipoperoxidation, evaluated by MDA, was only observed in those groups which received creatine supplementation. These results are in contrast to those found by Kingsley and colleagues [29], who sought to evaluate serum lipid peroxidation in

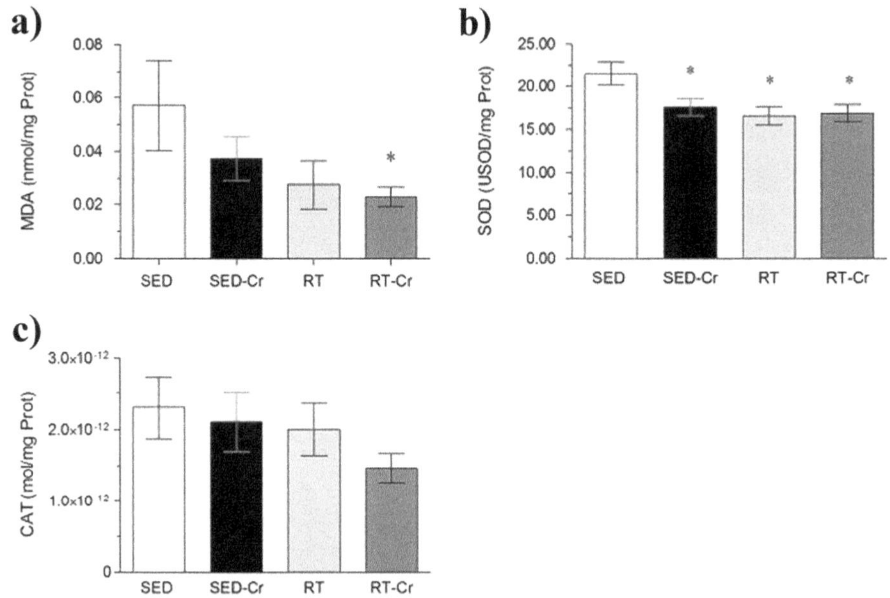

Figure 5 Oxidative stress in gastrocnemius after 8 weeks of intervention. Concentrations of **a)** MDA in gastrocnemius; **b)** SOD activity in gastrocnemius; and **c)** CAT activity in gastrocnemius. Values in mean ± SD; n = 10 for all groups. SED, sedentary rats; SED-Cr, sedentary supplemented with creatine rats; RT, resistance training rats; RT-Cr, resistance training supplemented with creatine rats. Two way ANOVA, followed by the *post hoc* test of Student Newman-Keuls. *$P < 0.05$ vs. SED.

humans submitted to two tests until exhaustion using a cycloergometer and did not observe any influence from creatine supplementation on this marker of oxidative stress. In the previous study, the volunteers were physically active and only familiarized to an exhaustive exercise protocol. However, in our work, we submitted the animals to a resistance training program which led to different muscular and metabolic adaptations. Deminice and colleagues [30] evaluated the acute effect of creatine supplementation for 7 days on plasma oxidative stress in humans submitted to sprint exercise; no antioxidant effect was observed. The divergence from the results presented here might be explained by the different types of exercise, such as the hemodynamic response and the predominant energetic metabolism related to resistance exercise compared to that reported for sprinting or cycling. In another study, rats submitted to 1-h of swimming (load of 4% of body weight) and supplemented with creatine (2% of diet) for a period of 28 days, showed a reduction in plasmatic TBARS immediately after exercise, and 2 h and 6 h after the swimming exercise [31]. It is possible that a longer loading phase of creatine supplementation can increase the antioxidant status, rather than a shorter period of loading. However, when it is associated with a training regimen, higher effects were observed for plasma lipoperoxidation [32]. Interestingly, similar results were observed in the present study. In this way, this antioxidant effect of creatine supplementation associated with RT in plasma oxidative stress corroborated our findings.

Since the SED-Cr group presented a reduction in plasma activity of SOD enzyme and lower lipoperoxidation, it is possible that the creatine may have acted as an ROS scavenger. In the same way, supplemented groups showed no increase in CAT activity; this only occurred in the group submitted to RT. CAT is an enzyme that is highly modulated by physical training, especially by endurance training, where the formation of ROS by the leakage of superoxide radicals in the electron transporter chain is much higher due to the greater utilization of the oxidative pathway [33-35]. Since, in our results, plasmatic CAT activity was higher in the RT group, it is possible that it is necessary to increase this antioxidant enzyme (due to the lack of non-enzymatic antioxidants like creatine) in order to reduce the plasma lipoperoxidation in this group.

Creatine has been considered a cytoplasmic antioxidant of direct action that would mainly promote the scavenging of ROS superoxide radicals [36]. Recently, Lygate and colleagues [37] sought to assess a possible protective effect of creatine in the ischemia-reperfusion process in mice submitted to acute myocardial infarction. The cardiomyocytes were exposed to an oxidant agent, H_2O_2, in order to evaluate the antioxidant action in the fluorescent pigment. Creatine treatment was not able to attenuate the damage promoted by H_2O_2.

However, in our work, a reduction of lipoperoxidation was demonstrated in the heart tissue of creatine supplemented groups, suggesting a possible direct antioxidant effect in the suppression of superoxide radicals in the heart, probably due to its chemical affinity as an antioxidant, being higher with this specific ROS [5,6].

An interesting finding of our study was that, in the heart, SOD activity was reduced in the sedentary group that was supplemented with creatine, in comparison to both the control group and the RT creatine supplemented group. This was in accordance with Siu and colleagues [38], where low intensity exercise (walking) for 8 and 20 weeks was not able to increase SOD activity in the heart of rats. Resistance exercise is characterized by a pressure overload in the heart during its execution, causing an increase in cardiac muscle mass [39]. This suggests that, in part, the RT-Cr group increased SOD activity as an adaptive response to a higher formation of anion superoxide in this tissue under physical training conditions, and that the increased production of this ROS occurs through the xanthine oxidase pathway [40,41]. Creatine supplementation may have exerted a synergistic effect with RT in relation to SOD activity modulation in the heart. In chronic-progressive stress conditions, and in RT, supplementation appears to exert a synergistic effect with regard to adaptation to RT with creatine supplementation, involving the cellular signaling enzymatic adaptation of SOD in cardiac tissue. This mechanism occurs via activation of the NAD(P)H oxidase system that, through vasoactive (angiotensin II) and inflammatory mediators (IL-6, TNF-α), modulates the expression of antioxidant enzymes in a short period [42,43].

CAT activity in cardiac tissue seems to be modulated by the interaction of creatine supplementation with RT, as observed by McClung and colleagues [44], who evaluated the effect of the association of creatine with high intensity exercise on cardiac function in rats and found that this interaction was able to up-regulate the cardiac functional capacity. These results indicate a possible direct or indirect enzymatic modulation of creatine in synergism with training.

As creatine is not synthesized exclusively in the kidney and in the pancreas, but at higher proportions in the liver, and is then mainly transported to the skeletal muscle, we investigated the liver with the aim of developing a hypothesis about the redox state of this organ in the presence of supplementation, either associated or not with resistance training. Our results are different to those found by Radak and colleagues [45], who reported an attenuation of lipoperoxidation levels in the animals submitted to treadmill running training which was adapted for rats. The difference in training protocols, age and animal species may have directly influenced the difference between the results obtained and those of our study.

Studies that have evaluated the effect of creatine supplementation on oxidative stress in different structures are very limited. In our study, we found lower SOD activity in both heart and liver. Botezelli and colleagues [32] evaluated lipid peroxidation, SOD and CAT activity in the liver following three different training protocols (aerobic, strength and concurrent). However, the training did not have any influence on antioxidant enzymatic activity. Creatine seems to have the same response in different tissues, since the increased production of ROS and RNS at the expense of strength exercise possibly acted upon cellular signaling to increase antioxidant enzymatic defenses [46].

When we analyzed the lipoperoxidation in skeletal muscle, we observed that only the RT-Cr group showed lower oxidative damage compared to the SED group. Similar results were found by Guimaraes-Ferreira and colleagues [36], since creatine supplementation associated or not with RT did not change the CAT and SOD activity in skeletal muscle. In this tissue, creatine seems to exert a scavenging antioxidant effect and does not act as an antioxidant enzymatic activity modulator. In a model of spontaneously hypertensive rats submitted to a creatine supplementation protocol, it has been demonstrated that this supplementation does not promote the attenuation of oxidative stress in skeletal muscle [47].

Lastly, this was one of the first studies to evaluate the effects of isolated creatine supplementation or that associated with RT on oxidative stress. As a limitation of this work, it can be noted that a few antioxidant enzymes (e.g. glutathione peroxidase, glutathione reductase, peroxiredoxin), non-enzymatic antioxidants (e.g. glutathione, GSH/GSSG ratio, total antioxidant capacity), biomarkers of oxidative damage (protein carbonyl, 8-OH-dG) and/or activity of ROS and RNS were not analyzed, but this could clarify certain results obtained in the present study.

Conclusions

The supplementation of creatine monohydrate along with 8-week RT was able to reduce oxidative stress. In addition, SOD activity was positively influenced by creatine supplementation in all of the organs analyzed. The supplementation did not influence CAT activity in all organs similarly, except for in the heart. However, further *in vivo* studies associating creatine supplementation with RT are necessary to confirm the findings of this study.

Competing interests

The authors declare that they have no competing interests.

Authors' contributions

SGP, NRB, DZA, AJP conception and design of research; SGP, NRB, DZA, AJP, POM, DDM performed experiments; SGP, NRB, DZA, AJP, POM, DDM, RRC, LPD analyzed data; SGP, NRB, DZA, AJP, POM, DDM, RRC, LPD interpreted results of experiments; SGP, NRB, DZA, AJP prepared figures; SGP, NRB, DZA, AJP, POM, DDM, RRC, LPD drafted manuscript; SGP, NRB, DZA, AJP, POM, DDM, RRC, LPD edited and revised manuscript; SGP, NRB, DZA, AJP, POM, DDM, RRC, LPD approved final version of manuscript. All authors read and approved the final manuscript.

Acknowledgments

This work was funded by the Universidade Federal de Ciências da Saúde de Porto Alegre, Rio Grande do Sul, Brazil.

Author details

[1]Laboratório de Fisiologia - UFCSPA/Porto Alegre, Rua Sarmento Leite, 245, 900050-170 Porto Alegre, RS, Brazil. [2]Laboratório de Poluição Atmosférica e Estresse Oxidativo - UFCSPA/Porto Alegre, Porto Alegre, RS, Brazil. [3]Programa de Pós Graduação em Ciências da Reabilitação - UFCSPA/Porto Alegre, Porto Alegre, RS, Brazil.

References

1. Volek JS, Duncan ND, Mazzetti SA, Staron RS, Putukian M, Gomez AL, Pearson DR, Fink WJ, Kraemer WJ: **Performance and muscle fiber adaptations to creatine supplementation and heavy resistance training.** *Med Sci Sports Exerc* 1999, **31**(8):1147–1156.
2. Volek JS, Rawson ES: **Scientific basis and practical aspects of creatine supplementation for athletes.** *Nutrition* 2004, **20**(7–8):609–614.
3. Willoughby DS, Rosene J: **Effects of oral creatine and resistance training on myosin heavy chain expression.** *Med Sci Sports Exerc* 2001, **33**(10):1674–1681.
4. Persky AM, Brazeau GA: **Clinical pharmacology of the dietary supplement creatine monohydrate.** *Pharmacol Rev* 2001, **53**(2):161–176.
5. Lawler JM, Barnes WS, Wu G, Song W, Demaree S: **Direct antioxidant properties of creatine.** *Biochem Biophys Res Commun* 2002, **290**(1):47–52.
6. Sestili P, Martinelli C, Bravi G, Piccoli G, Curci R, Battistelli M, Falcieri E, Agostini D, Gioacchini AM, Stocchi V: **Creatine supplementation affords cytoprotection in oxidatively injured cultured mammalian cells via direct antioxidant activity.** *Free Radic Biol Med* 2006, **40**(5):837–849.
7. Sestili P, Martinelli C, Colombo E, Barbieri E, Potenza L, Sartini S, Fimognari C: **Creatine as an antioxidant.** *Amino Acids* 2011, **40**(5):1385–1396.
8. Aoi W, Naito Y, Tokuda H, Tanimura Y, Oya-Ito T, Yoshikawa T: **Exercise-induced muscle damage impairs insulin signaling pathway associated with IRS-1 oxidative modification.** *Physiol Res* 2012, **61**(1):81–88.
9. Syu GD, Chen HI, Jen CJ: **Severe exercise and exercise training exert opposite effects on human neutrophil apoptosis via altering the redox status.** *PLoS One* 2011, **6**(9):e24385.
10. Turner JE, Bosch JA, Drayson MT, Aldred S: **Assessment of oxidative stress in lymphocytes with exercise.** *J Appl Physiol* 2011, **111**(1):206–211.
11. Hudson MB, Hosick PA, McCaulley GO, Schrieber L, Wrieden J, McAnulty SR, Triplett NT, McBride JM, Quindry JC: **The effect of resistance exercise on humoral markers of oxidative stress.** *Med Sci Sports Exerc* 2008, **40**(3):542–548.
12. Kyparos A, Vrabas IS, Nikolaidis MG, Riganas CS, Kouretas D: **Increased oxidative stress blood markers in well-trained rowers following two thousand-meter rowing ergometer race.** *J Strength Cond Res* 2009, **23**(5):1418–1426.
13. Zembron-Lacny A, Ostapiuk J, Slowinska-Lisowska M, Witkowski K, Szyszka K: **Pro-antioxidant ratio in healthy men exposed to muscle-damaging resistance exercise.** *J Physiol Biochem* 2008, **64**(1):27–35.
14. Bloomer RJ, Goldfarb AH: **Anaerobic exercise and oxidative stress: a review.** *Can J Appl Physiol* 2004, **29**(3):245–263.
15. Krisan AD, Collins DE, Crain AM, Kwong CC, Singh MK, Bernard JR, Yaspelkis BB 3rd: **Resistance training enhances components of the insulin signaling cascade in normal and high-fat-fed rodent skeletal muscle.** *J Appl Physiol* 2004, **96**(5):1691–1700.
16. Barauna VG, Magalhaes FC, Krieger JE, Oliveira EM: **AT1 receptor participates in the cardiac hypertrophy induced by resistance training in rats.** *Am J Physiol Regul Integr Comp Physiol* 2008, **295**(2):R381–387.
17. Tamaki T, Uchiyama S, Nakano S: **A weight-lifting exercise model for inducing hypertrophy in the hindlimb muscles of rats.** *Med Sci Sports Exerc* 1992, **24**(8):881–886.
18. Barauna VG, Batista ML Jr, Costa Rosa LF, Casarini DE, Krieger JE, Oliveira EM: **Cardiovascular adaptations in rats submitted to a resistance-training model.** *Clin Exp Pharmacol Physiol* 2005, **32**(4):249–254.

19. Kregel KCAD, Booth FW, Fleshner MR, Henriksen EJ, Musch TI, O'Leary DS, Parks CM, Poole DC, Ra'anan AW, Sheriff DD, Sturek MS, Toth LA: *Resource Book for the Design of Animal Exercise Protocols*. Bethesda: American Physiological Society; 2006.
20. Buford TW, Kreider RB, Stout JR, Greenwood M, Campbell B, Spano M, Ziegenfuss T, Lopez H, Landis J, Antonio J: **International Society of Sports Nutrition position stand: creatine supplementation and exercise.** *J Int Soc Sports Nutr* 2007, **4**:6.
21. Neves CMM: *Lipoperoxidação no encéfalo de rato submetido à isquemia global transitória*. Porto Alegre: Universidade Federal do Rio Grande do Sul; 1997.
22. Schleicher E, Wieland OH: **Changes of human glomerular basement membrane in diabetes mellitus.** *J Clin Chem Clin Biochem* 1984, **22**(3):223–227.
23. Buege JA, Aust SD: **Microsomal lipid peroxidation.** *Methods Enzymol* 1978, **52**:302–310.
24. Marklund S, Marklund G: **Involvement of the superoxide anion radical in the autoxidation of pyrogallol and a convenient assay for superoxide dismutase.** *Eur J Biochem* 1974, **47**(3):469–474.
25. Aebi H: **Catalase in vitro.** *Methods Enzymol* 1984, **105**:121–126.
26. Branch JD: **Effect of creatine supplementation on body composition and performance: a meta-analysis.** *Int J Sport Nutr Exerc Metab* 2003, **13**(2):198–226.
27. Rawson ES, Volek JS: **Effects of creatine supplementation and resistance training on muscle strength and weightlifting performance.** *J Strength Cond Res* 2003, **17**(4):822–831.
28. Volek JS, Ratamess NA, Rubin MR, Gomez AL, French DN, McGuigan MM, Scheett TP, Sharman MJ, Hakkinen K, Kraemer WJ: **The effects of creatine supplementation on muscular performance and body composition responses to short-term resistance training overreaching.** *Eur J Appl Physiol* 2004, **91**(5–6):628–637.
29. Kingsley M, Cunningham D, Mason L, Kilduff LP, McEneny J: **Role of creatine supplementation on exercise-induced cardiovascular function and oxidative stress.** *Oxid Med Cell Longev* 2009, **2**(4):247–254.
30. Deminice R, Rosa FT, Franco GS, Jordao AA, de Freitas EC: **Effects of creatine supplementation on oxidative stress and inflammatory markers after repeated-sprint exercise in humans.** *Nutrition* 2013, **29**(9):1127–1132.
31. Deminice R, Jordao AA: **Creatine supplementation reduces oxidative stress biomarkers after acute exercise in rats.** *Amino Acids* 2012, **43**(2):709–715.
32. Botezelli JD, Cambri LT, Ghezzi AC, Dalia RA, M Scariot PP, Ribeiro C, Voltarelli FA, Mello MA: **Different exercise protocols improve metabolic syndrome markers, tissue triglycerides content and antioxidant status in rats.** *Diabetol Metabol Syndr* 2011, **3**:35.
33. Lambertucci RH, Levada-Pires AC, Rossoni LV, Curi R, Pithon-Curi TC: **Effects of aerobic exercise training on antioxidant enzyme activities and mRNA levels in soleus muscle from young and aged rats.** *Mech Ageing Dev* 2007, **128**(3):267–275.
34. Laughlin MH, Simpson T, Sexton WL, Brown OR, Smith JK, Korthuis RJ: **Skeletal muscle oxidative capacity, antioxidant enzymes, and exercise training.** *J Appl Physiol* 1990, **68**(6):2337–2343.
35. Leeuwenburgh C, Fiebig R, Chandwaney R, Ji LL: **Aging and exercise training in skeletal muscle: responses of glutathione and antioxidant enzyme systems.** *Am J Physiol* 1994, **267**(2 Pt 2):R439–445.
36. Guimaraes-Ferreira L, Pinheiro CH, Gerlinger-Romero F, Vitzel KF, Nachbar RT, Curi R, Nunes MT: **Short-term creatine supplementation decreases reactive oxygen species content with no changes in expression and activity of antioxidant enzymes in skeletal muscle.** *European journal of applied physiology* 2012, **112**(11):3905–3911.
37. Lygate CA, Bohl S, ten Hove M, Faller KM, Ostrowski PJ, Zervou S, Medway DJ, Aksentijevic D, Sebag-Montefiore L, Wallis J, *et al*: **Moderate elevation of intracellular creatine by targeting the creatine transporter protects mice from acute myocardial infarction.** *Cardiovasc Res* 2012, **96**(3):466–475.
38. Siu PM, Pei XM, Teng BT, Benzie IF, Ying M, Wong SH: **Habitual exercise increases resistance of lymphocytes to oxidant-induced DNA damage by upregulating expression of antioxidant and DNA repairing enzymes.** *Exp Physiol* 2011, **96**(9):889–906.
39. Pluim BM, Zwinderman AH, van der Laarse A, van der Wall EE: **The athlete's heart. A meta-analysis of cardiac structure and function.** *Circulation* 2000, **101**(3):336–344.
40. Bellinger BM, Bold A, Wilson GR, Noakes TD, Myburgh KH: **Oral creatine supplementation decreases plasma markers of adenine nucleotide degradation during a 1-h cycle test.** *Acta Physiol Scand* 2000, **170**(3):217–224.
41. Souza Junior TP, Pereira B: **Creatina: auxílio ergogênico com potencial antioxidante?** *Rev Nutr Campinas* 2008, **21**(3):349–353.
42. Valko M, Leibfritz D, Moncol J, Cronin MT, Mazur M, Telser J: **Free radicals and antioxidants in normal physiological functions and human disease.** *Int J Biochem Cell Biol* 2007, **39**(1):44–84.
43. Zhao X, Bey EA, Wientjes FB, Cathcart MK: **Cytosolic phospholipase A2 (cPLA2) regulation of human monocyte NADPH oxidase activity. cPLA2 affects translocation but not phosphorylation of p67(phox) and p47 (phox).** *J Biol Chem* 2002, **277**(28):25385–25392.
44. McClung JM, Hand GA, Davis JM, Carson JA: **Effect of creatine supplementation on cardiac muscle of exercise-stressed rats.** *Eur J Appl Physiol* 2003, **89**(1):26–33.
45. Radak Z, Chung HY, Naito H, Takahashi R, Jung KJ, Kim HJ, Goto S: **Age-associated increase in oxidative stress and nuclear factor kappaB activation are attenuated in rat liver by regular exercise.** *FASEB J* 2004, **18**(6):749–750.
46. Powers SK, Jackson MJ: **Exercise-induced oxidative stress: cellular mechanisms and impact on muscle force production.** *Physiol Rev* 2008, **88**(4):1243–1276.
47. Alves CRR, Murai IH, Ramona P, Nicastro H, Bechara LRG, Lancha AH Jr, Brum PC, Irigoyen MC, Gualano B: **No effect of creatine supplementation on oxidative stress and cardiovascular parameters in spontaneously hypertensive rats.** *J Int Soc Sports Nutr* 2012, **9**(13):1–4.

β-alanine supplementation improves tactical performance but not cognitive function in combat soldiers

Jay R Hoffman[1*], Geva Landau[2], Jeffrey R Stout[1], Matan Dabora[2], Daniel S Moran[2,3], Nurit Sharvit[4], Mattan W Hoffman[2], Yuval Ben Moshe[2], William P McCormack[1], Gil Hirschhorn[2] and Ishay Ostfeld[2]

Abstract

Background: There are no known studies that have examined β-alanine supplementation in military personnel. Considering the physiological and potential neurological effects that have been reported during sustained military operations, it appears that β-alanine supplementation may have a potential benefit in maintaining physical and cognitive performance during high-intensity military activity under stressful conditions. The purpose of this study was to examine the effect of 28 days of β-alanine ingestion in military personnel while fatigued on physical and cognitive performance.

Methods: Twenty soldiers (20.1 ± 0.9 years) from an elite combat unit were randomly assigned to either a β-alanine (BA) or placebo (PL) group. Soldiers were involved in advanced military training, including combat skill development, navigational training, self-defense/hand-to-hand combat and conditioning. All participants performed a 4-km run, 5-countermovement jumps using a linear position transducer, 120-m sprint, a 10-shot shooting protocol with assault rifle, including overcoming a misfire, and a 2-min serial subtraction test to assess cognitive function before (Pre) and after (Post) 28 days of supplementation.

Results: The training routine resulted in significant increases in 4-km run time for both groups, but no between group differences were seen ($p = 0.597$). Peak jump power at Post was greater for BA than PL ($p = 0.034$), while mean jump power for BA at Post was 10.2% greater ($p = 0.139$) than PL. BA had a significantly greater ($p = 0.012$) number of shots on target at Post (8.2 ± 1.0) than PL (6.5 ± 2.1), and their target engagement speed at Post was also significantly faster ($p = 0.039$). No difference in serial subtraction performance was seen between the groups ($p = 0.844$).

Conclusion: Results of this study indicate that 4-weeks of β-alanine ingestion in young, healthy soldiers did not impact cognitive performance, but did enhance power performance, marksmanship and target engagement speed from pre-ingestion levels.

Keywords: Military performance, Marksmanship, Power, Physical performance, Supplements

Background

Investigations examining β-alanine ingestion in both recreational and competitive athletic populations have been consistent in demonstrating significantly greater performance during high-intensity physical activity than when these athletes are consuming a placebo [1-7]. The efficacy of β-alanine ingestion appears centered on its ability to enhance the quality of a workout by delaying skeletal muscle fatigue. The ergogenic properties of β-alanine by itself appear to be very limited. However, when β-alanine is absorbed into skeletal muscle it combines with histidine to form carnosine. It is carnosine which appears to provide the ergogenic benefit [8]. The primary role of carnosine is the maintenance of acid–base homeostasis through enhanced intra-muscular hydrogen ion (H^+) buffering capacity [9]. Increasing intra-muscular carnosine concentration through β-alanine supplementation has been demonstrated to have ergogenic potential

* Correspondence: jay.hoffman@ucf.edu
[1]Institute of Exercise Physiology and Wellness, Sport and Exercise Science, University of Central Florida, Orlando, FL, USA
Full list of author information is available at the end of the article

for maximal exercise lasting 60 sec - 240 sec [10]. Because carnosine is located in other excitable tissues other than skeletal muscle (such as the brain and heart), it may also have additional physiological roles [11-13].

Carnosine's biological role as an antioxidant, antiglycating and ion-chelating agent suggests that it may have a potential role during oxidative stress, serving as a neuroprotector [11-13]. However, only one study has examined the effect of β-alanine ingestion on changes in carnosine concentrations in the brain [14]. Daily ingestion of 22.5 $mmol{\cdot}kg^{-1}$ of β-alanine in mice under stressful conditions resulted in an increase in carnosine concentrations in the cerebral cortex and hypothalamus, and an increase in brain derived neurotrophic factor in the hippocampus. In addition a decrease in 5-hydroxyindoleacetic acid concentrations, a metabolite of serotonin, was seen in the hippocampus. These changes, which also included improved time in a maze that contained anxiolytic compounds, resulted in the authors suggesting that β-alanine ingestion may have possible anxiolytic-like effects [14]. Although this has not been examined in a human model, it does provide an interesting basis for study. If β-alanine ingestion can increase brain carnosine concentrations in humans, it may provide a benefit in maintaining focus, alertness and cognitive function during highly fatiguing, high intense activity.

During prolonged, high-intensity military training or simulated combat exercises, significant decreases in physical and cognitive performance measures are often reported [15-18]. To compensate for the physiological and psychological fatigue associated with military training and combat, a number of pharmacological interventions have been examined. However, a recent commentary among the Medical Corps of the United States military has expressed a need to examine non-pharmacological alternatives to counteract the fatigue associated with military combat [19]. The use of dietary supplements among military personnel appears to be quite common. A recent study indicated that up to 72% of the Marines deployed to Afghanistan used a dietary supplement [20], while 53% of the soldiers at various military installations around the world (outside of the combat theater) indicated that they used dietary supplements on a regular basis [21]. However, little is known regarding the efficacy of many of these supplements as they relate to specific military performance.

To date, there are no known studies that have examined β-alanine supplementation in military personnel. Considering the physiological and potential neurological effects, it appears that β-alanine supplementation could have a potential benefit in preparation for prolonged, high intense military activity that requires maintaining high levels of physical performance, focus, and decision making ability under stressful conditions. The purpose of this study was to examine the effect of 28 days of β-alanine ingestion in military personnel while fatigued on physical and cognitive performance.

Methods

Subjects

Twenty male soldiers from an elite combat unit of the Israel Defense Forces (IDF) volunteered to participate in this double-blind study. Following an explanation of all procedures, risks and benefits, each participant provided his informed consent to participate in the study. The Helsinki Committee of the IDF Medical Corp approved this research study. Subjects were not permitted to use any additional dietary supplementation and did not consume any androgens or any other performance enhancing drugs. Screening for performance enhancing drug use and additional supplementation was accomplished via a health questionnaire completed during participant recruitment. Participants were from the same unit, but were from three different squads. Volunteers from each squad were randomly assigned to one of two groups. The randomization procedure involved that each volunteer from the same squad to be alternatively assigned to each group. Two participants dropped from the study, one participant fractured his leg during training, while the other participant no longer wished to participate. Each participant was from a separate group. Thus, a total of 18 participants were used in the final analysis. Using the procedures described by Gravettier and Wallnau [22] for estimating samples sizes for repeated measures designs, a minimum sample size of $n = 8$ was required for each group to reach a statistical power (1-β) of 0.80 based on the jump power changes reported by Hoffman et al. [4] The first group; (BA; age 20.1 ± 0.7 years; height: 1.79 ± 0.07 m; body mass: 78.3 ± 9.7 kg) consumed 6.0 g of β-alanine per day, while the second group (PL; age 20.2 ± 1.1 years; height: 1.80 ± 0.05; body mass: 79.6 ± 7.8 kg) consumed 6 g of placebo (rice flour). During the 4-week study period all participants from all squads participated in the same advanced military training tasks that included combat skill development, physical work under pressure, navigational training, self-defense/hand-to-hand combat and conditioning.

Testing protocol

This randomized, double-blind, placebo controlled investigation was conducted at the unit's training facilities, under the unit's regular training protocols and safety regulations. Data collection occurred before (Pre) and after (Post) 28 days of supplementation. To create an acute fatigued state, each session required all participants to perform a 4 km run dressed in shorts, T-shirt and running shoes. Immediately following the 4 km run participants performed five countermovement jumps (CMJ). Participants then proceeded to put on their operational gear and weapon (12 kg) and ran a 120 m sprint. Following the sprint, participants proceeded as quickly as possible onto the shooting range and performed a 10-shot shooting protocol with their assault rifle. During the shooting, a planned misfire occurred that required the participant to correct and resume shooting. Immediately following the shooting drill all participants completed a serial subtraction test to assess cognitive function in a fatigued state.

Performance measurements

Global positioning system

All participants were provided with an individual global positioning system (GPS) that they wore in a vest underneath their shirt. The GPS unit (MinimaxX, V4.3, Catapult Innovations, Victoria, Australia) was positioned in a posterior pocket on the vest situated between the participant's right and left scapula in the upper-thoracic spine region. Information on velocity patterns was recorded during the 4 km run. Peak velocity, mean velocity, distance covered running at slow - moderate speed (< 4.44 m·sec^{-1}), distance covered running at high speed (4.44+ m·sec^{-1}), and the percent of total distance run at slow-moderate and high speeds were downloaded from the GPS receiver/transmitters. Data were collected at 10 Hz and all analysis was performed with the system software provided by the manufacturer. The validity and reliability of the GPS technology has been previously demonstrated [23].

Jump power

To quantify vertical jump power, participants performed five consecutive CMJ. During each CMJ participants stood with their hands on their waist at all times and were instructed to maximize the height of each jump, while minimizing the contact time with the ground between jumps. During each jump the participant wore a belt connected to a Tendo™ Power Output Unit (Tendo Sports Machines, Trencin, Slovak Republic). The Tendo™ unit consists of a linear position transducer attached to the end of the belt which measured linear displacement and time. Subsequently, the velocity of each jump was calculated and power determined. The average peak and mean power outputs for all five jumps were recorded. Intraclass correlations for the Tendo Unit and peak and mean vertical jump power in our laboratory has been R = 0.98, (SEM =106.2 W) and R =0.94 (SEM = 100.3 W), respectively.

Shooting performance

Targets were set at a 40-m distance from the firing line and were all headshots. Each shot that hit the target was considered accurate. Twenty targets were set up on the range. All participants were notified prior to the start of data collection which target they were required to shoot at. Immediately following the 120-m sprint, participants continued onto the shooting range and shot five times while kneeling and five times from a prone position with their assault rifle. Participants were instructed to shoot rapidly and accurately. While shooting each participant was required to handle a misfire in their weapon. The misfire was prearranged by the investigative team, which involved placing an empty bullet randomly into weapon's magazine (weapon's ammunition storage and feeding device). This required the participant to recognize and correct the misfire (clear the bullet) and continue to deliver fire at the designated target. The designed misfire was set to increase the stress of the shooting, with the participants already fatigued from the 4 km run, jumps and sprint with full gear. The number of accurate shots and the time required to perform these shots was recorded.

Cognitive function

A modified version of the original Serial Sevens Test was employed to analyze cognitive function [24]. The test consisted of a two-minute timed written test in which participants were required to subtract the number 7 from a randomly generated four digit number, in order to measure how quickly and accurately they can compute a simple mathematical problem. The four digit number appeared on the top of the first column of a three column sheet of paper. Participants were provided the sheet of paper and asked to complete as many calculations as possible in the two-minute period. Participant and timer/scorer sat opposite each other during testing. The answers to the calculations were written underneath the initial number. Regardless of answer provided, participants were then required to subtract the number 7 from that new number. Participants were not told if their answer was correct or not. The number of correct answers was recorded. Intraclass correlations for this assessment has been determined in our laboratory to be $R > 0.81$ [25].

Supplement schedule

The β-alanine supplement (CarnoSyn™) was obtained from Natural Alternatives International (San Marcos, CA, USA). Both the supplement and placebo were in tablet form and were similar in appearance. Participants in the supplement group were provided with 2 tablets of sustained-release β-alanine at a dose of (2 g per serving) three times per day (total β-alanine intake was 6 g per day) and subjects in the placebo group were provided with an equivalent amount of rice powder. Participants were instructed to consume the supplement following their meals with water. Each participant was provided with a bottle containing a week's supply of tablets. All bottles were returned at the end of the week. All tablets left in the bottle were counted, recorded, and the next week's bottle was provided to the participant. Supplementation occurred every day over a 28-day period.

Statistical analysis

Data were analyzed using a 2 × 2 [treatment (BA, PL) × time (pretest, posttest)] mixed factorial ANOVA. Differences in the mean posttest performance values were determined by using analysis of covariance, with pretest values serving as the covariate. One-Way Analysis of Covariance (ANCOVA) was utilized to analyze differences between treatment groups. For effect size (ES), the partial eta squared statistic was reported and according to Green and colleagues [26] 0.01, 0.06, and 0.14 represents small, medium, and large effect sizes, respectively. An alpha level of $p < 0.05$ was used to determine statistical significance. Data were analyzed using SPSS v20 software (SPSS Inc., Chicago, IL).

Results

Compliance for consuming the supplement or placebo was 97%. Four subjects within BA reported isolated incidences of paresthesia. Upon review, it was discovered that each of these soldiers combined 2 – 3 supplement doses for that day. No adverse events were reported in these participants or in any other participant consuming the supplement during the required time points. During the 4-week training period the decrease in body mass in BA (−1.3 ± 1.0 kg) was significantly greater ($p = 0.014$, ES = 0.34) than PL (−0.2 ± 0.6 kg).

Comparison of performance measures between BA and PL during the 4-km run is shown in Table 1. When collapsed across groups a significant increase ($p = 0.019$) in time for the 4-km run was observed from Pre to Post in both groups combined. However, no significant interactions were noted between the groups. Significant main effects for time were also noted for both peak ($p = 0.045$) and mean ($p = 0.005$) velocity (both variables decreased, meaning that the soldiers ran slower) during the 4-km run, and no significant interactions were observed between the groups in either velocity measure. The distance run at low to moderate velocities was significantly greater at Post than Pre ($p = 0.010$) for both groups combined, however no significant interactions were seen between the groups. The distance run at high velocity was significantly reduced for both BA and PL ($p = 0.022$), and no significant interaction was noted. The percent distance ran at low to moderate velocity was significantly increased ($p = 0.021$), while the percent distance ran at high-intensity was significantly lower, for both groups combined ($p = 0.019$). No between group differences were observed in either variable.

Comparisons of vertical jump relative peak and mean power performances are shown in Figures 1 and 2, respectively. Relative peak power at Post was significantly greater for BA than PL ($p = 0.034$, ES = 0.27), while relative mean power for BA at Post (14.1 ± 1.7 $w \cdot kg^{-1}$) was 10.2% greater ($p = 0.139$) than that observed for PL (12.8 ± 1.5 $w \cdot kg^{-1}$). Although differences in mean jump power were not significantly different between the groups, the effect size of 0.14 is suggestive of a large effect due to the intervention (BA). No significant change in 120 m sprint velocity was seen from pre to post in either BA (4.65 ± 0.53 $m \cdot sec^{-1}$ and 4.45 ± 0.56 $m \cdot sec^{-1}$, respectively) or PL (4.49 ± 0.56 $m \cdot sec^{-1}$ and 4.35 ± 0.40 $m \cdot sec^{-1}$, respectively), and no differences between the groups were noted.

The effect of the supplement on shooting accuracy and time per shot on target can be seen in Figures 3 and 4,

Table 1 Running velocities during 4-km run

Variable	Group	Pre	Post	p value	ES	95% Confidence interval
Peak velocity ($m \cdot sec^{-1}$)	BA	5.84 ± 0.63	5.46 ± 0.26	0.597	.02	5.16 – 5.71
	PL	5.69 ± 0.46	5.51 ± 0.50			5.26 – 5.80
Average velocity ($m \cdot sec^{-1}$)	BA	4.25 ± 0.22	4.13 ± 0.27	0.729	.01	3.96 – 4.24
	PL	4.18 ± 0.19	4.11 ± 0.19			3.99 – 4.28
Low – moderate running velocity (< 4.4 $m \cdot sec^{-1}$)	BA	2811 ± 605	2957 ± 672	0.224	.10	2571 – 3354
	PL	2827 ± 482	3297 ± 590			2900 - 3683
High running velocity (> 4.4 $m \cdot sec^{-1}$)	BA	1166 ± 610	1009 ± 675	0.364	.06	604 - 1399
	PL	1143 ± 485	748 ± 541			358 - 1153
% Distance run at low to moderate running velocity	BA	70.8 ± 16.2	74.3 ± 18.3	0.351	.06	64.4 – 84.6
	PL	71.3 ± 12.8	81.1 ± 14.4			70.9 – 91.0
% Distance run at high running velocity	BA	29.3 ± 16.1	25.4 ± 18.0	0.361	.06	15.4 – 35.2
	PL	28.8 ± 13.0	18.9 ± 14.4			9.1 – 29.0
4 K run time (sec)	BA	942.4 ± 39.3	962.6 ± 65.0	0.864	.002	929.4 – 1001.2
	PL	949.9 ± 46.2	963.9 ± 44.3			925.2 – 997.1

ES = Effect size.

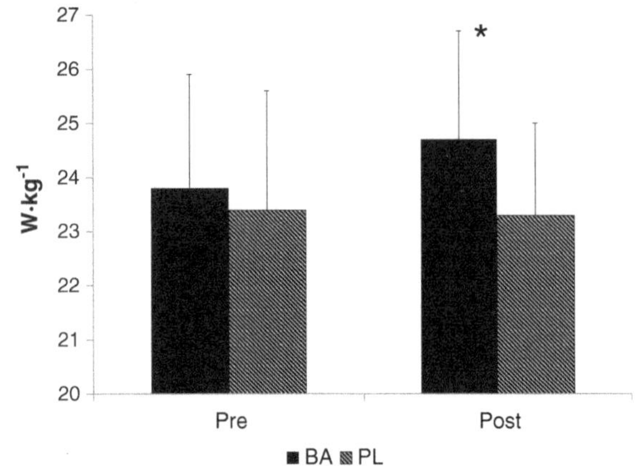

Figure 1 Vertical jump relative peak power performance. * = Significant difference between groups. W · kg^{-1} = Watts per kilogram body mass.

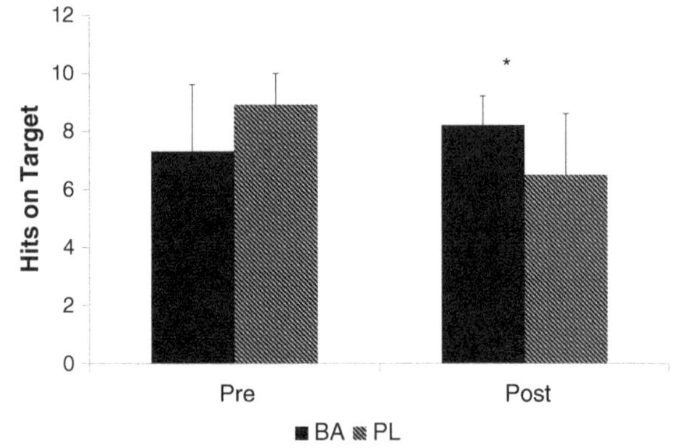

Figure 3 Shooting accuracy reported as shots on target. * = Significant difference between groups.

respectively. A significantly greater ($p = 0.012$, ES = .38) number of shots on target was seen at Post for BA (8.2 ± 1.0) compared to PL (6.5 ± 2.1). The time per shot on target at Post was also significantly faster for BA than PL ($p = 0.039$, ES .27). When collapsed across groups, significant improvements in the serial subtraction test was seen from Pre to Post ($p = 0.014$), but no differences (see Figure 5) between the groups were seen ($p = 0.844$, ES = .003).

Discussion

Results of this study demonstrate that 4 weeks of β-alanine supplementation during an intense military training period was effective in enhancing lower-body jump power and psychomotor performance (shooting accuracy) in soldiers of an elite IDF Combat unit, but did not appear to have any significant effects on cognitive function or running performance. While the benefits of β-alanine for athletic performance enhancement have been demonstrated in numerous studies [10,27,28], this investigation appears to be the first to provide evidence of β-alanine's potential efficacy in military specific tasks.

During the 4 week study period all participants were participating in advanced military training that included combat skill development, physical work under pressure, navigational training, self-defense/hand-to-hand combat and conditioning. This training program, as expected, appeared to be quite fatiguing as significant performance decrements were seen in 4-km run performance for both groups. Previous research has shown that intense military training from one to eight weeks can result in significant decreases in strength and power [16,18]. In addition to the physical performance decrements associated with intense military training, decreases in shooting performance [29] and cognitive function [30] have also been reported. To defend against the physical and cognitive performance decrements related to intense and sustained military action, several studies have examined the efficacy of various stimulants and other pharmacological

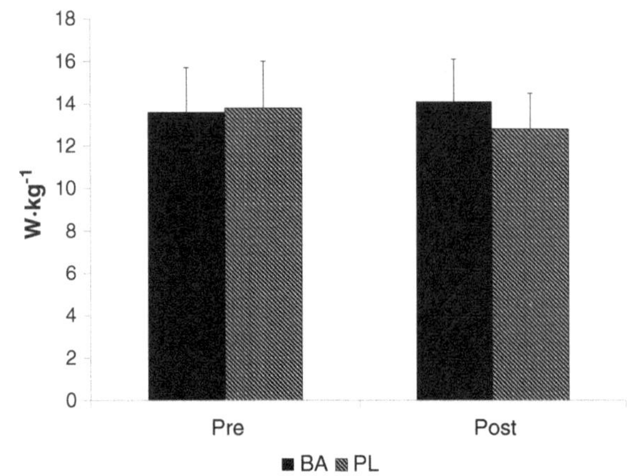

Figure 2 Vertical jump relative mean power performance. W · kg^{-1} = Watts per kilogram body mass.

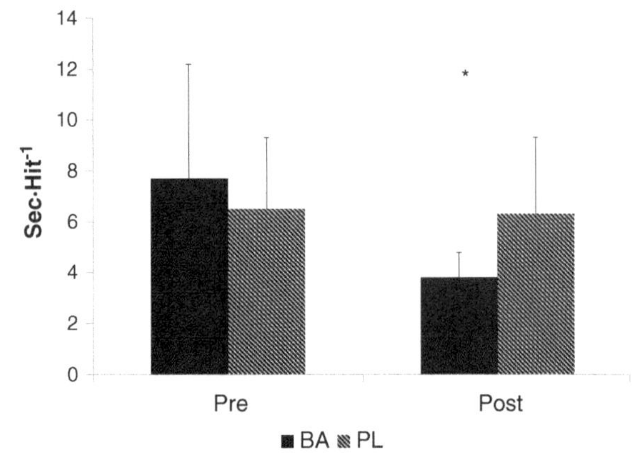

Figure 4 Time per shot on target reported as seconds per accurate hit. * = Significant difference between groups.

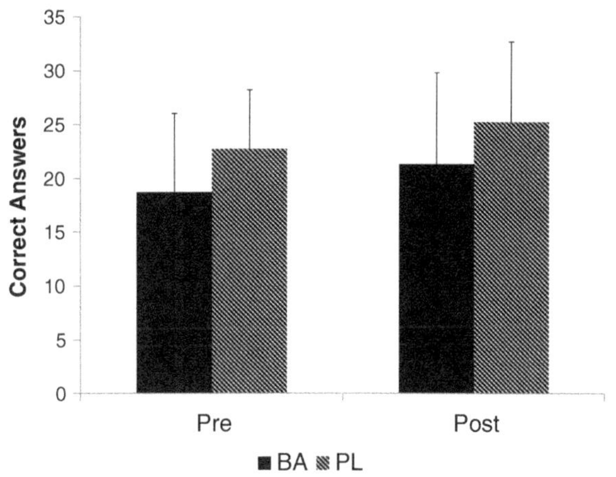

Figure 5 Serial subtraction test reported as number of correct responses.

agents [15,31,32]. These studies have shown that such interventions can be very effective in sustaining military performance. For instance, Lieberman and colleagues [15] reported that caffeine ingestion following 72 hours of sleep deprivation was able to maintain cognitive function and mood, while Estrada et al., [31] noted that helicopter pilots provided 3 doses of modafinil (a vigilance promoting drug used to treat sleepiness) at 4-hour intervals during a 40-hour period of sustained wakefulness were able to maintain alertness, cognitive function and feelings of well-being. However, concerns have been raised regarding the safety and potential side effects associated with pharmaceutical agents, and calls for a greater effort in exploring non-pharmacological alternatives for military populations have been published [19]. Despite the popularity of dietary supplements in both deployed and garrisoned soldiers [20,21], little is known regarding the efficacy of many of these supplements as they relate to specific military performance. The results of the present study demonstrate the ergogenic benefits of β-alanine ingestion on enhancing tactical performance in elite combat solders.

Four weeks of β-alanine ingestion with dosages similar to the one used in the present study has been shown to elevate muscle carnosine concentrations by 60% [1]. Elevations in muscle carnosine has been demonstrated to enhance intracellular muscle buffering capacity and delay fatigue during high-intensity anaerobic exercise [9,10], but its benefits during endurance activity has proved to be inconclusive. During the 4-km run performed in this study we were unable to show any significant advantage related to β-alanine ingestion. There have only been a limited number of studies examining the effects of β-alanine ingestion and endurance performance. Jordan and colleagues [33] reported that following 4 weeks of β-alanine ingestion in participants who were not training aerobically during the supplement period a delay in blood lactate accumulation was seen, but a decrease in aerobic capacity was also noted. The physiological role of carnosine in muscle does not provide a strong mechanism for enhancing aerobic exercise performance. However, it may increase the time spent running at higher velocities. Although our results do not support this statistically, a 34.9% difference was seen between BA and PL in the distance run at a high velocity, which warrants further exploration with larger sample sizes. Regardless, the 4-km run performed in this investigation was primarily done to increase the fatigue of the soldiers prior to the shooting and cognitive function measures.

Following the 4-km run, subjects were required to perform a jump power test. The greater power performance observed in BA compared to PL was consistent with other studies demonstrating the fatigue resistant effects of β-alanine during high-intensity activity [34-36]. Derave and colleagues [34] reported that 4 weeks of β-alanine supplementation (4.8 g·day^{-1}) was able to delay fatigue during repeated bouts of isokinetic exercise and Van Thienen and colleagues [36] noted improved 30-sec sprint performance following a 110-min time trial. Each of those studies demonstrated a delay in fatigue following an acute exhaustive exercise protocol. Kern and Robinson [35] reported enhanced anaerobic exercise performance following a prolonged period (8-weeks) of high-intensity training in athletes supplementing with β-alanine compared to a placebo. The present study provides additional support of the benefits associated with 4-weeks of β-alanine supplementation in delaying fatigue.

Shooting performance has been shown to be sensitive to acute fatiguing activity [29,32]. Gillingham and colleagues [32] demonstrated that caffeine intake before and following exhaustive exercise (2.5-hr loaded march and 1.0-hr sandbar wall construction) improve target detection, marksmanship and engagement speed during simulated combat. This present study is the first to demonstrate that the fatigue resistant effects afforded by β-alanine ingestion can also improve marksmanship and target engagement speed following fatiguing exercise. Considering that this study did not measure muscle or brain carnosine concentrations, it is unclear if this played any role in the improvements observed or whether another mechanism associated with β-alanine ingestion may be responsible for the improvement in target acquisition and marksmanship.

Fatigue during sustained and highly intense combat situations may jeopardize rapid judgment in differentiating friend from foe. The subjects in the present study were required to overcome a misfire in their weapon, and then following their shooting performance complete mathematical problems while seated. The participants in BA were able to perform their 10 shots (30.2 ± 5.8 sec) faster than PL (37.7 ± 13.9 sec), but this 24.8% difference between the groups was not statistically different ($p = 0.161$). However, when the time was calculated relative to the number of shots on target, BA was significantly faster than PL. Whether this was related to an improved neurological benefit is not clear; however it is clear that β-alanine supplementation directly led to enhanced marksmanship and rate of target acquisition, suggestive of improved psychomotor performance. Furthermore, the misfire in the weapon was similar for all participants and similar in both Pre and Post assessment periods. It is possible that the familiarity with how to handle the misfire for both groups also contributed to the similar completion time for the 10 shots.

There were several limitations with this study. Considering that no previous studies examined the role of β-alanine on cognitive function, the statistical power analysis used to determine subject size was based upon previous studies examining physical performance. In regards to the cognitive aspects of this study, the statistical power may not have been appropriate. In addition, the benefits of performing a field study are often offset by the inability to control all aspects of the participant's daily activity. For instance, the structure of the training did not provide an opportunity to control or record the participant's diet. However, considering that participants were provided the same meals we made certain assumptions that the dietary intake would be similar between groups. The training schedule also forced several volunteers to miss their scheduled ingestion time for the supplement or placebo. It was in those situations where incidences of paresthesia occurred when the volunteer ingested multiple doses at the same time. Although volunteers were required to show the empty bottle and receive the following week's supply at the end of each week, the daily control for ingestion during meals was not possible. However, this study provided a unique opportunity to examine the efficacy of this supplement under real-life conditions involving military operations. This opportunity is not common and the results provided important information for potential dietary interventions on sustaining tactical performance in stressful conditions.

Conclusions

The results of this study did not provide any evidence in support of β-alanine's role on enhancing cognitive function in fatigued soldiers. It is likely that the serial subtraction test performed with participants seated was not sufficient to ascertain the potential effects that β-alanine may have in improving cognitive performance following fatiguing activity. This study demonstrated that β-alanine ingestion for 4 weeks in young, healthy soldiers in an elite combat unit can enhance jump power performance, marksmanship and target engagement speed. These improvements occurred following 4 weeks of highly intense training and an acute fatiguing event (4-km run). The results of this study were unable to support any cognitive benefits from the 4-week supplement period. In consideration of the highly intense and fatiguing nature of sustained combat and prolonged military training, ingestion of β-alanine does appear to provide specific benefits for military personnel.

Competing interests

All authors declare that they have no competing interests.

Authors' contributions

JRH, GL and IO were the primary investigators, supervised all study recruitment and data analysis. JRH, GL, MD, JRS, YBM, GH and IO assisted in the design of the study, JRH and JRS performed the statistical analysis, JRH supervised the manuscript preparation, JRS, JRH, DSM, and IO helped draft the manuscript. JRH, GL, DSM, NS, MWH, WPM and IO assisted with data collection and data analysis. All authors read and approved the final manuscript.

Acknowledgements

The authors would like to thank Natural Alternatives International (San Marcos, CA, USA) for providing support for this study.

Author details

[1]Institute of Exercise Physiology and Wellness, Sport and Exercise Science, University of Central Florida, Orlando, FL, USA. [2]Israel Defense Force, Medical Corps, Tel Hashomer, Israel. [3]School of Health Science, Ariel University, Center of Samaria, Ariel, Israel. [4]Israel Defense Forces, Combat Fitness Branch, Netanya, Israel.

References

1. Hill CA, Harris RC, Kim HJ, Harris BD, Sale C, Boobis LH, Kim CK, Wise JA: **Influence of β-alanine supplementation on skeletal muscle carnosine concentrations and high intensity cycling capacity.** *Amino Acids* 2007, **32:**225–233.
2. Hoffman JR, Ratamess NA, Kang J, Mangine G, Faigenbaum AD, Stout JR: **Effect of creatine and β-alanine supplementation on performance and endocrine responses in strength/power athletes.** *Int J Sport Nutr Exerc Metab* 2006, **16:**430–446.
3. Hoffman JR, Ratamess NA, Faigenbaum AD, Ross R, Kang J, Stout JR, Wise JA: **Short-duration β-alanine supplementation increases training volume and reduces subjective feelings of fatigue in college football players.** *Nutr Res* 2008, **28:**31–35.
4. Hoffman JR, Ratamess NA, Ross R, Kang J, Magrelli J, Neese K, Faigenbaum AD, Wise JA: **β-Alanine and the hormonal response to exercise.** *Int J Sports Med* 2008, **29:**952–958.
5. Kendrick IP, Harris RC, Kim HJ, Kim CK, Dang VH, Lam TQ, Bui TT, Smith M, Wise JA: **The effects of 10 weeks of resistance training combined with beta-alanine supplementation on whole body strength, force production, muscular endurance and body composition.** *Amino Acids* 2008, **34:**547–554.
6. Stout JR, Cramer JT, Mielke M, O'Kroy J, Torok DJ, Zoeller RF: **Effects of twenty-eight days of β-alanine and creatine monohydrate supplementation on the physical working capacity at neuromuscular fatigue threshold.** *J Strength Cond Res* 2006, **20:**928–931.
7. Stout JR, Cramer JT, Zoeller RF, Torok D, Costa P, Hoffman JR, Harris RC, O'Kroy J: **Effects of β-alanine supplementation on the onset of neuromuscular fatigue and ventilatory threshold in women.** *Amino Acids* 2007, **32:**381–386.
8. Dunnett M, Harris RC: **Influence of oral beta-alanine and L-histidine supplementation on the carnosine content of the gluteus medius.** *Equine Vet J Suppl* 1999, **30:**499–504.
9. Harris RC, Tallon MJ, Dunnett M: **The absorption of orally supplied β-alanine and its effect on muscle carnosine synthesis in human vastus lateralis.** *Amino Acids* 2006, **30:**279–289.

10. Hobson RM, Saunders B, Ball G, Harris RC, Sale C: **Effects of beta-alanine supplementation on exercise performance: a meta-analysis.** *Amino Acids* 2012, **43:**25–37.
11. Boldyrev AA, Stvolinsky SL, Fedorova TN, Suslina ZA: **Carnosine as a natural antioxidant and geroprotector: from molecular mechanisms to clinical trials.** *Rejuvenation Res* 2010, **13:**156–158.
12. Hipkiss AR, Worthington VC, Himsworth DTJ, Herwig W: **Protective effects of carnosine against protein modification mediated by malondialdehyde and hypochlorite.** *Biochim Biophys Acta* 1998, **1380:**46–54.
13. Kohen R, Yamamoto Y, Cundy KC, Ames BN: **Antioxidant activity of carnosine, homocarnosine and anserine present in muscle and brain.** *Proc Natl Acad Sci* 1988, **85:**3175–3179.
14. Murakami T, Furuse M: **The impact of taurine- and beta-alanine-supplemented diets on behavioral and neurochemical parameters in mice: antidepressant versus anxiolytic-like effects.** *Amino Acids* 2010, **39:**427–434.
15. Lieberman HR, Tharion WJ, Shukitt-Hale B, Speckman KL, Tulley R: **Effect of caffeine, sleep loss, and stress on cognitive performance and mood during U.S. Navy SEAL training.** *Psychopharmacol* 2002, **164:**250–261.
16. Nindl BC, Barnes BR, Alemany JA, Frykman PN, Shippee RL, Friedl KE: **Physiological consequences of U.S. army ranger training.** *Med Sci Sports Exerc* 2007, **39:**1380–1387.
17. Weeks SR, McAuliffe CL, DuRussel D, Pasquina PF: **Physiological and psychological fatigue in extreme conditions: the military example.** *Phys Med Rehab* 2010, **2:**438–441.
18. Welsh TT, Alemany JA, Montain SJ, Frykman PN, Young AJ, Nindl BC: **Effects of intensified military field training on jumping performance.** *Int J Sports Med* 2008, **29:**45–52.
19. Russo MB, Arnett MV, Thomas ML, Caldwell JA: **Ethical use of cogniceuticals in the militaries of democratic nations.** *Amer J Bioethics* 2008, **8:**39–49.
20. Cassler NM, Sams R, Cripe PA, McGlynn AF, Perry AB, Banks BA: **Patterns and perceptions of supplement use by U.S. Marines deployed to Afghanistan.** *Mil Med* 2013, **178:**659–664.
21. Lieberman HR, Stavinoha TB, McGraw SM, White A, Hadden LS, Marriott BP: **Use of dietary supplements among active-duty US Army soldiers.** *Am J Clin Nutr* 2010, **92:**985–995.
22. Gravettier FJ, Wallnau LB: *Statistics for the Behavioral Sciences (4th Ed.).* St. Paul, MN: West Publishing Co; 1996:250–255.
23. Varley MC, Fairweather IH, Aughey RJ: **Validity and reliability of GPS for measuring instantaneous velocity during acceleration, deceleration, and constant motion.** *J. Sports Sci.* 2012, **30:**121–127.
24. Hayman M: **Two minute clinical test for measurement of intellectual impairment in psychiatric disorders.** *Arch Neuro Psychiatry* 1942, **47:**454–464.
25. Wells AJ, Hoffman JR, Gonzalez AM, Stout JR, Fragala MS, Mangine GT, McCormack WP, Jajtner AR, Townsend JR, Robinson EH 4th: **Phosphatidylserine and caffeine attenuates post-exercise mood disturbance and perception of fatigue in humans.** *Nutr Res* 2013, **33:**464–472.
26. Green SB, Salkind NJ, Akey TM: *Using SPSS for Windows: Analyzing and Understanding Data.* 2nd edition. Upper Saddle River, NJ: Prentice Hall; 2000.
27. Artioli GG, Gualano B, Smith A, Stout JR, Junior AHL: **The role of β-alanine supplementation on muscle carnosine and exercise performance.** *Med Sci Sports Exerc* 2010, **42:**1162–1173.
28. Hoffman JR, Emerson NS, Stout JR: **β-alanine supplementation.** *Curr Sports Med Rep* 2012, **11:**189–195.
29. Evans RK, Scoville CR, Ito MA, Mello RP: **Upper body fatiguing exercise and shooting performance.** *Mil Med* 2003, **168:**451–456.
30. Lieberman HR, Bathalon GP, Falco CM, Kramer FM, Morgan CA 3rd, Niro P: **Severe decrements in cognition function and mood induced by sleep loss, heat, dehydration, and undernutrition during simulated combat.** *Biol Psychiatry* 2005, **57:**422–429.
31. Estrada A, Kelley AM, Webb CM, Athy JR, Crowley JS: **Modafinil as a replacement for dextroamphetamine for sustaining alertness in military helicopter pilots.** *Aviat Space Environ Med* 2012, **83:**556–564.
32. Gillingham RL, Keefe AA, Tikuisis P: **Acute caffeine intake before and after fatiguing exercises improves target shooting engagement time.** *Aviat Space Environ Med* 2004, **75:**865–871.
33. Jordan T, Lukaszuk J, Misic M, Umoren J: **Effects of beta-alanine supplementation on the onset of blood lactate accumulation (OBLA) during treadmill running: pre/post 2 treatment experimental design.** *J Int Soc Sports Nutr* 2010, **7:**20–27.
34. Derave W, Ozdemir MS, Harris RC, Pottier A, Reyngoudt H, Koppo K, Wise JA, Achten E: **Beta-alanine supplementation augments muscle carnosine content and attenuates fatigue during repeated isokinetic contraction bouts in trained sprinters.** *J Appl Physiol* 2007, **103:**1736–1743.
35. Kern BD, Robinson TL: **Effects of β-alanine supplementation on performance and body composition in collegiate wrestlers and football players.** *J Strength Cond Res* 2011, **25:**1804–1815.
36. Van Thienen R, Van Proeyen K, Vanden Eynde B, Puype J, Lefere T, Hespel P: **Beta-alanine, improves sprint performance in endurance cycling.** *Med Sci Sports Exerc* 2009, **41:**898–903.

The effect of almond consumption on elements of endurance exercise performance in trained athletes

Muqing Yi[1*], Jinde Fu[1], Lili Zhou[1*], Hong Gao[1], Chenguang Fan[2], Jing Shao[1], Baohua Xu[1], Qirong Wang[1], Juntao Li[1], Guangwei Huang[3], Karen Lapsley[3], Jeffrey B Blumberg[4] and C-Y Oliver Chen[4]

Abstract

Background: Almonds are a healthy tree nut food with high nutrient density. Their consumption has been shown to ameliorate oxidative stress, inflammation, etc. The objective of the study was to examine the effect of almonds on elements of endurance exercise performance in trained athletes.

Methods: A 10-week crossover, placebo controlled study was conducted. Eight trained male cyclists and two triathletes were randomly assigned to consume 75 g/d whole almonds (ALM) or isocaloric cookies (COK) with equal subject number. They consumed the assigned food for 4 wks and then the alternate food for another 4 wks. They underwent 3 performance tests including 125-min steady status exercise (SS) and 20-min time trial (TT) on an indoor stationary trainer at the start of the study (BL) and at the end of each intervention phase. Venous blood was collected in the morning prior to the performance test for biochemical measurements and finger blood during the test for glucose determination. Carbohydrate and fat oxidation, energy expenditure, and oxygen use were calculated using respiratory gas analysis.

Results: ALM increased cycling distance during TT by 1.7 km as compared BL (21.9 vs. 20.2 km, $P = 0.053$) and COK increased 0.6 km (20.8 vs. 20.2 km, $P > 0.05$). ALM, but not COK, led to higher CHO and lower fat oxidation and less oxygen consumption during TT than BL ($P < 0.05$), whereas there was no significant difference in heart rate among BL, ALM and COK. ALM maintained higher blood glucose level after TT than COK ($P < 0.05$). ALM had higher vitamin E and haemoglobin and lower serum free fatty acid ($P < 0.05$), slightly elevated serum arginine and nitric oxide and plasma insulin ($P > 0.05$) than BL, and a higher total antioxidant capacity than COK ($P < 0.05$).

Conclusions: Whole almonds improved cycling distance and the elements related to endurance performance more than isocaloric cookies in trained athletes as some nutrients in almonds may contribute to CHO reservation and utilization and effective oxygen utilization. The results suggest that almonds can be incorporated into diets of those who undertake exercise training for performance improvement.

Keywords: Almonds, Exercise performance, Substrate oxidation, Antioxidant defense capacity

Background

Almonds (*Prunus dulcis*) are nutrient dense because they are an excellent source of α-tocopherol, riboflavin, magnesium, and manganese, and a good source of dietary fiber, protein, copper and phosphorus [1,2]. Further, almonds are rich in arginine, a substrate for synthesis of the endothelial dilator, nitric oxide [3]. Almonds are also a source of monounsaturated fats, containing over 9 g per oz (~28 g) [4]. A diverse array of phenolic and polyphenolic compounds, predominantly including flavonoids, e.g., isorhamnetin-3-O-rutinoside and catechin, have been characterized in almonds [5]. This nutrient profile plays an important role in human studies that showed almond consumption was linked to amelioration in biomarkers of oxidative stress [6,7] and inflammation [8,9] and enhancement in LDL resistance against oxidation [10], and improvement

* Correspondence: Muqingyi@163.com; lilizhou666@163.com
[1]Center for Sports Nutrition, National Institute of Sports Medicine, 1st Anding Road, Chaoyang District, Beijing 100029, China
Full list of author information is available at the end of the article

in dyslipidemia [11-15]. In July 2003, the U.S. Food and Drug Administration (FDA) approved a qualified health claim stating, "Scientific evidence suggests but does not prove that eating 1.5 ounces per day of most nuts, such as almonds, as part of a diet low in saturated fat and cholesterol may reduce the risk of heart disease."

Intense, prolonged physical exertion is linked to an increased production of reactive oxygen species (ROS) via oxidative flux into the mitochondrial respiration chain, phagocytic respiratory bursts, and other sources [16]. Such overproduction of ROS overwhelms antioxidant defense capacities, disturbs the balance of immune and endocrine systems, impairs exercise performance, and induces exercise fatigue [17,18]. As almonds are a good source of unsaturated fatty acids, antioxidants and some micronutrients, they may help maintain and/or enhance exercise performance by modulating fuel utilization and strengthening antioxidant defenses. For example, quercetin [19-22] and arginine [23-27] present in almonds may help augment the training effectiveness on exercise performance by upregulating mitochondrial biogenesis and oxygen sparing capacity and facilitating oxygen delivery to skeletal muscle, and decreasing ammonia liberation.

As of today, the effect of almond consumption on elements of exercise performance in trained athletes remains unknown. We hypothesized that almond consumption could improve exercise performance in trained endurance athletes. The main objective of the study was to investigate whether consumption of almonds would improve elements related to exercise performance as compared to isocaloric cookies in trained athletes participating in annual winter training.

Methods

Subjects

Ten trained, male professional athletes (8 cyclists and 2 triathletes) from the same sports team (club) were recruited to participate in the study throughout winter season training in a training camp in the south of China following their training in the north of China. The biometrics of the training subjects are shown in Table 1. Their mean training period was 6.3 ± 1.6 years. They ranked in the top 20 percent of national competition records, and even were champions in Asian games. As professional athletes they trained for 5-6 days a week, and basically participated in national and Asian competitions such as Taiwan/Hong Kong/Hainan/Qinghai Lake bicycle races each year.

The study was approved by the Ethical Board of National Institute of Sports Medicine (NISM) and was in compliance with the WMA Declaration of Helsinki. The study protocol was approved by the Review Board of NISM. All athletes signed the consent form before the study.

Table 1 Biometrics of the training subjects

Biometrics	Participants (n = 10)	Cyclists (n = 8)	Triathletes (n = 2)
Age (years)	22.3 ± 1.6	23.2 ± 0.8	20.3 ± 0.6
Height (cm)	180.6 ± 7.2	184.0 ± 2.0	172.7 ± 0.6
BM (kg)	74.2 ± 7.7	77.5 ± 2.3	66.5 ± 0.5
VO_2max (mL/kg/min)	70.3 ± 4.6	70.4 ± 5.6	70.2 ± 0.6
Training years	6.3 ± 1.6	7.2 ± 0.8	4.3 ± 0.6

Key: BM, body mass.
Age (years), height (cm), BM (kg), VO_2max (mL/kg/min), and Training years (years) for cyclists and triathletes separately and combined.

Study design, VO_2max test and food consumption

A 10-week self-controlled, crossover design with two 4-week phases of consuming whole almonds and isocaloric cookies in a randomized feeding trial fashion and a 2-week washout period between two phases was conducted (Figure 1). Eight cyclists and two triathletes were randomly assigned to almond- (ALM) and cookies-consuming (COK) groups with equal athlete number after the baseline (BL) performance test.

The individual VO_2max test was determined using an incremental workload (Watts) on a cycling ergometer (Lode Excalibur Sport, Groningen, Netherlands) 1 week prior to BL performance test. A 100-watt initial workload and 25-watt increment per minute were applied. Respiratory gas was measured using a Cortex MetaMax® 3B remote-controlled system (Cortex Biophysik, Germany), which provides a reliable gas exchange analysis based on the principle of breath-by-breath analysis [28,29]. The system was calibrated with a calibration gas (5% CO_2, 15%

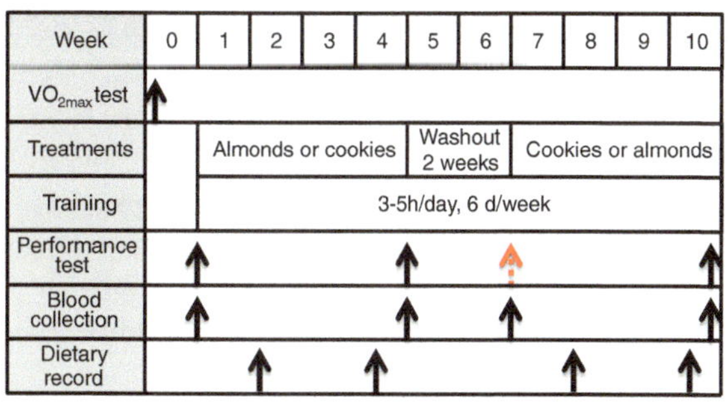

Figure 1 Study design. Ten trained male athletes (8 cyclists and 2 triathletes) participated in a 10-week self-controlled, crossover trial during winter season training with training for 3-5 hours per day, 5-6 days a week (see the section of Exercise training regimen and Additional file 4). Dietary treatments consisted of two intervention phases of 75 g raw whole almonds or 90 g isocaloric cookies per day for four weeks each, and a 2-week washout period between two phases. VO_2max test was undertaken one week prior to the baseline performance test. The time points for performance tests, blood collection and dietary record are indicated with black arrows. The red arrow shows the missed necessary performance test due to modification of athletes' training plan.

O_2, BAL. N_2) (Air Liquide Healthcare America Corporation, Plumsteadville, PA, USA) prior to the VO_2max test and each performance test.

After the BL performance test, subjects began to consume raw whole almonds (75 g/d as described by Xiao et al. [30]) as 1.8 times the FDA's claim considered to meet the athletes' need for intensive training or isocaloric starch-based commercial cookies (90 g/d), which was split equally into three portions fed before three main meals. We chose cookies as the placebo because they are carbohydrate-containing convenient snacks beneficial to exercise training and commonly used by the subjects. Additionally, 90 g of isocaloric cookies have a similar weight but a very different nutritional profile as 75 g of almonds (Additional file 1). In consideration of the unknown effective dosage of almonds for athletes we did not use a lower feeding of almonds. We recognized that the subjects were also aware of almonds as a kind of healthy food, while they seldom had it as snacks due to relative high cost.

Almonds were generously provided by the Almond Board of California. Nutrition information for 75 g almonds and 90 g cookies are presented in Additional file 1.

Exercise performance test

Subjects stopped their regular training one day before performance test. They reported to testing room either at 8:30 am or 2:30 pm, 1.5 h after standard breakfast or lunch. Each subject used the same indoor stationary bicycle trainer in all 3 performance tests and followed the same testing protocol with the same settings (Additional file 2, a representative video). The same trainer was also used for their routine training. The test consisted of 10 min of warm-up at 30% VO_2max, 115 min of steady-state (SS) cycling at 50-60% VO_2max, 20 min of time trial (TT) at all-out effort following a 10-min relaxation (for collection of urine). Expired gas composition and temperature, HR, ambient temperature and humidity during whole TT were monitored using Cortex MetaMax® 3B System and Polar 725 heart rate monitor. Carbohydrate (CHO) and fat utilization was calculated based on the equation built in the software by selecting an assumed 15% total energy expenditure derived from protein.

The rating of perceived exertion (RPE) using the 6-20 Borg scale was surveyed at 20-min intervals throughout the test. The pre- and post-testing body mass (BM) with removal of their racing suit was checked using an electronic BM scale. Urine sample was collected during 10-min relax time of the performance test for volume determination. To ensure subjects were enthusiastic about the test and performed at their highest level, they were informed at the beginning of the test that a prize would be awarded to the winner cycling the longest distance during TT.

Blood samples collection and biochemical measurements

Venous blood was collected from anticubital arm vein into vacutainer tubes before the performance tests. Heparin plasma and serum were obtained after centrifugation at 3000 × *g* for 10 min. Samples were stored at -80°C until analyses. Finger blood was obtained via puncture for glucose determination at 0, 60, 125 and 155 min during the test.

Free fatty acid (FFA), pyruvic acid (PA), and total antioxidant capacity (TAOC) in plasma were determined using commercial kits (Randox Laboratories Ltd, Crumlin, UK), and an auto-biochemical analyzer (Hitachi, Tokyo, Japan). Plasma VE, malondialdehyde (MDA) and arginine levels, xanthine oxidase (XOD) and glutathione peroxidase (GPx) and superoxide dismutase (SOD) and creatine kinase (CK) activities, and blood urea nitrogen (BUN) and nitric oxide (NO) were measured using spectrophotometric kits (Jiancheng Bioengineering Institute, Nanjing, China). Serum insulin (Ins) and cortisol (Cor) concentrations were measured using radioimmunoassay kit (Jiuding Diagnostic, Tianjin, China). Blood glucose (BG) was determined using handheld blood glucose analyzer (One Touch, LifeScan, Inc. Milpitas, CA).

Diet and dietary record

All subjects lived in a winter training camp and dined in the same canteen throughout the study, and were advised by a registered dietician to follow a diet with 60% total calories from CHO, 15% from protein, and 25% from fat for 2 days before each performance test. Generally subjects had a typical Chinese breakfast consisting of one chicken egg, two servings of steamed breads or noodles, deep-fried dough sticks, rice congee, bean milk, some meat, some vegetables and appetizers, and lunch and dinner consisting of meat, steamed rice, steamed breads, noodles, soup, milk, fruit and vegetables, etc.

To assess dietary intake throughout the study, a 2-day food record was conducted at week 2, 4, 8, and 10. Chinese food database (issued by Chinese Society of Nutrition) was used for nutritional analysis (Additional file 3). During the regular training, subjects were allowed to drink 6% CHO-electrolytes-vitamins (without VE) beverage (Competitor, Beijing, China) with an average amount of 1500 ml/d. Ten minutes prior to the performance test, subjects checked their BM after emptying bladder, and ingested 2.0% CHO-electrolytes-vitamins (without VE) beverage at 6 mL/kg BM for the pre-testing hydration, 2.5 mL/kg/15 min during SS. No beverage was provided during TT. Subjects did not take any other dietary supplements throughout the study.

Exercise training regimen

Basically, all subjects had their road cycling training together, whereas two triathletes had their run and swim training in the same training site throughout the study. Briefly, based on their training plan, subjects trained 5-6 days a week with incremental increase in training amount and intensity throughout the study. Detailed content of daily and weekly training was made by coaches on each weekend. The typical daily cycling training regimen consisted of 60-200 km (even 220-250 km) road endurance cycling, 2-3 km*N (N = 2-8) timing sprint cycling on the flat road and sloping fields. Exercise intensity was monitored by HR. Eight cyclists had a weekly road cycling distance of 2840 km and 3110 km during two phases, respectively (Additional file 4). Two triathletes had an average 380-km of road cycling weekly during two phases.

Limitation of the present study

The original study design included four performance tests performed by subjects before and after each intervention phase during the study. Regretfully, subjects did not undergo VO_2max test prior to the 2nd intervention phase and the performance test at the beginning of week 7 due to a modified training arrangement. Thus, baseline values of the performance test at the start of the 2nd phase were not available. However, the following 4 points may be helpful to support that the drawback should not affect significance of study outcomes observed at the end of the intervention phases. First, we originally had a crossover design, that is to say, when ALM or COK was compared with BL, there were 5 subjects in each group at the first intervention phase. Second, we had blood biochemistry tests at the end of washout (the end of 6th week). With the exception of a higher FFA, biochemical outcomes after washout at 6th week (MDA 3.7 ± 0.4; XOD 12.5 ± 0.8; TAOC 15.5 ± 1.6; GPx 0.39 ± 0.02; SOD 55.8 ± 0.6; VE 25.2 ± 2.2; CK 237.3 ± 46.4; Cor 19.3 ± 0.8; Hb 143.6 ± 2.7; PA 0.49 ± 0.07; FFA 0.20 ± 0.02; arginine 0.076 ± 0.003; NO 96.7 ± 13.2; Ins 5.0 ± 0.9) were not statistically different from the BL values (see Table 2, their units are the same as shown in Table 2 presented, n = 10). Third, half-life of some nutrients or primarily functional components present in almonds supports that the carry-over effect of the first intervention should be minimal if there was any, e.g, the half-life of α-tocopherol, quercetin, diverse polyphenols and arginine is 57 h [31], 11-25 h [32,33], 1-18 h [34] and 1.5-2.0 h [35], respectively. Finally, subjects all lived and trained in the same training camp throughout the study.

Statistical analysis

According to the balanced crossover design we combined the data of the same treatment in two phases for statistical analysis.

All results are expressed as mean ± SE except when specified elsewhere. Two-way ANOVA was performed to analyze the differences among groups. Significance was analyzed using post hoc least significant difference (LSD) test. All statistical analyses were performed using SPSS 13.0 software. Differences were considered significant at P < 0.05.

Table 2 Blood biochemistries pre-performance tests

Biomarkers	BL	COK	ALM
Antioxidant status			
MDA (μmol/L)	3.9 ± 0.15	3.2 ± 0.5	3.2 ± 0.3
XOD (U/L)	13.3 ± 0.4	13.1 ± 0.9	12.4 ± 1.0
TAOC (U/ml)	16.1 ± 0.5	12.8 ± 1.0*	16.3 ± 0.9#
GPx (U/ml)	0.41 ± 0.01	0.45 ± 0.05	0.43 ± 0.05
SOD (U/ml)	58.7 ± 1.4	61.2 ± 1.4	59.5 ± 1.4
VE (μmol/L)	19.8 ± 1.8	25.6 ± 1.7	28.7 ± 2.5*
Training, recovery and oxygen-carrying capacity			
CK (U/L)	224.2 ± 32.9	354.7 ± 62.9	288.3 ± 81.1
BUN (mmol/L)	6.5 ± 0.5	7.3 ± 0. 7	6.6 ± 0.6
Hb (g/L)	136.6 ± 2.5	143.2 ± 3.7	145.7 ± 2.7*
Carbohydrate and lipid metabolism production			
BG (mmol/L)	5.6 ± 0.2	5.3 ± 0.3	5.4 ± 0.2
PA (mmol/L)	0.42 ± 0.05	0.44 ± 0.07	0.44 ± 0.07
FFA (mmol/L)	0.22 ± 0.04	0.16 ± 0.03	0.11 ± 0.01*
Metabolism-regulating factors			
Arginine (mmol/L)	0.073 ± 0.005	0.089 ± 0.011	0.113 ± 0.031
NO (μmol/L)	99.6 ± 10.6	113.1 ± 15.3	136.0 ± 18.1
Ins (μIU/ml)	5.5 ± 0.9	5.3 ± 1.6	9.4 ± 2.3
Cor (mmol/L)	20.3 ± 0.9	22.3 ± 2.3	22.0 ± 1.7

MDA, malondialdehyde (μmol/L), XOD, xanthine oxidase (U/L), TAOC, total antioxidant capacity (U/ml), GPx, glutathione peroxidise (U/ml), SOD, superoxide dismutase (U/ml), VE, vitamine E (μmol/L), CK, creatine kinase (U/ml), BUN (blood urea nitrogen (mmol/L), Hb, haemoglubin (g/L), BG, blood glucose (mmol/L), PA, pyruvic acid (mmol/L), FFA, free fatty acid (mmol/L), NO, nitric oxide (μmol/L), Ins, insulin (μIU/ml), Cor, cortisol (mmol/L).
*significantly different from BL at P < 0.05.
#significantly different from COK at P < 0.05.

Results

Cycling distance

The mean cycling distance during SS phase among BL, ALM and COK was not significantly different (BL, COK and ALM: 80.1 ± 1.3, 82.4 ± 2.0 and 83.1 ± 1.3 km, P > 0.05), while ALM's distance during TT was 1.7 km (+8.4%) more than BL's one (21.9 ± 0.4 vs 20.2 ± 0.4 km, P = 0.053), and 1.1 km (+5.3%) longer (21.9 ± 0.4 vs 20.8 ± 0.6 km) than COK (P > 0.05) (Figure 2).

Rate of perceived exertion

BL showed a higher RPE score at several time points during SS than COK and ALM. No difference among BL, ALM and COK during TT was noted (Figure 3).

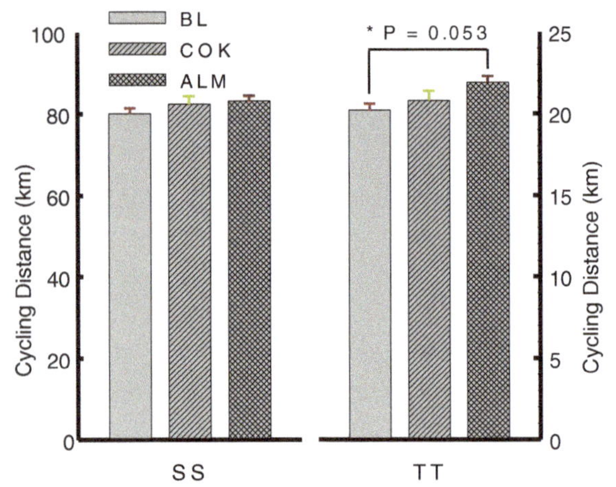

Figure 2 Cycling distance during TT. A 20-min time trial at all-out effort was undertaken during TT following a 115-min riding on indoor stationary bicycle trainer at 50%-60% VO_2max during SS and a 10-min relaxation for urine collection. Cycling distance was recorded by Polar 725 heart rate monitor equipped with a telemeter. ALM (not COK) performed a more cycling distance during TT than BL (*$P = 0.053$) and COK ($P > 0.05$). No difference in cycling distance during SS was noted among BL, COK and ALM.

Ambient temperature and humidity, and expired gas temperature

Mean ambient temperature during the performance test at BL was about ~1.3°C higher than COK and ALM (26.9 ± 0.4 vs 25.6 ± 0.3 and 25.6 ± 0.2°C, $P < 0.05$). The humidity during the performance test at BL was higher than COK and ALM (68.5 ± 1.4 vs 53.2 ± 2.0 and 52.7 ± 1.4%, $P < 0.05$). Mean expired gas temperature during the performance test at BL was 0.6°C higher than COK and ALM (BL vs COK and ALM: 32.6 ± 0.1 vs 32.0 ± 0.1 and 32.1 ± 0.1°C, $P < 0.05$).

BM loss

Mean pre-test BM among BL, COK and ALM was not different. Three groups had a significant BM loss post-test. COK and ALM had a larger magnitude of exercise-induced BM loss post-test than BL (Table 3).

Physiological indicators and gas exchange analysis

Mean HR, VO_2, energy expenditure (EE) during TT were not significantly different among BL, COK and ALM. The CHO oxidation during TT in COK and ALM was increased, FAT oxidation and oxygen use rate in both groups was decreased compared with BL. However the change reached a statistical significance only in ALM (Figure 4).

Blood biochemistries

Blood glucose was decreased with the progression of SS exercise by ~17% in BL, COK and ALM ($P < 0.005$). After the 10-min relaxation, blood glucose was increased by 14% and 9% from the end of SS in both BL and COK ($P < 0.05$), 7% in ALM ($P > 0.05$). At the end of TT, blood glucose in BL and COK went down as compared with that at the end of SS ($P < 0.05$), while that in ALM went up ($P < 0.05$), The difference at the end of TT between ALM and COK tended to be significant ($P = 0.054$) (Figure 5).

Among the biomarkers reflecting subjects' antioxidant status, TAOC in COK was decreased, while ALM's level, which was higher than that in COK, was not changed as compared to BL. ALM, not COK, had a higher blood VE than BL (Table 2). Other indicators were not significantly changed (Table 2).

The indicators of training and recovery, CK and BUN, were not affected by the interventions. Hb in ALM was higher than BL (Table 2).

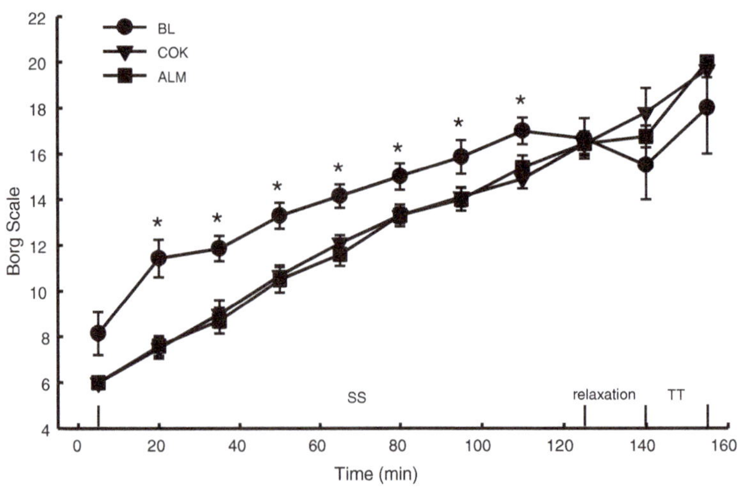

Figure 3 Time curve of RPE. RPE (rating of perceived exertion) assessed using a 6-20 Borg scale was recorded every 15 min during performance tests. BL had higher values at some time-points than ALM and COK. No difference between ALM and COK was observed at any time points.

Table 3 Change in BM post-performance tests

Groups	Pre-test (kg)	Post-test (kg)	BM loss (kg)
BL	73.9 ± 2.6	72.6 ± 2.6[&]	1.3 ± 0.2
COK	74.7 ± 2.1	72.7 ± 2.1[&]	2.0 ± 0.2*
ALM	74.9 ± 2.4	72.8 ± 2.4[&]	2.1 ± 0.2*

Key: BM, body mass.
[&]significantly different from pre-test in the same group at P < 0.05.
*significantly different from BL at P < 0.05.

Serum FFA, but not BG and PA in ALM, which are indicative of carbohydrate and fat metabolic production, were lower than BL (Table 2).

Some metabolism-regulating factors like arginine, NO and Ins, were not different among BL, COK and ALM, whereas ALM had slightly higher levels than COK (Table 2).

Nutritional intake

The dietary intakes of energy, carbohydrate, total fat (including saturated and mono- and multi-unsaturated fatty acids), protein, total VE and arginine were not different between COK and ALM (Additional file 3).

Discussion

The present study showed that 4-week consumption of both 75 g/d whole almonds and isocaloric cookies during the winter training season improved cycling distance of time trial and elements of exercise performance relative to BL, with a greater change in the ALM, even though BL's performance was likely partially affected by relatively high ambient temperature and humidity.

The data suggests that a few notable nutrients/compounds abundant in almonds might improve the effectiveness of the training in a synergistic way via modulating CHO reservation/utilization (by improving glucose transport into skeletal muscle and glycogen synthesis [36,37]), antioxidant capacity [6,7], oxygen transportation/utilization and metabolism regulation [19-26] through slightly raised arginine, insulin, and NO, and statistically increased VE, TAOC and Hb level (Table 2) without greatly affecting fluid balance (Table 3).

In general, training elevates fat-derived energy contribution to an endurance competition [38]. A continuous supply of fatty acids is crucial to athletes participating in distance/endurance competition at moderate intensity, whereas CHO serves as the main fuel during an intense exercise, especially during sprint of a competition [36,39]. Thus, CHO preloading and loading prior to or during a race are essential strategies for athletes participating in an endurance competition [40]. Statistically, our study showed that there were no differences in VO_2, CHO and fat oxidation during TT between COK and ALM. However ALM had lower VO_2 and higher CHO oxidation and lower fat oxidation than BL while ALM did not change HR and EE as compared to BL

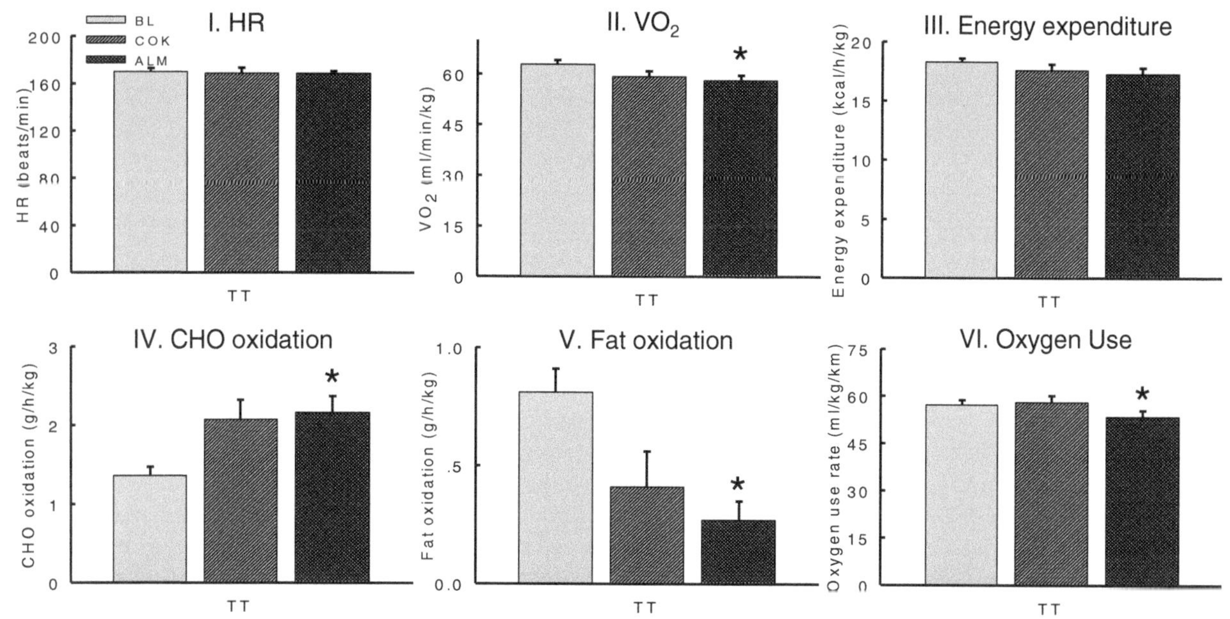

Figure 4 Main physiological records and gas exchange analysis throughout TT. Several main physiological parameters (HR, heart rate, and VO_2, oxygen uptake) throughout TT were recorded as described in the Methods. Energy expenditure (EE), carbohydrate and fat oxidation, and oxygen use were calculated as described in the Methods. No significant differences in HR and EE among BL, ALM and COK (P > 0.05) were found. ALM (not COK) had higher carbohydrate (CHO) oxidation, lower oxygen uptake (VO_2), fat oxidation and oxygen use as compared with BL (*P < 0.05), whereas there were no difference in VO_2, CHO and fat oxidation and oxygen use between ALM and COK.

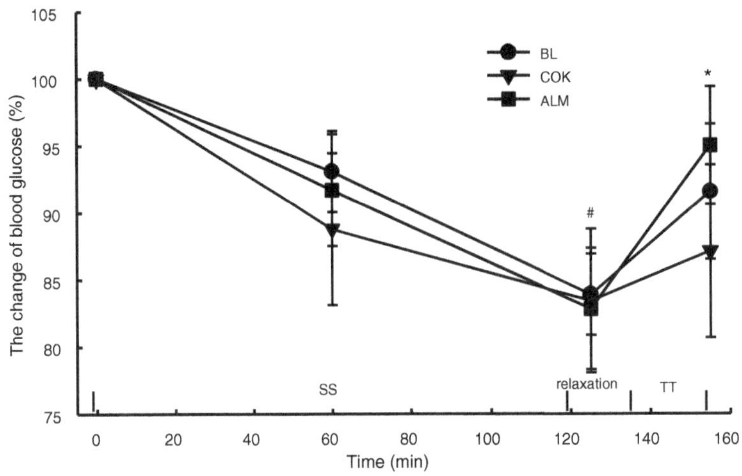

Figure 5 Change in blood glucose during performance tests. Blood glucose was tested at 0, 60 min and at the end of SS and TT. The values at the end of SS in BL, ALM and COK were lower than at the start of performance test ($^{\#}P < 0.05$). ALM had greater increased percentage at the end of TT than BL and COK as compared to that at the end of SS and a higher level than COK ($^{*}P < 0.05$) at the end of TT.

(Figure 3). It should be noted that ALM (not COK) had lower oxygen consumption during TT (Figure 3), lower blood FFA and higher blood glucose at the end of exercise than BL (Figure 5, Table 2), suggesting almonds might help athletes to mobilize more previously reserved CHO, instead of breaking down fat as an energy source during training and the intense exercise [41]. A higher Hb level in ALM might also help athletes transport more oxygen to skeletal muscles during exercise.

L-arginine, the natural precursor of NO, may stimulate insulin secretion [42], decrease oxygen consumption [23,25] and ammonia liberation [27] during exercise and regulate vascular dilation [43,44]. A clinical trial showed that a combined arginine and antioxidant supplement improved exercise performance in the elderly [26]. Insulin facilitates glucose transfer to skeletal muscle tissues and subsequent glycogen synthesis [42,45,46]. Our results suggest that almond consumption may contribute to an improvement in cycling performance- related elements via the effect of arginine on insulin secretion and muscle glycogen synthesis without enhancing insulin sensitivity via down-regulated insulin levels noted in patients with diabetes [14,47,48]. Unsatisfactorily, we did not observe a statistical difference in blood arginine and NO (Table 2) because daily arginine intake from almonds (about 2 g excluding that from the diet) provided ~100 mg/kg BM which was less than that administered in other's studies [25,27]; athletes had a larger need and utilization (metabolism) of arginine due to intensive exercise; there was a large inter-individual variation; arginine may work with other almond nutrients in a synergistic or additive manner.

Several studies had shown that quercetin alone or plus antioxidants improved mitochondrial biogenesis, VO_2max, and exercise capacity [19-22]. Therefore, the effect of quercetin on mitochondrial biogenesis and oxygen consumption might also be linked to almond consumption in this study.

Human studies demonstrated that almond consumption increases circulating α-tocopherol concentration in a dose-dependent manner [4,12], decreases biomarkers of oxidative stress in smokers and hypercholesterlemic patients [1,49]. Phenolics in almonds have shown to exert antioxidant action against reactive radicals in humans [6,7]. Thus, a diverse array of phenolic and polyphenolic compounds in almonds might contribute to improving antioxidant capacity in the athletes. Even though ALM (not COK) had a higher blood VE than BL and higher TAOC than COK, we did not find other significant changes related to the antioxidant effects of almond consumption in trained athletes. It is worth noting that the antioxidant effect by almonds was not a predominant factor in improving the elements associated with endurance performance in trained athletes due to their good adaptation to intensive training. Further, one of benefits exerted by almonds might be attributed to decreased inflammation markers (not determined in the study) [8].

Conclusions

The study showed that almond consumption at 75 g/d for 4 weeks improved time trial distance and the elements related to endurance performance more than did isocaloric cookie consumption in trained Chinese cyclists and triathletes during winter season training when compared to those at the beginning of the training season. Some nutrients/compounds present in almonds like arginine and quercetin might contribute to reserving and using more CHO and enhancing more effective oxygen utilization. Our study suggests that almonds can be incorporated into diets of those who are undertaking exercise training for performance improvement.

Additional files

Additional file 1: Nutritional facts of 75 g almonds and isocaloric 90 g cookies.

Additional file 2: A representative video during performance test. Individual athlete completed three performance tests following the same protocol by riding on the same indoor stationary bicycle trainer using their own training bicycle with the same setting.

Additional file 3: Main profiles of dietary nutritional intake for two groups during two phases.

Additional file 4: Cyclists's road cycling training distance during two phases.

Competing interests
The authors declare that they have no competing interest and that the results of the present study do not constitute endorsement by JISSN.

Authors' contributions
MY and LZ were responsible for study design, data collection, statistical analysis, and manuscript preparation. JF, HG, CF, QW, JS, BX, and JL were responsible for biochemical work, dietary record and calculation, data collection/entry, and assistance with manuscript preparation. GH and KL participated in formulating study design. JB and COC helped draft the manuscript. All authors read and approved the final manuscript.

Acknowledgements
The study was supported by the Almond Board of California. The authors thank the coaches and physicians for the Chinese Bayi Cycling and Triathlon Team for their support on training and performance test arrangement and dietary information collection.

Author details
[1]Center for Sports Nutrition, National Institute of Sports Medicine, 1st Anding Road, Chaoyang District, Beijing 100029, China. [2]Chinese Baiyi Cycling Team, Fengtai District, Beijing 100072, China. [3]Almond Board of California, Modesto, CA 95354, USA. [4]Antioxidants Research Laboratory, Jean Mayer USDA Human Nutrition Research Center on Aging, Tufts University, Boston, MA, USA.

References
1. Chen CY, Lapsley K, Blumberg J: **A nutrition and health perspective on almonds.** *J Sci Food Agric* 2006, **86:**2245–2250.
2. Kornsteiner M, Wagner K-H, Elmadfa I: **Tocopherols and total phenolics in 10 different nut types.** *Food Chem* 2006, **98:**381–387.
3. Sabaté J, Haddad E, Tanzman JS, Jambazian P, Rajaram S: **Serum lipid response to the graduated enrichment of a Step I diet with almonds: a randomized feeding trial.** *Am J Clin Nutr* 2003, **77:**1379–1384.
4. Maguire LS, O'Sullivan SM, Galvin K, O'Connor TP, O'Brien NM: **Fatty acid profile, tocopherol, squalene and phytosterol content of walnuts, almonds, peanuts, hazelnuts and the macadamia nut.** *Int J Food Sci Nutr* 2004, **55:**171–178.
5. Milbury PE, Chen CY, Dolnikowski GG, Blumberg JB: **Determination of flavonoids and phenolics and their distribution in almonds.** *J Agric Food Chem* 2006, **54:**5027–5033.
6. Chen CY, Blumberg JB: **In vitro activity of almond skin polyphenols for scavenging free radicals and inducing quinone reductase.** *J Agric Food Chem* 2008, **56:**4427–4434.
7. Jenkins DJ, Kendall CW, Marchie A, Josse AR, Nguyen TH, Faulkner DA, Lapsley KG, Blumberg J: **Almonds reduce biomarkers of lipid peroxidation in older hyperlipidemic subjects.** *J Nutr* 2008, **138:**908–913.
8. Rajaram S, Connell KM, Sabaté J: **Effect of almond-enriched high-monounsaturated fat diet on selected markers of inflammation: a randomised, controlled, crossover study.** *Br J Nutr* 2010, **103:**907–912.
9. Mandalari G, Bisignano C, Genovese T, Mazzon E, Wickham MS, Paterniti I, Cuzzocrea S: **Natural almond skin reduced oxidative stress and inflammation in an experimental model of inflammatory bowel disease.** *Int Immunopharmacol* 2011, **11:**915–924.
10. Chen CY, Milbury PE, Lapsley K, Blumberg JB: **Flavonoids from almond skins are bioavailable and act synergistically with vitamins C and E to enhance hamster and human LDL resistance to oxidation.** *J Nutr* 2005, **135:**1366–1373.
11. Jenkins DJ, Kendall CW, Marchie A, Parker TL, Connelly PW, Qian W, Haight JS, Faulkner D, Vidgen E, Lapsley KG, Spiller GA: **Dose response of almonds on coronary heart disease risk factors: blood lipids, oxidized low-density lipoproteins, lipoprotein(a), homocysteine, and pulmonary nitric oxide: a randomized, controlled, crossover trial.** *Circulation* 2002, **106:**1327–1332.
12. Jambazian PR, Haddad E, Rajaram S, Tanzman J, Sabaté J: **Almonds in the diet simultaneously improve plasma alpha-tocopherol concentrations and reduce plasma lipids.** *J Am Diet Assoc* 2005, **105:**449–454.
13. Lovejoy JC, Most MM, Lefevre M, Greenway FL, Food JC: **Effect of diets enriched in almonds on insulin action and serum lipids in adults with normal glucose tolerance or type 2 diabetes.** *Am J Clin Nutr* 2002, **76:**1000–1006.
14. Li SC, Liu YH, Liu JF, Chang WH, Chen CM, Chen CY: **Almond consumption improved glycemic control and lipid profiles in patients with type 2 diabetes mellitus.** *Metabolism* 2011, **60:**474–479.
15. Jenkins DJ, Kendall CWC, Josse AR, Salvatore S, Brighenti F, Augustin LS, Ellis PR, Vidgen E, Rao AV: **Almonds decrease postprandial glycemia, insulinemia, and oxidative damage in healthy individuals.** *J Nutr* 2006, **136:**2987–2992.
16. Finaud J, Lac G, Filaire E: **Oxidative stress: relationship with exercise and training.** *Sports Med* 2006, **36:**327–358.
17. Powers SK, Jackson MJ: **Exercise-induced oxidative stress: cellular mechanisms and impact on muscle force production.** *Physiol Rev* 2008, **88:**1243–1276.
18. Reid MB: **Free radicals and muscle fatigue: Of ROS, canaries, and the IOC.** *Free Radic Biol Med* 2008, **44:**169–179.
19. Davis JM, Murphy EA, Carmichael MD, Davis B: **Quercetin increases brain and muscle mitochondrial biosynthesis and exercise tolerance.** *Am J Physiol Regul Integr Comp* 2009, **296:**R1071–R1077.
20. Davis JM, CarlsteTT CJ, Chen S, Carmichael MD, Murphy EA: **The dietary flavonoid quercetin increases VO2max and endurance capacity.** *Int J Sport Nutr Exerc Metab* 2010, **20:**56–62.
21. MacRae HSH, Mefferd KM: **Dietary antioxidant supplementation combined with quercetin improves cycling time trial performance.** *Int J Sport Nutr Exer Metab* 2006, **16:**405–419.
22. Nieman DC, Williams AS, Shanely RA, Jin F, McAnulty SR, Triplett NT, Austin MD, Henson DA: **Quercetin's influence on exercise performance and muscle mitochondrial biogenesis.** *Med Sci Sports Exerc* 2010, **42:**338–345.
23. Campbell BI, Bounty PML, Roberts M: **The ergogenic potential of arginine.** *J Int Soc Sports Nutr* 2004, **1:**35–38.
24. Doutreleau S, Rouyer O, Di Marco P, Lonsdorfer E, Richard R, Piquard F, Geny B: **L-arginine supplementation improves exercise capacity after a heart transplant.** *Am J Clin Nutr* 2010, **91:**1261–1267.
25. Bailey SJ, Winyard PG, Vanhatalo A, Blackwell JR, DiMenna FJ, Wilkerson DP, Jones AM: **Acute L-arginine supplementation reduces the O_2 cost of moderate-intensity exercise and enhances high-intensity exercise tolerance.** *J Appl Physiol* 2010, **109:**1394–1403.
26. Chen S, Kim W, Henning SM, Carpenter CL, Li Z: **Arginine and antioxidant supplement on performance in elderly male cyclists: a randomized controlled trial.** *J Int Soc Sports Nutr* 2010, **7:**13.
27. Gonçalves LC, Bessa A, Freitas-Dias R, Luzes R, Werneck-de-Castro JP, Bassini A, Cameron LC: **A sportomics strategy to analyze the ability of arginine to modulate both ammonia and lymphocyte levels in blood after high-intensity exercise.** *J Int Soc Sports Nutr* 2012, **9:**30.
28. Meyer T, Georg T, Becker C, Kindermann W: **Reliability of gas exchange measurements from two different spiroergometry systems.** *Int J Sports Med* 2001, **22:**593–597.
29. Schulz H, Helle S, Heck H: **The validity of the telemetric system CORTEX X1 in the ventilatory and gas exchange measurement during exercise.** *Int J Sports Med* 1997, **18:**454–457.
30. Ying X, Jun-bo W, Shao-fang Y: **Study on effect of nut rich in monounsaturated fatty acid on serum lipids in hyperlipidemia patients.** *Chin Publ Health* 2002, **18:**931–932.
31. Leonard SW, Paterson E, Atkinson JK, Ramakrishnan R, Cross CE, Traber MG: **Studies in humans using deuterium-labeled α- and γ-tocopherol**

demonstrate faster plasma g-tocopherol disappearance and greater g-metabolite production. *Free Radic Biol Med* 2005, **38**:857–866.
32. Graefe EU, Wittig J, Mueller S, Riethling AK, Uehleke B, Drewelow B, Pforte H, Jacobasch G, Derendorf H, Beit M: **Pharmacokinetics and bioavailability of quercetin glycosides in humans.** *J Clin Pharmacol* 2001, **41**:492–499.
33. Lamson DW, Brignall MS: **Antioxidants and cancer, part 3: Quercetin.** *Altern Med Rev* 2000, **5**:196–208.
34. Manach C, Williamson G, Morand C, Scalbert A, Rémésy C: **Bioavailability and bioefficacy of polyphenols in humans. I. Review of 97 bioavailability studies.** *Am J Clin Nutr* 2005, **81**(suppl):230S–242S.
35. Böger RH, Bode-Böger SM: **The clinical pharmacology of L-arginine.** *Annu Rev Pharmacol Toxicol* 2001, **41**:79–99.
36. Thomas EJ, Richter EA: **Regulation of glucose and glycogen metabolism during and after exercise.** *J Physiol* 2012, **590**(Pt 5):1069–1076.
37. American Dietetic Association, Dietitians of Canada, American College of Sports Medicine, Rodriguez NR, Di Marco NM, Langley S: **American College of Sports Medicine position stand. Nutrition and Athletic Performance.** *Med Sci Sports Exerc* 2009, **41**:709–731.
38. Bergman BC, Butterfield GE, Wolfel EE, Casazza GA, Lopaschuk GD, Brooks GA: **Evaluation of exercise and training on muscle lipid metabolism.** *Am J Physiol* 1999, **276**(1 Pt 1):E106–E117.
39. Ivy JL: **Role of carbohydrate in physical activity.** *Clin Sports Med* 1999, **18**:469–484.
40. Dumke CL, McBride JM, Nieman DC, Gowin WD, Utter AC, McAnulty SR: **Effect of duration and exogenous carbohydrate on gross efficiency during cycling.** *J Strength Cond Res* 2007, **21**:1214–1219.
41. Hawley JA, Burke LM, Phillips SM, Spriet LL: **Nutritional modulation of training-induced skeletal muscle adaptations.** *J Appl Physiol* 2011, **110**:834–845.
42. Burke ER: *Optimal Muscle Performance and Recovery.* New York: Avery; 2003:91–99.
43. Valko M, Leibfritz D, Moncol J, Cronin MT, Mazur M, Telser J: **Free radicals and antioxidants in normal physiological functions and human disease.** *Int J Biochem Cell Biol* 2007, **39**:44–84.
44. Guzik TJ, Korbut R, Adamek-Guzik T: **Nitric oxide and superoxide in inflammation and immune regulation.** *J Physiol Pharmacol* 2003, **54**:469–487.
45. Illario M, Monaco S, Cavallo AL, Esposito I, Formisano P, D'Andrea L, Cipolletta E, Trimarco B, Fenzi G, Rossi G, Vitale M: **Calcium-calmodulin-dependent kinase II (CaMKII) mediates insulin-stimulated proliferation and glucose uptake.** *Cell Signal* 2005, **21**:786–792.
46. Khan AH, Pessin JE: **Insulin regulation of glucose uptake: a complex interplay of intracellular signalling pathways.** *Diabetologia* 2002, **45**:1475–1483.
47. Wien M, Bleich D, Raghuwanshi M, Gould-Forgerite S, Gomes J, Monahan-Couch L, Oda K: **Almond consumption and cardiovascular risk factors in adults with prediabetes.** *J Am Coll Nutr* 2010, **29**:189–197.
48. Cohen AE, Johnston CS: **Almond ingestion at mealtime reduces postprandial glycemia and chronic ingestion reduces hemoglobin A(1c) in individuals with well-controlled type 2 diabetes mellitus.** *Metabolism* 2011, **60**:1312–1317.
49. Li N, Jia X, Chen CY, Blumberg JB, Song Y, Zhang W, Zhang X, Ma G, Chen J: **Almond consumption reduces oxidative DNA damage and lipid peroxidation in male smokers.** *J Nutr* 2007, **137**:2717–2722.

Relationships between body image, nutritional supplement use, and attitudes towards doping in sport among adolescent boys: implications for prevention programs

Zali Yager[1*] and Jennifer A O'Dea[2]

Abstract

Background: Reports of high levels of use of protein powders and nutritional supplements among young men is a concern because these substances may act as a gateway for the use of drugs and illegal substances to enhance appearance or sports performance. The aim of this study was to investigate the relationship between body dissatisfaction, weight change behaviors, supplement use, and attitudes towards doping in sport among an adolescent male sample.

Methods: Participants were 1148 male adolescents (age range 11-21 years) in Australia who completed a self-report questionnaire that measured weight change behaviors, supplement use, body dissatisfaction (Male Body Attitudes Scale; MBAS) and attitudes towards doping in sport (Performance Enhancing Attitudes Survey; PEAS).

Results: There was a positive correlation between MBAS total and PEAS scores ($r = .19$, $p < .001$), indicating that the young men who were more dissatisfied with their bodies were more likely to support the use of doping in sport. Young men who were currently attempting weight loss or weight gain, and those currently consuming energy drinks ($\eta p^2 = .01$, $p < .01$) and vitamin/mineral supplements ($\eta p^2 = .01$, $p < .01$) were also significantly more supportive of doping in sport. However, those involved in weight lifting, and using protein powders were not ($p > .05$).

Conclusions: These findings suggest that body dissatisfaction, weight change behaviors, and supplement use are related to more lenient attitudes towards doping in sport among adolescent boys. Future research might examine whether combining educational content for the prevention of body dissatisfaction and the use of drugs in sport may have a greater preventive impact than current programs aimed at young men.

Keywords: Body image, Performance-enhancing drugs, Image-enhancing drugs, Nutritional supplements, Doping, Male adolescent

Background

The most recent decade of research has revealed that body image is an issue for young men [1,2]. Around two-thirds of adolescent boys are dissatisfied with their bodies, and this is equally split between those who desire weight loss and those who want to gain muscle [3-6]. The most recent prevalence study, conducted in Greece, indicated that the levels of body dissatisfaction were similar for adolescent boys and girls [1]. An early Australian study reported that 59.4% of adolescent boys were 'currently trying to build up their body' and 74% believed that they should 'develop their muscles' [7]. Interviews with adolescent boys revealed that half wanted to change their body weight, and the majority of participants thought that body size, shape and muscularity was important [8]. Body dissatisfaction is known to lead to the adoption of deleterious weight change strategies such as excessive exercise, and the use of supplements, some of which may be drugs and/or substances that are banned in sports competitions [9]. Cross-sectional and longitudinal research has confirmed that body dissatisfaction and drive for muscularity predict the consumption of nutritional

* Correspondence: zali.yager@vu.edu.au
[1]College of Education, Victoria University, Melbourne, Australia
Full list of author information is available at the end of the article

supplements such as protein powders, as well as anabolic steroids [10-12].

The consumption of these substances is a concern due to the immediate harms of use, but also the potential that they will eventually act as a gateway to more serious substances and illegal drug use. Gateway theory proposes that adolescents who use legal substances such as alcohol and cigarettes are more likely to progress to using more and more serious, illegal drugs, in a predictable pattern [13]. There is some recent evidence to suggest that the same progression also occurs for performance and image enhancing supplements, in that the use of protein powders and supplements predicts the use of anabolic steroids [14,15]. In a study of 212 male and female competitive adolescent athletes, those who were taking nutritional supplements were 3.5 times more likely to report doping, and had significantly more positive attitudes towards the use of drugs in sport [14]. Users of anabolic-adrenergic steroids [AAS] have also been found to be more likely to engage in the consumption of alcohol and other drugs [16,17].

Doping, as defined by the World Anti-Doping Agency, is any violation of the rules set out in the Anti-Doping Code, which range from possession, use, and trafficking of illegal substances to engaging in behaviors associated with illegal substances, and refusing, or tampering with sample collection for drug testing (WADA, 2009). These behaviors are also known as the use of performance enhancing drugs, and ergogenic aids. These actions are strongly governed among the athlete community, however there is sound evidence that doping behaviors are becoming more prevalent among the general population [18,19]. Male non-athletes have been found to have the highest usage levels of doping and ergogenic aids, followed by recreational athletes - while elite athletes report the lowest rates of use [20]. Males in the general population report using these substances to gain muscle in order to increase strength, improve their physical performance, and enhance their appearance [18]. In addition, the main reasons given for desired weight gain among male adolescents are to increase physical strength, protect themselves, and improve sports performance [7]. Young men want to succeed in physical endeavors regardless of their level of competition. The difference is that the use of supplements among elite athletes is heavily regulated; however in recreational settings, those who use these supplements are not penalized, and use may therefore occur freely, regardless of the impacts on health [18].

The Internet has increased accessibility to information about, and sales of, weight gain supplements. Young males are aware of the products and substances that are available via the Internet for performance and image enhancement [18]. However, knowledge of negative side effects of supplement use is generally poor, as evidenced by one study, in which none of the adolescents could name any potential risks or negative side effects of the supplements and nutritional products that they were consuming [21]. Research from the USA reported that 14.7% of young males in grades 8–12 stated that they would take a pill or potion that was guaranteed to help them meet their fitness goals, even if it would harm their health and 8.6% indicated that they would do so even if it shortened their life [22]. Nilsson and colleagues (2005) also found that those Swedish young men who had taken steroids were less likely to believe that these drugs were harmful [16]. Laboratory studies have demonstrated that at least one in five protein supplements is contaminated [23], and the American Academy of Pediatrics (2005) reports that the harm of performance and image enhancing drug use by adolescents is relatively unexplored and unknown [24]. Side effects of supplement and doping use in adults have also not been fully explored, but can include psychiatric symptoms, aggression, renal failure, increased blood pressure, cardiovascular disease and death [25].

Previous research has focused on investigating the prevalence of supplement use and the relationship between doping and body dissatisfaction among elite athletes [14,26] and university students [15]. However, no prior studies have explored the relationship between body dissatisfaction, use of weight gain supplements, and attitudes towards performance enhancing drugs in sport among adolescent boys. This research aimed to examine the relationship between body dissatisfaction and attitudes towards drug use in sport in order to inform education and health promotion programs.

We hypothesized that:

- 1) adolescent boys with higher levels of body dissatisfaction will be more likely to report using products and supplements for weight gain;
- 2) adolescents who use nutritional products and are engaged in weight lifting will be more likely to endorse the use of performance enhancing drugs in sport; and that
- 3) adolescent boys with increased body dissatisfaction will have positive attitudes towards drug use in sport.

Methods

Data collection took place as a part of a 12-year cross-sectional follow –up of early work by the second author [7]. Following institutional (University of Sydney) and departmental (NSW Department of Education) ethics approval, schools were recruited through contact with the principal. All males enrolled in school years 7–12 in each of the consenting schools were invited to participate in the study during their regular class time. Boys gave their signed consent to participate in the study, as did their parents. The questionnaire was introduced and explained to the students by the researchers, who supervised the session to ensure that the boys completed their own work in silence. Participant's height and weight were measured and recorded by the researchers using calibrated digital scales and a portable stadiometer. In total, data were collected from 1148 male students in 28 public, private and catholic schools in NSW, Australia.

The questionnaire used in this study was based on the initial instrumentation that was used in the year 2000 [27], with additional items and standardized scales [28,29] added to collect a wider range of data and reflect the changing nature of measurement and methodologies in public health. The questionnaire was not changed significantly enough to warrant pilot testing. Table 1 provides the details of the measures used in this study.

Quantitative data were entered into SPSS and cleaned. Height and weight were used to calculate Body Mass Index [BMI] (weight divided by height squared), and weight status was determined using BMI cutoffs appropriate for each age group [30]. Standardized measures of body image [MBAS] and attitudes towards doping [PEAS] were scored in accordance with the instructions of those who designed the measures and mean scores were generated. Higher scores on these measures indicate higher levels of body dissatisfaction [MBAS], and more lenient attitudes towards doping in sport [PEAS]. Significant Kolmogov-Smirnov statistics indicated that total scores on subscales and final scales for these measures were not normally distributed. Transforming these scores using square root did not restore normality, so non-parametric versions of tests were used wherever possible. ANOVA and t-tests were used to determine the difference between the adolescent boys' use of weight gain strategies, supplements and attitudes towards doping by age. These were checked with Kruskal-Wallace tests, the nonparametric alternative. There is no non-parametric alternative for ANCOVA, which was used to determine the difference in mean scores on MBAS and PEAS scales by other participant characteristics, controlling for age. We used Pearson's correlations to determine the strength and direction of the relationship between MBAS and PEAS scores. Effect sizes (partial eta squared) are also reported. Descriptive statistics were used to determine results for the items using direct questioning. Open-ended written responses were analyzed by determining categories and tallying responses in order to present frequencies of these comments.

Results

Demographics

A total of $N = 1148$ young men completed the survey. Age ranged from 11.08-21.08 years and the mean age was 14.56 [SD = 1.48]. The majority of participants reported their ethnic/cultural background as Caucasian/ Northern European (53.3%, $n = 610$). Other cultural backgrounds included Southern European (25.1%, $n = 287$), South East Asian/Chinese (10%, $n = 114$), Middle Eastern/ Arabic (3.8%, $n = 44$), Aboriginal/ Torres Straight Islander (2.9%, $n = 33$), Polynesian/Maori (2.5%, $n = 29$), Indian or Sri Lankan (1.5%, $n = 17$) and African (1%, $n = 11$). The Socio-Economic Status [SES] of each school was ranked as low/medium/high using the Australian national government school data [31]. Participants were distributed by SES as follows: low SES (37.3%, $n = 428$); middle SES 35.9% ($n = 412$) and high SES 26.8% ($n = 307$).

The majority of participants (68.3%, $n = 784$) were classified as being within the healthy weight range, according to their BMI. A further 19.5% ($n = 224$) of participants were considered to be overweight, 7.7% ($n = 88$) were classified as obese, and 4.5% ($n = 52$) were underweight.

Body image

In response to the direct questions about body image and body dissatisfaction, 77.7% ($n = 883$) of adolescent boys indicated that they would describe their body as 'about right', while 9.8% ($n = 111$) selected 'too thin' and

Table 1 Measures used to assess body image, supplement use, and attitudes towards doping in sport

Variable	Measure
Body image	Direct questioning: (*Do you think you are: Too fat/ just right/ too thin*) and (*"Would you like to be: A little lighter, A lot lighter, The same as it is now, Heavier, A lot heavier"*) [6]
Current attempts to gain or lose weight	Direct questioning *'Are you currently trying to gain weight' (Yes/No)* and *'Are you currently trying to lose weight' (Yes/No)* [6].
Sports participation	Direct questioning about participation in weight lifting asked participants to indicate their levels of sports involvement [*Not involved, Recreational, Serious, Weight lifting or Body building*]
Supplement use	Direct questioning about the use of sports drinks, vitamins and minerals, energy drinks, protein powders, herbal supplements, and creatine in the past two weeks (*yes/no*)
Body dissatisfaction	Male Body Attitudes Scale [MBAS] [28]. Participants responded on a likert-type scale [*Never* = *1*, to *Always* = *6*] includes three subscales of dissatisfaction with height (2 items), fatness (12 items), muscle (14 items), and a total score (24 items). Chronbach's Alpha was .92.
Attitudes towards performance enhancing drugs	Performance Enhancement Attitudes Scale [PEAS] [29]. Participants respond to 17-items on a Likert scale [Strongly disagree = 1, to Strongly agree = 6]. Chronbach's Alpha was .89.

12.5% ($n = 142$) selected 'too fat'. In contrast, for the question about body dissatisfaction, only 35.2% ($n = 400$) of adolescent boys indicated that they would like to be their present weight, with 30.0% ($n = 341$) indicating that they would like to be a little lighter, and 27.6% ($n = 314$) indicated that they wanted to be a little heavier.

Previous research indicates that levels of body image and dissatisfaction vary according to age. We therefore analyzed the differences in MBAS subscale scores according to participants' age category. These data are presented in Table 2.

Total MBAS scores, and dissatisfaction with muscularity increased with age. Males older than 16 years of age were significantly more likely to have higher scores on the muscularity subscale and the total MBAS indicating greater levels of body dissatisfaction. Dissatisfaction with height and fatness were relatively stable across age groups. In contrast, there was no significant difference in mean PEAS scores by age group. The mean (SD) total score on the PEAS was 38.25 [13.93] for the whole cohort.

Body image by use of products

We asked participants whether they had consumed certain nutritional products or supplements in the past 2 weeks. Almost half (49.9%) of the participants had consumed sports drinks such as Gatorade and Powerade, and 37.0% had taken vitamins or minerals. Almost one – third of the boys had consumed 'energy drinks' such as Red Bull, and a quarter had used protein powder such as Sustagen (24.8%). The following table (Table 3) provides the MBAS scores of those who had, or had not recently used these products, after controlling for the effect of age.

Hypothesis one was supported. Adolescent boys who had taken vitamins and minerals, protein powder, sports drinks and energy drinks were significantly more likely to be dissatisfied with their muscularity. Those participants who had used protein powders in the last two weeks had significantly higher scores on all of the MBAS subscales, indicating that they had higher levels of body dissatisfaction. Age was significant in some, but not all, of these analyses, as shown in Table 3.

In the open-ended questions, we asked participants to indicate why they had consumed these products. Most (37.3%, n = 426) indicated that they had used them to improve their sports performance, while only 4.8% (n = 55) indicated that they used them to gain weight. Many young men (38.6%, n = 441) indicated that they had used them for other reasons, which included 'wanting to' or 'liking it', 'needing energy', and consuming them for 'taste'. Others indicated that they consumed them for 'energy, health, to recover from illness', or 'because their doctor told them to'.

Relationship between doping attitudes, body dissatisfaction and weight change behaviours

The following table (Table 4) provides the PEAS scores of men who had, or had not engaged in a range of weight change strategies.

Hypothesis two was partially supported. Adolescent boys who indicated that they were currently trying to lose weight and currently trying to gain weight were significantly more likely to have higher scores on the PEAS, indicating more lenient attitudes towards doping in sport. Participants who indicated that they had taken vitamins and minerals, and consumed energy drinks in the past two weeks were significantly more likely to have higher scores on the PEAS measures, indicating that they were more supportive of doping in sport. However, there was no significant difference in the PEAS scores of young men who had recently used protein powder and sports drinks, or were involved in weight lifting. The effect of age was not significant in any of the ANCOVA analyses.

Relationship between body dissatisfaction and attitudes towards doping in sport

We utilized Pearson's correlations to examine the relationship between participants' body dissatisfaction and

Table 2 Male Body Attitudes Survey [MBAS] scores by age

	12 year olds and under ($n = 176$)	13 year olds ($n = 262$)	14 year olds ($n = 286$)	15 year olds ($n = 215$)	16 year olds and over ($n = 205$)	Total group ($n = 1148$)	ANOVA
	Mean [SD]	Mean [SD]	Mean [SD]	Mean [SD]	Mean [SD]	Mean [SD]	
MBAS height (Score out of 12)	6.25 [3.05]	6.41 [2.83]	6.27 [2.78]	5.91 [2.67]	6.49 [2.78]	6.26 [2.82]	$F(4,1101) = 1.32$
MBAS fat (score out of 48)	19.72 [8.75]	19.34 [8.28]	19.56 [8.31]	19.12 [8.42]	19.18 [8.77]	19.40 [8.45]	$F(5,1002) = 0.64$
MBAS muscle (score out of 60)	25.81 [9.85]	26.72 [9.91]	27.17 [9.70]	28.37 [9.20]	31.30 [10.55]	27.64 [9.91]	$F(4, 993) = 9.79$***
MBAS total score (score out of 144)	62.61 [22.18]	61.52 [20.01]	62.67 [20.50]	64.17 [20.27]	67.06 [21.82]	63.31 [20.84]	$F(4, 888) = 3.79$**

Note: **$p < 0.01$; ***$p < 0.001$.

Table 3 Male Body Attitudes Scale [MBAS] subscale scores of adolescent boys using certain products and supplements in the past two weeks

	Used	Not used	ANCOVA[a]	Effect size	Effect of age
	Mean [*SD*]	Mean [*SD*]		ηp²	
Vitamins and Minerals					
• MBAS height	6.37 [2.85]	6.24 [2.82]	F(1,1100) = 0.60	.001	NS
• MBAS fatness	19.82 [9.01]	19.52 [8.36]	F(1,1001) = 0.41	.000	NS
• MBAS muscularity	31.34 [11.25]	29.92 [10.69]	F(1,992) = 5.37*	.005	***
• MBAS total score	65.12 [22.17]	63.31 [20.34]	F(1,887) = 1.90	.002	***
Protein powder					
• MBAS height	6.68 [2.74]	6.15 [2.85]	F(1,1100) = 6.77*	.006	NS
• MBAS fatness	21.09 [9.20]	19.16 [8.35]	F(1,1001) = 8.63**	.009	NS
• MBAS muscularity	33.41 [10.99]	29.48 [10.72]	F(1,992) = 20.94***	.02	***
• MBAS total score	69.89 [21.85]	62.04 [20.40]	F(1,887) = 20.89***	.02	***
Sports drinks (eg., Gatorade, Powerade)					
• MBAS height	6.32 [2.80]	6.25 [2.86]	F(1,1100) = .18	.000	NS
• MBAS fatness	19.55 [8.51]	19.71 [8.70]	F(1,1001) = .08	.000	NS
• MBAS muscularity	31.79 [10.72]	29.08 [10.94]	F(1,992) = 16.44***	.02	***
• MBAS total score	65.19 [20.59]	62.62 [21.40]	F(1,887) = 3.30	.00	***
Energy drinks (e.g., Red Bull, V, Mother)					
• MBAS height	6.44 [2.66]	6.22 [2.90]	F(1,1100) = 1.28	.00	NS
• MBAS fatness	20.26 [8.92]	19.36 [8.45]	F(1,1001) = 1.39	.00	NS
• MBAS muscularity	33.38 [10.76]	29.16 [10.74]	F(1,992) = 22.07***	.02	***
• MBAS total score	68.06 [20.18]	62.17 [21.16]	F(1,887) = 10.26**	.01	**

Note: $^*p < 0.05$; $^{**}p < 0.01$; $^{***}p < 0.001$ [a]ANCOVA controlled for age in these analyses.

attitudes towards doping in sport. Table 5 presents these data.

There were significant correlations between participants' scores on MBAS subscales. There were also significant, positive relationships between PEAS total scores, total MBAS scores, and MBAS subscales of dissatisfaction with fat and muscularity. This indicates that those participants who had higher levels of body dissatisfaction were more likely to support doping in sport, indicating that hypothesis three was supported. Although these correlations were significant, the strength of the correlation was still small according to Cohen's guidelines [small = .10-.29; medium = .30-.49; large = .50-1.0] [32].

Discussion

This research provides evidence of a significant relationship between body image, use of weight change products, and attitudes towards the use of doping. We found that the adolescent boys who reported using supplements and dietary products such as vitamins and minerals, protein powders,

Table 4 Relationship between doping attitudes [PEAS scores], weight change, weightlifting, and nutritional product use in the past two weeks

	Yes	No	ANCOVA[a]	Effect size
	Mean [*SD*]	Mean [*SD*]		ηp²
Current weight gain	42.95 [15.38]	37.67 [13.93]	F(1,669) = 11.82**	.02
Energy drinks	41.09 [16.03]	37.36 [13.19]	F(1,672) = 9.81**	.01
Vitamins and minerals	40.46 [15.21]	37.47 [13.54]	F(1,672) = 6.87**	.01
Current weight loss	40.81 [13.16]	37.69 [14.41]	F(1,667) = 5.93*	.009
Sports drinks	39.50 [13.86]	37.48 [14.41]	F(1,672) = 3.42	.005
Protein powder	40.33 [15.51]	37.94 [13.75]	F(1,672) = 3.19	.005
Weightlifting	41.09 [17.90]	38.17 [14.76]	F(1,673) = 2.49	.004

Note: $^*p < 0.05$; $^{**}p < 0.01$; [a]ANCOVA controlled for age in these analyses.

Table 5 Pearson's correlations between measures of body dissatisfaction and attitudes towards doping in sport

	MBAS height	MBAS fatness	MBAS muscularity	MBAS total score	PEAS total score
MBAS height	-	.19***	.30***	.42***	.04
MBAS fatness		-	.53***	.84***	.16***
MBAS muscularity			-	.88***	.20***
MBAS total score				-	.19***
PEAS total score					-

***p < .0001 (2-tailed).

sports drinks and energy drinks were more likely to have higher levels of body dissatisfaction. Those participants who had used vitamins and minerals, and energy drinks (but not those who had used sports drinks and protein powders) were also more likely to have more lenient attitudes towards the use of drugs in sport. Furthermore, this research is the first study to report a significant, positive correlation that indicates that adolescent boys who have higher levels of body dissatisfaction are also more likely to be more supportive of the use of drugs in sport.

Our findings reflect those of previous work in this area. Male adolescents who reported using steroids have been found to have poorer body image [33] and to engage in disordered eating behaviors [11]. Recent work also reported significantly more positive attitudes towards doping among older adolescent male competitive athletes who reported using nutritional supplements [14]. Our findings add evidence of positive attitudes towards doping in sport among a universal sample of adolescent males who are attempting weight change, dissatisfied with their body (and in particular, their muscularity) and using products such as vitamins and minerals, and energy drinks.

This relationship has a wide range of implications for education, health promotion and drug prevention programs. School-based programs aiming to reduce body dissatisfaction among adolescent boys have not been widely successful [34]. This may be because the nature of body image prevention programming that focuses on discussions about the influence of peers and the media, and was designed for young girls, is not particularly appealing for adolescent boys. While young girls are primarily interested in becoming thinner for aesthetic reasons [35] males are interested in the functional aspects of their body [36], and state that they take supplements, and engage in weight change behaviors for the purposes of gaining strength and improving sports performance [7]. Therefore, body image prevention programming that focuses on body acceptance ignores one of the primary drivers for men engaging in weight change behaviors.

Similarly, interventions to prevent the use of steroids among adolescents have not targeted body dissatisfaction. Nilsson and colleagues recognized the necessity of targeting appearance in interventions to reduce steroid use, and trialed a program in Sweden, but did not use standardized measures in their evaluation [37].

The Athletes Training and Learning to Avoid Steroids [ATLAS] program [38] represents exemplary practice in the prevention of anabolic steroid use among high school athletes in the USA. This program has undergone two decades of systematic testing with extensive follow-up periods. The most recent trial involved 3207 male adolescent football players in the USA, who participated in a program that included nutrition information, role plays of drug refusal, analysis of media influences, and discussion of alternate strategies to improve performance. This theory-based session was supported by a weights session in the gym each week. Classes were conducted by coaches and trainers, and achieved significant increases in self esteem, knowledge about, attitudes towards, and intentions to use anabolic steroids [38]. Further research could investigate whether there are any long term outcomes from such interventions and whether future drug use attitudes or behaviors are associated with educational initiatives that are delivered consistently from a young age.

It is suggested that programs aiming to prevent the development of body dissatisfaction and the use of performance and image-enhancing drugs could be combined due to the potential to target shared risk factors. It is likeley that content focusing on alternatives to the use of performance and image-enhancing products and doping could make body image programming more relevant for young males. Materials could include information about the potential harmful effects of using protein supplements and other image and performance-enhancing drugs in the same way that we discuss the dangers of dieting for girls. Programs could then provide information about safe and effective ways to achieve increases in strength and sports performance without the use of products and doping. Similarly, the inclusion of evidence-based body image materials, such as media literacy, and cognitive dissonance activities, in doping prevention programs could enhance the impact of these interventions.

One final element of a combined intervention program could revolve around the theme of fair play. Some researchers suggest that doping prevention needs to go beyond health education, to examine the moral and ethical basis for decision making in relation to doping in sport

[39], and report that trials comparing the effects of a decision-making intervention with traditional psycho-educational approaches are underway [39]. WADA's prevention and education program *'Play True Generation'* includes a range of materials aimed at engaging young athletes with the moral issues surrounding doping in sport [40]. The *Play True Challenge*, an online game where players are able to practice making decisions about doping in sport, and see the consequences of these actions, could easily be incorporated into prevention programming, and the high school health and physical education curriculum.

This research offers new insight into the relationships between body image, nutritional product use, and attitudes towards doping in sport. Strengths included the large sample, and the use of standardized measures to assess body image and attitudes towards doping in sport. However, there were also some limitations. Very few adolescent men reported using performance enhancing drugs, and we don't know if this was due to the lack of comfort they felt in reporting this information. In addition, adolescent men might have misinterpreted the meaning of some of the words and concepts in this questionnaire, which might have resulted in inaccurate reporting. We suggest that future research tracks these relationships longitudinally in order to determine whether body dissatisfaction predicts the use of drugs in sport.

Conclusions

This research suggests that there is a relationship between body image, use of supplements, and attitudes towards the use of drugs in sport. These findings suggest that health educators, sports professionals and administrators could take a different preventive approach that combines the prevention of doping with complementary interventions to prevent body dissatisfaction. Universal and targeted prevention that takes this approach for males is likely to improve the physical and psychological health of young boys in the short term, as they are less likely to suffer from body dissatisfaction, and the negative side effects of using supplements and anabolic steroids. Widespread dissemination of this approach to prevention could then have flow-on effects for reducing doping behaviors in competitive sports.

Competing interests

The authors declare that they have no competing interests.

Authors' contributions

J O'D and ZY obtained grant funding for this project. J O'D conducted data collection and instructed research assistants in data entry. ZY prepared data files and conducted data analysis. ZY and J O'D prepared this manuscript for publication. Both authors read and approved the final manuscript.

Acknowledgements

This research was funded by the Australian Government 2010-2011 Australian Anti-doping Research Program [ADRP] as 17-USYD-2010-2011 *Nutritional Supplements and weight gain behaviors in male adolescents from 2000–2010: Implications for anti-doping interventions and school education.* ZY was based at La Trobe University when this grant was awarded, and conducted data analysis while on a Postdoctoral Fellowship funded by the Leverhulme Foundation, to spend one year at the Centre for Appearance Research at the University of the West of England in the UK.

Author details

[1]College of Education, Victoria University, Melbourne, Australia. [2]Faculty of Education and Social Work, University of Sydney, Sydney, Australia.

References

1. Adamidou E, Zisi V, Chasandra M, Chroni S: **Body image in 13–17 years Old adolescents: gender and physical activity effects.** *Inquiries Sport Phys Educ Psychol Rev* 2013, **11**(1):65–75.
2. McCabe MP, Fuller-Tyszkiewicz M, Mellor D, Ricciardelli LA, Skouteris H, Mussap A: **Body satisfaction among adolescents in eight different countries.** *J Health Psychol* 2011, **17**(5):693–701.
3. Furnham A, Calnan A: **Eating disturbance, self-esteem, reasons for exercising and body weight dissatisfaction in adolescent males.** *Eur Eat Disord Rev* 1998, **6**:58–72.
4. O'Dea J, Yager Z: **Body Image and Eating Disorders in Male Adolescents and Young men.** In *New Developments in Eating Disorders Research. edn.* Edited by Swain P. New York: Nova; 2005.
5. McCabe MP, Ricciardelli LA: **Body image dissatisfaction among males accross the lifespan: a review of past literature.** *J Psychosom Res* 2004, **56**:675–685.
6. Finne E, Bucksch J, Lampert T, Kolip P: **Age, puberty, body dissatisfaction, and physical activity decline in adolescents. Results of the German Health Interview and Examination Survey (KiGGS).** *Int J Behav Nutr Phys Act* 2011, **8**:119–133.
7. O'Dea J, Rawstorne P: **Male adolescents identify their weight gain practices, reasons for desired weight gain and sources of weight gain information.** *J Am Diet Assoc* 2001, **11**:105–107.
8. McCabe MP, Ricciardelli LA: **Body image and body change techniques among young adolescent boys.** *Eur Eat Disord Rev* 2001, **9**:335–347.
9. McCabe MP, Ricciardelli LA: **Body image and strategies to lose weight and increase muscle among boys and girls.** *Health Psychol* 2003, **22**(1):39–46.
10. Field AE, Austin B, Carmargo CA, Barr Taylor C, Striegel-Moore R, Loud K, Colditz GA: **Exposure to mass media, body shape concerns, and use of supplements to improve weight and shape among male and female adolescents.** *Pediatrics* 2005, **116**(2):214–220.
11. Irving LM, Wall MM, Neumark Sztainer D, Story M: **Steroid use among adolescents: findings from project EAT.** *J Adolesc Health* 2002, **30**:243–252.
12. van den Berg P, Neumark Sztainer D, Cafri G, Wall M: **Steroid use among adolescents: longitudinal findings from project EAT.** *Pediatrics* 2007, **119**(3):476–477.
13. Kandel D: **Stages in adolescent involvement in drug-use.** *Science* 1975, **190**:912–914.
14. Backhouse S, Whitaker L, Petroczi A: **Gateway to doping? Supplement use in the context of preferred competitive situations, doping attitude, beliefs, and norms.** *Scand J Med Sci Sports* 2013, **23**:244–252.
15. Hildebrandt T, Harty S, Langenbucher JW: **Fitness supplements as a gateway substance for anabolic-androgenic steroid use.** *Psychol Addict Behav* 2012, **26**(4):955–962.
16. Nilsson S, Spak F, Marklund B, Baigi A, Allebeck P: **Attitudes and behaviors with regards to androgenic anabolic steroids among male adolescents in a County of Sweden.** *Subst Use Misuse* 2005, **40**(1):1–12.
17. Dunn M, White V: **The epidemiology of anabolic-androgenic steroid use among Australian secondary school students.** *J Sci Med Sport* 2011, **14**(1):10–14.
18. Lippi G, Franchini M, Guidi GC: **Doping in competition or doping in sport?** *Br Med Bull* 2008, **86**(1):95–107.
19. Baron DA, Martin DM, Abol Magd S: **Doping in sports and its spread to at-risk populations: an international review.** *World Psychiatry* 2007, **6**:118–123.
20. Wanjek B, Rosenthal J, Strauss B, Gabriel HH: **Doping, drugs and drug abuse among adolescents in the state of Thuringia (Germany): prevalence, knowledge and attitudes.** *Int J Sports Med* 2007, **28**:346–353.

21. O'Dea J: **Consumption of nutritional supplements among adolescents: usage and perceived benefits.** *Health Educ Res* 2003, **18**(1):98–107.
22. Hoffman JR, Faigenbaum AD, Ratamess NA, Ross R, Kang J, Tenenbaum G: **Nutritional supplementation and anabolic steroid use in adolescents.** *Med Sci Sports Exerc* 2008, **40**(1):15–24.
23. Baume N, Kamber M, Mangin P, Saugy M: **Research of stimulants and anabolic steroids in dietary supplements.** *Scand J Med Sci Sports* 2004, **16**:41–48.
24. American Academy of Pediatrics: **Use of performance enhancing substances.** *Pediatrics* 2005, **115**:1103–1106.
25. Turillazzi E, Perilli G, Di Paolo M, Riezzo I, Fineschi V: **Side effects of AA abuse: an overview.** *Mini Rev Med Chem* 2011, **11**(5):374–389.
26. Bloodworth AJ, Petrocczi A, Bailey R, McNamee MJ: **Doping and supplementation: the attitudes of talented young athletes.** *Scand J Med Sci Sports* 2012, **22**:293–301.
27. O'Dea J, Rawstorne P: **Consumption of dietary supplements and energy drinks by schoolchildren.** *Med J Aust* 2000, **173**(2):389.
28. Tylka TL, Bergeron D, Schwartz JP: **Development and psychometric evaluation of the male body attitudes scale (MBAS).** *Body Image* 2005, **2**:161–175.
29. Petroczi A, Aidman EV, Nepusz T: *Capturing Doping Attitudes by Self-Report Declarations and Implicit Assessment: A Methodology Study.* Prevention and Policy: Substance Abuse Treatment; 2008:3(9).
30. Cole TJ, Bellizzi MC, Flegal KM, Dietz W: **Establishing a standard definition for child overweight and obesity worldwide: international survey.** *Br Med J* 2000, **320**:1240–1246.
31. **MySchool website.** [http://www.myschool.edu.au/]
32. Pallant J: *SPSS Survival Manual.* Crows Nest: Allen & Unwin; 2007.
33. Smolak L, Murnen SK, Thompson JK: **Sociocultural influences and muscle building in adolescent boys.** *Psychol Men Masculinity* 2005, **6**(4):227–239.
34. Yager Z, Diedrichs PC, Ricciardelli LA, Halliwell E: **What works in secondary schools? A systematic review of classroom-based body image programs.** *Body Image* 2013, **10**:271–281.
35. Tiggemann M, Gardiner M, Slater A: **"I would rather be size 10 than have straight A's": a focus group study of adolescent girls' wish to be thinner.** *J Adolesc* 2000, **23**:645–659.
36. McCabe MP, Ricciardelli LA, Ridge D: **"Who thinks I need a perfect body? Perceptions and internal dialogue among adolescents about their bodies.** *Sex Roles* 2006, **55**:409–419.
37. Nilsson S, Allebeck P, Marklund B, Baigi A, Fridlund B: **Evaluation of a health promotion programme to prevent the misuse of androgenic anabolic steroids among Swedish adolescents.** *Health Promot Int* 2004, **19**(1):61–68.
38. Goldberg L, MacKinnon DP, Elliott DL, Moe EL, Clarke G, Cheong J: **The adolescents training and learning to avoid steroids program.** *Arch Pediatr Adolesc Med* 2000, **154**:322–338.
39. Melzer M, Elbe A, Brand R: **Moral and ethnical decision-making: a chance for doping prevention in sports?** *Nordic J Appl Ethics* 2010, **4**(1):69–85.
40. Cieret L: **The role of anti-doping education in delivering WADA's mission.** *Int J Sport Policy Politics* 2011, **3**(2):271–277.

Supplementation with Silk Amino Acids improves physiological parameters defining stamina in elite fin-swimmers

Igor Z Zubrzycki[1,3*†], Zbigniew Ossowski[1†], Stanislaw Przybylski[1], Magdalena Wiacek[1], Anna Clarke[2] and Bartosz Trabka[1]

Abstract

Background: Previous animal study has shown that supplementation with silk amino acid hydrolysate (SAA) increases stamina in mice. The presented study was the first formal evaluation of the influence of SAA supplementation on parameters defining physiological fitness level in humans.

Methods: It was a randomized controlled trial with a parallel-group design on elite male fin-swimmers. The experimental group was supplemented with 500 mg of SAA per kg of body mass, dissolved in 250 ml of a Carborade Drink®; the control group with Carborade Drink® alone; 3 times a day, 30 minutes prior to the training session.

Results: Changes discerned in the experimental group were more pronounced than those observed in the control group. For example, the change in the serum lactic acid concentration observed in the experimental group was sevenfold less than in the control group [21.8 vs. -3.7 L% for the control and experimental groups, respectively]. An analysis of a lactate profile as a function of a maximal swimming velocity exposed a statistically significant positive shift in the swimming velocity of 0.05 m/s, at the lactate concentration of 4 mmol/L in the experimental group. There was also a positive, although statistically insignificant, increase of 2.6 L% in serum testosterone levels in the experimental group.

Conclusions: This study showed that a 12-day SAA supplementation combined with an extensive and rigorous training schedule was sufficient to increase an aerobic stamina. However, this phenomenon was associated with an augmented level of muscular damage (an increased level of creatine phosphokinase in the experimental group).

Keywords: Silk amino acids, Stamina, Testosterone, Human

Introduction

A shorter running time, a longer jump, or a longer distance run during a specific time, are results of not only a rigorous training regime but also of an increase of understanding of human physiology combined with modern nutritional techniques.

Recently, a hydrolysate of silk amino acids (SAA) from silk of silkworms (*Bombyx mori*) comprising of peptides of a length of 18 to 19 amino acids, has become very popular among people performing leisure and competition sports.

According to a variety of findings employing animal models, SAA exerts a vista of physiological actions including, among others, anti-diabetic [1], anti-oxidant [2], and anti-tumor [3] properties. One study had even shown that SAA may also influence levels of blood triglycerides [4].

Although some study indicated that branched-chain amino acids (BCAA) supplementation (300 mg/kg of body mas/day) may enhance exercise capacity [5] recent studies on an animal model, performed by South Korean scientists, showed that high doses of SAA, i.e., 800 mg/kg of body-mass [6] or 500 mg/kg [7] also enhance stamina.

* Correspondence: igorzubrzycki@yahoo.com
†Equal contributors
[1]Jędrzej Śniadecki Academy of Physical Education and Sport ul, Kazimierza Górskiego 1, Gdańsk 80-336, Poland
[3]School of Health and Applied Sciences, Polytechnic of Namibia, Private Bag 13388, 13 Storch Street, Windhoek, Namibia
Full list of author information is available at the end of the article

The latter also shows a clear augmentation of testosterone production.

Although, as stated above, SAA and BCAA evoke similar physiological response, i.e., enhancement of exercise capacity, the obvious differences in their amino acid compositions – BCAA comprises of Leu, Ile, and Val whereas SAA: Ala, Gly, Ser, Val, and Thr - enforces, most probably, different modes of their metabolic action. It is known that BCAAs are mainly oxidized in skeletal muscle and that exercises promote oxidation of BCAA [8]. The mode of action of SAA is currently not established, although there are some indications that its oxidation will occur mainly in liver and the main amino acid, playing the paramount role in its physiological function, is L-alanine -through its conversion to beta-alanine [9].

Since SAA is already on shelves of many sport nutrition shops, we undertook the task of verifying its stamina-enhancing viability on a human model. The presented study was a randomized controlled trial with a parallel-group design on male competitive fin-swimmers.

Methods

Ethics

All procedures used in this study were in accordance with the ethical standards of the regional medical chamber. A written consent was obtained in writing from participants and/or guardians of participants under the age of 18 years.

Study subjects

We conducted a randomized controlled trial with a parallel-group design of competitive male fin-swimmers. All participants were recruited from the national fin-swimmer team.

Both samples' size was eight (i.e., the control and the experimental sample), and the age means and standard deviations were 17.6 ± 3.78 and 20.71 ± 4.82, respectively.

Training program

The training camp, during which the experiment was performed, was a microcycle lasting 12 days and comprising three training units daily: (1) 7:00–9:30 am swimming, (2) 11:00–1:00 pm walking and/or running, every other day stretching, and (3) 3:00–5:00 pm swimming.

Within this microcycle, each of the competitors performed 30 training units constituting of total 65training hours. Each of the subjects swam, on average, 7 km per day.

Supplementation

All the required supplements were bought directly from a distributor (Fitness Authority®, http://www.fanutrition.pl/en) without an indication of the purpose of the purchase. According to the producer, the supplement contained 85.95 g of SAA (alanine, glycine, serine, valine, and threonine) per 100 g of dry mass. A required daily amount of SAA, comprising total of 500 mg SAA per kg of body mass, was dissolved in 250 ml of a Carborade Drink® containing 6.3 g of carbohydrates, 0.046 g of sodium, 2.4 mg of niacin, 1.8 mg Vitamin E, 0.9 g pantothenic acid, 0.21 g Vitamin B6, and 7.5 µg of Biotin per 750 ml. A respective nutrition, i.e., a mixture of SAA and Carborade Drink®, and Carborade Drink® alone was served through a straw in lidded cups to both the experimental and the control groups three times a day30 minutes before each training session [10]. It has to be stressed that all drinks were prepared by a person who did not have an access to competitors.

During the study, we also monitored the total calories, proteins, carbohydrates, and lipids consumed by the control and the experimental groups, stratified into breakfast, lunch, and supper.

Data acquisition

A fasting blood draw was completed to measure the following parameters: (1) creatine phosphokinase (CPK), (2) aspartate aminotransferase (AS), (3) alanine transaminase (ALT), (4) lactate dehydrogenase (LDH), (5) serum creatinine (SCr), (6) lactic acid (LH), (7) serum glucose (Gluc), (8) total blood protein (TBP), (9) corticosterone (C), (10) testosterone (T), and (11) blood urea nitrogen (BUN). All laboratory analyses were performed using the ARCHITECT ci8200 Integrated System, Abbott Diagnostic.

Lactate profiling protocol

The incremental 7 × 200 m step test was used to provide objective information on the aerobic fitness of a swimmer. All testing was conducted in a 50 m pool. Individualized target times, based on the personal best time for each swimmer, were calculated before each test. The final swim was set to be for maximum effort. The time for each 100 m split and the total 200 m was recorded manually. After completion of each 200 m, heart rate was measured with a Polar Sports Tester PE (Polar Electro Oy, Kempele, Finland) and a 25 mL capillary blood sample was taken from the earlobe or finger tip and analyzed for lactate concentration using the Accusport Blood Lactate Meter (Boehringer Mannheim, Germany). Lactate tolerance was assessed graphically on a plot of swimming velocity (swimming pace, m/s over the distance of 200 m) versus lactate concentration.

Statistical analysis

Changes induced by the training period in experimental and control groups were examined using the Wilcoxon signed-rank test. Differences between the groups were evaluated using the Wilcoxon rank sum test using the P-value of 0.05 as the statistical threshold.

Relative changes induced by the experiment were measured using the "natural" relative difference, employing the natural logarithm, which was denoted as log percent (L%) [11]: L% =100 * ln (after/before).

Results

The basic statistics of the baseline and the experimental period are shown in Table 1.

An analysis of changes induced by SAA supplementation in experimental and control groups revealed the lack of statistically significant changes. However, the majority of changes observed in the experimental group are more pronounced than those observed in the control group.

A statistical comparison of the total calories, proteins, carbohydrates, and lipids consumed during the breakfast, lunch, and supper, revealed the lack of significant differences between the control and experimental group.

A concentration of serum lactic acid in the control group elevated (21.8 L%), and decreased (–3.7 L%) in experiment group.

Corticosterone concentration decreased in the control group (–2.0 %L) while in the experimental group, it increased (10.9 L%). Analogous, although not so pronounced, a decrease of –6.1 L% and an increase of 2.6 L% of testosterone levels in the control and experimental groups was observed. It has to be noted that in the previous study an increase of only 1.3 L% in mean testosterone levels after 44 days of exercise program was observed [7].

An increase of 47.7 L% in the control group versus the lack of any changes in the experimental group was observed for ALT. AST concentration increased in both groups, and an increase in the control group was more pronounced than in the experimental group.

There was also a substantial increase in serum creatine kinase levels in both control and experimental groups.

An analysis of a lactate profile, Figure 1A-B, as a function of a maximal swimming velocity, exposed a statistically significant positive shift of swimming velocity, at the reference of the lactate concentration of 4 mmol/L, between the experimental group and the control group.

Conclusions

A search for novel supplements, other than anabolic steroids, lead to founding of a well-prospering industry, providing amateur and professional sportsmen with a vista of nutrition increasing muscular gain and stamina.

Among them, SAA has become very popular due to their supposed positive influence on physical stamina. Unfortunately, the popularity of this supplement is rendered rather by claims of a manufacturer and not lucid scientific reports on human models. To address this shortcomings we performed this study, which is the first ever attempt to analyze an impact of SAA supplementation on physical stamina in humans.

Taking into account the current literature on translation of drugs dose from animal to human [12], we primarily contemplated the use of ~41 mg of SAA per kg of body mass/day, not 500 mg/kg/day as presented in this study. However, we did not consider SAA as drugs, *per se*, but only as a nutritional supplement. Additionally a limited duration of an experiment i.e., 12-day training regime, and demands of team coaches inclined us to employ a very high dose of SAA. i.e., 500 mg/kg body mass/day.

In this study, performed on a group of competitive male swimmers, we confirmed the earlier finding, that indicated SAA induced increase in physical stamina; *vide* an increase of a maximal swimming velocity at the lactate threshold of 4 mmol/L [13,14] in the experimental group.

Table 1 Differences in physiological parameters at baseline and after 12-days training program in SAA supplemented group and a control group

Variable	Cont (0)	Ex (0)	Cont (12)	Ex (12)	L% Cont	L% Ex
LA	0.82 (0.76,0.9)	1.1 (0.98,1.1)	1.02 (0.92,1.15)	1.06 (0.905,1.2)	21.8	−3.7
G	94 (92,101)	90 (90,93)	80 (74,81)	85 (80,87)	−16.1	−5.7
CPK	195 (168,215)	168 (113,368)	290 (288,297)	413 (331,568.5)	39.7	89.9
LDH	310 (272,314)	298 (266,310)	389 (303,391)	339 (305.5,398.5)	22.7	12.9
AST	18 (17,18)	21 (15,26)	29 (21,29)	27 (25,32.5)	47.7	25.1
TBP	6.7 (6.5,6.9)	6.8 (6.8,7)	6.5 (6.4,6.8)	6.6 (6.5,6.7)	−3.0	−3.0
ALT	17 (15,20)	22 (15,29)	25.5 (22.75,28.75)	22 (20.5,27)	40.6	0
SCr	1.08 (1.01,1.08)	1.19 (1.16,1.27)	0.93 (0.91,0.99)	1.26 (1.165,1.32)	−15.0	5.7
BUN	28 (26,29)	32 (30,32)	24 (24,27)	27 (26,30)	−15.4	−17.0
C	39.7 (30.3,50.3)	52.3 (40.8,53)	38.9 (33.8,39.2)	58.3 (52.2,64.55)	−2.0	10.9
T	23.92 (21.01,28.07)	20.57 (19.43,26.64)	22.51 (21.49,22.8)	21.12 (15.73,24.69)	−6.1	2.6

Ex = experimental group; Cont = control group; LA = Lactic Acid (mmol/L); G = blood glucose (mg/dL); CPK = creatine kinase (U/L); LDH = lactate dehydrogenase (U/L); AST = aspartate aminotransferase (U/L); TBP = Total Blood Protein (g/dL); ALT = alanine transaminase (U/L); SCr = Serum creatinine (mg/dL); BUN = blood urea nitrogen (mg/dL), C = corticosterone (nmol/L); T = Testosterone (nmol/L). The values are presented as a median and an inter-quartile range.

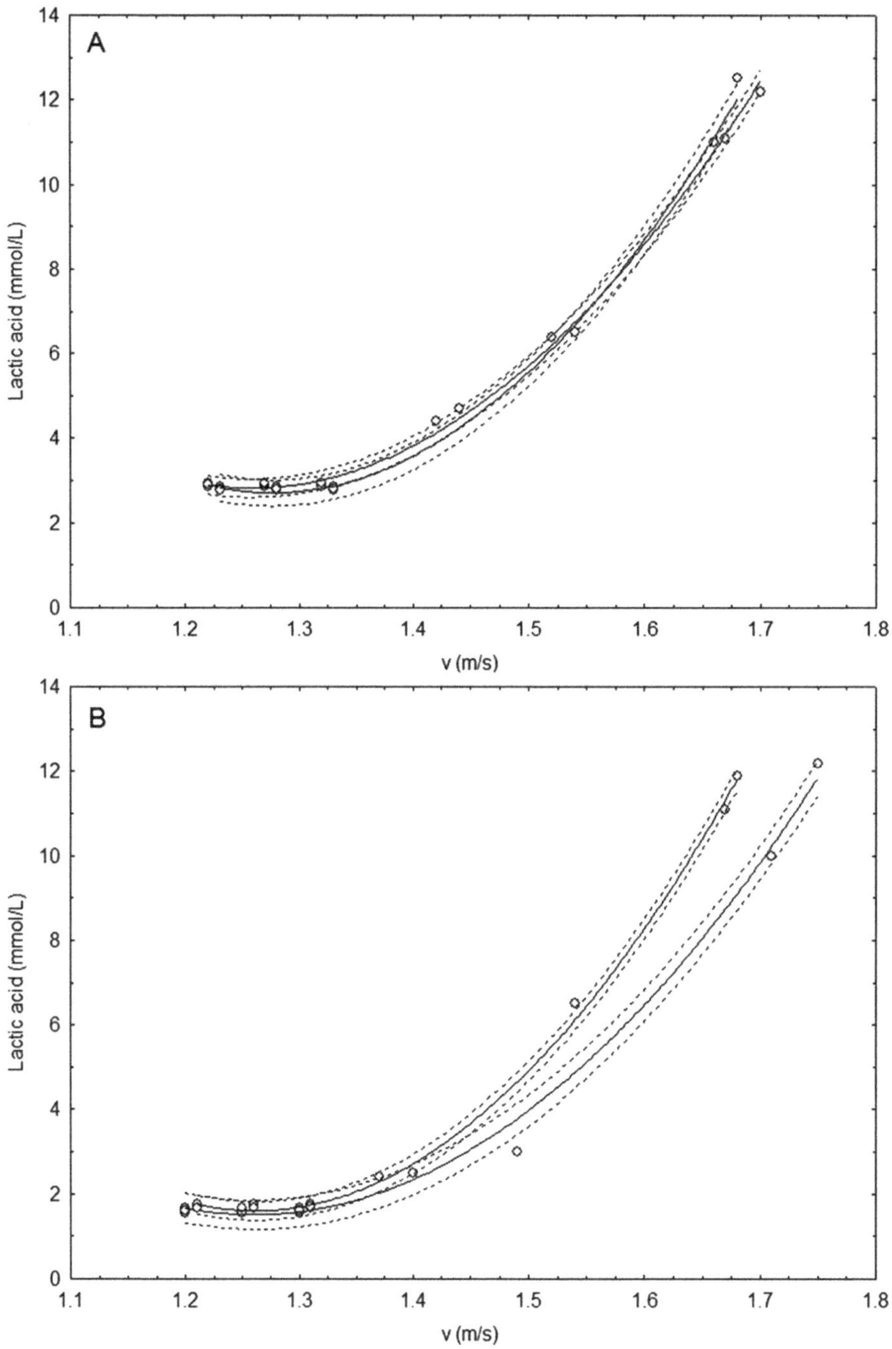

Figure 1 Blood Lactic Acid (mmol/L) concentration in the control group (A) and the experimental group (B) of elite male fin-swimmers athletes before and after 12 days training microcycle.

Although the previous study showed a positive influence of SAA supplementation on the elevation of testosterone levels on the 44th day program, in which mice were administered to a weight-loaded (5% of body weight) forced swimming, this study, i.e., a 12-day SAA supplementation program combined with an extensive and rigorous training program, resulted only in an slight increase in serum testosterone levels.

There is a significant discrepancy regarding the levels of creatine phosphokinase (CPK), a marker of muscle damage, between this report and the previous one [7]. Opposite to the animal model study, this analysis shows a perspicacious increase in CPK levels in the experimental group as compared to the control group; a change of 36.7 L% in the former versus 89.9 L% in the latter. This observation allows us to conjecture that

SAA supplementation induces a higher stamina, but it does not prevent a muscular damage caused by an extensive training effort. However, an analysis of the current literature indicated that supplementation with branched-chain amino acids and taurine-the supplement diminishing or preventing muscular damage caused by extensive training-may be the right direction for utilizing the whole potential of SAA supplementation [15].

The weak point of this study is small sample size, which may be responsible for the lack of more pronounced changes induced by SAA supplementation. Nevertheless, a comparison of our study's data with those performed on an animal model [7], where the study sample comprised only 10 animals, supported the practical viability of the obtained results.

Competing interests

The authors declare that they have no competing interests.

Authors' contributions

Significant manuscript writers: IZZ, SP, and MW. Concept and design: IZZ, ZO, and SP. Data analysis and interpretation: IZZ, AZ, and AC. Statistical expertise: IZZ. All authors read and approved the final manuscript.

Acknowledgements

The authors gratefully acknowledge the financial support of the grant RSA2 053 52.

Author details

[1]Jędrzej Śniadecki Academy of Physical Education and Sport ul, Kazimierza Górskiego 1, Gdańsk 80-336, Poland. [2]Department of Microbiology and Biochemistry, University of Fort Hare, P/B X1314, Alice 5700, South Africa. [3]School of Health and Applied Sciences, Polytechnic of Namibia, Private Bag 13388, 13 Storch Street, Windhoek, Namibia.

References

1. Kim J, Kyung J, Kim D, Choi EK, Bang P, Park D, Kim YB: **Anti-obesity effects of Rapha diet(R) preparation in mice fed a high-fat diet.** *Lab Anim Res* 2012, **28**:265–271.
2. Zhaorigetu S, Yanaka N, Sasaki M, Watanabe H, Kato N: **Silk protein, sericin, suppresses DMBA-TPA-induced mouse skin tumorigenesis by reducing oxidative stress, inflammatory responses and endogenous tumor promoter TNF-alpha.** *Oncol Rep* 2003, **10**:537–543.
3. Moore AJ, Devine DA, Bibby MC: **Preliminary experimental anticancer activity of cecropins.** *Pept Res* 1994, **7**:265–269.
4. Sugiyama K, Mizuno M, Muramatsu K: **Effect of individual amino acids on plasma cholesterol level in rats fed a high cholesterol diet.** *J Nutr Sci Vitaminol* 1986, **32**:623–633.
5. Gualano AB, Bozza T, Lopes De Campos P, Roschel H, Dos Santos Costa A, Luiz Marquezi M, Benatti F, Herbert Lancha Junior A: **Branched-chain amino acids supplementation enhances exercise capacity and lipid oxidation during endurance exercise after muscle glycogen depletion.** *J Sports Med Phys Fitness* 2011, **51**:82–88.
6. Shin S, Park D, Yeon S, Jeon JH, Kim TK, Joo SS, Lim WT, Lee JY, Kim YB: **Stamina-enhancing effects of silk amino acid preparations in mice.** *Lab Anim Res* 2009, **25**:127–134.
7. Shin S, Yeon S, Park D, Oh J, Kang H, Kim S, Joo SS, Lim WT, Lee JY, Choi KC, Kim KY, Kim SU, Kim JC, Kim YB: **Silk amino acids improve physical stamina and male reproductive function of mice.** *Biol Pharm Bull* 2010, **33**:273–278.
8. Rennie MJ: **Influence of exercise on protein and amino acid metabolism.** In *Handbook of Physiology.* Edited by Rowell LB, Shepherd JT. Bethesda, MD: American Physiological Society; 1996:995–1035.
9. Harris RC, Sale C: **Beta-alanine supplementation in high-intensity exercise.** *Med Sport Sci* 2012, **59**:1–17.
10. Tipton KD: **Role of protein and hydrolysates before exercise.** *Int J Sport Nutr Exerc Metab* 2007, **17**(Suppl):S77–86.
11. Tornqvist L, Vartia P, Vartia YO: **How Should Relative Changes Be Measured.** *Am Stat* 1985, **39**:43–46.
12. Reagan-Shaw S, Nihal M, Ahmad N: **Dose translation from animal to human studies revisited.** *FASEB J* 2008, **22**:659–661.
13. Sjodin B, Jacobs I: **Onset of blood lactate accumulation and marathon running performance.** *Int J Sports Med* 1981, **2**:23–26.
14. Tanaka K, Matsuura Y, Kumagai S, Matsuzaka A, Hirakoba K, Asano K: **Relationships of anaerobic threshold and onset of blood lactate accumulation with endurance performance.** *Eur J Appl Physiol Occup Physiol* 1983, **52**:51–56.
15. Ra SG, Miyazaki T, Ishikura K, Nagayama H, Komine S, Nakata Y, Maeda S, Matsuzaki Y, Ohmori H: **Combined effect of branched-chain amino acids and taurine supplementation on delayed onset muscle soreness and muscle damage in high-intensity eccentric exercise.** *J Int Soc Sports Nutr* 2013, **10**:51.

Effect of an herbal/botanical supplement on strength, balance, and muscle function following 12-weeks of resistance training: a placebo controlled study

Jonathan Furlong[1], Corey A Rynders[2], Mark Sutherlin[1], James Patrie[1], Frank I Katch[1], Jay Hertel[1] and Arthur Weltman[1*]

Abstract

Background: StemSport (SS; StemTech International, Inc. San Clemente, CA) contains a proprietary blend of the botanical Aphanizomenon flos-aquae and several herbal antioxidant and anti-inflammatory substances. SS has been purported to accelerate tissue repair and restore muscle function following resistance exercise. Here, we examine the effects of SS supplementation on strength adaptations resulting from a 12-week resistance training program in healthy young adults.

Methods: Twenty-four young adults (16 males, 8 females, mean age = 20.5 ± 1.9 years, mass = 70.9 ± 11.9 kg, stature = 176.6 ± 9.9 cm) completed the twelve week training program. The study design was a double-blind, placebo controlled parallel group trial. Subjects either received placebo or StemSport supplement (SS; mg/day) during the training. 1-RM bench press, 1-RM leg press, vertical jump height, balance (star excursion and center of mass excursion), isokinetic strength (elbow and knee flexion/extension) and perception of recovery were measured at baseline and following the 12-week training intervention.

Results: Resistance training increased 1-RM strength ($p < 0.008$), vertical jump height ($p < 0.03$), and isokinetic strength ($p < 0.05$) in both SS and placebo groups. No significant group-by-time interactions were observed (all p-values >0.10).

Conclusions: These data suggest that compared to placebo, the SS herbal/botanical supplement did not enhance training induced adaptations to strength, balance, and muscle function above strength training alone.

Keywords: Anti-oxidant, Blue-green Algae, Strength exercise

Introduction

Various nutritional supplements have been investigated for accelerating recovery from resistance exercise. For example, carbohydrate ingestion within 1 to 2 hours following a strength training session promotes glycogen re-synthesis and decreases muscle recovery time [1,2]. Protein supplementation stimulates protein synthesis, which may aid recovery, thus leading to enhanced strength gains with resistance training [3,4]. Several herbal supplements with anti-inflammatory and/or anti-oxidant properties also purport to enhance recovery from resistance exercise and enhance strength gains. There is no consensus in the literature concerning how herbal supplements impact the magnitude of their performance enhancing benefits [5].

We recently examined the effects of a dietary supplement containing a blend of herbal antioxidants/anti-inflammatory substances including the fresh water blue-green algae Aphanizomenon flos-aquae (StemSport; SS, StemTech International, Inc. San Clemente, CA) on the severity and time course of delayed onset muscle soreness (DOMS) following an acute bout of eccentric upper arm exercise

* Correspondence: alw2v@virginia.edu
[1]Department of Kinesiology Exercise Physiology Core Laboratory, University of Virginia, 203 Memorial Gymnasium, Charlottesville 22904, Virginia, USA
Full list of author information is available at the end of the article

(Rynders et al., In Review, JISSN). Our study reported that compared to a placebo, SS supplementation had no effect on muscle swelling, isometric strength, muscle pain and tenderness, and swelling measured 24 h, 48 h, 72 h, and 168 h (1 week) post-eccentric exercise (Rynders et al., In Review, JISSN). There were no differences in measures of recovery between SS and placebo after DOMS, yet it is possible that the amount of muscle tissue damage elicited by the DOMS protocol negated any beneficial effect of the supplement. If a less dramatic overload were utilized such as strength training, it is possible that the supplement would enhance recovery and performance in a subsequent exercise bout. This would lead to a greater cumulative training response (i.e. greater total work completed per workout session).

The present placebo-controlled study examined the effects of SS supplementation on the adaptations to strength, balance, and muscle function resulting from a 12-week resistance training program in healthy young adults. We hypothesized that SS would accelerate the rate of recovery from each training session, allowing for a greater overload in subsequent training sessions, and an enhanced training response.

Methods

Experimental approach to the problem

This was a randomized, double blind, placebo-controlled, parallel group design to examine the effects of SS supplementation on training adaptations following a 12-week resistance training program. Independent variables included supplement type (SS or Placebo) and measurement period (pre- and post- 12 weeks of training). Dependent variables included 1 repetition max (1RM) bench press and 1RM leg press; vertical jump; Star Excursion Balance Test (SEBT); static balance; isokinetic concentric phase peak torque and average power for knee and elbow flexion and extension; and perception of recovery.

Subjects

The University Institutional Review Board approved the study and subjects provided written informed consent prior to participation. Thirty-five healthy male and female undergraduate and graduate students were recruited from Lifetime Physical Activity weight training classes. All participants were enrolled in an introductory strength training class, and had not participated in more than 1 day/week of resistance training prior to study enrollment. All participants provided written informed consent and a medical history. Exclusion criteria included a history of kidney disease, vascular disease, circulatory insufficiencies, or cancer; use of anti-depressants, warfarin, or any protein/muscle building supplements; and self-reported pregnancy, drug use, or smoking.

SS and placebo supplementation

Subjects were randomly assigned to receive either the active SS supplement (n = 17) or placebo (n = 18). The SS ingredient list is presented in Table 1. Subjects were instructed to adhere to the following dosing schedule according to manufacturer recommendations: 1000 mg of Aphanizomenon flos-aquae extract 3 times per day (breakfast, lunch, and dinner) and 1575 mg of a proprietary herbal/botanical blend twice per day (breakfast and dinner). One additional dose of Aphanizomenon flos-aquae and one additional dose of the herbal/botanical blend were consumed before exercise and after exercise according to manufacture instructions. The placebo consisted of 1000 mg of encapsulated corn starch. Subjects were required to maintain a pill diary throughout the study and were instructed to forfeit any capsules not ingested during the study period. Supplements (SS and placebo) were dispensed weekly by the University investigational pharmacy. Over-the-counter analgesic and anti-inflammatory medications (i.e. Tylenol, Advil, Ibuprofen, Motrin, Bextra, Celebrex, etc.) were prohibited during the supplementation period.

Two subjects in the SS condition and one subject in the placebo condition withdrew prior to beginning the training intervention. Five subjects in the SS condition withdrew during the 12-week training program due to injury (n = 1), an adverse reaction to the supplement (n = 1), or time constraints (n = 3). Three subjects in the placebo condition withdrew during the intervention period due to time constraints. Twenty-four subjects completed the twelve week training program.

Procedures

Pre- and post-training (12-weeks) testing consisted of 1RM bench press and 1RM leg press, isokinetic concentric phase peak torque and average power for knee and elbow flexion and extension, vertical jump, SEBT, and static balance.

1RM testing

The IRM testing was performed using the National Strength and Conditioning Association ARM protocol [6]. Participants began the 1RM bench press and leg press assessments by warming up with repetitions on the bench press using a 20.5-kg bar and free weights or dumbbells, and multiple repetitions on the leg press machine (Hammer Strength, Schiller Park, IL, USA). The goal was to build to the 1RM load within five attempts. For the bench press, a successful repetition was scored if the weight was lowered to the chest and raised to full arm extension without losing foot, hip, back, or shoulder contact with the bench of the floor without help provided by a spotter. For the leg press, a successful repetition was scored if the weight was lowered such that

Table 1 StemSport ingredient list and purported benefits

Ingredient	Amount per serving	Purported benefit
1. Aphanizomenon flos-aquae extract	1000mg	Increase the number of circulating stem cells
2. Proprietary herbal/botanical blend	1575mg	
Cats claw	–	Antioxidant
Mangosteen	–	Antioxidant
Rehmannia	–	Anti-inflammatory
Berry extracts	–	Antioxidant
Nattokinase	–	Anti-inflammatory/fibrinolytic
Serrapeptase	–	Anti-inflammatory/fibrinolytic
Curcumin	–	Antioxidant/anti-inflammatory

knees created a 90° angle and raised to full leg extension without the subject losing back or shoulder contact with the machine and without spotter assistance. Two failed attempts at a given weight or voluntary termination ended each test.

Isokinetic strength testing

A Biodex System 3 multijoint dynamometer (Shirley, NY) was used for isokinetic assessments. Subjects performed 3 sets of 5 repetitions for each of the isokinetic exercises, with a 90 second rest interval between sets. Verbal encouragement was given for each repetition, and testing was preceded with 10 to 15 practice repetitions to familiarize the subject with the isokinetic device. Each exercise was conducted at angular velocities of 60 and 180 degrees per second (deg.sec^{-1}). The isokinetic knee flexion and extension tests were performed from full knee extension (0°) to 90° flexion. The isokinetic elbow flexion and extension tests were performed from full elbow extension (0°) to 160° of flexion. For all tests, the seatback angle was set at 85°, and the hips were in 90° of flexion. For each motion, peak torque and average power from the 3 sets were averaged prior to statistical analysis.

Static balance

Static balance was assessed using an Accusway force plate (AMTI, Watertown, MA). Subjects performed three trials of single-limb stance on their dominant leg with eyes open and then closed for 15 seconds. Subjects were instructed to stand as still as possible with arms folded across their chest, holding the opposite limb at 45° of knee flexion and 30° of hip flexion. If the subject touched down with the non-stance limb, made contact with the stance limb, or was unable to maintain standing posture during the 15-s trial, the trial was terminated and repeated. Traditional center of pressure (COP) based measures of the mean velocity of COP excursions (total COP excursion length in centimeters divided by the 10-s trial time) and the area of the 95% confidence ellipse of COP excursions were calculated via computer software. The mean of each measure for the three eyes-open and eyes-closed trials were used for statistical analysis.

Star excursion balance test

A trained investigator assessed anterior, posteromedial, and posterolateral components of the SEBT. Subjects maintained single limb stance on the test limb while reaching as far as possible with the contralateral limb in the given direction, made a light touch on the line at their point of maximum reach, and returned to the starting position. Subjects performed 5 practice trials in each reach direction. The reach distances of three trials in each direction were recorded. Trials were repeated if a subject bore excessive weight on the reaching limb, removed the stance foot from the starting position, or lost balance. Reach distance were normalized to subject leg length in accordance to previously established methods using the mean of three trials for each direction [7].

Vertical jump

Subjects performed three trials of a counter-movement vertical jump using a Vertec Jump Measurement System (JumpUSA, Sunnyvale, CA). The highest attained value was used for analysis.

Training intervention

Subjects performed supervised resistance training exercises 3 times a week for 12 weeks. Subjects performed 2 sets of 10 exercises using a combination of free weights and machines. When the subject was able to successfully perform 2 sets of 10 repetitions for an exercise, the weight was increased by 5 to 25 pounds at the next training session. The same 10 exercises were performed each training session for 4 weeks, and then modified (i.e. lunges to split squats). Examples of exercises performed included bench press, leg press, seated row, overhead press, knee extension, hamstring curls, biceps curls, triceps extensions, and lunges, calf raises. Subjects maintained training logs, recording the weights and repetitions completed during each session.

Perception of recovery

Perception of recovery from strength training was assessed using a visual analog scale throughout the 12-week training program at weeks 1, 2, 4, 6, 8, 10, and 12. Subjects were instructed to make a vertical line at the position on the scale to represent their perceived recovery from training, with the left end point labeled "completely recovered" and the right end point "not recovered at all". The measured distance of the marked position from the left end point served as the score and normalized by dividing by total scale length.

Statistical analyses

Data were evaluated for normality using the Shapiro-Wilk Test. Variables that violated the normality assumption (Shapiro-Wilk p-value < 0.05) were log transformed for analysis. Separate 2-factor analysis of variance (ANOVA) with repeated measures over time was executed with the treatment group (SS or placebo) as the independent variable. For the performance tests, the dependent variable was the respective outcome measure. Thus, there was 1 between-subjects factor (treatment group) and 1 within-subjects factor (time). For the perception of recovery scale, the dependent variable was the normalized score calculated as the distance from the left endpoint divided by the total length of the scale. Scales were completed at weeks 1, 2, 4, 6, 8, 10, and 12; thus there was 1 between-subjects factor (treatment group) and 7 within-subjects factors. Where significant main effects were observed, post hoc procedures were applied to examine within group changes over time. Independent samples t-tests were conducted to examine differences in adherence to training, where the number of training sessions completed served as the dependent variable, and the percentage of pills consumed to verify adherence to supplement consumption. The threshold for significance for all tests was set at $p < 0.05$.

Results

Adherence to training

There was no significant difference between groups in adherence to training assessed by the number of training sessions completed (30.3 sessions for placebo, 29.8 sessions for SS, p = 0.50), or adherence to treatment assessed by the percentage of pills ingested (92.9% of pills in placebo, 86.3% of pills in SS, p = 0.10).

1-RM

Figures 1 and 2 display the individual and mean responses for 1 RM bench press and 1 RM leg press. Bench press 1-RM increased by 18.2% (p = 0.008) with placebo and 11.0% with S (p = 0.001). Leg press 1-RM increased by 48.6% with placebo (p < 0.001) and by 50.5% with SS (p < 0.001). There were no differences in 1-RM improvement (bench press and leg press) between placebo and SS conditions (p-values > 0.28). Similar results were observed when the values were normalized for body weight (data shown in Table 2).

Vertical jump

Vertical jump increased 7.2% with placebo (p = 0.03) and 10.6% with SS (p =0.001), but no significant between group differences (p > 0.05; Table 2).

Isokinetic strength

Seven of the eight measures of isokinetic elbow flexion and extension strength improved in the placebo condition compared to only two measures in the SS condition (Table 2). No pre- to post-training improvements were observed for the measures of isokinetic knee extension and flexion strength. Post hoc tests revealed decrements in of two of the eight measures of isokinetic knee extension and flexion strength in the SS condition (Table 2).

Balance

There was a significant improvement in eyes open center of pressure excursion velocity in the placebo condition,

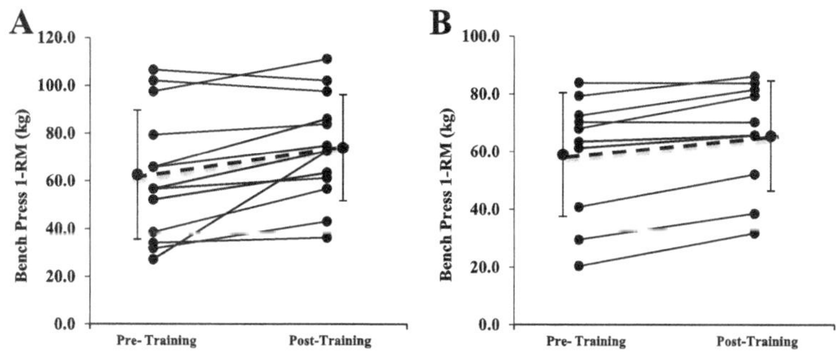

Figure 1 Individual and mean (±SD) responses in 1RM bench press in (A) placebo condition and (B) StemSport condition. Both groups improved significantly with training ($p < 0.01$), but there was no time × condition interaction ($p = 0.28$).

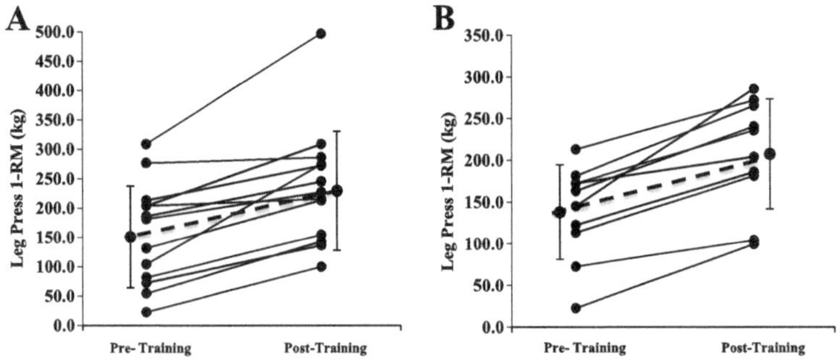

Figure 2 Individual and mean (±SD) responses in 1RM leg press in (A) placebo condition and (B) StemSport condition. Both groups improved significantly with training ($p < 0.001$), but there was no time × condition interaction ($p = 0.652$).

Table 2 Mean (±SD) pre- and post-training values for strength, balance, and muscle function in the StemSport and Placebo supplementation conditions

Parameter	StemSport		Placebo	
	Pre	Post	Pre	Post
Weight Adjusted Bench Press 1RM*	0.84 ± 0.25	0.95 ± 0.21	0.83 ± 0.28	1.00 ± 0.22
Weight Adjusted Leg Press 1RM*	1.95 ± 0.71	2.97 ± 0.64	2.10 ± 0.85	3.19 ± 0.94
Height Adjusted Vertical Jump*	0.28 ± 0.06	0.31 ± 0.06	0.27 ± 0.04	0.29 ± 0.04
Anterior SEBT	0.70 ± 0.11	0.70 ± 0.07	0.71 ± 0.07	0.68 ± 0.06
Posteromedial SEBT	0.91 ± 0.10	0.91 ± 0.60	0.92 ± 0.10	0.89 ± 0.09
Posterolateral SEBT	0.86 ± 0.11	0.86 ± 0.08	0.87 ± 0.11	0.85 ± 0.10
Eyes Open COM Excursion Velocity (cm/sec)†	4.49 ± 1.36	4.50 ± 1.16	4.71 ± 2.02	4.05 ± 1.15
Eyes Open COM Excursion Area	6.24 ± 2.76	5.79 ± 2.82	6.24 ± 2.49	5.40 ± 2.09
Eyes Closed COM Excursion Velocity (cm/sec)	9.91 ± 2.90	10.30 ± 3.33	11.33 ± 3.94	9.65 ± 2.98
Eyes Closed COM Excursion Area	32.85 ± 13.6	33.87 ± 12.0	32.54 ± 11.1	28.28 ± 8.36
Elbow Extension Peak Torque @ 60°/sec (N · m)*	46.79 ± 14.2	51.64 ± 13.4	47.09 ± 14.4	60.04 ± 22.6
Elbow Extension Peak Torque @ 180°/sec (N · m)†	30.65 ± 11.7	32.48 ± 9.7	30.65 ± 8.5	34.55 ± 10.5
Elbow Extension Average Power @ 60°/sec (W)†	42.82 ± 15.0	46.58 ± 13.1	42.43 ± 13.2	54.68 ± 20.3
Elbow Extension Average Power @ 180°/sec (W)†	60.11 ± 28.3	63.58 ± 25.1	54.80 ± 22.0	68.03 ± 25.0
Elbow Flexion Peak Torque @ 60°/sec (N · m)†	47.94 ± 11.7	54.98 ± 14.4	48.26 ± 15.6	58.05 ± 20.1
Elbow Flexion Peak Torque @ 180°/sec (N · m)†	32.99 ± 8.8	38.35 ± 11.6	32.90 ± 11.9	39.05 ± 13.08
Elbow Flexion Average Power @ 60°/sec (W)*	44.1 ± 11.0	51.05 ± 14.4	45.21 ± 16.1	56.40 ± 20.3
Elbow Flexion Average Power @ 180°/sec (W)	58.27 ± 19.7	68.42 ± 27.0	58.97 ± 31.0	70.09 ± 28.2
Knee Extension Peak Torque @ 60°/sec (N · m)Ω	122.5 ± 32.8	103.9 ± 25.6	124.99 ± 42.8	114.7 ± 44.6
Knee Extension Peak Torque @ 180°/sec (N · m)	83.7 ± 21.5	76.2 ± 15.9	85.24 ± 28.7	74.82 ± 29.5
Knee Extension Average Power @ 60°/sec (W)Ω	101.5 ± 27.6	88.9 ± 21.5	106.4 ± 37.3	94.8 ± 25.5
Knee Extension Average Power @ 180°/sec (W)	157.6 ± 46.9	146.0 ± 30.3	173.3 ± 76.7	139.7 ± 59.9
Knee Flexion Peak Torque @ 60°/sec (N · m)	64.4 ± 14.6	57.1 ± 12.9	71.0 ± 24.8	64.8 ± 24.9
Knee Flexion Peak Torque @ 180°/sec (N · m)	48.2 ± 14.2	45.4 ± 9.4	56.1 ± 21.6	46.9 ± 21.4
Knee Flexion Average Power @ 60°/sec (W)	56.4 ± 15.8	53.5 ± 14.6	66.5 ± 26.6	61.1 ± 24.8
Knee Flexion Average Power @ 180°/sec (W)	89.5 ± 36.7	84.2 ± 23.6	114.0 ± 54.1	92.5 ± 46.2

1-RM = 1 repetition maximum; SEBT = Star excursion balance test; COM = center of mass; kg = kilogram; cm = centimeter; sec = second; N·m = newton meter; W = watts. * = Significant improvement with training in both conditions, $p < 0.05$. † = Significant improvement with training in placebo condition only, $p < 0.05$. Ω = Significant decrement with training in StemSport condition only, $p < 0.05$.

but not for SS. SEBT measures did not improve post-training in either group (Table 2).

Perception of recovery

Figure 3 presents the weekly mean perception of recovery scores for both conditions. There was a significant effect of time ($p < 0.001$) on perception of recovery, but no significant group by time interaction effects ($p = 0.895$).

Discussion

The manufacturer of StemSport claims that usage of the product "may play a role in assisting the recovery process, thus reducing recovery time and enhancing the natural renewal process" [8]. In the present study we tested the manufacturer claims and hypothesized that if the claims were accurate, enhanced recovery in response to the SS supplement would improve performance in subsequent exercise training sessions and ultimately lead to a greater cumulative training response and larger strength gains. The major findings of the present study were, 1) twelve weeks of strength training significantly improved muscle strength and function and 2) compared to placebo, SS supplementation did not provide additional benefits above resistance training alone.

To our knowledge, this is the first study evaluating the effects of SS supplementation in response to strength training. SS is a commercially available nutritional product purported to increase the concentration of circulating stem cells, while reducing oxidative and inflammatory stress, which the manufacturers suggest will accelerate post-exercise recovery.

The primary ingredient of SS includes an extract of the fresh water botanical Aphanizomenon flos-aquae (AFA). AFA has been shown to increase the circulating

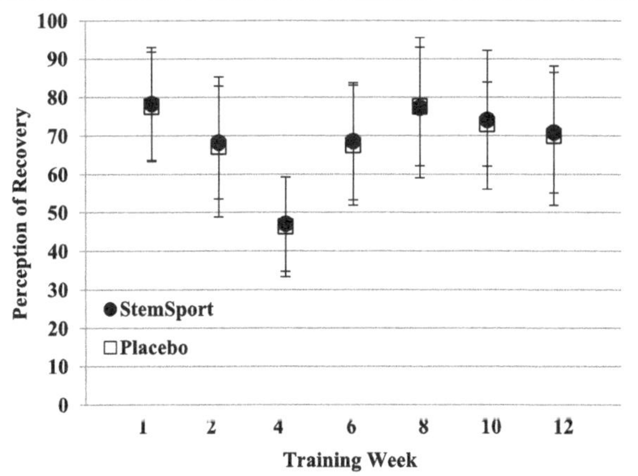

Figure 3 Weekly mean (±SD) perception of recovery. ANOVA analyses revealed a significant main effect of time on perception of recovery ($p < 0.001$), but no significant condition × time interaction ($p = 0.895$).

level of human bone marrow derived stem cells [9,10]. Significant increases in the proliferation of cultures of both human bone marrow cells and human CD34+ stem cell with in vitro administration of AFA [10]. In a randomized double-blind placebo controlled crossover study, oral administration of SS produced transient but significant increase in in vivo concentrations of circulating human CD34+ stem cells, peaking at 25% above baseline at 1 hour, with only minor fluctuations observed in a placebo condition [9].

No measurements of circulating stem cells were collected in the present study, and thus the role of stem cells in the recovery from resistance training remains unclear. The supplementation protocol failed to produce any improvements with resistance training above placebo, suggesting that the transient increase in circulating stem cells associated with SS was inadequate to promote accelerated post-exercise recovery. It seems reasonable to suggest that elevated levels of stem cells above those typically observed do not play a significant role in recovery from resistance training, or that SS did not adequately increase circulating stem cells.

StemSport contains a proprietary blend of natural and herbal substances, with documented anti-oxidative, anti-inflammatory, and fibrinolytic effects [11-16]. The manufacturers suggest that by reducing oxidative and inflammatory stress while promoting fibrinolysis, SS would promote post-exercise recovery. No previous studies have examined the effects of SS on recovery from resistance training, although the effects of other anti-oxidative and anti-inflammatory substances on resistance training have been explored [17-19]. Bloomer et al. [17] examined the effects of anti-oxidant supplementation on the acute recovery from an eccentric strength training bout. Anti-oxidant supplementation was not associated with any improvements in blood markers of recovery, perceived muscle soreness, or muscle function. Similarly, no difference in strength gains with vitamin C and E supplementation compared to placebo occurred after 6 months of resistance training in older adults [18]. Antioxidant supplementation may blunt the endogenous adaptive responses to exercise-induced oxidative stress such as improvements in insulin sensitivity [20]. The consequences of these effects remain unclear, yet the limited data demonstrate no ergogenic benefit associated with antioxidant supplementation during resistance training [17,18].

Studies regarding the effects of anti-inflammatory agents on resistance training have focused primarily on non-steroidal anti-inflammatories (NSAIDs). A counterbalanced, double-blind, randomized trial, comparing adaptations to resistance training with ibuprofen supplementation versus placebo in young adults showed no changes in strength or hypertrophy, or in reported muscle soreness [20]. Animal models suggest that the inhibition of cyclo-oxygenase activity associated with NSAIDs may impair muscle hypertrophy [21]. Although not measured in the present study, a prior study using the DOMS model indicated that SS had no effect on circulating inflammatory markers (IL-6 and hsCRP) (Rynders et al. JSCR, In Review).

A secondary finding of the present study demonstrated significant reductions in the perception of recovery from resistance training after 4 weeks, with only minor fluctuations observed throughout the rest of the 12 week period. Flann et al. [22] reported a similar observation in untrained subjects during an eccentric strength training protocol, although their program intentionally utilized a three week "ramp up" period.

An unexpected finding of the present study was the lack of significant change in most measures of knee isokinetic strength or power, with both groups demonstrating small decrements after the training period (Table 2). This observation is inconsistent (and surprising) with previous results from our lab [23] given the significant improvement in leg press performance (Figure 2). All testing for each subject was performed in the same order during the pre- and post-testing sessions, yet the possibility exists that subjects may have been more fatigued from the 1RM testing during the post-training tests compared to the pre-testing sessions.

Limitations to the present study include: 1) diet, which can have a significant impact on the adaptations to resistance training [1,3,24], was not controlled, and 2) by design, the sample consisted of untrained subjects, and whether SS would be more effective at producing strength gains in more advanced athletes, where tissue repair may be more important compared to novice exercisers, cannot be addressed.

Conclusions

Many supplements are commercially available; however, these supplements are often promoted without conclusive research demonstrating their efficacy. A recent review of 250 commercially advertised supplements found only 6 had been examined in randomized, placebo-controlled studies greater than 3 weeks in duration [5]. The present study demonstrates that twelve weeks of resistance training results in significant improvements in most measures of muscle strength and function, but the SS supplement did not lead to improvements above strength training alone.

Competing interests

The authors declare that they have no competing interests. The study was funded in part by an urestricted gift to the Curry School of Education Exercise Physiology Fund from StemTech International, Inc. San Clemente, CA. FIK, JH, and AW served as scientific consultants for StemTech International.

Author's contributions

JF, CAR, JH, FIK, and AW contributed to the study conception and design, JF and MS acquired the data, JP performed the data analysis, JF, CAR, JH, FIK, and AW interpreted the data; All authors were involved in drafting the manuscript and have given final approval of the published version.

Acknowlegments

The authors would like to thank the subjects for their participation in the study.

Author details

[1]Department of Kinesiology Exercise Physiology Core Laboratory, University of Virginia, 203 Memorial Gymnasium, Charlottesville 22904, Virginia, USA. [2]Department of Human Movement Sciences, Human Performance Laboratory, Old Dominion University, Norfolk, VA, USA.

References

1. Roy BD, Tarnopolsky MA: **Influence of differing macronutrient intakes on muscle glycogen resynthesis after resistance exercise.** *J Appl Physiol* 1998, **84**:890–6.
2. Conley MS, Stone MH: **Carbohydrate ingestion/supplementation or resistance exercise and training.** *Sports Med* 1996, **21**:7–17.
3. Biolo G, Tipton KD, Klein S, Wolfe RR: **An abundant supply of amino acids enhances the metabolic effect of exercise on muscle protein.** *Am J Physiol* 1997, **273**:E122–9.
4. Tipton KD, Ferrando AA, Phillips SM, Doyle D Jr, Wolfe RR: **Postexercise net protein synthesis in human muscle from orally administered amino acids.** *Am J Physiol* 1999, **276**:E628–34.
5. Nissen SL, Sharp RL: **Effect of dietary supplements on lean mass and strength gains with resistance exercise: a meta-analysis.** *J Appl Physiol* 2003, **94**:651–9.
6. Baechle TRE, Roger W: *Essentials of Strength Training and Conditioning.* Champaign, IL: Human Kinetics; 2001.
7. Gribble PA, Hertel J, Plisky P: **Using the star excursion balance test to assess dynamic postural-control deficits and outcomes in lower extremity injury: a literature and systematic review.** *J Athl Train* 2012, **47**:339–57.
8. **StemSport® Advanced Formula.** http://www.stemtechbiz.com/StemSport.aspx.
9. Jensen GS, Hart AN, Zaske LA, Drapeau C, Gupta N, Schaeffer DJ, Cruickshank JA: **Mobilization of human CD34+ CD133+ and CD34+ CD133(−) stem cells in vivo by consumption of an extract from Aphanizomenon flos-aquae–related to modulation of CXCR4 expression by an L-selectin ligand?** *Cardiovasc Revasc Med* 2007, **8**:189–202.
10. Shytle DR, Tan J, Ehrhart J, Smith AJ, Sanberg CD, Sanberg PR, Anderson J, Bickford PC: **Effects of blue-green algae extracts on the proliferation of human adult stem cells in vitro: a preliminary study.** *Med Sci Monit* 2010, **16**:BR1–5.
11. Weecharangsan W, Opanasopit P, Sukma M, Ngawhirunpat T, Sotanaphun U, Siripong P: **Antioxidative and neuroprotective activities of extracts from the fruit hull of mangosteen (Garcinia mangostana Linn.).** *Med Princ Pract* 2006, **15**:281–7.
12. Pilarski R, Zielinski H, Ciesiolka D, Gulewicz K: **Antioxidant activity of ethanolic and aqueous extracts of Uncaria tomentosa (Willd.) DC.** *J Ethnopharmacol* 2006, **104**:18–23.
13. Purdy Lloyd KL, Wasmund W, Smith L, Raven PB: **Clinical Effects of a Dietary Antioxidant Silicate Supplement, Microhydrin((R)), on Cardiovascular Responses to Exercise.** *J Med Food* 2001, **4**:151–9.
14. Goud VK, Polasa K, Krishnaswamy K: **Effect of turmeric on xenobiotic metabolising enzymes.** *Plant Foods Hum Nutr* 1993, **44**:87–92.
15. Sumi H, Hamada H, Nakanishi K, Hiratani H: **Enhancement of the fibrinolytic activity in plasma by oral administration of nattokinase.** *Acta Haematol* 1990, **84**:139–43.
16. Kubo M, Asano T, Shiomoto H, Matsuda H: **Studies on rehmanniae radix. I. Effect of 50% ethanolic extract from steamed and dried rehmanniae radix on hemorheology in arthritic and thrombosic rats.** *Biol Pharm Bull* 1994, **17**:1282–6.
17. Bloomer RJ, Falvo MJ, Schilling BK, Smith WA: **Prior exercise and antioxidant supplementation: effect on oxidative stress and muscle injury.** *J Int Soc Sports Nutr* 2007, **4**:9.
18. Bobeuf F, Labonte M, Dionne IJ, Khalil A: **Combined effect of antioxidant supplementation and resistance training on oxidative stress markers, muscle and body composition in an elderly population.** *J Nutr Health Aging* 2011, **15**:883–9.

19. Ristow M, Zarse K, Oberbach A, Kloting N, Birringer M, Kiehntopf M, Stumvoll M, Kahn CR, Bluher M: **Antioxidants prevent health-promoting effects of physical exercise in humans.** *Proc Natl Acad Sci U S A* 2009, **106:**8665–70.
20. Krentz JR, Quest B, Farthing JP, Quest DW, Chilibeck PD: **The effects of ibuprofen on muscle hypertrophy, strength, and soreness during resistance training.** *Appl Physiol Nutr Metab* 2008, **33:**470–5.
21. Novak ML, Billich W, Smith SM, Sukhija KB, McLoughlin TJ, Hornberger TA, Koh TJ: **COX-2 inhibitor reduces skeletal muscle hypertrophy in mice.** *Am J Physiol Regul Integr Comp Physiol* 2009, **296:**R1132–9.
22. Flann KL, LaStayo PC, McClain DA, Hazel M, Lindstedt SL: **Muscle damage and muscle remodeling: no pain, no gain?** *J Exp Biol* 2011, **214:**674–9.
23. Dannelly BD, Otey SC, Croy T, Harrison B, Rynders CA, Hertel JN, Weltman A: **The effectiveness of traditional and sling exercise strength training in women.** *J Strength Cond Res* 2011, **25:**464–71.
24. Willoughby DS, Stout JR, Wilborn CD: **Effects of resistance training and protein plus amino acid supplementation on muscle anabolism, mass, and strength.** *Amino Acids* 2007, **32:**467–77.

Effects of dietary intervention in young female athletes with menstrual disorders

Karolina Łagowska[1*], Karina Kapczuk[2], Zbigniew Friebe[2] and Joanna Bajerska[1]

Abstract

Background: The aim of this study was to evaluate the influence of three months of dietary intervention on menstrual cycle in young female athletes with amenorrhea or oligomenorrhea.

Methods: From forty-five female professional athletes with menstrual irregularity that were recruited thirty-one, aged 18.1 ± 2.6 years, completed the study and were analyzed. Hyperprolactinemia, thyroid dysfunction, primary ovarian failure and hyperandrogenism were excluded in the study participants. The subjects started intense training at the age of 11.2 ± 3.5 years and continued during next 6.8 ± 3.3 years. Energy and nutrients intake, total energy expenditure, energy availability and body composition as well as serum concentrations of LH, FSH, 17 – beta estradiol and progesterone were measured at the beginning of the study and after three months of individualized dietary intervention.

Results: Following three months of dietary intervention significant increase in energy intake (2354 ± 539 vs. 258 8 ± 557 kcal, P = 0.004) and energy availability (28.3 ± 9.2 vs. 35.8 ± 12.3 kcal/kg FFM/d, P = 0.011) was observed as well as improved energy balance (−288 ± 477 vs. -51 ± 224 kcal/d, P = 0.002). Though no changes in BMI and body composition were noted but significant rise in LH concentrations (3.04 ± 1.63 vs. 4.59 ± 2.53 mIU/ml, P = 0.009) and LH to FSH ratio (0.84 ± 0.56 vs. 0.96 ± 0.52, P = 0.001) was achieved, but no restoration of menstrual cyclicity.

Conclusions: This report provides further support for the role of energy deficiency in menstrual disorders among young female athletes and the benefits of an adequate energy intake and energy availability on hormones concentration. Continuation controlled dietary intervention is needed to assess the extent to which long-term improvement in the nutritional status results in improvements in the hormonal status of female athletes, to an extent that would allow the regulation of the menstrual cyclity.

Keywords: Menstrual disorders, Female athletes, Nutritional habits, Nutritional status, Dietary intervention

Background

The strenuous physical activity of professional female athletes may generate serious health problems. It is estimated that between 16% [1] and 61% [2] of female athletes suffer from hypothalamic-pituitary menstrual disorders. In studies conducted by Torstveit et al. [3], the frequency of menstrual disorders among elite female athletes was 34.5% in aesthetic disciplines, 30.9% in endurance disciplines, 23.5% in weight class disciplines, 17.6% in anti-gravitation disciplines, 16.7% in technical disciplines, 12.8% in ball game and power sport disciplines.

There is a disturbingly low level of knowledge among athletes of different sports disciplines regarding the potential health effects of untreated menstrual dysfunctions [4,5]. Young female athletes are not aware that a long-term negative energy balance, inadequate nutrient intake, and endocrine disorders including the hypothalamic-pituitary-ovarian axis are particularly dangerous in the period of achieving the peak bone mass and may contribute to metabolism disturbances in the skeletal tissue. Christo et al. [6] observed significantly lower BMD values in the lumbar spine area among athletes with menstrual disorders compared to physically active and sedentary women with regular cycles. The study of Nicolas et al. [7] also showed a significantly decreased bone density in athletes suffering from amenorrhea and oligomenorrhea. Studies of athletes with amenorrhea and low bone mass showed that even after the restoration of the menstrual

* Correspondence: karolina@up.poznan.pl
[1]Department of Human Nutrition and Hygiene, Dietetic Division, University of Life Sciences, Wojska Polskiego 28 str, 60-637 Poznań, Poland
Full list of author information is available at the end of the article

cycle bone density remained significantly lower compared to the average value of women in this age group [8].

Prolonged menstrual disorders have a negative effect on the quality and quantity of plasma lipoproteins, which favors the formation of atherosclerotic lesions. Significant differences in blood lipid parameters in athletes with amenorrhea compared to athletes with regular cycles have been demonstrated. In the study of Rickenlund et al. [9], athletes with amenorrhea had significantly higher levels of total and LDL cholesterol compared to athletes and sedentary women with regular cycles. The increase in the LDL levels was higher when the energy intake was lower.

Taking the afore mentioned into account it seemed appropriate to take steps to limit menstrual disorders and their negative health effects. The aim of this study was to evaluate nonpharmacological dietary interventions on the menstrual disorders in young female athletes.

Methods

Subjects

Forty-five well-trained female athletes with menstrual disorders (18 rowers, 12 synchronized swimmers, 15 triathlonists) were recruited from different sports club in Poznań and thirty-one the (12 rowers, 8 synchronized swimmers, 11 triathlonists) completed a dietary intervention. The inclusion criteria were: menstrual irregularity within the last 12 months, a training period of at least 3 years, training session > 4/wk, no serious medical conditions, no use of hormonal contraception or other medications that might interfere with the hypothalamic-pituitary-gonadal axis activity, no clinical diagnosis of an eating disorders, no history of clinical diagnosis of primary ovarian failure, hyperprolactinemia, thyroid dysfunction or polycystic ovary syndrome and non-smoking.

Written informed consent was obtained from all participants or their parents. The study was approved by the Poznań Medical Ethics Committee (no. 334/09).

Menstrual status

Each subject completed a two-part medical questionnaire. The questions in the first part concerned menstruation: age at menarche, length of the menstrual cycles, and history of amenorrhea. Part two of the questionnaire referred to sport activities: age at the beginning of training, training period, number of training session per week, hours of training per day and per week.

Primary amenorrhea was diagnosed where there was no onset of menses by 15 years, while secondary amenorrhea was diagnosed when there was no menstruation for 6 months, or for more than three times the previous cycle length. Menstrual periods that occurred more than 35 days apart were described as oligomenorrhea [10].

Each participant underwent gynecological evaluation, including a pelvic ultrasound and measurements of luteinizing hormone (LH), follicle-stimulating hormone (FSH), progesterone (P), 17β - estradiol (E2), prolactin (PRL), thyroid-stimulating hormone (TSH), testosterone (T), and sex-hormone-binding globulin (SHBG) serum concentration, in order to exclude independent causes of amenorrhea or oligomenorrhea (such as pregnancy, primary ovarian failure, hyperprolactinemia, thyroid dysfunction or polycystic ovary syndrome).

Blood sampling and biochemical analyses

Blood samples were obtained in menstruating subjects between days 2 and 5 of the menstrual cycle (in the early follicular phase), and at random in amenorrheic subjects. Blood serum samples were taken between 6.00 a.m. and 9.00 a.m. following overnight fasting and rest. The athletes were instructed to abstain from caffeine and alcohol for 24 hours prior to the blood sampling, and to refrain from performing strenuous exercise on the day of sampling.

Serum concentration of LH, FSH, E2, P, PRL, TSH, T and SHBG were measured by immunochemical methods using Chemiluminescent Microparticle Immunoassay (CMIA) and Microparticle Chemiflex Flexible interassay protocols and making use of diagnostic sets and an ARCHITECT automatic analyzer. Serum leptin levels were estimated using Human Leptin Elisa by LINCO Research. All hormones concentrations were determined in duplicated.

Body weight and body composition measurements

In order to evaluate the nutritional status, the anthropometrical indices, height and weight were measured using an anthropometer coupled with a WPT 200 OC verified medical scale (Rad Wag). BMI (kg/m^2) was calculated as body weight divided by squared body height. The participants were dressed in minimal clothing during the measurements, which were rounded to the nearest 0.5 kg and 0.5 cm. Analysis of body fat mass (FM) and fat-free mass (FFM) was performed in the morning, following an overnight fast, with the subjects lying in a supine position, using BODYSTAT 1500, as described by Heyward et al. [11].

Resting metabolic rate

Resting metabolic rate (RMR) was assessed by using a portable indirect calorimeter for 25 minutes (Cosmed K4b2, Cosmed, Italy). A face mask (Hans Rudolph, Kansas City, MO) covering the mouth and nose of the participant was attached to a bidirectional digital turbine flow-meter and fastened to the participant using a mesh hairnet with Velcro straps. To guarantee an airtight seal, a disposable gel seal (Hans Rudolph) was positioned between the inside of the face mask and the skin. The Cosmed K4b2 system was calibrated prior to each individual test according to the manufacturer's guidelines. Breath-by-breath O_2 and CO_2 gas exchange was measured and recorded in the portable unit's computer system. On completion of each test, the stored data were transferred to the Cosmed K4b2 version 6 computer software running on a Windows-based laptop computer. The data were then averaged over 15 second intervals and transferred to Microsoft *Excel* for further analysis. The morning before the RMR measurements, the Cosmed K4b2 was calibrated with a calibration gas mixture (16% O_2, 5% CO_2). The test was carried out with the participant in a comfortable supine position, at an environmental temperature of 21–22°C. All measurements were done in the morning (between 6 and 9 a.m.) following a 12 hours fast and a minimum of 8 hours of rest. The results of the RMR measurement were compared with the RMR predicted by the Harris-Benedict equation [12] and the RMR(kcal)/FFM(kg) ratio was also calculated.

Energy and nutrients intake

Seven consecutive days of dietary records were obtained under the supervision of dieticians. Athletes had a regularly contact with registered dietitian who teach them and control how to record nutrition intake. All meals (including recipes and item masses), nonmeal foods, beverages, and fluids were recorded in diary form using a photographic album of dishes [13]. The daily diets were analyzed for their energy and nutrient levels (fat, protein, carbohydrate, dietary fiber, calcium, phosphorus, iron, zinc, vitamins A, D, B_1, B_2, niacin, B_6, B_{12}, foliate and vitamin C) using the *Dietician* computer software package, based on Polish food composition tables [14].

Total energy expenditure and energy availability

For three days, each subject wore a heart-rate monitor (HR) (Polar Sport Tester, RS 400, Finland) in order to estimate total energy expenditure (TEE). For each subject, the relationship between HR and VO_2 was established. The measurements were carried out two or more hours after meals, and after the subject had rested for 30 min, having arriving at the laboratory. Results were obtained by simultaneous measurement of HR and VO_2 for the following activities carried out sequentially: lying in supine position, sitting quietly, standing quietly, and continuous graded exercise on a cycle ergometer. After preliminary editing to remove spurious HR data, the total energy expenditure (TEE) was calculated using the Flex-HR method. This method requires the definition of a Flex-HR for each subject, above which there is a good correlation between HR and VO_2, but below which there is a poor correspondence between the two parameters. The Flex-HR was calculated as the mean of the highest HR for the resting activities (supine, sitting, and standing) and the lowest HR of the exercise activities. At the end of the measurement session, researchers transferred the minute-by-minute records of the last twenty-four hours from the instrument to a database. The 24-hour energy balance (EB) was calculated as the difference between the means of seven consecutive days of 24-hour energy intake and the TEE as a mean of three days. Energy availability (EA) was calculated by subtracting exercise energy expenditure (EEE) from total daily energy intake, and was adjusted for FFM kg [10].

Dietary intervention

After the evaluation of the participants' nutritional habits, all the athletes were informed of nutritional mistakes in their current diets and of the health consequences of dietary deficiencies. Then, for each of the athletes who was qualified for the study, we prepared an individual diet. Taking into account the energy balance and the energy availability, the daily energy intake was established on the basis of the individual energy requirements that had been calculated from the total energy expenditure data. The recommended level of protein intake was determined in accordance with the recommendations of the American College of Sports Medicine Female Athlete Triad Position Stand (ACSM) [10], taking into account 1.2–1.6 g/kg/d intake. Using the recommendations of Manore et al. [15], the level of carbohydrates and fat intake was determined, which respectively amounted to a minimum of 55% and 25–30% of the daily energy intake. Adequate daily intake for calcium (1000–1300 mg) and vitamin D (400–800 IU or 10–20 mcg) are based on the ACSM recommendations [10] and on Roupas et al. [16] results. The recommended intake of other vitamins and minerals was established in accordance with Recommended Dietary Allowances for girls aged 16–18 years and women over 19 years, in accordance with Jarosz et al. [17]. The dietary counseling session also included a discussion of special foods for athletes, sports drink, supplements, shopping tips, low-fat and low-calorie food, food preparation, dining out, iron, calcium and vitamins in foods. After first and second month of non-pharmacological dietary intervention, the control of following dietary intervention was conducted. Repeated assessments of total energy expenditure (1 day), energy availability, and the energy and nutrient values of daily diets (3 days) were conducted (data no shown). After third month the control of effect of dietary intervention was conducted and then total energy expenditure (3 day), energy availability, and the energy and nutrient values of the athlete's daily diets (7 days), LH, FSH, E2 and P serum concentration were repeated by measured. To statistical analysis we used data from baseline of study and after third month of dietary intervention.

Statistical analysis

Means and standard deviations of the quantitative variables were calculated. The normality of the distribution was checked. Comparisons between data from before and after the three-month dietary intervention were carried out using a *t*-test for independent variables. Connection between energy availability and LH serum concentration were carried out using Spearman's rank correlation test. Statistical analyses were performed using *Statistica 8.0* software (StatSoft, 2008). *P*-values of less than 0.05 were considered statistically significant.

Results

Subjects characteristic

The subject characteristics of those who completed the study are shown in Table 1. The investigated group consisted of 5 secondary amenorrheic subjects and 26 oligomenorrheic subjects.

Effect of the three month dietary intervention on energy and nutrient intake, energy balance, energy availability, body weight and composition

Three months of dietary intervention changed dietary habits of the study participants and resulted in significant increase in energy (mean 234 kcal/d), protein (mean 8 g/d), carbohydrate (mean 66.8 g/d), calcium (mean 146 mg/d), magnesium (mean 56 mg/d), vitamin A (450.9 mg/d), vitamin D (0.67 μg/d), foliate (mean 49.2 μg/d) and vitamin C (mean 53.9 mg/d) intake. EB and EA before and after the intervention differed significantly in the study subjects (mean 237 kcal/d and 7.5 kcal/kg FFM/d, respectively) (Table 2). No significant changes in athletes' body weight, BMI and body composition were observed (Table 3).

Table 1 Baseline group characteristics M ± SD

Parameters	
Baseline characteristics	
Age (years)	18.1 ± 2.6
Age at menarche (years)	13.0 ± 1.2
Age at the beginning of training (years)	11.2 ± 3.5
Training period (years)	6.8 ± 3.3
Number of training session per week (n/d)	5.2 ± 1.1
Hours of training per day (hours/d)	4.0 ± 1.8
Hours of training per week (hours/wk)	19.5 ± 7.2
RMR predicted (kcal/d)	1458 ± 56
RMR measured (kcal/d)	1354 ± 151
RMR measured/predicted*100%	92.8 ± 10.0
RMR measured - RMR predicted (kcal/d)	−105.0 ± 146.8
RMR/FFM (kcal/kg)	29.0 ± 3.6
Hormonal parameters	
TSH (0.35 –4.94 μlU/ml)	1.74 ± 0.80 (0.74–4.37)
PRL (5.18–26.53 ng/ml)	13.0 ± 9.33 (3.71–50.5)
T (10–90 ng/dl)	37.28 ± 21.85 (0.15–90.0)
SHBG (19.80–155.20 nmol/l)	62.79 ± 41.91 (18.0–228.4)

Effect of the dietary intervention on hormonal parameters

Neither resumption of regular cycles nor improved menstrual frequency was observed in the athletes during the three month study period. However, LH concentration and LH to FSH ratio measured after three months of dietary intervention were found to be significantly higher than at the beginning of the study (mean 41.55 mlU/ml and 0.12, respectively) (Table 4). A positive correlation between EA and LH concentrations appeared ($r = 0.26$, $p < 0.05$) (Figure 1).

Discussion

In the study, the authors evaluated the effects of an individualized dietary intervention, providing an appropriate energy availability, energy balance and an adequate intake

Table 2 Energy and nutrients intake at 0 and 3 measurement points M ± SD

Energy and nutrients	0	3	p - value*
Energy (kcal)	2354 ± 539	2588 ± 557	0.041
Fat (g)	92.2 ± 27.5	84.2 ± 20.4	NS
Protein (g)	75.6 ± 14.8	85.5 ± 15.6	0.004
Carbohydrate (g)	305.4 ± 78.0	372.2 ± 86.3	< 0.001
Dietary fiber (g)	20.1 ± 5.4	21.8 ± 5.4	NS
Calcium (mg)	816.3 ± 232.9	963.3 ± 247.5	0.021
Phosphors (mg)	1442.0 ± 333.9	1435.1 ± 327.4	NS
Iron (mg)	11.1 ± 3.3	12.8 ± 3.2	NS
Zink (μg)	10.1 ± 3.0	11.0 ± 2.8	NS
Magnesium (mg)	275.0 ± 87.5	331.0 ± 80.7	0.003
Vitamin A (μg)	645.0 ± 234.8	1095.9 ± 655.1	< 0.001
Vitamin D (μg)	2.34 ± 1.42	3.01 ± 1.04	0.040
Vitamin E (mg)	9.9 ± 4.2	9.2 ± 3.4	NS
Vitamin B_1 (mg)	1.20 ± 0.56	1.28 ± 0.26	NS
Vitamin B_2 (mg)	1.80 ± 0.50	1.72 ± 0.46	NS
Niacin (mg)	12.5 ± 4.1	14.3 ± 3.3	NS
Vitamin B_6 (mg)	1.80 ± 0.73	2.35 ± 0.94	NS
Foliate (μg)	202.7 ± 62.4	251.9 ± 64.4	0.014
Vitamin B_{12} (μg)	2.78 ± 1.47	3.67 ± 1.61	NS
Vitamin C (mg)	57.3 ± 24.4	111.2 ± 87.1	0.002
TEE (kcal/d)	2642 ± 348	2638 ± 421	NS
EB (kcal/d)	−288 ± 477	−51 ± 224	0.002
EEE (kcal/d)	959 ± 174	905 ± 337	NS
EA (kcal/kg FFM/d)	28.3 ± 9.2	35.8 ± 12.3	0.011

*Before dietary intervention (0) vs. after three months of dietary intervention (3).

Table 3 Anthropometric characteristics at 0 and 3 measurement points M ± SD

Parameters	0	3	p-value*
Body weight (kg)	59.3 ± 5.3	59.6 ± 5.3	NS
BMI (kg/m^2)	20.6 ± 1.4	20.7 ± 1.5	NS
FM (%)	20.6 ± 3.7	21.0 ± 3.5	NS
FM (kg)	12.2 ± 2.4	12.5 ± 2.4	NS
FFM (%)	79.4 ± 3.7	79.0 ± 3.7	NS
FFM (kg)	47.1 ± 4.9	47.1 ± 4.8	NS

*Before nutritional intervention (0) vs. after three months of dietary intervention (3).

of minerals and vitamins, on the menstrual cycle in young female athletes. Diets were planned by taking into account the total energy expenditure, nutritional status and the current training period, in the expectation that an individualized diet will help reduce menstrual dysfunctions without decreasing total energy expenditure, training volume and hormonal treatment. The planned study period was nine months, and this study provides results obtained after three months, the first time-point, post dietary intervention start.

Our results concerning energy and nutritional intakes, obtained before the start of the above dietary intervention, were similar to our previous results [18,19]. They were also comparable to those obtained by Hoch et al. [20] and Tomten et al. [21], who also demonstrated energy availability below 30 kcal/kg FFM/d and the negative energy balance in athletes with menstrual disorders. Furthermore, similarly to studies by Manore [15], Hoogenboom et al. [22], Quah et al. [23] and Woolf et al. [24], daily diet values for most vitamins and minerals indicated deficiency. In study participants, the RMR was also lower than predicted value. Similar to Mallinson et al. [25], we used the RMR/pRMR ratio as an indicator of the energy status. The mean value obtained was 92.8 with a range of 72.3-115.5, potentially indicating an energy deficiency in some part of study participants. Many authors suggested that body weight alone and an intensive physical activity are not sufficient to explain the onset of menstrual disorders. Many authors suggested that menstrual dysfunction occurs only in the presence of relative caloric deficiency resulting from inadequate nutritional intake precluding achievement of an appropriate energy expenditure. They also emphasize that this is the most important factor leading to menstrual disorders development [26,27]. Results presented by Thong et al. [28] also showed an inadequate energy intake among female athletes with amenorrhea. In the above case, energy availability was 50% lower compared to regularly menstruating women (16 kcal/d/kg FFM and 30 kcal/d/kg FFM, respectively). The relationship between normal functioning of the hypothalamic-pituitary-gonadal axis and an adequate energy intake under stress conditions was already demonstrated in the 1980s. In runners, Kaiserrauer et al. [29] showed that the use of a low-energy diet, deficient in protein and fat, may contribute to progesterone serum concentrations reduction and the luteal phase shortening.

Table 4 Hormones concentration at 0 and 3 measurement points M ± SD

Hormones (reference values)	0	3	p-value*
LH (2.39–6.60 mIU/ml)	3.04 ± 1.63	4.59 ± 2.53	0.009
FSH (3.03–8.08 mIU/ml)	5.01 ± 2.37	5.00 ± 2.08	NS
E2 (21–251 pg/ml)	36.5 ± 19.4	36.2 ± 15.3	NS
P (0.1–0.3 ng/ml)	0.54 ± 0.99	0.68 ± 0.77	NS
LH/FSH (0.6–1.2)	0.84 ± 0.56	0.96 ± 0.52	0.001

*Before dietary intervention (0) vs. after three months of dietary intervention (3).

In athletes' daily diets, the control of energy and nutrients intakes demonstrate significant variations. Despite mean values showing an increase of energy and nutrients intakes, the high standard deviation indicates that not all study participants adhere to the recommendations of the dietary intervention. This situation demonstrates how difficult it is to implement an individual diet in this group of subjects. During a three-month dietary intervention, an increased energy availability in the studied athletes was also observed. Additionally, the energy availability exceeded the critical value of 30 kcal/kg FFM/d. In athletes with menstrual disorders, Nattiv et al. [10] and DeSouza [30] indicated that an increased energy availability, and not the weight gain alone, is the most important factor for the restoration of regular menstrual cycles. Loucks et al. [25] suggested that the pulsatile secretion of LH depends on the energy availability, which was also confirmed in this paper (significant relationship between LH and energy availability). In our paper, despite the fact that after three months of non-pharmacological dietary intervention none of study participants resumed regular menses, LH and LH to FSH ratio significantly increased. In athletes, a surprising lack of changes in body weight and composition may be explained by decreased level of baseline RMR resulting from the long-term energy deficiency. Moreover, diets implemented during this dietary intervention aimed to provide a sustainable energy balance, thus to avoid weight gain.

In athletes, Dueck et al. [31] and Kopp-Woodroffe et al. [32] demonstrated the resumption of menses after approximately 6 months and 9–12 weeks, respectively. Competitive athletes should be counseled that the sustained resumption of menses (involving regular menstrual cycles of 36 days or less occurring in the period of 3 months or more) may take longer than one year, when non-pharmacological therapy is implemented. Arends et al. [33] found that the restoration of regular menstrual

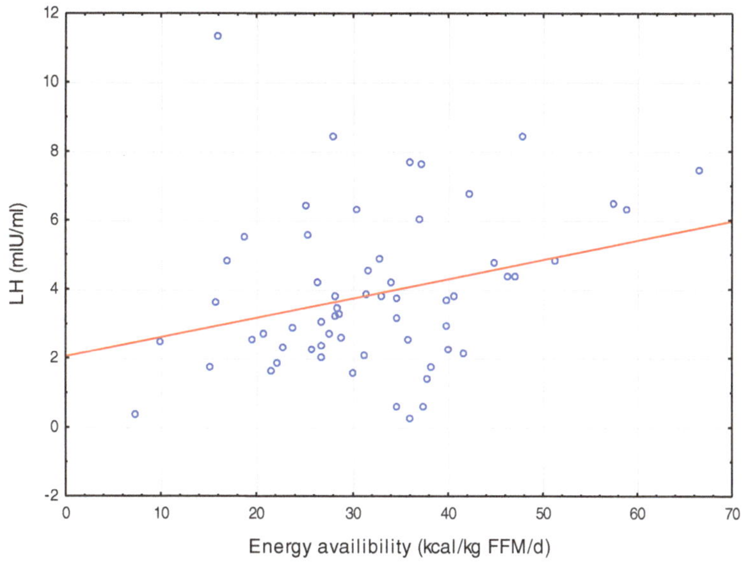

Figure 1 Correlation between energy availability and LH levels.

cycles in female athletes is possible after increasing the energy value of daily meals contributing to body weight and BMI increase. In the group of 373 female athletes, after five-year non-pharmacological dietary therapy, regular menstrual periods returned in 17.6% subjects. Moreover, in this group, a significant increase in BMI, from 20.8 ± 0.5 kg/m^2 to 22.7 ± 0.6 kg/m^2 ($p < 0.005$), as well as in body weight, from 58.0 ± 2.0 kg to 63.3 ± 2.3 kg ($p < 0.005$), were also observed. However, no information on body composition of the athletes from the above group were obtained. Dueck et al. [31] showed LH pulsatility accompanied by the weight gain of approximately 3 kg and a 6% body fat increase. In contrast, Loucks et al. [34,35] have suggested that body weight changes are not associated with menstrual disturbances in athletes, probably due to adaptive energy-conserving mechanisms development allowing for the maintenance of body weight despite poor energy availability. Mallinson et al. [25] compared and contrasted responses of two exercising women with amenorrhea of varying duration to an intervention of increased energy intake. This study was very similar to ours due to implementation of a non-pharmacological dietary intervention without reducing the energy expenditure or the intensity and volume of training. In the case study conducted by Mallinson et al. [25], resumption of menses occurred 23 and 74 days into the intervention for the women with short-term and long-term amenorrhea, respectively. Recovery of regular menses and onset of ovulation coincided closely with increases in energy intake, weight gain and improvements in the metabolic environment.

In female athletes, difficulties in the restoration of regular menstrual cycles may result from multiple overlapping causes of such disorders. Bruni et al. [36] reported that inadequate dietary habits, extensive physical activity and stress are key factors differentiating women with menstrual disorders. The above situation demonstrates that an eventual use of a homogenous treatment in the population of women with menstrual disturbances or amenorrhea is impossible. Potential factors affecting menstrual cycle include various genetic, neuroendocrine and metabolic aspects. It seems that in the specific population included in our studies, all above mentioned factors, predisposing to such disorders, are present. Nattiv et al. [10] and Manore et al. [15] emphasized that an appropriately balanced diet with reduced training volume and intensity is the only possible way to alleviate menstrual disorders in female athletes. The present study is valuable because it is based on an individual, non-pharmacological diet intervention taking into account everyday burden of an intense physical effort without reduction of intensity and volume of everyday activities, which could be, according to authors' knowledge, a potential cause of subject's withdrawal from the study. In case of female athletes aiming to achieve desired results, the limitation of training sessions intensity is potentially difficult to accept intervention, therefore it was not suggested to study participants.

This study has several limitations. Firstly, LH and FSH concentrations were assessed only once before the start of dietary intervention, and then after three months. We did not determinate the pulsatile nature of those hormones, thus an assessment of the presence of ovulatory cycles in menstruating women was impossible. Secondly, the body composition was determined using the electrical bioimpedance method, which potentially raises some controversies. However, DEXA method was not used due to young age of study participants, tests frequency, and potential adverse (UV) effects.

Conclusion

This report provides further support for the role of energy deficiency in menstrual disorders among young female athletes and the benefits of an adequate energy intake and energy availability on hormones concentration. Continuation controlled dietary intervention is needed to assess the extent to which long-term improvement in the nutritional status results in improvements in the hormonal status of female athletes, to an extent that would allow the regulation of the menstrual cyclity.

Competing interests

The authors declare that they have no competing interests.

Authors' contributions

KŁ (corresponding author) was responsible for the study design, the statistical analysis, execution of the measurements and the writing of the manuscript. KK was involved in the execution of the measurements and the writing of the manuscript. ZF provided assistance in the study design and JB provided assistance in the editing of the manuscript. All authors read and approved the final manuscript.

Acknowledgement

The project was financed by Ministry of Science and Higher Education under a number N N312 239738.

Author details

[1]Department of Human Nutrition and Hygiene, Dietetic Division, University of Life Sciences, Wojska Polskiego 28 str, 60-637 Poznań, Poland.
[2]Department of Perinatology and Gynecology, Division of Gynecology, Karol Marcinkowski University of Medical Sciences in Poznań, Polna 33 str, 60-535 Poznań, Poland.

References

1. Mudd LM, Fornetti W, Pivarnik JM: **Bone mineral density in collegiate female athletes comparisons among sports.** *J Athl Train* 2007, **42**(3):403–408.
2. Klentrou P, Plyley M: **Onset of puberty, menstrual frequency, and body fat in elite rhythmic gymnasts compared with normal controls.** *Br J Sports Med* 2003, **37**:490–494.
3. Torstveit MK, Sundgot-Borgen J: **Participation in leanness sports but not training volume is associated with menstrual dysfunction: a national survey of 1276 elite athletes and controls.** *Br J Sports Med* 2005, **39**:141–147.
4. Miller SM, Kukuljan S, Turner AI, van der Pligt P, Ducher G: **Energy deficiency, menstrual disturbances, and low bone mass: what do exercising Australian women know about the female athlete triad?** *Int J Sport Nutr Exerc Metab* 2012, **22**(2):131–138.
5. Feldmann JM, Belsha JP, Eissa MA, Middleman AB: **Female adolescent athletes' awareness of the connection between menstrual status and bone health.** *J Pediatr Adolesc Gynecol* 2011, **24**(5):311–314.
6. Christo K, Prabhakaran R, Lamparello B, Cord J, Miller KK, Goldstein MA, Gupta N, Herzog DB, Klibanski A, Misra M: **Bone metabolism in adolescent athletes with amenorrhea, athletes with eumenorrhea and control subjects.** *Pediatrics* 2008, **121**:1127–1136.
7. Nicholas JF, Rauh MJ, Barrack MT, Hava-Shoshana Barkai HS, Pernick Y: **Disordered eating and menstrual irregularity in high school athletes in lean-build and nonlean-build sports.** *Int J Sport Nutr Exerc Metab* 2007, **17**:364–377.
8. Hind K: **Recovery of bone mineral density and fertility in a former amenorrheic athlete.** *J Sports Sci Med* 2008, **7**:415–418.
9. Rickenlund A, Eriksson MJ, Schenck-Gustafsson K, Hirschberg AL: **Amenorrhea in female athletes is associated with endothelial dysfunction and unfavorable lipid profile.** *J Clin Endocrinol Metab* 2005, **90**(3):1354–1359.
10. Nattiv A, Loucks AB, Manore MM, Sanborn CF, Sundgot-Borgen J, Warren MP: **American College of Sports Medicine. The female athlete triad. Position stand.** *Med Sci Sports Exerc* 2007, **39**:1867–1881.
11. Heyward VH, Wagner DL: *Applied body composition assessment.* Champaign, IL: Human Kinetics; 2003.
12. Harris JA, Benedict FA: *A Biometric Study of Basal Metabolic Rate in man.* Washington, DC: Carnegie Institute of Washington, DC (Pub No 279); 1919:370–373.
13. Szponar L, Wolnicka K, Rychlik E: *Album fotografii produktów i potraw.* Wydawnictwo IŻŻ: Warsaw; 2000.
14. Kunachowicz H, Nadolna I, Przygoda B, Ivanow K: *Tables of Nutritional Value of Foodstuffs and Dishes. 3rd extended and updated edition.* Warsaw: Instytut Żywności i Żywienia; 2005.
15. Manore MM, Kam LC, Loucks AB: **The female athlete triad: components, nutrition issues, and health consequences.** *J Sports Sci* 2007, **25**:61–71.
16. Roupas ND, Georgopoulos NA: **Menstrual function in sports.** *Hormones* 2011, **10**(2):104–116.
17. Jarosz M, Bułhak-Jachymczyk B: *Normy Żywienia Człowieka. Podstawy prewencji otyłości i chorób niezakaźnych.* Warsaw: Instytut Żywności i Żywienia: Wydawnictwo Lekarskie PZWL; 2008.
18. Łagowska K, Jeszka J, Bajerska J: **The evaluation of nutritional habits, nutritional status triathlon with and without menstrual disorders.** *Med Sportiva* 2010, **14**(4):204–208.
19. Łagowska K, Jeszka J: **Are young female athletes at risk of amenorrhoea? Analysis of body composition, nutritional and endocrine factors.** *ACTA Sci Polonorum* 2011, **10**(2):227–232.
20. Hoch AZ, Pajewski NM, Moraski L, Carrera GF, Wilson CR, Hoffmann RG, Schimke JE, Gutterman DD: **Prevalence of the female athlete triad in high school athletes and sedentary students.** *Clin J Sport Med* 2009, **19**(5):421–428.
21. Tomten SE, Høstmark AT: **Energy balance in weight stable athletes with and without menstrual disorders.** *Scand J Med Sci Sports* 2006, **16**(2):127–133.
22. Hoogenboom BJ, Morris J, Morris C, Schaefer K: **Nutritional knowledge and eating behaviors of female, collegiate swimmers.** *N Am J Sports Phys Ther* 2009, **4**(3):139–148.
23. Quah YV, Poh BK, Ng LO, Noor MI: **The female athlete triad among elite Malaysian athletes: prevalence and associated factors.** *Asia Pac J Clin Nutr* 2009, **18**(2):200–208.
24. Woolf K, Manore MM: **B-vitamins and exercise: does exercise alter requirements?** *Int J Sport Nutr Exerc Metab* 2006, **16**(5):453–484.
25. Mallinson RJ, Williams NI, Olmsted MP, Scheid JL, Riddle ES, De Souza MJ: **A case report of recovery of menstrual function following a dietary intervention in two exercising women with amenorrhea of varying duration.** *J Int Soc Sports Nutr* 2013, **10**(1):34.
26. Loucks AB, Verdun M, Heath EM: **Low energy availability, not stress of exercise, alters LH pulsatility in exercising women.** *J Appl Physiol* 1998, **84**:37.
27. Laughlin GA, Dominguez CE, Yen SS: **Nutritional and endocrine-metabolic aberrations in women with functional hypothalamic amenorrhea.** *J Clin Endocrinol Metab* 1998, **83**:25.
28. Thong FSL, McLean C, Graham TE: **Plasma leptin in female athletes: relationship with body fat, reproductive, nutritional, and endocrine factors.** *J Appl Physiol* 2000, **88**(6):2037–2044.
29. Kaiserauer S, Synder AC, Sleeper M, Zierath J: **Nutritional, physiological and menstrual status of distance runners.** *Med Sci Sports Exerc* 1989, **21**:120–125.
30. De Souza MJ, Lee DK, VanHesst JI, Scheid JL, West SL, Williams NI: **Severity of energy-related menstrual disturbances increases in proportion to indices of energy conservation in exercising women.** *Fertil Steril* 2007, **88**:971–975.
31. Dueck CA, Matt KS, Manore MM, Skinner JS: **Treatment of athletic amenorrhea with a diet and training intervention program.** *Int J Sport Nutr* 1996, **6**:24–40.
32. Kopp-Woodroffe SA, Manore MM, Dueck CA, Skinner JS, Matt KS: **Energy and nutrient status of amenorrheic athletes participating in a diet and exercise training intervention program.** *Int J Sport Nutr* 1999, **9**:70–88.
33. Arends JC, Cheung MY, Barrack MT, Nattiv A: **Restoration of menses with nonpharmacologic therapy in collegiate athletes with menstrual disturbances: A 5 year Retrospective Study.** *Int J Sport Nutr Exerc Metab* 2012, **22**(2):98–108.

34. Loucks AB, Thuma JR: **Luteinizing hormone pulsatility is disrupted at a threshold of energy availability in regularly menstruating women.** *J Clin Endocrinol Metab* 2003, **88**(1):297–311.
35. Loucks AB, Laughlin GA, Mortola JF, Girton L, Nelson JC, Yen SS: **Hypothalamic-pituitary-thyroidal function in eumenorrheic and amenorrheic athletes.** *J Clin Endocrinol Metab* 1992, **75**:514–518.
36. Bruni V, Dei M, Morelli C, Schettino MT, Balzi D, Nuvolone D: **Body composition variables and leptin levels in functional hypothalamic amenorrhea and amenorrhea related to eating disorders.** *J Pediatr Adolesc Gynecol* 2011, **24**:347–352.

Evidence-based recommendations for natural bodybuilding contest preparation: nutrition and supplementation

Eric R Helms[1*], Alan A Aragon[2] and Peter J Fitschen[3]

Abstract

The popularity of natural bodybuilding is increasing; however, evidence-based recommendations for it are lacking. This paper reviewed the scientific literature relevant to competition preparation on nutrition and supplementation, resulting in the following recommendations. Caloric intake should be set at a level that results in bodyweight losses of approximately 0.5 to 1%/wk to maximize muscle retention. Within this caloric intake, most but not all bodybuilders will respond best to consuming 2.3-3.1 g/kg of lean body mass per day of protein, 15-30% of calories from fat, and the reminder of calories from carbohydrate. Eating three to six meals per day with a meal containing 0.4-0.5 g/kg bodyweight of protein prior and subsequent to resistance training likely maximizes any theoretical benefits of nutrient timing and frequency. However, alterations in nutrient timing and frequency appear to have little effect on fat loss or lean mass retention. Among popular supplements, creatine monohydrate, caffeine and beta-alanine appear to have beneficial effects relevant to contest preparation, however others do not or warrant further study. The practice of dehydration and electrolyte manipulation in the final days and hours prior to competition can be dangerous, and may not improve appearance. Increasing carbohydrate intake at the end of preparation has a theoretical rationale to improve appearance, however it is understudied. Thus, if carbohydrate loading is pursued it should be practiced prior to competition and its benefit assessed individually. Finally, competitors should be aware of the increased risk of developing eating and body image disorders in aesthetic sport and therefore should have access to the appropriate mental health professionals.

Keywords: Hypertrophy, Calories, Frequency, Nutrient, Body fat, Resistance training, Competition

Introduction

The popularity of natural bodybuilding is increasing rapidly. In the United States, over 200 amateur natural (drug tested) bodybuilding contests occurred during 2013 and the number of contests is expected to increase in 2014 [1]. Preparation for bodybuilding competition involves drastic reductions in body fat while maintaining muscle mass. This is typically achieved through a decreased caloric intake, intense strength training, and increased cardiovascular exercise. Competitors partake in numerous dietary and supplementation strategies to prepare for a contest. Some have a strong scientific basis; however, many do not. Therefore, the purpose of this article is to review the scientific literature on topics relevant to nutrition and supplementation for bodybuilding competition preparation. Dietary modifications during the last week to enhance muscle definition and fullness (peaking) and psychosocial issues will also be covered. Ultimately, evidence-based recommendations will be made for nutrition, supplementation, and "peak week" strategies for natural bodybuilders. As a final note, this paper does not cover training recommendations for natural bodybuilding and the training methodology used will interact with and modify the effects of any nutritional approach.

* Correspondence: eric.helms@aut.ac.nz
[1]Sport Performance Research in New Zealand (SPRINZ) at AUT Millennium Institute, AUT University, 17 Antares Place, Mairangi Bay, Auckland 0632, New Zealand
Full list of author information is available at the end of the article

Methods

PubMed, MEDLINE, SPORTDiscus and CINAHL electronic databases were searched online. Each author was assigned a portion of the manuscript to write specific to their area(s) of expertise. Authors performed searches for key words associated with their portion(s) of the manuscript; calories and macronutrients, nutrient timing and meal frequency, dietary supplementation, psychosocial issues and "peak week" were the selected topics. The publications obtained were carefully screened for studies that included healthy humans or humans in a caloric deficit. Long-term human studies focusing on hypertrophy and body fat loss were preferentially selected; however, acute studies and/or studies using animal models were selected in the absence of adequate long-term human studies. In addition, author names and reference lists were used for further search of the selected papers for related references. As this review is intended to be an evidence-based guide and the available data relevant to natural bodybuilding is extremely limited, a narrative review style was chosen.

Nutrition

Calories and macronutrients

Competitive bodybuilders traditionally follow two to four month diets in which calories are decreased and energy expenditure is increased to become as lean as possible [2-6]. In addition to fat loss, muscle maintenance is of primary concern during this period. To this end, optimal caloric intakes, deficits and macronutrient combinations should be followed while matching the changing needs that occur during competition preparation.

Caloric intake for competition

To create weight loss, more energy must be expended than consumed. This can be accomplished by increasing caloric expenditure while reducing caloric intake. The size of this caloric deficit and the length of time it is maintained will determine how much weight is lost. Every pound of pure body fat that is metabolized yields approximately 3500 kcals, thus a daily caloric deficit of 500 kcals theoretically results in fat loss of approximately one pound per week if the weight loss comes entirely from body fat [7]. However, a static mathematical model does not represent the dynamic physiological adaptations that occur in response to an imposed energy deficit [8]. Metabolic adaptation to dieting has been studied in overweight populations and when observed, reductions in energy expenditure amount to as little as 79 kcal/d [9], to as much as 504 kcal/d beyond what is predicted from weight loss [10]. Metabolic adaptations to bodybuilding contest preparation have not been studied however; non-overweight men who consumed 50% of their maintenance caloric intake for 24 weeks and lost one fourth of their body mass experienced a 40% reduction in their baseline energy expenditure. Of that 40% reduction 25% was due to weight loss, while metabolic adaptation accounted for the remaining 15% [11]. Therefore, it should be expected that the caloric intake at which one begins their preparation will likely need to be adjusted over time as body mass decreases and metabolic adaptation occurs. A complete review of metabolic adaptation to dieting in athletes is beyond the scope of this review. However, coaches and competitors are encouraged to read the recent review on this topic by Trexler et al. [12] which covers not only the physiology of metabolic adaptation, but also potential methods to mitigate its negative effects.

In determining an appropriate caloric intake, it should be noted that the tissue lost during the course of an energy deficit is influenced by the size of the energy deficit. While greater deficits yield faster weight loss, the percentage of weight loss coming from lean body mass (LBM) tends to increase as the size of the deficit increases [7,13-15]. In studies of weight loss rates, weekly losses of 1 kg compared to 0.5 kg over 4 weeks resulted in a 5% decrease in bench press strength and a 30% greater reduction in testosterone levels in strength training women [16]. Weekly weight loss rates of 1.4% of bodyweight compared to 0.7% in athletes during caloric restriction lasting four to eleven weeks resulted in reductions of fat mass of 21% in the faster weight loss group and 31% in the slower loss group. In addition, LBM increased on average by 2.1% in the slower loss group while remaining unchanged in the faster loss group. Worthy of note, small amounts of LBM were lost among leaner subjects in the faster loss group [13].

Therefore, weight loss rates that are more gradual may be superior for LBM retention. At a loss rate of 0.5 kg per week (assuming a majority of weight lost is fat mass), a 70 kg athlete at 13% body fat would need to be no more than 6 kg to 7 kg over their contest weight in order to achieve the lowest body fat percentages recorded in competitive bodybuilders following a traditional three month preparation [4,6,17-20]. If a competitor is not this lean at the start of the preparation, faster weight loss will be required which may carry a greater risk for LBM loss.

In a study of bodybuilders during the twelve weeks before competition, male competitors reduced their caloric intake significantly during the latter half and subsequently lost the greatest amount of LBM in the final three weeks [21]. Therefore, diets longer than two to four months yielding weight loss of approximately 0.5 to 1% of bodyweight weekly may be superior for LBM retention compared to shorter or more aggressive diets. Ample time should be allotted to lose body fat to avoid an aggressive deficit and the length of preparation should be tailored to the competitor; those leaner dieting for shorter periods than those with higher body fat percentages. It must also be taken into consideration that the leaner the competitor becomes the greater the risk for LBM loss

[14,15]. As the availability of adipose tissue declines the likelihood of muscle loss increases, thus it may be best to pursue a more gradual approach to weight loss towards the end of the preparation diet compared to the beginning to avoid LBM loss.

Determining macronutrient intake

Protein Adequate protein consumption during contest preparation is required to support maintenance of LBM. Athletes require higher protein intakes to support increased activity and strength athletes benefit from higher intakes to support growth of LBM [5,22-28]. Some researchers suggest these requirements increase further when athletes undergo energy restriction [13,16,22,28-33]. Furthermore, there is evidence that protein requirements are higher for leaner individuals in comparison to those with higher body fat percentages [7,33,34].

The collective agreement among reviewers is that a protein intake of 1.2-2.2 g/kg is sufficient to allow adaptation to training for athletes whom are at or above their energy needs [23-28,35-38]. However, bodybuilders during their contest preparation period typically perform resistance and cardiovascular training, restrict calories and achieve very lean conditions [2-6,17-21]. Each of these factors increases protein requirements and when compounded may further increase protein needs [33]. Therefore, optimal protein intakes for bodybuilders during contest preparation may be significantly higher than existing recommendations.

In support of this notion, Butterfield et al. [22] found that male athletes running five to 10 miles per day during a slight caloric deficit were in a significant negative nitrogen balance despite consuming 2 g/kg of protein daily. Celejowa et al. [39] showed that five out of 10 competitive weight lifters achieved a negative nitrogen balance over the course of a training camp while consuming an average protein intake of 2 g/kg. Out of these five, as many as three were in a caloric deficit. The authors concluded that a protein intake of 2–2.2 g/kg under these conditions only allows for a small margin of error before nitrogen losses occur.

Walberg et al. [32] examined the effects of two energy restricted isocaloric diets of differing protein intakes in 19 lean (9.1-16.7% body fat), male, non-competitive body builders. One group consumed a protein intake of 0.8 g/kg and higher carbohydrates, while the other consumed 1.6 g/kg of protein with lower carbohydrates. The length of the intervention was only one week, but nonetheless nitrogen losses occurred only in the lower protein group and LBM decreased by a mean of 2.7 kg in the 0.8 g/kg protein group and by a mean of 1.4 kg in the 1.6 g/kg protein group. While the high protein group mitigated LBM losses compared to the low protein group, they were not eliminated.

A recent study by Mettler et al. [29] employed the same basic methodology as Walberg et al. [32]. However, one group consumed a protein intake of 1 g/kg, while the other consumed 2.3 g/kg. The high-protein group lost significantly less LBM (0.3 kg) over the course of the two week intervention compared to the low-protein group (1.6 kg). Unlike Walberg et al. [32] calorie balance between diets was maintained by reducing dietary fat as opposed to carbohydrate to allow for the increase in protein.

While it appears that the 2.3 g/kg protein intervention in Mettler et al. [29] was superior for maintaining LBM compared to 1.6 g/kg in Walberg et al. [32] a recent study by Pasiakos et al. [40] found a trend towards the opposite. In this study, a non-significant trend of greater LBM retention occurred when subjects consumed 1.6 g/kg of protein compared to 2.4 g/kg of protein. However, the participants were intentionally prescribed low volume, low intensity resistance training "to minimize the potential of an unaccustomed, anabolic stimulus influencing study outcome measures". Thus, the non-anabolic nature of the training may not have increased the participants' protein requirements to the same degree as the participants in Mettler et al. [29] or to what would be expected among competitive bodybuilders.

Maestu et al. [6] did not observe a significant loss of LBM in a group of drug free bodybuilders consuming 2.5-2.6 g/kg of protein during the 11 weeks prior to competition. These results when considered alongside the works by Walberg et al. [32] and Mettler et al. [29] imply that the higher the protein intake, the lower the chance for LBM loss. However, it should be noted that this study did not include a low protein control and not all studies show a linear increase in LBM preservation with increases in protein [40]. Furthermore, two subjects did lose significant amounts of LBM (1.5 kg and 1.8 kg), and the authors noted that these specific bodybuilders were among the leanest of the subjects. These two subjects lost the majority of their LBM (approximately 1 kg) during the latter half of the intervention as their percentage of calories from protein increased from 28% to 32-33% by the end of the study. The group as a whole progressively decreased their calories by reducing all three macronutrients throughout the investigation. Thus, the two subjects uniquely increased their proportion of protein, possibly reducing fat and carbohydrate to the point of detriment [6]. That said it is also plausible that the lost LBM seen by these two subjects was necessary in order to achieve their low levels of body fat. It is unknown whether or not the lost LBM influenced their competitive outcome and it is possible that had the competitors not been as lean, they may have retained more LBM but also not have placed as well.

In a review by Phillips and Van Loon [28], it is suggested that a protein intake of 1.8-2.7 g/kg for athletes training in hypocaloric conditions may be optimal. While this is one of the only recommendations existing that targets athletes during caloric restriction, this recommendation is not given with consideration to bodybuilders performing concurrent endurance and resistance training at very low levels of body fat. However, the recently published systematic review by Helms et al. [33] on protein intakes in resistance-trained, lean athletes during caloric restriction suggests a range of 2.3-3.1 g/kg of LBM, which may be more appropriate for bodybuilding. Moreover, the authors suggest that the lower the body fat of the individual, the greater the imposed caloric deficit and when the primary goal is to retain LBM, the higher the protein intake (within the range of 2.3-3.1 g/kg of LBM) should be.

Carbohydrate High carbohydrate diets are typically thought to be the athletic performance standard. However, like protein, carbohydrate intake needs to be customized to the individual. Inadequate carbohydrate can impair strength training [41] and consuming adequate carbohydrate prior to training can reduce glycogen depletion [42] and may therefore enhance performance.

While it is true that resistance training utilizes glycogen as its main fuel source [43], total caloric expenditure of strength athletes is less than that of mixed sport and endurance athletes. Thus, authors of a recent review recommend that carbohydrate intakes for strength sports, including bodybuilding, be between 4–7 g/kg depending on the phase of training [26]. However, in the specific case of a bodybuilder in contest preparation, achieving the necessary caloric deficit while consuming adequate protein and fat would likely not allow consumption at the higher end of this recommendation.

Satiety and fat loss generally improve with lower carbohydrate diets; specifically with higher protein to carbohydrate ratios [44-49]. In terms of performance and health, low carbohydrate diets are not necessarily as detrimental as typically espoused [50]. In a recent review, it was recommended for strength athletes training in a calorically restricted state to reduce carbohydrate content while increasing protein to maximize fat oxidation and preserve LBM [28]. However, the optimal reduction of carbohydrate and point at which carbohydrate reduction becomes detrimental likely needs to be determined individually.

One comparison of two isocaloric, energy restricted diets in bodybuilders showed that a diet that provided adequate carbohydrate at the expense of protein (1 g/kg) resulted in greater LBM losses compared to a diet that increased protein (1.6 g/kg) through a reduction of carbohydrate [32]. However, muscular endurance was degraded in the lower carbohydrate group. In a study of athletes taking in the same amount of protein (1.6 g/kg) during weight loss, performance decrements and LBM losses were avoided when adequate carbohydrate was maintained and dietary fat was lowered [13]. Mettler, et al. [29] also found that a caloric reduction coming from dietary fat while maintaining adequate carbohydrate intake and increasing protein to 2.3 g/kg maintained performance and almost completely eliminated LBM losses in resistance trained subjects. Finally, in Pasiakos et al. [40] participants undergoing an equal calorie deficit and consuming the same amount of protein as those observed in Mettler et al. [29] lost three times the amount of LBM over the same time period (0.9 kg in the first two weeks of energy restriction observed by Pasiakos versus 0.3 kg observed by Mettler). One key difference between these studies was the highest protein group in Mettler et al. [29] consumed a 51% carbohydrate diet while the comparable group in Pasiakos et al. [40] consumed a 27% carbohydrate diet. While performance was not measured, the participants in Pasiakos et al. [40] performing sets exclusively of 15 repetitions very likely would have experienced decrements in performance due to this carbohydrate intake level [32]. The difference in training protocols or a nutritionally mediated decrement in training performance could have either or both been components that lead to the greater losses of LBM observed by Pasiakos et al. [40].

While it appears low carbohydrate, high protein diets can be effective for weight loss, a practical carbohydrate threshold appears to exist where further reductions negatively impact performance and put one at risk for LBM losses. In support of this notion, researchers studying bodybuilders during the final 11 weeks of contest preparation concluded that had they increased carbohydrate during the final weeks of their diet they may have mitigated metabolic and hormonal adaptations that were associated with reductions in LBM [6].

Therefore, once a competitor has reached or has nearly reached the desired level of leanness, it may be a viable strategy to reduce the caloric deficit by an increase in carbohydrate. For example, if a competitor has reached competition body fat levels (lacking any visible subcutaneous fat) and is losing half a kilogram per week (approximately a 500 kcals caloric deficit), carbohydrate could be increased by 25-50 g, thereby reducing the caloric deficit by 100-200 kcals in an effort to maintain performance and LBM. However, it should be noted that like losses of LBM, decrements in performance may not affect the competitive outcome for a bodybuilder. It is possible that competitors who reach the leanest condition may experience unavoidable drops in performance.

Fat The importance of carbohydrate and protein in sports nutrition is often emphasized over that of dietary fat. Subsequently, recommendations typically focus on maintaining adequate fat intake while emphasizing carbohydrate to fuel performance and protein to build and repair LBM. However, there is evidence that dietary fat influences anabolic hormone concentrations which may be of interest to bodybuilders attempting to maintain LBM while dieting [5,26,51,52].

Reductions in the percentage of dietary fat in isocaloric diets from approximately 40% to 20% has resulted in modest, but significant, reductions in testosterone levels [53,54]. However, distinguishing the effects of reducing total dietary fat on hormonal levels from changes in caloric intake and percentages of saturated and unsaturated fatty acids in the diet is difficult [51,52,55]. In a study by Volek et al. [51], correlations were found between testosterone levels, macronutrient ratios, types of lipids, and total dietary fat, illustrating a complex interaction of variables. In a similar study of resistance trained males, correlations were found between testosterone, protein, fat and saturated fat which lead the researchers to conclude that diets too low in fat or too high in protein might impair the hormonal response to training [52].

Competing bodybuilders must make an obligatory caloric reduction. If a reduction in fat is utilized, it may be possible to attenuate a drop in testosterone by maintaining adequate consumption of saturated fat [5]. However, a drop in testosterone does not equate to a reduction in LBM. In direct studies of resistance trained athletes undergoing calorically restricted high protein diets, low fat interventions that maintain carbohydrate levels [13,29] appear to be more effective at preventing LBM loses than lower carbohydrate, higher fat approaches [32,40]. These results might indicate that attempting to maintain resistance training performance with higher carbohydrate intakes is more effective for LBM retention than attempting to maintain testosterone levels with higher fat intakes.

Body composition and caloric restriction may play greater roles in influencing testosterone levels that fat intake. During starvation, a reduction in testosterone occurs in normal weight, but not obese, males [56]. In addition, rate of weight loss may influence testosterone levels. Weekly target weight loss rates of 1 kg resulted in a 30% reduction in testosterone compared to target weight loss rates of 0.5 kg per week in resistance trained women of normal weight [16]. Additionally, an initial drop in testosterone occurred in the first six weeks of contest preparation in a group of drug free bodybuilders despite various macronutrient percentages [6]. Finally, in a one year case study of a natural competitive bodybuilder, testosterone levels fell to one fourth their baseline values three months into the six month preparation period. Levels then fully recovered three months into the six month recovery period. Testosterone did not decline further after the initial drop at the three month mark despite a slight decrease in fat intake from 27% to 25% of calories at the six month mark. Furthermore, the quadrupling of testosterone during the recovery period from its suppressed state back to baseline was accompanied by a 10 kg increase in body mass and a 1000 kcal increase in caloric intake. However, there was only a minor increase in calories from fat (percentage of calories from fat during recovery was between (30 and 35%) [57]. Finally, these testosterone changes in men appear mostly related to energy availability (body fat content and energy balance), and not surprisingly low-levels of sustained energy availability are also the proposed cause of the hormonal disturbance "athletic amenorrhea" in women [58]. Thus, the collective data indicates that when extremely lean body compositions are attained through extended, relatively aggressive dieting, the caloric deficit and loss of body fat itself may have a greater impact on testosterone than the percentage of calories coming from dietary fat.

While cogent arguments for fat intakes between 20 to 30% of calories have been made to optimize testosterone levels in strength athletes [59], in some cases this intake may be unrealistic in the context of caloric restriction without compromising sufficient protein or carbohydrate intakes. While dieting, low carbohydrate diets may degrade performance [32] and lead to lowered insulin and IGF-1 which appear to be more closely correlated to LBM preservation than testosterone [6]. Thus, a lower end fat intake between 15-20% of calories, which has been previously recommended for bodybuilders [5], can be deemed appropriate if higher percentages would reduce carbohydrate or protein below ideal ranges.

Ketogenic diets and individual variability

Some bodybuilders do use very-low carbohydrate, "ketogenic diets" for contest preparation [60,61]. While these diets have not been sufficiently studied in bodybuilders, some study of ketogenic diets has occurred in resistance trained populations. In an examination of the effects of a 1 week ketogenic diet (5.4% of calories from carbohydrate) in subjects with at least 2 years of resistance training experience, Sawyer et al. [62] observed slight decreases in body fat among female participants and maintenance or slight increases in measures of strength and power among both male and female participants. However, it is difficult to draw conclusions due to the very short term nature of this study and due to an ad libitum implementation of the ketogenic diet. As implemented in this study, besides a reduction in carbohydrate and an increase in dietary fat, the ketogenic diet resulted in an average reduction of 381 calories per day and an increase of 56 g of protein per day compared to the participants' habitual diets. Thus, it is unclear whether the improvements in body composition and performance can be attributed to the low-carbohydrate and high-fat nature of the diets or rather a decrease in calories and an increase in protein. At least with regards to weight loss, previous research indicates that the often concomitant increase in protein observed in very low carbohydrate diets may actually be the key to their success [63].

The only research on strength athletes following ketogenic diets for longer periods is a study of gymnasts in which they were observed to maintain strength performance and lose more body fat after 30 days on a ketogenic diet in comparison to 30 days on a traditional western diet [64]. However, this study's sample size was limited (n = 8) and it was not a controlled study of an intentional fat-loss phase such as seen among bodybuilders during competition preparation. Therefore, more study is needed in resistance trained populations and bodybuilders before definitive recommendations can be made to support ketogenic diets.

However, the research that does exist challenges traditional views on carbohydrate and anaerobic performance. Despite the common belief that carbohydrate is the sole fuel source for weight training, intramuscular triglyceride is used during short term heavy resistance training [65] and likely becomes an increasingly viable fuel source for those adapted to high-fat low-carbohydrate diets. While some might suggest that this implies a ketogenic diet could be a viable option for contest preparation, a trend of decreased performance and impaired maintenance of FFM is associated with lower carbohydrate intakes in the majority of studies included in this review.

While it is our contention that the majority of the evidence indicates that very-low carbohydrate diets should be avoided for contest preparation (at least until more research is performed), it must be noted that there is a high degree of variability in the way that individuals respond to diets. Carbohydrate and fat utilization as a percentage of energy expenditure at rest and various intensities has as much as a four-fold difference between individual athletes; which is influenced by muscle fiber-composition, diet, age, training, glycogen levels and genetics [66]. Additionally, individuals that are more insulin sensitive may lose more weight with higher-carbohydrate low-fat diets while those more insulin resistant may lose more weight with lower-carbohydrate higher-fat diets [67].

Due to this individual variability, some popular commercial bodybuilding literature suggests that somatotype and/or body fat distribution should be individually assessed as a way of determining macronutrient ratios. However, there is no evidence of any relationships with bone structure or regional subcutaneous fat distribution with any response to specific macronutrient ratios in bodybuilders or athletic populations. Bodybuilders, like others athletes, most likely operate best on balanced macronutrient intakes tailored to the energy demands of their sport [68].

In conclusion, while the majority of competitors will respond best to the fat and carbohydrate guidelines we propose, the occasional competitor will undoubtedly respond better to a diet that falls outside of these suggested ranges. Careful monitoring over the course of a competitive career is required to determine the optimal macronutrient ratio for pre-contest dieting.

Macronutrient recommendations summary

After caloric intake is established based on the time frame before competition [69], body composition of the athlete [14,15,34], and keeping the deficit modest to avoid LBM losses [13,16], macronutrients can be determined within this caloric allotment. Table 1 provides an overview of these recommendations.

If training performance degrades it may prove beneficial to decrease the percentage of calories from dietary fat within these ranges in favor of a greater proportion of carbohydrate. Finally, while outside of the norm, some competitors may find that they respond better to diets that are higher in fat and lower in carbohydrate than recommended in this review. Therefore, monitoring of individual response over a competitive career is suggested.

Nutrient timing

Traditional nutrient timing guidelines are typically based on the needs of endurance athletes. For example, it is common lore that post-exercise carbohydrate must elicit a substantial glycemic and insulinemic response in order to optimize recovery. The origin of this recommendation can be traced back to 1988, when Ivy et al. [70] put fasted subjects through a glycogen-depleting cycling bout and compared the rate of glycogen resynthesis from a carbohydrate solution (2 g/kg) consumed either immediately after, or two hours after the bout. Glycogen storage was 2–3 times faster in the immediate condition during four hours post-exercise resulting in greater glycogen storage at four hours.

These findings initiated the faster-is-better post-exercise guideline for carbohydrate. However, complete glycogen resynthesis to pre-trained levels can occur well within 24 hours given sufficient total carbohydrate intake. Jentjens and Jeukendrup [71] suggest that a between-bout period of eight hours or less is grounds for maximally

Table 1 Dietary recommendations for bodybuilding contest preparation

Diet component	Recommendation
Protein (g/kg of LBM)	2.3-3.1 [33]
Fat (% of total calories)	15-30% [5,59]
Carbohydrate (% of total calories)	remaining
Weekly weight loss (% of body weight)	0.5-1% [13,16]

expediting glycogen resynthesis. Therefore, the urgency of glycogen resynthesis is almost an exclusive concern of endurance athletes with multiple glycogen-depleting events separated by only a few hours. Bodybuilders in contest preparation may exceed a single training bout per day (e.g., weight-training in the morning, cardio in the evening). However, bodybuilders do not have the same performance objectives as multi-stage endurance competition, where the same muscle groups are trained to exhaustion in a repeated manner within the same day. Furthermore, resistance training bouts are typically not glycogen-depleting. High-intensity (70-80% of 1 RM), moderate-volume (6–9 sets per muscle group) bouts have been seen to reduce glycogen stores by roughly 36-39% [72,73].

A more relevant question to bodybuilding may be whether protein and/or amino acid timing affect LBM maintenance. With little exception [74], acute studies have consistently shown that ingesting protein/essential amino acids and carbohydrate near or during the training bout can increase muscle protein synthesis (MPS) and suppress muscle protein breakdown [75-79]. However, there is a disparity between short- and long-term outcomes in studies examining the effect of nutrient timing on resistance training adaptations.

To-date, only a minority of chronic studies have shown that specific timing of nutrients relative to the resistance training bout can affect gains in muscular size and/or strength. Cribb and Hayes [80] found that timing a supplement consisting of 40 g protein, 43 g carbohydrate, and 7 g creatine immediately pre- and post-exercise resulted in greater size and strength gains than positioning the supplement doses away from the training bout. Additionally, Esmarck et al. [81] observed greater hypertrophy in subjects who ingested a supplement (10 g protein, 8 g carbohydrate, 3 g fat) immediately post-exercise than subjects who delayed the supplement 2 hours post-exercise.

In contrast, the majority of chronic studies have not supported the effectiveness of timing nutrients (protein in particular) closely around the training bout. Burk et al. [82], found that a *time-divided* regimen (two 35 g protein doses consumed at far-off points in the morning and evening away from the afternoon training bout) caused slightly better gains in squat strength and fat-free mass than the *time-focused* regimen, where the protein supplement doses were consumed in the morning, and then again immediately prior to the resistance training bout. Hoffman et al. [83] found no significant differences in strength gains or body composition when comparing an immediate pre- and post-exercise supplement ingestion (each dose provided 42 g protein) with the supplement ingested distantly separate from each side of the training bout. This lack of effect was attributed to the subjects' sufficient daily protein consumption combined with their advanced lifting status. Wycherley et al. [84] examined the effects of varying nutrient timing on overweight and obese diabetics. A meal containing 21 g protein consumed immediately before resistance training was compared with its consumption at least two hours after training. No significant differences in weight loss, strength gain, or cardio metabolic risk factor reductions were seen. Most recently, Weisgarber et al. [85] observed no significant effect on muscle mass and strength from consuming whey protein immediately before or throughout resistance training.

It's important to note that other chronic studies are referred to as nutrient timing studies, but have not matched total protein intake between conditions. These studies examined the effect of additional nutrient content, rather than examining the effect of different temporal placement of nutrients relative to the training bout. Thus, they cannot be considered true timing comparisons. Nevertheless, these studies have yielded inconsistent results. Willoughby et al. [86] found that 10 weeks of resistance training supplemented with 20 g protein and amino acids 1 hour pre- and post-exercise increased strength performance and MPS compared to an energy-matched carbohydrate placebo. Hulmi et al. [87] found that 21 weeks of supplementing 15 g of whey before and after resistance training increased size and altered gene expression favorably towards muscle anabolism in the vastus lateralis. In contrast to the previous 2 studies, Verdijk et al. [88] found no significant effect of 10 g protein timed immediately before and after resistance training over a 12-week period. The authors attributed this lack of effect to an adequate total daily protein intake. Recently, a 12-week trial by Erksine et al. [89] reported a lack of effect of 20 g protein taken pre- and post-exercise compared to placebo.

The disparity of outcomes between the acute and chronic studies could also potentially be due to a longer "anabolic window" than traditionally thought. Burd and colleagues [90] found that resistance training to failure can cause an increased anabolic response to protein feedings that can last up to 24 hours. Demonstrating the body's drive toward equilibrium, Deldicque et al. [91] observed a greater intramyocellular anabolic response in fasted compared to fed subjects given a post-exercise carbohydrate/protein/leucine mixture. This result suggests that the body is capable of anabolic supercompensation despite the inherently catabolic nature of fasted resistance training. These data, in addition to the previously discussed chronic studies, further support the idea that macronutrient totals by the end of the day may be more important than their temporal placement relative to the training bout.

There are additional factors that might explain the lack of consistent effectiveness of nutrient timing in chronic studies. Training status of the subjects could influence outcomes since novice trainees tend to respond similarly to a wider variety of stimuli. Another possible explanation for the lack of timing effects is the protein dose used, 10–20 g, which may not be sufficient to elicit a maximal anabolic response. MPS rates have been shown to plateau with a post-exercise dose of roughly 20 g of high-quality protein [92]. However, in subsequent research on older subjects, Yang et al. [93] observed that an even higher post-exercise protein dose (40 g) stimulated MPS to a greater extent than 10 g or 20 g.

In addition to the paucity of studies using ample protein doses, there is a lack of investigation of protein-carbohydrate combinations. Only Cribb and Hayes [80] have compared substantial doses of both protein (40 g) and carbohydrate (43 g) taken immediately surrounding, versus far apart from both sides of the training bout. Nearly double the lean mass gains were seen in the proximally timed compared to the distally timed condition. However, acute studies examining the post-exercise anabolic response elicited by co-ingesting carbohydrate with protein have thus far failed to show significant effects given a sufficient protein dose of approximately 20–25 g [94,95]. These results concur with previous data indicating that only moderate insulin elevations (15–30 mU/L) are required to maximize net muscle protein balance in the presence of elevated plasma amino acids [96]. Koopman et al. [97] observed a similar lack of carbohydrate-mediated anabolic effect when protein was administered at 0.3 g/kg/hr in the post-exercise recovery period.

Questions remain about the utility of consuming protein and/or carbohydrate during bodybuilding-oriented training bouts. Since these bouts typically do not resemble endurance bouts lasting 2 hours or more, nutrient consumption during training is not likely to yield any additional performance-enhancing or muscle -sparing benefits if proper pre-workout nutrition is in place. In the exceptional case of resistance training sessions that approach or exceed two hours of exhaustive, continuous work, it might be prudent to employ tactics that maximize endurance capacity while minimizing muscle damage. This would involve approximately 8–15 g protein co-ingested with 30–60 g carbohydrate in a 6-8% solution per hour of training [98]. Nutrient timing is an intriguing area of study that focuses on what might clinch the competitive edge. In terms of practical application to resistance training bouts of typical length, Aragon and Schoenfeld [99] recently suggested a protein dose corresponding with 0.4-0.5 g/kg bodyweight consumed at both the pre- and post-exercise periods. However, for objectives relevant to bodybuilding, the current evidence indicates that the global macronutrient composition of the diet is likely the most important nutritional variable related to chronic training adaptations. Figure 1 below provides a continuum of importance with bodybuilding-specific context for nutrient timing.

Meal frequency

Previous optimal meal frequency studies have lacked structured resistance training protocols. Moreover, there are no studies that specifically examined meal frequency in bodybuilders, let alone during contest preparation conditions. Despite this limitation, the available research has consistently refuted the popular belief that a grazing pattern (smaller, more frequent meals) raises energy expenditure compared to a gorging pattern (larger, less frequent meals). Disparate feeding patterns ranging from two to seven meals per day have been compared in tightly controlled studies using metabolic chambers, and no significant differences in 24-hour thermogenesis have been detected [100,101]. It should be noted that irregular feeding patterns across the week, as opposed to maintaining a stable daily frequency, has been shown to decrease post-prandial thermogenesis [102] and adversely affect insulin sensitivity and blood lipid profile [103]. However, relevance of the latter findings might be limited to sedentary populations, since regular exercise is well-established in its ability to improve insulin sensitivity and blood lipids.

Bodybuilders typically employ a higher meal frequency in an attempt to optimize fat loss and muscle preservation. However, the majority of chronic experimental studies have failed to show that different meal frequencies have different influences on bodyweight or body composition [104-108]. Of particular interest is the research examining the latter, since the preservation of muscle mass during fat loss is a paramount concern in the pre-contest phase. A recent review by Varady [109] examined 11 daily caloric restriction (CR) studies and 7 intermittent calorie restriction (ICR) studies. CR involved a linear consumption of 15-60% of baseline needs every day, while ICR alternated ad libitum 'feed' days with 'fast' days involving partial or total food intake restriction. It was concluded that although both types have similar effects on total bodyweight reduction, ICR has thus far been more effective for retaining lean mass. Three of the ICR studies showed no significant decrease in LBM, while all of the CR studies showed decreased LBM. However, the majority of the ICR trials used bio-electrical impedance analysis (BIA) to measure body composition, while the majority of CR studies used dual X-ray absorptiometry (DXA) or magnetic resonance imaging (MRI). These methods have been shown to have greater accuracy than BIA [110-112], so the results of Varady's [109] analysis should be interpreted with caution. Along these lines, Stote et al. [113] found that compared to three meals per day, one meal per day caused slightly more weight and fat loss. Curiously, the one meal per day group also showed a slight gain in lean mass, but this could have been due to the inherent error in BIA for body composition assessment.

	MINIMAL IMPORTANCE	VARIABLE IMPORTANCE	MAXIMAL IMPORTANCE
Carbohydrate	▪ Non-fasted, low-to-moderate-intensity resistance-training lasting 1 hr or less.	▪ Training that occurs shortly after an overnight fast. ▪ Exhaustive/continuous training that significantly exceeds 1 hour, especially training that approaches 2 hours.	▪ Training involving more than one glycogen-depleting bout in a single day, for example a day in which legs are trained with moderate volume followed or preceded by a high intensity cardiovascular training session. ▪ Training that significantly exceeds 2 hours; especially training that approaches or exceeds 3 hours.
Protein	▪ Timing in relation to cardiovascular training sessions.	▪ Timing in relation to resistance training in a fed state (after a meal containing adequate protein).	▪ Timing in relation to resistance training in a fasted state (occurring after a meal consumed more than 3 hours prior, especially approaching or exceeding 4 hours prior).
Supplements	▪ Specific timing of creatine, beta-alanine, or other such supplements used for chronic muscular adaptations rather than acute ergogenic effects.		▪ Specific timing of CHO/electrolyte sports beverages, caffeine, or other such supplements used for acute ergogenic effects rather than chronic muscular adaptations.

Figure 1 Continuum of nutrient & supplement timing importance.

To-date, only two experimental studies have used trained, athletic subjects. Iwao et al. [114] found that boxers consuming six meals a day lost less LBM and showed lower molecular measures of muscle catabolism than the same diet consumed in two meals per day. However, limitations to this study included short trial duration, subpar assessment methods, a small sample size, and a 1200 kcal diet which was artificially low compared to what this population would typically carry out in the long-term. It is also important to note that protein intake, at 20% of total kcal, amounted to 60 g/day which translates to slightly under 1.0 g/kg. To illustrate the inadequacy of this dose, Mettler et al. [29] showed that protein as high as 2.3 g/kg and energy intake averaging 2022 kcal was still not enough to completely prevent LBM loss in athletes under hypocaloric conditions. The other experimental study using athletic subjects was by Benardot et al. [115], who compared the effects of adding three 250 kcal between-meal snacks with the addition of a noncaloric placebo. A significant increase in anaerobic power and lean mass was seen in the snacking group, with no such improvements seen in the placebo group. However, it is not possible to determine if the superior results were the result of an increased meal frequency or increased caloric intake.

A relatively recent concept with potential application to meal frequency is that a certain minimum dose of leucine is required in order to stimulate muscle protein synthesis. Norton and Wilson [116] suggested that this threshold dose is approximately 0.05 g/kg, or roughly 3 g leucine per meal to saturate the mTOR signaling pathway and trigger MPS. A related concept is that MPS can diminish, or become 'refractory' if amino acids are held at a constant elevation. Evidence of the refractory phenomenon was shown by Bohé et al. [117], who elevated plasma amino acid levels in humans and observed that MPS peaked at the 2-hour mark, and rapidly declined thereafter despite continually elevated blood amino acid levels. For the goal of maximizing the anabolic response, the potential application of these data would be to avoid spacing meals too closely together. In addition, an attempt would be made to reach the leucine threshold with each meal, which in practical terms would be to consume at least 30–40 g high-quality protein per meal. In relative agreement, a recent review by Phillips and Van Loon [28] recommends consuming one's daily protein requirement over the course of three to four isonitrogenous meals per day in order to maximize the acute anabolic response per meal, and thus the rate of muscle gain.

It is important to note that the leucine threshold and the refractory nature of MPS are not based on human feeding studies that measure concrete outcomes over the long-term. These ideas are largely based on mechanistic studies whose data was derived via steady intravenous infusion of amino acids [117,118]. Long-term studies are needed to determine if the refractory nature of MPS seen in acute infusion data would have any real impact on the gain or preservation of LBM at various meal frequencies.

Munster and Saris [119] recently shed further light on what might be optimal in the context of pre-contest dieting. Lean, healthy subjects underwent 36-hour periods in a respiration chamber. Interestingly, three meals per day resulted in higher protein oxidation and RMR, along with lower overall blood glucose concentrations than an isoenergetic diet composed of 14 meals per day. The lower glucose AUC observed in this study is in agreement with previous research by Holmstrup et al. [120], who reported lower 12-hour glucose concentrations as a result of consuming three high-carbohydrate meals compared to the equivalent distributed over the course of six meals. Another interesting finding by Munster and Saris [119] was lower hunger and higher satiety ratings in the lower meal frequency condition. This finding concurred with previous work by Leidy et al. [121], who compared varying protein levels consumed across either three or six meals per day. Predictably, the higher-protein level (25% vs. 14%) promoted greater satiety. Interestingly, the higher meal frequency led to lower daily fullness ratings regardless of protein level. Meal frequency had no significant impact on ghrelin levels, regardless of protein intake. PYY, a gut peptide associated with satiety, was 9% lower in the higher meal frequency condition. However, Arciero et al. [122] recently found that six meals per day in a high-protein condition (35% of total energy) were superior to three meals with a high-protein or traditional protein intake (15% of total energy) for improving body composition in overweight subjects. The discrepancy between Leidy et al's short-term effects and Arciero's chronic effects warrants further study, preferably in subjects undergoing progressive resistance training.

Other common meal frequencies (i.e., 4 or 5 meals per day) have eluded scientific investigation until very recently. Adechian et al. [123] compared whey versus casein consumed in either a 'pulse' meal pattern (8/80/4/8%) or a 'spread' pattern (25/25/25/25%) over a six week hypocaloric period. No significant changes were seen in body composition between conditions. These outcomes challenge Phillips and Van Loon's recommendation for protein-rich meals throughout the day to be isonitrogenous (40). Moore et al. [124] compared evenly spaced distributions of two, four, and eight meals consumed after a fasted, acute bout of bilateral knee extension. A trend toward a small and moderate increase in net protein balance was seen in the four meal and eight meal conditions, respectively, compared to the two meal condition. Subsequent work by Areta et al. [125] using the same dosing comparison found that the four meal treatment (20 g protein per meal) caused the greatest increase in myofibrillar protein synthesis. A limitation of both of the previous studies was the absence of other macronutrients (aside from protein in whey) consumed during the 12-hour postexercise period. This leaves open questions about how a real-world scenario with mixed meals might have altered the outcomes. Furthermore, these short-term responses lack corroboration in chronic trials measuring body composition and/or exercise performance outcomes.

The evidence collectively suggests that extreme lows or highs in meal frequency have the potential to threaten lean mass preservation and hunger control during bodybuilding contest preparation. However, the functional impact of differences in meal frequency at moderate ranges (e.g., 3–6 meals per day containing a minimum of 20 g protein each) are likely to be negligible in the context of a sound training program and properly targeted total daily macronutrition.

Nutritional supplementation

When preparing for a bodybuilding contest, a competitor primarily focuses on resistance training, nutrition, and cardiovascular training; however, supplements may be used to further augment preparation. This section will discuss the scientific evidence behind several of the most commonly used supplements by bodybuilders. However, natural bodybuilding federations have extensive banned substance lists [126]; therefore, banned substances will be omitted from this discussion. It should be noted that there are considerably more supplements that are used by bodybuilders and sold on the market. However, an exhaustive review of all of the supplements commonly used by bodybuilders that often lack supporting data is beyond the scope of this paper. In addition, we have omitted discussion of protein supplements because they are predominantly used in the same way that whole food protein sources are used to reach macronutrient targets; however, interested readers are encouraged to reference the ISSN position stand on protein and exercise [127].

Creatine

Creatine monohydrate (CM) has been called the most ergogenic and safe supplement that is legally available [128]. Supplementation of healthy adults has not resulted in any reported adverse effects or changes in liver or kidney function [129]. Numerous studies have found significantly increased muscle size and strength when CM was added to a strength training program [130-134]. In many of these studies, 1-2 kg increases in total body mass were observed after CM loading of 20 g/day for 4–28 days [135]. However, the loading phase may not be necessary. Loading 20 g CM per day has been shown to increase muscle total creatine by approximately 20 percent and this level of muscle creatine was maintained with 2 g CM daily for 30 days [136]. However, the same study also observed a 20 percent increase in muscle creatine when 3 g CM was supplemented daily for 28 days, indicating the loading phase may not be necessary to increase muscle creatine concentrations.

Recently, alternative forms of creatine, such as creatine ethyl ester (CEE) and Kre Alkalyn (KA) have been marketed as superior forms of creatine to CM; however, as of this time these claims have not been supported by scientific studies. Tallon and Child [137,138] found that a greater portion of CEE and KA are degraded in the stomach than CM. Additionally, recent investigations have shown that 28–42 days of CEE or KA supplementation did not increase muscle creatine concentrations more than CM [139,140]. Thus, it appears that CM may be the most effective form of creatine.

Beta-alanine

Beta-alanine (BA) is becoming an increasingly popular supplement among bodybuilders. Once consumed, BA enters the circulation and is up-taken by skeletal muscle where it is used to synthesize carnosine, a pH buffer in muscle that is particularly important during anaerobic exercise such as sprinting or weightlifting [141]. Indeed, consumption of 6.4 g BA daily for four weeks has been shown to increase muscle carnosine levels by 64.2% [142]. Moreover, supplementation with BA for 4–10 weeks has been shown to increase knee extension torque by up to 6% [143], improve workload and time to fatigue during high intensity cardio [144-148], improve muscle resistance to fatigue during strength training [149], increase lean mass by approximately 1 kg [147] and significantly reduce perceptions of fatigue [150]. Additionally, the combination of BA and CM may increase performance of high intensity endurance exercise [151] and has been shown to increase lean mass and decrease body fat percentage more than CM alone [152]. However, not all studies have shown improvements in performance with BA supplementation [143,153,154]. To clarify these discrepancies, Hobson et al. [155] conducted a meta-analysis of 15 studies on BA supplementation and concluded that BA significantly increased exercise capacity and improved exercise performance on 60-240 s (ES = 0.665) and >240 s (ES = 0.368) exercise bouts.

Although BA appears to improve exercise performance, the long-term safety of BA has only been partially explored. Currently, the only known side effect of BA is unpleasant symptoms of parasthesia reported after consumption of large dosages; however, this can be minimized through consumption of smaller dosages throughout the day [142]. While BA appears to be relatively safe in the short-term, the long-term safety is unknown. In cats, an addition of 5 percent BA to drinking water for 20 weeks has been shown to deplete taurine and result in damage to the brain; however, taurine is an essential amino acid for cats but not for humans and it is unknown if the smaller dosages consumed by humans could result in similar effects [156]. BA may increase exercise performance and increase lean mass in bodybuilders and currently appears to be safe; however, studies are needed to determine the long-term safety of BA consumption.

HMB

Beta-hydroxy-beta-methylbutyrate (HMB) is a metabolite of the amino acid leucine that has been shown to decrease muscle protein catabolism and increase muscle protein synthesis [157,158]. The safety of HMB supplementation has been widely studied and no adverse effects on liver enzymes, kidney function, cholesterol, white blood cells, hemoglobin, or blood glucose have been observed [159-161]. Furthermore, two meta-analyses on HMB supplementation have concluded that HMB is safe and does not result in any major side effects [159,160]. HMB may actually decrease blood pressure, total and LDL cholesterol, especially in hypercholesterolemic individuals.

HMB is particularly effective in catabolic populations such as the elderly and patients with chronic disease [162]. However, studies on the effectiveness of HMB in trained, non-calorically restricted populations have been mixed. Reasons for discrepancies in the results of HMB supplementation studies in healthy populations may be due to many factors including clustering of data in these meta-analysis to include many studies from similar groups, poorly designed, non-periodized training protocols, small sample sizes, and lack of specificity between training and testing conditions [163]. However, as a whole HMB appears to be effective in a majority of studies with longer-duration, more intense, periodized training protocols and may be beneficial to bodybuilders, particularly during planned over-reaching phases of training [164]. While the authors hypothesize that HMB may be effective in periods of increased catabolism, such as during contest preparation, the efficacy of HMB on maintenance of lean mass in dieting athletes has not been investigated in a long-term study. Therefore, future studies are needed to determine the effectiveness of HMB during caloric restriction in healthy, lean, trained athletes.

Branched chain amino acids

Branched chain amino acids (BCAA's) make up 14-18% of amino acids in skeletal muscle proteins and are quite possibly the most widely used supplements among natural bodybuilders [165]. Of the BCAA's, leucine is of particular interest because it has been shown to stimulate protein synthesis to an equal extent as a mixture of all amino acids [166]. However, ingestion of leucine alone can lead to depletion of plasma valine and isoleucine; therefore, all three amino acids need to be consumed to prevent plasma depletion of any one of the BCAA's [167]. Recently, the safe upper limit of leucine was set at 550 mg/kg bodyweight/day in adult men; however, future studies are needed to determine the safe upper limit for both other populations and a mixture of all 3 BCAA's [168].

Numerous acute studies in animals and humans have shown that consumption of either essential amino acids, BCAA's, or leucine either at rest or following exercise increases skeletal muscle protein synthesis, decreases muscle protein degradation, or both [27,169-172]; however, there are few long-term studies of BCAA supplementation in resistance-trained athletes. Stoppani et al. [173] supplemented trained subjects with either 14 g BCAAs, whey protein, or a carbohydrate placebo for eight weeks during a periodized strength training routine. After training the BCAA group had a 4 kg increase in lean mass, 2% decrease in body fat percentage, and 6 kg increase in bench press 10 repetition maximum. All changes were significant compared to the other groups. However, it should be noted that this data is only available as an abstract and has yet to undergo the rigors of peer-review.

The use of BCAA's between meals may also be beneficial to keep protein synthesis elevated. Recent data from animal models suggest that consumption of BCAA's between meals can overcome the refractory response in protein synthesis that occurs when plasma amino acids are elevated, yet protein synthesis is reduced [174]. However, long-term human studies examining the effects of a diet in which BCAA's are consumed between meals on lean mass and strength have not been done to date. It should also be noted that BCAA metabolism in humans and rodents differ and the results from rodent studies with BCAA's may not translate in human models [175]. Therefore, long-term studies are needed in humans to determine the effectiveness of this practice.

Based on the current evidence, it is clear BCAA's stimulate protein synthesis acutely and one study [173] has indicated that BCAA's may be able to increase lean mass and strength when added to a strength training routine; however, additional long-term studies are needed to determine the effects of BCAA's on lean mass and strength in trained athletes. In addition, studies are needed on the effectiveness of BCAA supplementation in individuals following a vegetarian diet in which consumption of high-quality proteins are low as this may be population that may benefit from BCAA consumption. Furthermore, the effects of BCAA ingestion between meals needs to be further investigated in a long-term human study.

Arginine

"NO supplements" containing arginine are consumed by bodybuilders pre-workout in an attempt to increase blood flow to the muscle during exercise, increase protein synthesis, and improve exercise performance. However, there is little scientific evidence to back these claims. Fahs et al. [176] supplemented healthy young men with 7 g arginine or a placebo prior to exercise and observed no significant change in blood flow following exercise. Additionally, Tang et al. [177] supplemented either 10 g arginine or a placebo prior to exercise and found no significant increase in blood flow or protein synthesis following exercise. Moreover, arginine is a non essential amino acid and prior work has established that essential amino acids alone stimulate protein synthesis [178]. Based on these findings, it appears that arginine does not significantly increase blood flow or enhance protein synthesis following exercise.

The effects of arginine supplementation on performance are controversial. Approximately one-half of acute and chronic studies on arginine and exercise performance have found significant benefits with arginine supplementation, while the other one-half has found no significant benefits [179]. Moreover, Greer et al. [180] found that arginine supplementation significantly reduced muscular endurance by 2–4 repetitions on chin up and push up endurance tests. Based on these results, the authors of a recent review concluded that arginine supplementation had little impact on exercise performance in healthy individuals [181]. Although the effects of arginine on blood flow, protein synthesis, and exercise performance require further investigation, dosages commonly consumed by athletes are well below the observed safe level of 20 g/d and do not appear to be harmful [182].

Citrulline malate

Citrulline malate (CitM) has recently become a popular supplement among bodybuilders; however, there has been little scientific research in healthy humans with this compound. CitM is hypothesized to improve performance through three mechanisms: 1) citrulline is important part of the urea cycle and may participate in ammonia clearance, 2) malate is a tricarboxylic acid cycle intermediate that may reduce lactic acid accumulation, and 3) citrulline can be converted to arginine; however, as discussed previously, arginine does not appear to have an ergogenic effect in young healthy athletes so it is unlikely CitM exerts an ergogenic effect through this mechanism [179,183].

Supplementation with CitM for 15 days has been shown to increase ATP production by 34% during exercise, increase the rate of phosphocreatine recovery after exercise by 20%, and reduce perceptions of fatigue [184]. Moreover, ingestion of 8 g CitM prior to a chest workout significantly increased repetitions performed by approximately 53% and decreased soreness by 40% at 24 and 48 hours post-workout [183]. Furthermore, Stoppani et al. [173] in an abstract reported a 4 kg increase in lean mass, 2 kg decrease in body fat percentage, and a 6 kg increase in 10 repetition maximum bench press after consumption of a drink containing 14 g BCAA, glutamine, and CitM during workouts for eight weeks; although, it is not clear to what degree CitM contributed to the outcomes observed. However, not all studies have supported ergogenic effects of CitM. Sureda et al. [185] found no significant difference in race time when either 6 g CitM or a placebo were consumed prior to a 137 km cycling stage. Hickner et al. [186] found that treadmill time to exhaustion was significantly impaired, with the time taken to reach exhaustion occurring on average seven seconds earlier following CitM consumption.

Additionally, the long-term safety of CitM is unknown. Therefore, based on the current literature a decision on the efficacy of CitM cannot be made. Future studies are needed to conclusively determine if CitM is ergogenic and to determine its long term safety.

Glutamine

Glutamine is the most abundant non-essential amino acid in muscle and is commonly consumed as a nutritional supplement. Glutamine supplementation in quantities below 14 g/d appear to be safe in healthy adults [182]; however, at present there is little scientific evidence to support the use of glutamine in healthy athletes [187]. Acutely, glutamine supplementation has not been shown to significantly improve exercise performance [188,189], improve buffering capacity [189], help to maintain immune function or reduce muscle soreness after exercise [187]. Long-term supplementation studies including glutamine in cocktails along with CM, whey protein, BCAA's, and/or CitM have shown 1.5 – 2 kg increases in lean mass and 6 kg increase in 10RM bench press strength [173,190]. However, the role of glutamine in these changes is unclear. Only one study [191] has investigated the effects of glutamine supplementation alone in conjunction with a six week strength training program. No significant differences in muscle size, strength, or muscle protein degradation were observed between groups. Although the previous studies do not support the use of glutamine in bodybuilders during contest preparation, it should be noted that glutamine may be beneficial for gastrointestinal health and peptide uptake in stressed populations [192]; therefore, it may be beneficial in dieting bodybuilders who represent a stressed population. As a whole, the results of previous studies do not support use of glutamine as an ergogenic supplement; however, future studies are needed to determine the role of glutamine on gastrointestinal health and peptide transport in dieting bodybuilders.

Caffeine

Caffeine is perhaps the most common pre-workout stimulant consumed by bodybuilders. Numerous studies support the use of caffeine to improve performance during endurance training [193,194], sprinting [195,196], and strength training [197-199]. However, not all studies support use of caffeine to improve performance in strength training [200,201]. It should be noted that many of the studies that found increases in strength training performance supplemented with larger (5–6 mg/kg) dosages of caffeine. However, this dosage of caffeine is at the end of dosages that are considered safe (6 mg/kg/day) [202]. Additionally, it appears that regular consumption of caffeine may result in a reduction of ergogenic effects [203]. Therefore, it appears that 5–6 mg/kg caffeine taken prior to exercise is effective in improving exercise performance; however, caffeine use may need to be cycled in order for athletes to obtain the maximum ergogenic effect.

Micronutrients

Several previous studies have observed deficiencies in intakes of micronutrients, such as vitamin D, calcium, zinc, magnesium, and iron, in dieting bodybuilders [3,17,18,204,205]. However, it should be noted that these studies were all published nearly 2 decades ago and that micronutrient deficiencies likely occurred due to elimination of foods or food groups and monotony of food selection [3,205]. Therefore, future studies are needed to determine if these deficiencies would present while eating a variety of foods and using the contest preparation approach described herein. Although the current prevalence of micronutrient deficiencies in competitive bodybuilders is unknown, based on the previous literature, a low-dose micronutrient supplement may be beneficial for natural bodybuilders during contest preparation; however, future studies are needed to verify this recommendation.

Peak week

In an attempt to enhance muscle size and definition by reducing extracellular water content, many bodybuilders engage in fluid, electrolyte, and carbohydrate manipulation in the final days and hours before competing [2,60,206]. The effect of electrolyte manipulation and dehydration on visual appearance has not been studied, however it may be a dangerous practice [207]. Furthermore, dehydration could plausibly degrade appearance considering that extracellular water is not only present in the subcutaneous layer. A significant amount is located in the vascular system. Thus, the common practice of "pumping up" to increase muscle size and definition by increasing blood flow to the muscle with light, repetitive weight lifting prior to stepping on stage [208] could be compromised by dehydration or electrolyte imbalance. Furthermore, dehydration reduces total body hydration. A large percentage of muscle tissue mass is water and dehydration results in decreases in muscle water content [209] and therefore muscle size, which may negatively impact the appearance of muscularity.

In the final days before competing, bodybuilders commonly practice carbohydrate loading similar to endurance athletes in an attempt to raise muscle-glycogen levels and increase muscle size [4,18,60,208]. In the only direct study of this practice, no significant quantitative change in muscle girth was found to occur [208]. However, an isocaloric diet was used, with only a change in the percentage of carbohydrate contributing to the diet. If total calories had also been increased, greater levels of glycogen might have been stored which could have changed the outcome of this study. Additionally, unlike the subjects in this study bodybuilders prior to carbohydrate loading have reduced glycogen levels from a long calorically restricted diet and it is possible in this state that carbohydrate loading might effect a visual change. Furthermore, bodybuilding performance is measured subjectively, thus analysis of girth alone may not discern subtle visual changes which impact competitive success. Lastly, some bodybuilders alter the amount of carbohydrate loaded based on the visual outcome, increasing the amount if the desired visual change does not occur [60]. Thus, an analysis of a static carbohydrate load may not accurately represent the dynamic nature of actual carbohydrate loading practices.

In fact, in an observational study of competitive bodybuilders in the days before competition who loaded carbohydrates, subjects showed a 4.9% increase in biceps thickness the final day before competition compared to six weeks prior [4]. Although it is unknown if this was caused by increased muscle glycogen, it is unlikely it was due to muscle mass accrual since the final weeks of preparation are often marked by decreases not increases in LBM [6]. Future studies of this practice should include a qualitative analysis of visual changes and analyze the effects of concurrent increases in percentage of carbohydrates as well as total calories.

At this time it is unknown whether dehydration or electrolyte manipulation improves physique appearance. What is known is that these practices are dangerous and have the potential to worsen it. It is unclear if carbohydrate loading has an impact on appearance and if so, how significant the effect is. However, the recommended muscle-sparing practice by some researchers to increase the carbohydrate content of the diet in the final weeks of preparation [6] might achieve any proposed theoretical benefits of carbohydrate loading. If carbohydrate loading is utilized, a trial run before competition once the competitor has reached or nearly reached competition leanness should be attempted to develop an individualized strategy. However, a week spent on a trial run consuming increased carbohydrates and calories may slow fat loss, thus ample time in the diet would be required.

Psychosocial issues

Competitive bodybuilding requires cyclical periods of weight gain and weight loss for competition. In a study by Anderson et al. [207], it was found that 46% of a group of male drug free bodybuilders reported episodes of binge eating after competitions. One third to half reported anxiety, short tempers or anger when preparing for competition and most (81.5%) reported preoccupation with food.

Competitive male bodybuilders exhibit high rates of weight and shape preoccupation, binge eating and bulimia nervosa. However, they exhibit less eating-related and general psychopathology compared to men already diagnosed with bulimia nervosa [210]. Often they are more focused on muscle gain versus fat loss when compared to males with eating disorders [211]. That being said, this may change during preparation for competition when body builders need to reduce body fat levels.

Muscle dysmorphia is higher in male competitive natural bodybuilders than in collegiate football players and non-competitive weight trainers for physique [212]. However, the psychosocial profile of competitive bodybuilders is rather complex. Despite exhibiting greater risk for eating disturbances and a greater psychological investment in their physical appearance, they may have greater levels of physique satisfaction compared to non-competitive weight lifters and athletically active men [213]. Also, male bodybuilders are not a body-image homogenous group when experience is taken into account. Novice bodybuilders show greater levels of dissatisfaction with their muscle size and greater tendencies towards unhealthy and obsessive behavior [214]. Furthermore, the physical effects of semi-starvation in men can approximate the signs and symptoms of eating disorders such as anorexia nervosa and bulimia nervosa [11]. Thus, many of the psychosocial effects and behaviors seen in competitive bodybuilders may be at least partially the result of a prolonged diet and becoming very lean. When these factors are all considered it may indicate that at least in men, competitive bodybuilding drives certain psychosocial behaviors, in addition to those with prior existing behaviors being drawn to the sport.

However this may not be as much the case with female bodybuilders. Walberg [215] when comparing competitive bodybuilders to non-competitive female weight lifters, found that among bodybuilders 42% used to be anorexic, 67% were terrified of becoming fat, and 50% experienced uncontrollable urges to eat. All of these markers were significantly higher in bodybuilders than in non-competitors. Furthermore, it was found that menstrual dysfunction was more common among the bodybuilders. In agreement with this finding, Kleiner et al. [2] reported that 25% of female bodybuilding competitors reported abnormal menstrual cycles.

Competitive bodybuilders are not alone in their risk and disposition towards behaviors that carry health concerns. Elite athletes in aesthetic and weight-class sports as a whole share these risks [216]. In some sports, minimum body fat percentages can be established and minimum hydration levels for weighing in can be set. However, because bodybuilding performance is directly impacted by body fat percentage and not by weight per se, these regulatory changes to the sport are unlikely. Therefore, competitors and trainers should be aware of the potential psychosocial risks involved with competition. Open and frequent communication on these topics should be practiced and competitors and trainers should be aware of the signs and symptoms of unhealthy behaviors. Early therapeutic intervention by specialists with experience in competitive bodybuilding and eating disorders should occur if disordered eating patterns or psychological distress occurs.

Limitations

The primary limitation of this review is the lack of large-scale long-term studies on competitive natural bodybuilders. To circumvent this, long-term studies on skeletal muscle hypertrophy and body fat loss in athletic dieting human populations were preferentially selected. In the absence of such studies, acute studies and/or animal studies were selected.

Competing interests

The authors declare that they have no competing interests.

Authors' contributions

ERH developed the concept for this manuscript and wrote the sections on caloric intake, macronutrients, psychosocial issues and "peak week". AAA wrote the sections on nutrient timing and meal frequency. PJF wrote the abstract, methods, limitations, and the section on dietary supplementation. All authors read and approved the final manuscript.

Author details

[1]Sport Performance Research in New Zealand (SPRINZ) at AUT Millennium Institute, AUT University, 17 Antares Place, Mairangi Bay, Auckland 0632, New Zealand. [2]California State University, Northridge, CA, USA. [3]Division of Nutritional Sciences, University of Illinois, Urbana, IL, USA.

References

1. Scott BR, Lockie RG, Knight TJ, Clark AC, De Jonge XAKJ: **A comparison of methods to quantify the in-season training load of professional soccer players.** *Int J Sports Physiol Perform* 2013, **8**:195–202.
2. Kleiner SM, Bazzarre TL, Litchford MD: **Metabolic profiles, diet, and health practices of championship male and female bodybuilders.** *J Am Diet Assoc* 1990, **90**:962–967.
3. Sandoval WM, Heyward VH: **Food selection patterns of bodybuilders.** *Int J Sport Nutr* 1991, **1**:61–68.
4. Bamman MM, Hunter GR, Newton LE, Roney RK, Khaled MA: **Changes in body composition, diet, and strength of bodybuilders during the 12 weeks prior to competition.** *J Sports Med Phys Fitness* 1993, **33**:383–391.
5. Lambert CP, Frank LL, Evans WJ: **Macronutrient considerations for the sport of bodybuilding.** *Sports Med* 2004, **34**:317–327.
6. Maestu J, Eliakim A, Jurimae J, Valter I, Jurimae T: **Anabolic and catabolic hormones and energy balance of the male bodybuilders during the preparation for the competition.** *J Strength Cond Res* 2010, **24**:1074–1081.
7. Hall KD: **What is the required energy deficit per unit weight loss?** *Int J Obes* 2007, **32**:573–576.
8. MacLean PS, Bergouignan A, Cornier M-A, Jackman MR: **Biology's response to dieting: the impetus for weight regain.** *Am J Physiol Regul Integr Comp Physiol* 2011, **301**:R581–R600.
9. Camps SG, Verhoef SP, Westerterp KR: **Weight loss, weight maintenance, and adaptive thermogenesis.** *Am J Clin Nutr* 2013, **97**:990–994.
10. Johannsen DL, Knuth ND, Huizenga R, Rood JC, Ravussin E, Hall KD: **Metabolic slowing with massive weight loss despite preservation of fat-free mass.** *J Clin Endocrinol Metab* 2012, **97**:2489–2496.
11. University of Minnesota. Laboratory of Physiological Hygiene, Keys A: *The Biology Of Human Starvation.* Minneapolis: University of Minnesota Press; 1950.
12. Trexler E, Smith-Ryan A, Norton L: **Metabolic adaptation to weight loss: implications for the athlete.** *J Int Soc Sport Nutr* 2014, **11**:7.
13. Garthe I, Raastad T, Refsnes PE, Koivisto A, Sundgot-Borgen J: **Effect of two different weight-loss rates on body composition and strength and power-related performance in elite athletes.** *Int J Sport Nutr Exerc Metab* 2011, **21**:97–104.
14. Forbes GB: **Body fat content influences the body composition response to nutrition and exercise.** *Ann N Y Acad Sci* 2000, **904**:359–365.
15. Hall KD: **Body fat and fat-free mass inter-relationships: Forbes's theory revisited.** *Br J Nutr* 2007, **97**:1059–1063.
16. Mero AA, Huovinen H, Matintupa O, Hulmi JJ, Puurtinen R, Hohtari H, Karila T: **Moderate energy restriction with high protein diet results in healthier outcome in women.** *J Int Soc Sports Nutr* 2010, **7**:4.
17. Sandoval WM, Heyward VH, Lyons TM: **Comparison of body composition, exercise and nutritional profiles of female and male body builders at competition.** *J Sports Med Phys Fitness* 1989, **29**:63–70.
18. Walberg-Rankin J, Edmonds CE, Gwazdauskas FC: **Diet and weight changes of female bodybuilders before and after competition.** *Int J Sport Nutr* 1993, **3**:87–102.
19. Withers RT, Noell CJ, Whittingham NO, Chatterton BE, Schultz CG, Keeves JP: **Body composition changes in elite male bodybuilders during preparation for competition.** *Aust J Sci Med Sport* 1997, **29**:11–16.
20. van der Ploeg GE, Brooks AG, Withers RT, Dollman J, Leaney F, Chatterton BE: **Body composition changes in female bodybuilders during preparation for competition.** *Eur J Clin Nutr* 2001, **55**:268–277.
21. Newton LE, Hunter GR, Bammon M, Roney RK: **Changes in psychological state and self-reported diet during various phases of training in competitive bodybuilders.** *J Strength Cond Res* 1993, **7**:153–158.
22. Butterfield GE: **Whole-body protein utilization in humans.** *Med Sci Sports Exerc* 1987, **19**:S157–S165.
23. Lemon PW: **Beyond the zone: protein needs of active individuals.** *J Am Coll Nutr* 2000, **19**:513S–521S.
24. Phillips SM: **Dietary protein for athletes: from requirements to metabolic advantage.** *Appl Physiol Nutr Metab* 2006, **31**:647–654.
25. Phillips SM, Moore DR, Tang JE: **A critical examination of dietary protein requirements, benefits, and excesses in athletes.** *Int J Sport Nutr Exerc Metab* 2007, **17**(Suppl):S58–S76.
26. Slater G, Phillips SM: **Nutrition guidelines for strength sports: sprinting, weightlifting, throwing events, and bodybuilding.** *J Sports Sci* 2011, **29**:S67–S77.
27. Tipton KD, Wolfe RR: **Protein and amino acids for athletes.** *J Sports Sci* 2004, **22**:65–79.
28. Phillips SM, Van Loon LJ: **Dietary protein for athletes: from requirements to optimum adaptation.** *J Sports Sci* 2011, **29**(Suppl 1):S29–S38.
29. Mettler S, Mitchell N, Tipton KD: **Increased protein intake reduces lean body mass loss during weight loss in athletes.** *Med Sci Sports Exerc* 2010, **42**:326–337.
30. Millward DJ: **Macronutrient intakes as determinants of dietary protein and amino acid adequacy.** *J Nutr* 2004, **134**:1588S–1596S.
31. Stiegler P, Cunliffe A: **The role of diet and exercise for the maintenance of fat-free mass and resting metabolic rate during weight loss.** *Sports Med* 2006, **36**:239–262.
32. Walberg JL, Leidy MK, Sturgill DJ, Hinkle DE, Ritchey SJ, Sebolt DR: **Macronutrient content of a hypoenergy diet affects nitrogen retention and muscle function in weight lifters.** *Int J Sports Med* 1988, **9**:261–266.
33. Helms ER, Zinn C, Rowlands DS, Brown SR: **A systematic review of dietary protein during caloric restriction in resistance trained lean athletes: a case for higher intakes.** *Int J Sport Nutr Exerc Metab* 2013, Epub ahead of print.
34. Elia M, Stubbs RJ, Henry CJ: **Differences in fat, carbohydrate, and protein metabolism between lean and obese subjects undergoing total starvation.** *Obes Res* 1999, **7**:597–604.
35. Phillips SM: **Protein requirements and supplementation in strength sports.** *Nutrition* 2004, **20**:689–695.
36. Tarnopolsky MA: **Building muscle: nutrition to maximize bulk and strength adaptations to resistance exercise training.** *Eur J Sport Sci* 2008, **8**:67–76.
37. Tipton KD: **Protein for adaptations to exercise training.** *Eur J Sport Sci* 2008, **8**:107–118.
38. Wilson J, Wilson GJ: **Contemporary issues in protein requirements and consumption for resistance trained athletes.** *J Int Soc Sports Nutr* 2006, **3**:7–27.

39. Celejowa I, Homa M: **Food intake, nitrogen and energy balance in Polish weight lifters, during a training camp.** *Nutr Metab* 1970, **12**:259–274.
40. Pasiakos SM, Cao JJ, Margolis LM, Sauter ER, Whigham LD, McClung JP, Rood JC, Carbone JW, Combs GF Jr, Young AJ: **Effects of high-protein diets on fat-free mass and muscle protein synthesis following weight loss: a randomized controlled trial.** *FASEB J* 2013, **27**:3837–3847.
41. Leveritt M, Abernethy PJ: **Effects of carbohydrate restriction on strength performance.** *J Strength Cond Res* 1999, **13**:52–57.
42. Haff GG, Koch AJ, Potteiger JA, Kuphal KE, Magee LM, Green SB, Jakicic JJ: **Carbohydrate supplementation attenuates muscle glycogen loss during acute bouts of resistance exercise.** *Int J Sport Nutr Exerc Metab* 2000, **10**:326–339.
43. MacDougall JD, Ray S, Sale DG, McCartney N, Lee P, Garner S: **Muscle substrate utilization and lactate production.** *Can J Appl Physiol* 1999, **24**:209–215.
44. Layman DK, Boileau RA, Erickson DJ, Painter JE, Shiue H, Sather C, Christou DD: **A reduced ratio of dietary carbohydrate to protein improves body composition and blood lipid profiles during weight loss in adult women.** *J Nutr* 2003, **133**:411–417.
45. Layman DK, Baum JI: **Dietary protein impact on glycemic control during weight loss.** *J Nutr* 2004, **134**:968S–973S.
46. Halton TL, Hu FB: **The effects of high protein diets on thermogenesis, satiety and weight loss: a critical review.** *J Am Coll Nutr* 2004, **23**:373–385.
47. Veldhorst M, Smeets A, Soenen S, Hochstenbach-Waelen A, Hursel R, Diepvens K, Lejeune M, Luscombe-Marsh N, Westerterp-Plantenga M: **Protein-induced satiety: effects and mechanisms of different proteins.** *Physiol Behav* 2008, **94**:300–307.
48. Westerterp-Plantenga MS: **Protein intake and energy balance.** *Regul Pept* 2008, **149**:67–69.
49. Smeets AJ, Soenen S, Luscombe-Marsh ND, Ueland O, Westerterp-Plantenga MS: **Energy expenditure, satiety, and plasma ghrelin, glucagon-like peptide 1, and peptide tyrosine-tyrosine concentrations following a single high-protein lunch.** *J Nutr* 2008, **138**:698–702.
50. Cook CM, Haub MD: **Low-carbohydrate diets and performance.** *Curr Sports Med Rep* 2007, **6**:225–229.
51. Volek JS, Kraemer WJ, Bush JA, Incledon T, Boetes M: **Testosterone and cortisol in relationship to dietary nutrients and resistance exercise.** *J Appl Physiol* 1997, **82**:49–54.
52. Sallinen J, Pakarinen A, Ahtiainen J, Kraemer WJ, Volek JS, Häkkinen K: **Relationship between diet and serum anabolic hormone responses to heavy-resistance exercise in men.** *Int J Sports Med* 2004, **25**:627–633.
53. Hämäläinen EK, Adlercreutz H, Puska P, Pietinen P: **Decrease of serum total and free testosterone during a low-fat high-fibre diet.** *J Steroid Biochem* 1983, **18**:369–370.
54. Dorgan JF, Judd JT, Longcope C, Brown C, Schatzkin A, Clevidence BA, Campbell WS, Nair PP, Franz C, Kahle L, Taylor PR: **Effects of dietary fat and fiber on plasma and urine androgens and estrogens in men: a controlled feeding study.** *Am J Clin Nutr* 1996, **64**:850–855.
55. Hämäläinen EK, Adlercreutz H, Puska P, Pietinen P: **Diet and serum sex hormones in healthy men.** *J Steroid Biochem* 1984, **20**:459–464.
56. Suryanarayana BV, Kent JR, Meister L, Parlow AF: **Pituitary-gonadal axis during prolonged total starvation in obese men.** *Am J Clin Nutr* 1969, **22**:767–770.
57. Rossow LM, Fukuda DH, Fahs CA, Loenneke JP, Stout JR: **Natural bodybuilding competition preparation and recovery: a 12-month case study.** *Int J Sports Physiol Perform* 2013, **8**:582–592.
58. Loucks AB, Verdun M, Heath EM: **Low energy availability, not stress of exercise, alters LH pulsatility in exercising women.** *J Appl Physiol* 1998, **84**:37–46.
59. Bird SP: **Strength nutrition: maximizing your anabolic potential.** *Strength Cond J* 2010, **32**:80–86.
60. Shephard RJ: **Electrolyte manipulation in female body-builders.** *Br J Sports Med* 1994, **28**:60–61.
61. Too D, Wakayama EJ, Locati LL, Landwer GE: **Effect of a precompetition bodybuilding diet and training regimen on body composition and blood chemistry.** *J Sports Med Phys Fitness* 1998, **38**:245–252.
62. Sawyer JC, Wood RJ, Davidson PW, Collins SM, Matthews TD, Gregory SM, Paolone VJ: **Effects of a short-term carbohydrate-restricted diet on strength and power performance.** *J Strength Cond Res* 2013, **27**:2255–2262.
63. Soenen S, Bonomi AG, Lemmens SGT, Scholte J, Thijssen MAMA, van Berkum F, Westerterp-Plantenga MS: **Relatively high-protein or 'low-carb' energy-restricted diets for body weight loss and body weight maintenance?** *Physiol Behav* 2012, **107**:374–380.
64. Paoli A, Grimaldi K, D'Agostino D, Cenci L, Moro T, Bianco A, Palma A: **Ketogenic diet does not affect strength performance in elite artistic gymnasts.** *J Int Soc Sports Nutr* 2012, **9**:34.
65. Essen-Gustavsson B, Tesch PA: **Glycogen and triglyceride utilization in relation to muscle metabolic characteristics in men performing heavy-resistance exercise.** *Eur J Appl Physiol* 1990, **61**:5–10.
66. Goedecke JH, Gibson ASC, Grobler L, Collins M, Noakes TD, Lambert EV: **Determinants of the variability in respiratory exchange ratio at rest and during exercise in trained athletes.** *Am J Physiol Endocrinol Metab* 2000, **279**:E1325–E1334.
67. Cornier MA, Donahoo WT, Pereira R, Gurevich I, Westergren R, Enerback S, Eckel PJ, Goalstone ML, Hill JO, Eckel RH, Draznin B: **Insulin sensitivity determines the effectiveness of dietary macronutrient composition on weight loss in obese women.** *Obes Res* 2005, **13**:703–709.
68. Pendergast DR, Leddy JJ, Venkatraman JT: **A perspective on fat intake in athletes.** *J Am Coll Nutr* 2000, **19**:345–350.
69. Turocy PS, DePalma BF, Horswill CA, Laquale KM, Martin TJ, Perry AC, Somova MJ, Utter AC: **National athletic trainers' association position statement: safe weight loss and maintenance practices in sport and exercise.** *J Athl Train* 2011, **46**:322–336.
70. Ivy JL, Katz AL, Cutler CL, Sherman WM, Coyle EF: **Muscle glycogen synthesis after exercise: effect of time of carbohydrate ingestion.** *J Appl Physiol* 1988, **64**:1480–1485.
71. Jentjens R, Jeukendrup A: **Determinants of post-exercise glycogen synthesis during short-term recovery.** *Sports Med* 2003, **33**:117–144.
72. Robergs RA, Pearson DR, Costill DL, Fink WJ, Pascoe DD, Benedict MA, Lambert CP, Zachweija JJ: **Muscle glycogenolysis during differing intensities of weight-resistance exercise.** *J Appl Physiol* 1991, **70**:1700–1706.
73. Roy BD, Tarnopolsky MA: **Influence of differing macronutrient intakes on muscle glycogen resynthesis after resistance exercise.** *J Appl Physiol* 1998, **84**:890–896.
74. Fujita S, Dreyer HC, Drummond MJ, Glynn EL, Volpi E, Rasmussen BB: **Essential amino acid and carbohydrate ingestion before resistance exercise does not enhance postexercise muscle protein synthesis.** *J Appl Physiol* 2009, **106**:1730–1739.
75. Baty JJ, Hwang H, Ding Z, Bernard JR, Wang B, Kwon B, Ivy JL: **The effect of a carbohydrate and protein supplement on resistance exercise performance, hormonal response, and muscle damage.** *J Strength Cond Res* 2007, **21**:321–329.
76. Tipton KD, Elliott TA, Cree MG, Aarsland AA, Sanford AP, Wolfe RR: **Stimulation of net muscle protein synthesis by whey protein ingestion before and after exercise.** *Am J Physiol Endocrinol Metab* 2007, **292**:E71–E76.
77. Bird SP, Tarpenning KM, Marino FE: **Liquid carbohydrate/essential amino acid ingestion during a short-term bout of resistance exercise suppresses myofibrillar protein degradation.** *Metabolism* 2006, **55**:570–577.
78. Levenhagen DK, Gresham JD, Carlson MG, Maron DJ, Borel MJ, Flakoll PJ: **Postexercise nutrient intake timing in humans is critical to recovery of leg glucose and protein homeostasis.** *Am J Physiol Endocrinol Metab* 2001, **280**:E982–E993.
79. Tipton KD, Rasmussen BB, Miller SL, Wolf SE, Owens-Stovall SK, Petrini BE, Wolfe RR: **Timing of amino acid-carbohydrate ingestion alters anabolic response of muscle to resistance exercise.** *Am J Physiol Endocrinol Metab* 2001, **281**:E197–E206.
80. Cribb PJ, Hayes A: **Effects of supplement timing and resistance exercise on skeletal muscle hypertrophy.** *Med Sci Sports Exerc* 2006, **38**:1918–1925.
81. Esmarck B, Andersen JL, Olsen S, Richter EA, Mizuno M, Kjaer M: **Timing of postexercise protein intake is important for muscle hypertrophy with resistance training in elderly humans.** *J Physiol* 2001, **535**:301–311.
82. Burk A, Timpmann S, Medijainen L, Vahi M, Oopik V: **Time-divided ingestion pattern of casein-based protein supplement stimulates an increase in fat-free body mass during resistance training in young untrained men.** *Nutr Res* 2009, **29**:405–413.
83. Hoffman JR, Ratamess NA, Tranchina CP, Rashti SL, Kang J, Faigenbaum AD: **Effect of protein-supplement timing on strength, power, and body-composition changes in resistance-trained men.** *Int J Sport Nutr Exerc Metab* 2009, **19**:172–185.
84. Wycherley TP, Noakes M, Clifton PM, Cleanthous X, Keogh JB, Brinkworth GD: **Timing of protein ingestion relative to resistance exercise training**

does not influence body composition, energy expenditure, glycaemic control or cardiometabolic risk factors in a hypocaloric, high protein diet in patients with type 2 diabetes. *Diabetes Obes Metab* 2010, **12**:1097–1105.

85. Weisgarber KD, Candow DG, Vogt ES: **Whey protein before and during resistance exercise has no effect on muscle mass and strength in untrained young adults.** *Int J Sport Nutr Exerc Metab* 2012, **22**:463–469.
86. Willoughby DS, Stout JR, Wilborn CD: **Effects of resistance training and protein plus amino acid supplementation on muscle anabolism, mass, and strength.** *Amino Acids* 2007, **32**:467–477.
87. Hulmi JJ, Kovanen V, Selanne H, Kraemer WJ, Hakkinen K, Mero AA: **Acute and long-term effects of resistance exercise with or without protein ingestion on muscle hypertrophy and gene expression.** *Amino Acids* 2009, **37**:297–308.
88. Verdijk LB, Jonkers RA, Gleeson BG, Beelen M, Meijer K, Savelberg HH, Wodzig WK, Dendale P, van Loon LJ: **Protein supplementation before and after exercise does not further augment skeletal muscle hypertrophy after resistance training in elderly men.** *Am J Clin Nutr* 2009, **89**:608–616.
89. Erskine RM, Fletcher G, Hanson B, Folland JP: **Whey protein does not enhance the adaptations to elbow flexor resistance training.** *Med Sci Sports Exerc* 2012, **44**:1791–1800.
90. Burd NA, West DW, Moore DR, Atherton PJ, Staples AW, Prior T, Tang JE, Rennie MJ, Baker SK, Phillips SM: **Enhanced amino acid sensitivity of myofibrillar protein synthesis persists for up to 24 h after resistance exercise in young men.** *J Nutr* 2011, **141**:568–573.
91. Deldicque L, De Bock K, Maris M, Ramaekers M, Nielens H, Francaux M, Hespel P: **Increased p70s6k phosphorylation during intake of a protein-carbohydrate drink following resistance exercise in the fasted state.** *Eur J Appl Physiol* 2010, **108**:791–800.
92. Moore DR, Robinson MJ, Fry JL, Tang JE, Glover EI, Wilkinson SB, Prior T, Tarnopolsky MA, Phillips SM: **Ingested protein dose response of muscle and albumin protein synthesis after resistance exercise in young men.** *Am J Clin Nutr* 2009, **89**:161–168.
93. Yang Y, Breen L, Burd NA, Hector AJ, Churchward-Venne TA, Josse AR, Tarnopolsky MA, Phillips SM: **Resistance exercise enhances myofibrillar protein synthesis with graded intakes of whey protein in older men.** *Br J Nutr* 2012, **108**:1–9.
94. Hamer HM, Wall BT, Kiskini A, de Lange A, Groen BB, Bakker JA, Gijsen AP, Verdijk LB, van Loon LJ: **Carbohydrate co-ingestion with protein does not further augment post-prandial muscle protein accretion in older men.** *Nutr Metab (Lond)* 2013, **10**:15.
95. Staples AW, Burd NA, West DW, Currie KD, Atherton PJ, Moore DR, Rennie MJ, Macdonald MJ, Baker SK, Phillips SM: **Carbohydrate does not augment exercise-induced protein accretion versus protein alone.** *Med Sci Sports Exerc* 2011, **43**:1154–1161.
96. Greenhaff PL, Karagounis LG, Peirce N, Simpson EJ, Hazell M, Layfield R, Wackerhage H, Smith K, Atherton P, Selby A, Rennie MJ: **Disassociation between the effects of amino acids and insulin on signaling, ubiquitin ligases, and protein turnover in human muscle.** *Am J Physiol Endocrinol Metab* 2008, **295**:E595–E604.
97. Koopman R, Beelen M, Stellingwerff T, Pennings B, Saris WH, Kies AK, Kuipers H, van Loon LJ: **Coingestion of carbohydrate with protein does not further augment postexercise muscle protein synthesis.** *Am J Physiol Endocrinol Metab* 2007, **293**:E833–E842.
98. Kerksick C, Harvey T, Stout J, Campbell B, Wilborn C, Kreider R, Kalman D, Ziegenfuss T, Lopez H, Landis J, Ivy JL, Antonio J: **International Society of Sports Nutrition position stand: nutrient timing.** *J Int Soc Sports Nutr* 2008, **5**:17.
99. Aragon AA, Schoenfeld BJ: **Nutrient timing revisited: is there a post-exercise anabolic window?** *J Int Soc Sports Nutr* 2013, **10**:5.
100. Taylor MA, Garrow JS: **Compared with nibbling, neither gorging nor a morning fast affect short-term energy balance in obese patients in a chamber calorimeter.** *Int J Obes Relat Metab Disord* 2001, **25**:519–528.
101. de Venne WP V-v, Westerterp KR: **Influence of the feeding frequency on nutrient utilization in man: consequences for energy metabolism.** *Eur J Clin Nutr* 1991, **45**:161–169.
102. Farshchi HR, Taylor MA, Macdonald IA: **Decreased thermic effect of food after an irregular compared with a regular meal pattern in healthy lean women.** *Int J Obes Relat Metab Disord* 2004, **28**:653–660.
103. Farshchi HR, Taylor MA, Macdonald IA: **Regular meal frequency creates more appropriate insulin sensitivity and lipid profiles compared with irregular meal frequency in healthy lean women.** *Eur J Clin Nutr* 2004, **58**:1071–1077.
104. Harvie MN, Pegington M, Mattson MP, Frystyk J, Dillon B, Evans G, Cuzick J, Jebb SA, Martin B, Cutler RG, Son TG, Maudsley S, Carlson OD, Egan JM, Flyvbjerg A, Howell A: **The effects of intermittent or continuous energy restriction on weight loss and metabolic disease risk markers: a randomized trial in young overweight women.** *Int J Obes* 2011, **35**:714–727.
105. Soeters MR, Lammers NM, Dubbelhuis PF, Ackermans M, Jonkers-Schuitema CF, Fliers E, Sauerwein HP, Aerts JM, Serlie MJ: **Intermittent fasting does not affect whole-body glucose, lipid, or protein metabolism.** *Am J Clin Nutr* 2009, **90**:1244–1251.
106. Arnal MA, Mosoni L, Boirie Y, Houlier ML, Morin L, Verdier E, Ritz P, Antoine JM, Prugnaud J, Beaufrere B, Mirand PP: **Protein feeding pattern does not affect protein retention in young women.** *J Nutr* 2000, **130**:1700–1704.
107. Arnal MA, Mosoni L, Boirie Y, Houlier ML, Morin L, Verdier E, Ritz P, Antoine JM, Prugnaud J, Beaufrere B, Mirand PP: **Protein pulse feeding improves protein retention in elderly women.** *Am J Clin Nutr* 1999, **69**:1202–1208.
108. La Bounty PM, Campbell BI, Wilson J, Galvan E, Berardi J, Kleiner SM, Kreider RB, Stout JR, Ziegenfuss T, Spano M, Smith A, Antonio J: **International Society of Sports Nutrition position stand: meal frequency.** *J Int Soc Sports Nutr* 2011, **8**:4.
109. Varady KA: **Intermittent versus daily calorie restriction: which diet regimen is more effective for weight loss?** *Obes Rev* 2011, **12**:e593–e601.
110. Bosy-Westphal A, Later W, Hitze B, Sato T, Kossel E, Gluer CC, Heller M, Muller MJ: **Accuracy of bioelectrical impedance consumer devices for measurement of body composition in comparison to whole body magnetic resonance imaging and dual X-ray absorptiometry.** *Obes Facts* 2008, **1**:319–324.
111. Pateyjohns IR, Brinkworth GD, Buckley JD, Noakes M, Clifton PM: **Comparison of three bioelectrical impedance methods with DXA in overweight and obese men.** *Obesity (Silver Spring)* 2006, **14**:2064–2070.
112. Neovius M, Hemmingsson E, Freyschuss B, Udden J: **Bioelectrical impedance underestimates total and truncal fatness in abdominally obese women.** *Obesity (Silver Spring)* 2006, **14**:1731–1738.
113. Stote KS, Baer DJ, Spears K, Paul DR, Harris GK, Rumpler WV, Strycula P, Najjar SS, Ferrucci L, Ingram DK, Longo DL, Mattson MP: **A controlled trial of reduced meal frequency without caloric restriction in healthy, normal-weight, middle-aged adults.** *Am J Clin Nutr* 2007, **85**:981–988.
114. Iwao S, Mori K, Sato Y: **Effects of meal frequency on body composition during weight control in boxers.** *Scand J Med Sci Sports* 1996, **6**:265–272.
115. Benardot D, Martin DE, Thompson WR, Roman SB: **Between-meal energy intake effects on body composition, performance, and totol caloric consumption in athletes.** *Med Sci Sports Exerc* 2005, **37**:S339.
116. Norton LE, Wilson GJ: **Optimal protein intake to maximize muscle protein synthesis: examinations of optimal meal protein intake.** *Agro Food Industry Hi-Tech* 2009, **20**:54–57.
117. Bohe J, Low JF, Wolfe RR, Rennie MJ: **Latency and duration of stimulation of human muscle protein synthesis during continuous infusion of amino acids.** *J Physiol* 2001, **532**:575–579.
118. Atherton PJ, Etheridge T, Watt PW, Wilkinson D, Selby A, Rankin D, Smith K, Rennie MJ: **Muscle full effect after oral protein: time-dependent concordance and discordance between human muscle protein synthesis and mTORC1 signaling.** *Am J Clin Nutr* 2010, **92**:1080–1088.
119. Munsters MJ, Saris WH: **Effects of meal frequency on metabolic profiles and substrate partitioning in lean healthy males.** *PLoS One* 2012, **7**:e38632.
120. Holmstrup M, Owens CM, Fairchild TJ, Kanaley JA: **Effect of meal freqnency on glucose and insulin excursions over the course of a day.** *Eur e-J Clin Nutr Metab* 2010, **5**:277–280.
121. Leidy HJ, Armstrong CL, Tang M, Mattes RD, Campbell WW: **The influence of higher protein intake and greater eating frequency on appetite control in overweight and obese men.** *Obesity (Silver Spring)* 2010, **18**:1725–1732.
122. Arciero PJ, Ormsbee MJ, Gentile CL, Nindl BC, Brestoff JR, Ruby M: **Increased protein intake and meal frequency reduces abdominal fat during energy balance and energy deficit.** *Obesity (Silver Spring)* 2013, **21**:1357–1366.
123. Adechian S, Balage M, Remond D, Migne C, Quignard-Boulange A, Marset-Baglieri A, Rousset S, Boirie Y, Gaudichon C, Dardevet D, Mosoni L: **Protein feeding pattern, casein feeding or milk soluble protein feeding did not change the evolution of body composition during a short-term weight loss program.** *Am J Physiol Endocrinol Metab* 2012, **303**:E973–E982.

124. Moore DR, Areta J, Coffey VG, Stellingwerff T, Phillips SM, Burke LM, Cleroux M, Godin JP, Hawley JA: **Daytime pattern of post-exercise protein intake affects whole-body protein turnover in resistance-trained males.** *Nutr Metab (Lond)* 2012, **9**:91.
125. Areta JL, Burke LM, Ross ML, Camera DM, West DW, Broad EM, Jeacocke NA, Moore DR, Stellingwerff T, Phillips SM, Hawley JA, Coffey VG: **Timing and distribution of protein ingestion during prolonged recovery from resistance exercise alters myofibrillar protein synthesis.** *J Physiol* 2013, **591**:2319–2331.
126. **OCB/NANBF/IFPA Drug Testing Guidelines.** [http://www.thenaturalmusclenetwork.com/OCB/forms/DrugTestingGuidelines.pdf]
127. Campbell B, Kreider RB, Ziegenfuss T, La Bounty P, Roberts M, Burke D, Landis J, Lopez H, Antonio J: **International Society of Sports Nutrition position stand: protein and exercise.** *J Int Soc Sports Nutr* 2007, **4**:8.
128. Buford TW, Kreider RB, Stout JR, Greenwood M, Campbell B, Spano M, Ziegenfuss T, Lopez H, Landis J, Antonio J: **International Society of Sports Nutrition position stand: creatine supplementation and exercise.** *J Int Soc Sports Nutr* 2007, **4**:6.
129. Kim H, Kim C, Carpentier A, Poortmans J: **Studies on the safety of creatine supplementation.** *Amino Acids* 2011, **40**:1409–1418.
130. Becque MD, Lochmann JD, Melrose DR: **Effects of oral creatine supplementation on muscular strength and body composition.** *Med Sci Sports Exerc* 2000, **32**:654–658.
131. Volek JS, Duncan ND, Mazzetti SA, Staron RS, Putukian M, Gomez AL, Pearson DR, Fink WJ, Kraemer WJ: **Performance and muscle fiber adaptations to creatine supplementation and heavy resistance training.** *Med Sci Sports Exerc* 1999, **31**:1147–1156.
132. Willoughby DS, Rosene J: **Effects of oral creatine and resistance training on myosin heavy chain expression.** *Med Sci Sports Exerc* 2001, **33**:1674–1681.
133. Vandenberghe K, Goris M, Van Hecke P, Van Leemputte M, Vangerven L, Hespel P: **Long-term creatine intake is beneficial to muscle performance during resistance training.** *J Appl Physiol* 1997, **83**:2055–2063.
134. Stone MH, Sanborn K, Smith LL, O'Bryant HS, Hoke T, Utter AC, Johnson RL, Boros R, Hruby J, Pierce KC, Stone ME, Garner B: **Effects of in-season (5 weeks) creatine and pyruvate supplementation on anaerobic performance and body composition in American football players.** *Int J Sport Nutr* 1999, **9**:146–165.
135. Persky AM, Brazeau GA: **Clinical pharmacology of the dietary supplement creatine monohydrate.** *Pharmacol Rev* 2001, **53**:161–176.
136. Hultman E, Soderlund K, Timmons JA, Cederblad G, Greenhaff PL: **Muscle creatine loading in men.** *J Appl Physiol* 1996, **81**:232–237.
137. Tallon MJ, Child R: **Kre-alkalyn suppplementation has no beneficial effect on creatine-to-creatinine conversion rates.** In *Book Kre-alkalyn suppplementation has no beneficial effect on creatine-to-creatinine conversion rates.* City: 2007.
138. Child RT MJ: **Creatine ethyl ester rapidly degrades to creatinine in stomach acid.** In *Book Creatine ethyl ester rapidly degrades to creatinine in stomach acid*; 2007.
139. Spillane M, Schoch R, Cooke M, Harvey T, Greenwood M, Kreider R, Willoughby DS: **The effects of creatine ethyl ester supplementation combined with heavy resistance training on body composition, muscle performance, and serum and muscle creatine levels.** *J Int Soc Sports Nutr* 2009, **6**:6.
140. Jagim AR, Oliver JM, Sanchez A, Galvan E, Fluckey J, Riechman S, Greenwood M, Kelly K, Meininger C, Rasmussen C, Kreider RB: **A buffered form of creatine does not promote greater changes in muscle creatine content, body composition, or training adaptations than creatine monohydrate.** *J Int Soc Sports Nutr* 2012, **9**:43.
141. Artioli GG, Gualano B, Smith A, Stout J, Lancha AH Jr: **Role of beta-alanine supplementation on muscle carnosine and exercise performance.** *Med Sci Sports Exerc* 2010, **42**:1162–1173.
142. Harris RC, Tallon MJ, Dunnett M, Boobis L, Coakley J, Kim HJ, Fallowfield JL, Hill CA, Sale C, Wise JA: **The absorption of orally supplied beta-alanine and its effect on muscle carnosine synthesis in human vastus lateralis.** *Amino Acids* 2006, **30**:279–289.
143. Derave W, Ozdemir MS, Harris RC, Pottier A, Reyngoudt H, Koppo K, Wise JA, Achten E: **beta-Alanine supplementation augments muscle carnosine content and attenuates fatigue during repeated isokinetic contraction bouts in trained sprinters.** *J Appl Physiol* 2007, **103**:1736–1743.
144. Hill CA, Harris RC, Kim HJ, Harris BD, Sale C, Boobis LH, Kim CK, Wise JA: **Influence of beta-alanine supplementation on skeletal muscle carnosine concentrations and high intensity cycling capacity.** *Amino Acids* 2007, **32**:225–233.
145. Van Thienen R, Van Proeyen K, Vanden Eynde P, Puype J, Lefere T, Hespel P: **Beta-alanine improves sprint performance in endurance cycling.** *Med Sci Sports Exerc* 2009, **41**:898–903.
146. Sale C, Saunders B, Hudson S, Wise JA, Harris RC, Sunderland CD: **Effect of beta-alanine plus sodium bicarbonate on high-intensity cycling capacity.** *Med Sci Sports Exerc* 2011, **43**:1972–1978.
147. Smith AE, Walter AA, Graef JL, Kendall KL, Moon JR, Lockwood CM, Fukuda DH, Beck TW, Cramer JT, Stout JR: **Effects of beta-alanine supplementation and high-intensity interval training on endurance performance and body composition in men; a double-blind trial.** *J Int Soc Sports Nutr* 2009, **6**:5.
148. Stout JR, Cramer JT, Zoeller RF, Torok D, Costa P, Hoffman JR, Harris RC, O'Kroy J: **Effects of beta-alanine supplementation on the onset of neuromuscular fatigue and ventilatory threshold in women.** *Amino Acids* 2007, **32**:381–386.
149. Hoffman J, Ratamess NA, Ross R, Kang J, Magrelli J, Neese K, Faigenbaum AD, Wise JA: **Beta-alanine and the hormonal response to exercise.** *Int J Sports Med* 2008, **29**:952–958.
150. Hoffman JR, Ratamess NA, Faigenbaum AD, Ross R, Kang J, Stout JR, Wise JA: **Short-duration beta-alanine supplementation increases training volume and reduces subjective feelings of fatigue in college football players.** *Nutr Res* 2008, **28**:31–35.
151. Zoeller RF, Stout JR, O'Kroy JA, Torok DJ, Mielke M: **Effects of 28 days of beta-alanine and creatine monohydrate supplementation on aerobic power, ventilatory and lactate thresholds, and time to exhaustion.** *Amino Acids* 2007, **33**:505–510.
152. Hoffman J, Ratamess N, Kang J, Mangine G, Faigenbaum A, Stout J: **Effect of creatine and beta-alanine supplementation on performance and endocrine responses in strength/power athletes.** *Int J Sport Nutr Exerc Metab* 2006, **16**:430–446.
153. Kendrick IP, Harris RC, Kim HJ, Kim CK, Dang VH, Lam TQ, Bui TT, Smith M, Wise JA: **The effects of 10 weeks of resistance training combined with beta-alanine supplementation on whole body strength, force production, muscular endurance and body composition.** *Amino Acids* 2008, **34**:547–554.
154. Sweeney KM, Wright GA, Glenn Brice A, Doberstein ST: **The effect of beta-alanine supplementation on power performance during repeated sprint activity.** *J Strength Cond Res* 2010, **24**:79–87.
155. Hobson RM, Saunders B, Ball G, Harris RC, Sale C: **Effects of beta-alanine supplementation on exercise performance: a meta-analysis.** *Amino Acids* 2012, **43**:25–37.
156. Lu P, Xu W, Sturman JA: **Dietary beta-alanine results in taurine depletion and cerebellar damage in adult cats.** *J Neurosci Res* 1996, **43**:112–119.
157. Smith HJ, Mukerji P, Tisdale MJ: **Attenuation of proteasome-induced proteolysis in skeletal muscle by {beta}-hydroxy-{beta}-methylbutyrate in cancer-induced muscle loss.** *Cancer Res* 2005, **65**:277–283.
158. Eley HL, Russell ST, Baxter JH, Mukerji P, Tisdale MJ: **Signaling pathways initiated by beta-hydroxy-beta-methylbutyrate to attenuate the depression of protein synthesis in skeletal muscle in response to cachectic stimuli.** *Am J Physiol Endocrinol Metab* 2007, **293**:E923–E931.
159. Rathmacher JA, Nissen S, Panton L, Clark RH, Eubanks May P, Barber AE, D'Olimpio J, Abumrad NN: **Supplementation with a combination of beta-hydroxy-beta-methylbutyrate (HMB), arginine, and glutamine is safe and could improve hematological parameters.** *JPEN J Parenter Enteral Nutr* 2004, **28**:65–75.
160. Nissen S, Sharp RL, Panton L, Vukovich M, Trappe S, Fuller JC Jr: **beta-hydroxy-beta-methylbutyrate (HMB) supplementation in humans is safe and may decrease cardiovascular risk factors.** *J Nutr* 2000, **130**:1937–1945.
161. Gallagher PM, Carrithers JA, Godard MP, Schulze KE, Trappe SW: **Beta-hydroxy-beta-methylbutyrate ingestion, part II: effects on hematology, hepatic and renal function.** *Med Sci Sports Exerc* 2000, **32**:2116–2119.
162. Fitschen PJ, Wilson GJ, Wilson JM, Wilund KR: **Efficacy of beta-hydroxy-beta-methylbutyrate supplementation in elderly and clinical populations.** *Nutrition* 2013, **29**:29–36.
163. Wilson GJ, Wilson JM, Manninen AH: **Effects of beta-hydroxy-beta-methylbutyrate (HMB) on exercise performance and body composition across varying levels of age, sex, and training experience: a review.** *Nutr Metab (Lond)* 2008, **5**:1.

164. Wilson J, Fitschen P, Campbell B, Wilson G, Zanchi N, Taylor L, Wilborn C, Kalman D, Stout J, Hoffman J, Ziegenfuss T, Lopez H, Kreider R, Smith-Ryan A, Antonio J: **International Society of Sports Nutrition Position Stand: beta-hydroxy-beta-methylbutyrate (HMB).** *J Int Soc Sports Nutr* 2013, **10**:6.
165. Shimomura Y, Yamamoto Y, Bajotto G, Sato J, Murakami T, Shimomura N, Kobayashi H, Mawatari K: **Nutraceutical effects of branched-chain amino acids on skeletal muscle.** *J Nutr* 2006, **136**:529S–532S.
166. Garlick PJ, Grant I: **Amino acid infusion increases the sensitivity of muscle protein synthesis in vivo to insulin. Effect of branched-chain amino acids.** *Biochem J* 1988, **254**:579–584.
167. Balage M, Dardevet D: **Long-term effects of leucine supplementation on body composition.** *Curr Opin Clin Nutr Metab Care* 2010, **13**:265–270.
168. Pencharz PB, Elango R, Ball RO: **Determination of the tolerable upper intake level of leucine in adult men.** *J Nutr* 2012, **142**:2220S–2224S.
169. Biolo G, Tipton KD, Klein S, Wolfe RR: **An abundant supply of amino acids enhances the metabolic effect of exercise on muscle protein.** *Am J Physiol* 1997, **273**:E122–E129.
170. Tipton KD, Ferrando AA, Phillips SM, Doyle D Jr, Wolfe RR: **Postexercise net protein synthesis in human muscle from orally administered amino acids.** *Am J Physiol* 1999, **276**:E628–E634.
171. Louard RJ, Barrett EJ, Gelfand RA: **Effect of infused branched-chain amino acids on muscle and whole-body amino acid metabolism in man.** *Clin Sci* 1990, **79**:457–466.
172. Borsheim E, Tipton KD, Wolf SE, Wolfe RR: **Essential amino acids and muscle protein recovery from resistance exercise.** *Am J Physiol Endocrinol Metab* 2002, **283**:E648–E657.
173. Stoppani J, Scheett T, Pena J, Rudolph C, Charlebois D: **Consuming a supplement containing branched-chain amino acids during a resistance-traning program increases lean mass, muscle strength, and fat loss.** *J Int Soc Sports Nutr* 2009, **6**:P1.
174. Wilson GJ, Layman DK, Moulton CJ, Norton LE, Anthony TG, Proud CG, Rupassara SI, Garlick PJ: **Leucine or carbohydrate supplementation reduces AMPK and eEF2 phosphorylation and extends postprandial muscle protein synthesis in rats.** *Am J Physiol Endocrinol Metab* 2011, **301**:E1236–E1242.
175. Suryawan A, Hawes JW, Harris RA, Shimomura Y, Jenkins AE, Hutson SM: **A molecular model of human branched-chain amino acid metabolism.** *Am J Clin Nutr* 1998, **68**:72–81.
176. Fahs CA, Heffernan KS, Fernhall B: **Hemodynamic and vascular response to resistance exercise with L-arginine.** *Med Sci Sports Exerc* 2009, **41**:773–779.
177. Tang JE, Lysecki PJ, Manolakos JJ, MacDonald MJ, Tarnopolsky MA, Phillips SM: **Bolus arginine supplementation affects neither muscle blood flow nor muscle protein synthesis in young men at rest or after resistance exercise.** *J Nutr* 2011, **141**:195–200.
178. Volpi E, Kobayashi H, Sheffield-Moore M, Mittendorfer B, Wolfe RR: **Essential amino acids are primarily responsible for the amino acid stimulation of muscle protein anabolism in healthy elderly adults.** *Am J Clin Nutr* 2003, **78**:250–258.
179. Alvares TS, Meirelles CM, Bhambhani YN, Paschoalin VM, Gomes PS: **L-Arginine as a potential ergogenic aid in healthy subjects.** *Sports Med* 2011, **41**:233–248.
180. Greer BK, Jones BT: **Acute arginine supplementation fails to improve muscle endurance or affect blood pressure responses to resistance training.** *J Strength Cond Res* 2011, **25**:1789–1794.
181. McConell GK: **Effects of L-arginine supplementation on exercise metabolism.** *Curr Opin Clin Nutr Metab Care* 2007, **10**:46–51.
182. Shao A, Hathcock JN: **Risk assessment for the amino acids taurine, L-glutamine and L-arginine.** *Regul Toxicol Pharmacol* 2008, **50**:376–399.
183. Perez-Guisado J, Jakeman PM: **Citrulline malate enhances athletic anaerobic performance and relieves muscle soreness.** *J Strength Cond Res* 2010, **24**:1215–1222.
184. Bendahan D, Mattei JP, Ghattas B, Confort-Gouny S, Le Guern ME, Cozzone PJ: **Citrulline/malate promotes aerobic energy production in human exercising muscle.** *Br J Sports Med* 2002, **36**:282–289.
185. Sureda A, Cordova A, Ferrer MD, Perez G, Tur JA, Pons A: **L-citrulline-malate influence over branched chain amino acid utilization during exercise.** *Eur J Appl Physiol* 2010, **110**:341–351.
186. Hickner RC, Tanner CJ, Evans CA, Clark PD, Haddock A, Fortune C, Geddis H, Waugh W, McCammon M: **L-citrulline reduces time to exhaustion and insulin response to a graded exercise test.** *Med Sci Sports Exerc* 2006, **38**:660–666.
187. Gleeson M: **Dosing and efficacy of glutamine supplementation in human exercise and sport training.** *J Nutr* 2008, **138**:2045S–2049S.
188. Antonio J, Sanders MS, Kalman D, Woodgate D, Street C: **The effects of high-dose glutamine ingestion on weightlifting performance.** *J Strength Cond Res* 2002, **16**:157–160.
189. Haub MD, Potteiger JA, Nau KL, Webster MJ, Zebas CJ: **Acute L-glutamine ingestion does not improve maximal effort exercise.** *J Sports Med Phys Fitness* 1998, **38**:240–244.
190. Colker CM, Swain MA, Fabrucini B, Shi Q, Kalman DS: **Effects of supplemental protein on body composition and muscular strength in healthy athletic male adults.** *Curr Ther Res* 2000, **61**:19–28.
191. Candow DG, Chilibeck PD, Burke DG, Davison KS, Smith-Palmer T: **Effect of glutamine supplementation combined with resistance training in young adults.** *Eur J Appl Physiol* 2001, **86**:142–149.
192. Camilleri M, Madsen K, Spiller R, Van Meerveld BG, Verne GN: **Intestinal barrier function in health and gastrointestinal disease.** *Neurogastroenterol Motil* 2012, **24**:503–512.
193. Ivy JL, Kammer L, Ding Z, Wang B, Bernard JR, Liao YH, Hwang J: **Improved cycling time-trial performance after ingestion of a caffeine energy drink.** *Int J Sport Nutr Exerc Metab* 2009, **19**:61–78.
194. McNaughton LR, Lovell RJ, Siegler J, Midgley AW, Moore L, Bentley DJ: **The effects of caffeine ingestion on time trial cycling performance.** *Int J Sports Physiol Perform* 2008, **3**:157–163.
195. Carr A, Dawson B, Schneiker K, Goodman C, Lay B: **Effect of caffeine supplementation on repeated sprint running performance.** *J Sports Med Phys Fitness* 2008, **48**:472–478.
196. Glaister M, Howatson G, Abraham CS, Lockey RA, Goodwin JE, Foley P, McInnes G: **Caffeine supplementation and multiple sprint running performance.** *Med Sci Sports Exerc* 2008, **40**:1835–1840.
197. Green JM, Wickwire PJ, McLester JR, Gendle S, Hudson G, Pritchett RC, Laurent CM: **Effects of caffeine on repetitions to failure and ratings of perceived exertion during resistance training.** *Int J Sports Physiol Perform* 2007, **2**:250–259.
198. Woolf K, Bidwell WK, Carlson AG: **The effect of caffeine as an ergogenic aid in anaerobic exercise.** *Int J Sport Nutr Exerc Metab* 2008, **18**:412–429.
199. Duncan MJ, Oxford SW: **The effect of caffeine ingestion on mood state and bench press performance to failure.** *J Strength Cond Res* 2011, **25**:178–185.
200. Williams AD, Cribb PJ, Cooke MB, Hayes A: **The effect of ephedra and caffeine on maximal strength and power in resistance-trained athletes.** *J Strength Cond Res* 2008, **22**:464–470.
201. Hendrix CR, Housh TJ, Mielke M, Zuniga JM, Camic CL, Johnson GO, Schmidt RJ, Housh DJ: **Acute effects of a caffeine-containing supplement on bench press and leg extension strength and time to exhaustion during cycle ergometry.** *J Strength Cond Res* 2010, **24**:859–865.
202. Nawrot P, Jordan S, Eastwood J, Rotstein J, Hugenholtz A, Feeley M: **Effects of caffeine on human health.** *Food Addit Contam* 2003, **20**:1–30.
203. Tarnopolsky MA, Atkinson SA, MacDougall JD, Sale DG, Sutton JR: **Physiological responses to caffeine during endurance running in habitual caffeine users.** *Med Sci Sports Exerc* 1989, **21**:418–424.
204. Bazzarre TL, Kleiner SM, Litchford MD: **Nutrient intake, body fat, and lipid profiles of competitive male and female bodybuilders.** *J Am Coll Nutr* 1990, **9**:136–142.
205. Kleiner SM, Bazzarre TL, Ainsworth BE: **Nutritional status of nationally ranked elite bodybuilders.** *Int J Sport Nutr* 1994, **4**:54–69.
206. Hickson JF Jr, Johnson TE, Lee W, Sidor RJ: **Nutrition and the precontest preparations of a male bodybuilder.** *J Am Diet Assoc* 1990, **90**:264–267.
207. Andersen RE, Barlett SJ, Morgan GD, Brownell KD: **Weight loss, psychological, and nutritional patterns in competitive male body builders.** *Int J Eat Disord* 1995, **18**:49–57.
208. Balon TW, Horowitz JF, Fitzsimmons KM: **Effects of carbohydrate loading and weight-lifting on muscle girth.** *Int J Sport Nutr* 1992, **2**:328–334.
209. Costill DL, Cote R, Fink W: **Muscle water and electrolytes following varied levels of dehydration in man.** *J Appl Physiol* 1976, **40**:6–11.
210. Goldfield GS, Blouin AG, Woodside DB: **Body image, binge eating, and bulimia nervosa in male bodybuilders.** *Can J Psychiatry* 2006, **51**:160–168.
211. Mangweth B, Pope HG Jr, Kemmler G, Ebenbichler C, Hausmann A, De Col C, Kreutner B, Kinzl J, Biebl W: **Body image and psychopathology in male bodybuilders.** *Psychother Psychosom* 2001, **70**:38–43.

212. Baghurst T, Lirgg C: **Characteristics of muscle dysmorphia in male football, weight training, and competitive natural and non-natural bodybuilding samples.** *Body Image* 2009, **6**:221–227.
213. Pickett TC, Lewis RJ, Cash TF: **Men, muscles, and body image: comparisons of competitive bodybuilders, weight trainers, and athletically active controls.** *Br J Sports Med* 2005, **39**:217–222. discussion 217–222.
214. Jankauskiene R, Kardelis K, Pajaujiene S: **Muscle size satisfaction and predisposition for a health harmful practice in bodybuilders and recreational gymnasium users.** *Medicina (Kaunas)* 2007, **43**:338–346.
215. Walberg JL, Johnston CS: **Menstrual function and eating behavior in female recreational weight lifters and competitive body builders.** *Med Sci Sports Exerc* 1991, **23**:30–36.
216. Sundgot-Borgen J, Garthe I: **Elite athletes in aesthetic and Olympic weight-class sports and the challenge of body weight and body compositions.** *J Sports Sci* 2011, **29**(Suppl 1):S101–S114.

Effects of a dietary supplement on golf drive distance and functional indices of golf performance

Tim N Ziegenfuss[1*], Scott M Habowski[1], Robert Lemieux[2], Jennifer E Sandrock[1], A William Kedia[1], Chad M Kerksick[3] and Hector L Lopez[1]

Abstract

Background: Limited research exists examining the impact of nutrition on golfing performance. This study's purpose was to determine the impact of daily supplementation with an over-the-counter dietary supplement on golf performance.

Methods: Healthy men (30.3 ± 6.9 y, 183.1 ± 5.6 cm, 86.7 ± 11.9 kg), with a 5–15 handicap were assigned in a double-blind, placebo-controlled manner to ingest for 30 days either a placebo (PLA, n = 13) or a dietary supplement containing creatine monohydrate, *coffea arabica* fruit extract, calcium fructoborate and vitamin D (Strong Drive™, SD, n = 14). Subjects ingested two daily doses for the first two weeks and one daily dose for the remaining two weeks. Participants followed their normal dietary habits and did not change their physical activity patterns. Two identical testing sessions in a pre/post fashion were completed consisting of a fasting blood sample, anthropometric measurements, 1-RM bench press, upper body power and golf swing performance using their driver and 7-iron. Data were analyzed using two-way mixed factorial ANOVAs and ANCOVA when baseline differences were present. Statistical significance was established *a priori* at $p \leq 0.05$.

Results: ANCOVA revealed significantly greater (post-test) best drive distance ($p = 0.04$) for SD (+5.0% [+13.6 yards], ES = 0.75) as well as a tendency ($p = 0.07$) for average drive distance to increase (+8.4% [+19.6 yards], ES = 0.65), while no such changes were found with PLA (−0.5% [−1.2 yards], ES = 0.04 and +1.3% [+2.8 yards], ES = 0.08, respectively). Both groups experienced significant increases in body mass and 1-RM bench press ($p < 0.001$). No other significant group × time interactions were found. For the SD group only, within-group analysis confirmed significant improvements in set 1 average (+8.9%, $p = 0.001$) and peak velocity (+6.8%, p < =0.01). No changes were noted for reported adverse events, pain inventories, quality of life or any measured blood parameter.

Conclusions: SD supplementation for 30 days significantly improved best drive distance more than placebo. Supplementation was well tolerated and did not result in any clinically significant changes in markers of health or adverse events/side effect profiles.

Keywords: Golf, Performance, Creatine, Drive distance, Velocity, Driver

* Correspondence: tz@appliedhealthsciences.org
[1]The Center for Applied Health Sciences, 4302 Allen Road, Ste 120, Stow, OH 44224, USA
Full list of author information is available at the end of the article

Introduction

The sport of golf requires an intricate mix of physical, emotional and cognitive factors to achieve optimal performance [1]. The swing itself is a complex pattern of coordinated biomechanical movements that impact both the accuracy and distance with which the ball is struck. In its purest sense, the golf swing is a movement centered mostly upon the production of power; consequently, swings are considered to be largely anaerobic in nature [1].

As the popularity of golf rises, the development of ergogenic approaches have produced a seemingly endless array of clubs and other pieces of equipment intended to help improve performance. In light of the physical and cognitive challenges brought forth by golf, nutritional approaches may impact performance, but minimal effort, to date, has been made in this area.

The lack of nutritional considerations within the sport of golf is somewhat surprising. Currently, nutritional guidelines center upon prudent management of fluid and carbohydrate levels, but other demands found in golf present the need for additional nutritional concerns. For example, under certain environmental conditions the extended duration to complete a round of golf (~3 – 4 hours) can promote dehydration, reduced energy levels and mental fatigue [1]. When these factors are considered collectively, it makes intuitive sense that a nutritional formulation that can improve anaerobic performance and increase a golfer's focus and attention may impact performance. In this respect, one of the only published studies to examine the impact of a nutritional agent on golfing performance utilized phosphatidylserine supplementation to lower the stress hormone cortisol and improve shot-making during simulated golf swings [2]. SuperDrive™ (Purity Products, Plainview, NY) is a commercially available dietary supplement that combines creatine monohydrate, coffee arabica fruit extract, calcium fructoborate and vitamin D and is marketed to the golfing community to aid in performance and recovery from musculoskeletal complications associated with participation in golf [1].

Creatine monohydrate is one of the most popular and effective dietary supplements due to its ability to improve strength, power, lean mass and explosive performance. Creatine supplementation protocols are well established to significantly increase intramuscular levels of phosphocreatine and total creatine which, in the vast majority of studies, result in measureable improvements in a wide variety of high-intensity activities [3-8]. However, to our knowledge, no research is available that has examined the impact of creatine supplementation on golfing performance. In light of the fact that the golf swing is an anaerobic event [1], it is logical that creatine supplementation may have the potential to improve golf swing power.

Coffea arabica is a fruit extract (CoffeeBerry®) that is derived from the same plant as traditional coffee, thus making caffeine the primary active ingredient found within the extract. For years, scientific research has supported the use of caffeine as an ergogenic aid, primarily known for its positive impact on executive functions such as focus, attention and concentration, stimulation of fatty acid mobilization, improvements in endurance performance [9], and various direct effects on muscle function [10,11]. From a physical perspective, caffeine is known to antagonize adenosine receptors, thereby inhibiting the negative impact of adenosine on neurotransmission, arousal, and pain perception [12] in addition to reducing ratings of perceived exertion [13]. Beyond physical benefits, caffeine can also operate to enhance a number of cognitive aspects. Caffeine is commonly used and accepted for its ability to promote wakefulness as well as enhance focus and concentration, all attributes that would be of particular benefit to a golfer, while also preventing both peripheral and central manifestations of fatigue [10]. An excellent review by Glade summarized available literature on caffeine's impact of cognitive functioning and reported that caffeine in doses in modest amounts (30 – 50 mg) are able to favorably impact mental energy, but typical doses of 100 – 150 mg are needed to positively impact assessments of cognitive functioning [10]. Similarly, Einother and investigators expertly summarized the literature and concluded that caffeine favorably impacts both simple and complex tasks through both attention enhancement and optimized executive function [14].

A myriad of musculoskeletal problems can negatively impact golfing performance and strategies to minimize pain and joint discomfort while also promoting favorable bone and muscle health are important concerns for active golfers. The trace mineral boron is closely linked to improved rates of calcium retention and bone health. Although no recommended daily allowance for boron has been established, doses ranging from 1–4 mg have been shown to safely promote improvements in bone density [15,16]. Recent technology has produced calcium fructoborate (FruiteX-B®), a patented compound that results in calcium being bound to boron, forming a natural chelation and effective stabilization of the available boron. While relatively new, calcium fructoborate has been shown to exert strong anti-inflammatory functions [17] and pronounced antioxidant activity [18]. Interestingly, the compound can favorably impact hormonal regulation and vitamin D metabolism leading to its interest as a pain and bone/joint health aid. Specifically, unpublished research in mild and severe osteoporotic patients using an open-label approach indicated that eight weeks of supplementation with calcium fructoborate reduced pain and stiffness during walking and climbing stairs and improved joint mobility [19]. More recent published literature utilized a two-week double-blind, placebo-controlled supplementation approach on 116 osteoporotic patients and concluded that calcium fructoborate supplementation improved inflammatory markers for all groups [20].

Another ingredient that continues to get attention regarding its ability to favorably impact bone health [21] and healthy muscle metabolism [22-24] is vitamin D. The average adult American diet contains only 150–300 IU of vitamin D per day while recommended levels are 600–800 IU, despite multiple studies indicating that higher daily amounts may be optimal [21,25]. Currently, the Endocrine Society recommends 1,500 – 2,000 IU/day, with other reports recommending between 400 – 1,000 IU/day. To date, the impact of supplementation with vitamin D (either in isolation or as part of a multi-ingredient formula) on golf performance is unknown.

The primary purpose of this preliminary, proof-of-concept investigation was to examine the impact of a nutritional formulation containing creatine, *coffea arabica* fruit extract (CoffeeBerry®), calcium fructoborate (FruiteX-B®) and vitamin D on functional indices of golf swing performance, and upper-body strength/power. Secondary purposes were to assess changes in indices of quality of life, pain and standard blood-based markers of clinical safety and health.

Methods

Overview of research design

This study was completed as a randomized, double-blind, placebo-controlled trial. Over a 30 day period, eligible study participants who first signed an IRB-approved informed consent document were assigned in a randomized, double-blind, placebo-controlled fashion to ingest either a dietary supplement or a placebo. In an identical fashion, two daily supplement (or placebo) doses were ingested during the first two weeks and one daily dose was ingested during the final two weeks for 30 days total. Prior to testing, all study participants were instructed to refrain from heavy exercise for 48 hours and observe a 12 hour fast. To enhance reliability and minimize a learning effect, subjects were familiarized to all experimental procedures prior to testing. Participants then completed two identical testing sessions consisting of a fasting blood sample, anthropometric assessments, resting heart rate and blood pressure, muscular strength and power assessments, golf swing performance, and quality of life, pain and adverse event questionnaires. To determine indications of clinical safety, fasting blood samples were collected and analyzed for complete blood counts, clinical chemistry panels and other indicators of health and safety along with resting levels of heart and blood pressure. To assess changes in strength and power and evaluate the impact of supplementation, bench press 1-RM was determined along with bench press throw power, respectively. In addition to these accepted laboratory methods of upper body strength and power, functional performance was also assessed using three-dimensional analysis of a series of golf swings using participants' 7-iron and driver. Finally and as a general means to assess the impact of supplementation on potential changes in musculoskeletal health, self-assessments of pain, quality of life and other adverse outcomes were gleaned from all study participants.

Subjects

Twenty-seven healthy men (mean ± SD age, height, body mass: 30.3 ± 6.9 y, 183.1 ± 5.6 cm, 86.7 ± 11.9 kg) with a handicap index of 5–15 were recruited as participants in this study. Prior to any research-related activity, all study participants reviewed and signed an IRB approved informed consent document (Integreview, Austin, TX, Protocol #PUR-002, approval date: July 30, 2013). During their first laboratory visit, participants completed medical history paperwork and were screened for eligibility by a licensed physician. Inclusion criteria for this study required study participants to be in good health as determined by medical history review and baseline blood chemistries, normotensive (systolic blood pressure ≤ 140 mm Hg, diastolic blood pressure ≤ 90 mm Hg and resting heart rate ≤ 90 beats per minute) and have maintained a modest level of physical activity (defined as an average of two workouts per week) for at least one year. Participants were excluded if they had any metabolic disorder including known electrolyte abnormalities, diabetes, thyroid disease, hypogonadism, or a history of hepatic, renal, musculoskeletal, autoimmune, or neurologic disease. Exclusion criteria also included subjects with history of heart disease, hypertension, psychiatric disorders, cancer, benign prostatic hypertrophy, gastric ulcer, gastroesophegal reflux disease, or any other medical disorder deemed unsuitable for inclusion in the study by the investigators. Participants who reported a history of taking creatine or other dietary supplements were only allowed entry if they had not taken or had refrained from taking any dietary supplements containing these ingredients for at least 30 days prior to initiating the study (excluding a multi-vitamin/mineral) and agreed to only use their assigned supplement throughout the study protocol. Individuals who reported as regularly consuming caffeine (<200 mg/day) were instructed to not change their caffeine intake throughout the duration of the protocol; participants who consumed >200 mg caffeine were excluded. Participants currently prescribed any thyroid, antihyperlipidemic, hypoglycemic, antihypertensive, anticoagulant, or androgenic medications, nitrates/nitrate derivatives, or phosphodiesterase (PDE)-5 inhibitors were also excluded. Subjects who had admitted to using anabolic steroids, growth hormone, insulin-like growth factor (IGF)-1, or other hormone medication including oral contraceptives during the previous 12 months were also excluded, as were smokers and those with orthopedic limitations or injuries.

Procedures

Testing protocol

All study participants were first familiarized to all experimental procedures prior to completing their first testing session. Prior to arriving for all testing sessions, study participants were instructed to refrain from physically taxing exercise for 48 hours and to observe a 12 hour fast. Upon arrival for the initial testing session, physical activity and health history were determined using standardized questionnaires. Subjects then had their resting heart rate and blood pressure determined using an automated sphygmomanometer, standing height determined using a wall-mounted stadiometer, and body mass determined using a calibrated scale (Seca Medical Scale, Hanover, MD). On separate days thereafter, study participants completed a 1-RM test on the bench press, an upper-body power test (bench press throws) and an assessment of their golf swing performance.

Suggested Use: As a dietary supplement, mix one heaping scoop with 8 oz. of cold, pure water. For the first 15 days, take twice daily (optimally one serving in the morning and one in the afternoon).

Supplement Facts

Serving Size 1 Heaping Scoop (approx 7 grams)
Servings Per Container 30

Amount Per Serving		% Daily Value*
Calories	20	
Total Carbohydrate	<1 g	<1%*
Sugars	0.5 g	†
Vitamin D (as cholecalciferol)	1,000 IU	250%
Creapure® Creatine Monohydrate	5,000 mg	†
CoffeeBerry® (*Coffea arabica*) (fruit) extract (50 mg naturally occurring caffeine)	100 mg	†
Boron (FruiteX-B™ PhytoBoron)	3 mg	†

* Percent Daily Value based on a 2,000 calorie diet.
† Daily Value not established.

Other ingredients: Sucrose, maltodextrin, citric acid, beetroot juice powder, natural flavor, dextrose and silica.

Creapure® is a registered trademark of AlzChem Trostberg GmbH, Germany.
FruiteX-B™ is a trademark of FutureCeuticals, U.S. Patent #5,962,049.
CoffeeBerry® is a registered trademark of VDF FutureCeuticals, Inc.

Figure 1 Supplement Facts for Strong Drive™.

Supplementation protocol

In a double-blind, placebo-controlled fashion, study participants were instructed to ingest either a powdered dietary supplement containing creatine, *coffea arabica* fruit extract (CoffeeBerry®), calcium fructoborate (FruiteX-B®) and vitamin D (Strong Drive™, SD, n = 14) or an isocaloric placebo (PLA, n = 13). A representative Supplement Facts label of the investigational product is shown in Figure 1. Irrespective of group assignment, all study participants were instructed to take each serving of their assigned supplement with eight ounces of cold water. For the first two weeks of the study, one serving was consumed twice per day (with breakfast and lunch). During the final two weeks of the study, study participants consumed only one serving per day of their assigned supplement (with breakfast). This protocol was employed to match manufacturer guidelines; the protocol also corresponded with previous creatine supplementation literature showing effective increases in intramuscular creatine and phosphocreatine levels [3,6]. To ensure complete blinding, all study supplements were in powder form of similar color, texture and flavor while also being packaged in coded generic containers. Compliance to the supplementation protocol was monitored by having study participants complete a supplementation log. In addition, study participants were required to return their empty supplement containers and were reminded of details associated with the study protocols with weekly text messages and/or emails. Participants were instructed to refrain from using other supplemental courses of caffeine or creatine.

Blood collection and analysis

Whole blood and serum samples were collected using standard phlebotomy techniques on day 0 and day 30 of the study protocol. Whole blood samples were collected into K2-EDTA treated vacutainer tubes and upon collection were slowly inverted ten consecutive times prior to immediate refrigeration. Serum samples were collected in non-treated tubes and allowed to clot for 30 minutes at room temperature prior to being centrifuged (Horizon mini E Centrifuge, Drucker Diagnostics, Port Matilda, PA) for 15 minutes at 3200 rpm. Serum was extracted from all samples and aliquots were pipetted into cryovial storage tubes. All blood samples were analyzed for clinical chemistry analysis (plasma glucose, blood urea nitrogen [BUN], creatinine, aspartate aminotransaminase [AST], alanine aminotransaminase [ALT], creatine kinase, lactate dehydrogenase, total bilirubin, alkaline phosphatase [ALP], triacylglycerol [TG], total cholesterol [TC], LDL, HDL, uric acid, sodium, potassium, total protein, albumin, globulin, iron, complete blood cells, and platelet count) using automated clinical chemistry analyzers (LabCorp, Dublin, OH branch). All samples from the same day were batch analyzed with test-retest reliabilities commonly reported using internal quality control data from clinical laboratories and associated automated analyzers within a range of 3 – 5% [26].

Muscular strength and power determination

On day 0 and day 30, maximal upper body muscle strength was estimated by 1-RM bench press testing using protocols adapted from the National Strength and Conditioning Association [27]. Only upper-body strength was assessed in this study due to previous experience in our lab and others indicating greater reliability of upper-body vs. lower-body testing [28]. It is recognized that the bench press exercise acts primarily in the sagittal plane whereby the golf swing occurs through multiple planes at a wide range of accelerations and decelerations. In this respect, Marta and colleagues published a review of EMG studies involving the golf swing and they reported that the pectoralis muscle group experienced a great deal of activity during the golf swing movement [29]. Thus, our analytical approach in this styd was to combine a standardized, well-accepted measure of upper-body strength and power (1RM bench press and bench throws) along with a three-dimensional analysis of golf swing performance (described below) to assess the potential impact of nutritional supplementation. After a general warm-up of three to five minutes of light activity consisting of upper body ergometry and static stretching of the involved musculature, the subject performed a warm-up set of ten repetitions with only the bar, followed by eight repetitions at approximately 50% of their estimated 1-RM, followed by one set of three repetitions at 70% of their perceived 1-RM. Thereafter, study participants performed single repetition lifts at progressively increasing loads until 1-RM was determined. No more than five maximal attempts were completed in one testing session.

Upper body power production (average power [AP], average velocity [AV], peak power [PP], peak velocity [PV]) was assessed using the bench press exercise using a Tendo unit interfaced to a standard Smith machine rack. Previous studies have successfully incorporated the use of a Tendo into their study design [30] and Stock and colleagues [31] recently published data to indicate it is a reliable means of assessment. The unit consists of a position transducer that measures the rate of linear displacement providing velocity and acceleration in addition to power production. After 1RM determination, subjects rested for five minutes and completed three sets of three explosive repetitions (i.e. bench throws) with a load equal to 40% of their actual 1-RM on the bench press. Interset rest periods were strictly standardized at 90 seconds each. The reliability of our procedures using these procedures is similar to that previously reported [28,31].

Golf swing performance

On day 1 and day 30, golf swing performance was measured using a three-dimensional (3-D) swing analysis system (TRACKMAN PRO, Brighton, MI) by a NCAA Division I golf coach. Study participants completed a series of 10 successive swings using their 7-iron and driver. Although a wide variety of data is captured with this system (e.g. club delivery, ball launch, flight data) for the purpose of this study we chose to focus on peak and average club head speed, ball speed, as well as average and best distance for each club. Reliability was determined by having five representative participants complete five swings using both the 7-iron and driver clubs. Intraclass correlation coefficient and standard error of measurement using the 7-iron were calculated for ball speed ($ICC_{3,1}$: 0.934, SEM: 10.99 miles/hour), club speed ($ICC_{3,1}$: 0.991, SEM: 2.42 miles/hour) and total distance ($ICC_{3,1}$: 0.862, SEM: 41.74 yards). Identical measurements were made using the driver for ball speed ($ICC_{3,1}$: 0.975, SEM: 3.26 miles/hour) , club speed ($ICC_{3,1}$: 0.990, SEM: 2.28 miles/hour) and total distance ($ICC_{3,1}$: 0.967, SEM: 8.46 yards). All calculations and assumptions were made according to Weir 2005 [32].

Qualitative assessments

Study participants were asked to maintain their normal patterns of exercise and habitual physical activity. Assessment of physical activity was completed on day 0, day 1 and day 30 using the Yale Physical Activity Survey prior to the study protocol and again on the last day of testing [33]. The Brief Pain Inventory and Quality of Life (SF-12, version 2) were also administered on day 1 and day 30.

Dietary intake

No dietary restrictions or prescriptions were made as part of this study protocol. Subjects recorded their dietary intake over a three day period (two week days, one weekend day) according to instructions given by a research dietitian on day 0 and day 30. Each subject's baseline diet was analyzed by NutriBase IX software (CyberSoft, Inc., Phoenix, AZ) to determine average energy and macronutrient content as well as distribution. Additional three-day dietary records were collected and analyzed in an identical fashion at the end of the supplementation protocol (day 30). Twenty-four hours prior to post-testing on day 30, study participants duplicated their dietary intake using diet records from day 0.

Statistical analyses

Data were analyzed using a two-way mixed factorial ANOVA (treatment [PLA vs. SD] x time [pre vs. post]) with repeated measures on the time factor. ANCOVA was utilized when baseline differences were present using respective baseline scores as the covariate. Within-group main effects over time were fully decomposed using paired samples t-tests. Within-group effect sizes (ES) were also calculated (post mean – pre mean/pooled SD) for all variables and are reported in table format.

Normality was determined on all data using the Shapiro-Wilk statistics and visual inspection of standardized skewness and kurtosis scores. When the sphericity assumption was not met, the Huynh-Feldt correction was applied. Any non-normally distributed data were log-transformed prior to analysis. A p-value of less than or equal to 0.05 was used for determination of statistical significance. Trends were identified as p-values between 0.051 and 0.10. All statistical analyses were completed using SPSS software, version 21 (Cary, NC).

Results

Of the 45 people screened for this study, 30 met inclusion criteria and were randomized to the study protocol. Reasons for excluding participants included not achieving an adequate golf handicap score, taking medications for blood pressure and not wanting to cease current supplement use. Of the 30 people randomized into the protocol, three participants were dropped because one did not arrive for post-testing while two others failed to show for their final golf swing performance test. Thus, 27 people completed the study. Descriptive characteristics and baseline demographics are found in Table 1. No significant differences ($p > 0.05$) were found at baseline between groups for age, height, body mass, systolic blood pressure, or diastolic blood pressure. Resting heart rate values at baseline tended to be greater in the PLA group (PLA: 67.5 ± 8.4 vs. SD: 61.4 ± 7.4 beats/min, $p = 0.052$). In response to the intervention, no significant group × time interaction ($p > 0.05$) effects were revealed for body mass, systolic blood pressure, diastolic blood pressure or resting heart rate.

Data from maximal strength and power assessments are found in Table 2. Significant baseline differences ($p < 0.05$) were found for maximal strength and peak power production during all sets of the bench throws. As a result, ANCOVA was used to determine statistical differences for these variables during post-testing. Both the PLA and SD groups experienced similar significant increases in body mass (data not shown) and 1RM bench press across time ($p < 0.001$ in both groups) with but no between-group differences were present via ANCOVA ($p = 0.86$). Using ANCOVA, no between group differences ($p > 0.05$) were found for peak power production during all sets that were completed (Table 2). Using 2x2 mixed factorial ANOVA, no significant group × time interaction were found for peak velocity during set 2 and set 3 while the peak velocity tended ($p = 0.07$) to change for set 1 peak velocity (Table 2). Additionally, the SD group experienced a significant within-group increase (delta: 0.079 ± 0.089 miles/hour, $p = 0.005$; ES = 0.62) in peak velocity during the 1st set of bench throws. In contrast, within-group changes in the PLA group for peak velocity during set 1 of bench throws were not significant (delta: 0.015 ± 0.086, $p = 0.55$; ES = 0.11).

Golf performance data are shown in Table 3. Using 2×2 mixed factorial ANOVA, no significant ($p > 0.05$) group × time interaction effect was found for best 7-iron club speed, best 7-iron ball speed and best 7-iron distance. There was a significant difference at baseline ($p < 0.05$) in best driver distance, best driver club speed, and best driver ball speed, thus ANCOVA was used to compare post-test values for these variables. No between-group differences were noted for best driver club speed and best driver ball speed, but a significant difference was found for best driver distance (Table 3 and Figure 2) and there was a tendency for average driver distance to be different (PLA: 2.7 ± 25.2 vs. SD: 13.6 ± 24.5 yards, $p = 0.07$). In the SD group, a trend (delta: 13.6 ± 29.0 yards, $p = 0.10$, ES = 0.75) was identified for best drive distance. No within-group changes were seen in the PLA group for any of the golf performance parameters with the exception of a tendency for an increase in best 7-iron distance (+6.9 ± 13.2 yards, $p = 0.08$, ES = 0.31).

No significant group × time interaction effects were revealed for the following blood variables (Table 4): red blood cell count, hemoglobin, hematocrit, glucose, blood urea nitrogen (BUN), creatinine, BUN: creatinine, sodium, potassium, chloride, carbon dioxide, calcium, total protein, albumin, globulin, albumin: globulin, bilirubin, alkaline phosphatase, alanine aminotransferase, aspartate aminotransferase, total cholesterol, triglycerides, HDL

Table 1 Baseline anthropometric and hemodynamic characteristics of study participants

	PLA (n = 13)	SD (n = 14)	Between groups (*p*)
Age (years)	30.1 ± 7.9	30.5 ± 6.0	0.876
Height (cm)	182.1 ± 5.4	184.0 ± 5.7	0.392
Body mass (kg)	85.4 ± 9.0	87.8 ± 14.1	0.601
Systolic BP (mm Hg)	133.3 ± 15.0	129.6 ± 11.0	0.464
Diastolic BP (mm Hg)	81.5 ± 6.5	80.0 ± 6.9	0.556
Resting HR (beats/min)	67.5 ± 8.4	61.4 ± 7.4	0.052
1RM (kg)	85.1 ± 20.9	105.5 ± 25.0	0.031*

Values are mean ± SD. *Significant difference between groups via t-test, $p < 0.05$.

Table 2 Upper-body maximal strength and power characteristics

	Intervention			Comparison of change (p)		
	Pre	Post	Change	Effect size (*d*)	Within groups	Group × Time
Bench press 1RM (kg)						
PLA	85 ± 21	89 ± 22	3.8 ± 3.0	0.18	<0.01*	0.86§
SD	106 ± 25†	109 ± 25	3.7 ± 2.9	0.15	<0.01*	
Bench Press Throws Peak Power Set 1 (watts)‡						
PLA	396 ± 91	410 ± 105	14.5 ± 43.8	0.16	0.26	0.35§
SD	487 ± 124	517 ± 124	28.6 ± 26.7	0.23	<0.01*	
Bench Press Throws Peak Velocity Set 1 (m/s)‡						
PLA	1.20 ± 0.13	1.22 ± 0.12	0.015 ± 0.086	0.11	0.55	0.07
SD	1.17 ± 0.13	1.25 ± 0.11	0.079 ± 0.089	0.62	0.02*	
Bench Press Throws Peak Power Set 2 (watts)‡						
PLA	401 ± 86	422 ± 108	21.4 ± 44.7	0.25	0.11	0.36§
SD	504 ± 124	513 ± 129	8.7 ± 38.8	0.07	0.42	
Bench Press Throws Peak Velocity Set 2 (m/s)‡						
PLA	1.21 ± 0.10	1.24 ± 0.16	0.025 ± 0.132	0.26	0.52	0.86
SD	1.22 ± 0.15	1.24 ± 0.10	0.016 ± 0.096	0.11	0.53	
Bench Press Throws Peak Power Set 3 (watts)‡						
PLA	400 ± 95	416 ± 97	15.5 ± 36.8	0.16	0.15	0.75§
SD	515 ± 118	523 ± 126	8.5 ± 40.3	0.07	0.44	
Bench Press Throws Peak Velocity Set 3 (m/s)‡						
PLA	1.21 ± 0.10	1.24 ± 0.12	0.032 ± .109	0.31	0.31	0.61
SD	1.25 ± 0.14	1.27 ± 0.09	0.012 ± 0.093	0.08	0.63	

Values are mean ± SD. ‡= 3 sets × 3 reps of bench press throws @ 40% 1RM. § = Group differences assessed using ANCOVA with respective baseline scores as the covariate due to significant difference between groups at baseline. *= Significant within group change.

cholesterol, VLDL cholesterol, LDL cholesterol, vitamin D (25-hydroxy D) and C-reactive protein. Only a small number of blood variables experienced changes or seemed to exhibit within-group changes over time. In all situations, the magnitude of change was within clinically accepted normative ranges for these variables. Specifically, in the SD group significant changes ($p < 0.05$) were noted in diastolic blood pressure, carbon dioxide, and total cholesterol while in the PLA group significant changes were noted in sodium, potassium, and glucose. Both groups experienced significant changes in total protein, globulin, and albumin: globulin ratio. No significant group × time interaction effects were reported for any of the pain indices, physical activity or enjoyment scales (Table 5, $p > 0.05$).

Discussion

Golf is a unique sport that requires a challenging combination of physical, mental and emotional attributes. Nutritional formulations developed to enhance these attributes are lacking, but multiple ingredients are available that have been examined scientifically which may improve golfing performance. The primary findings from the present study were that, over a 4-week period of supplementation, a blend of ingredients found in SD (e.g. creatine monohydrate, coffea arabica fruit extract [CoffeeBerry®], calcium fructoborate [FruiteX-B®], and vitamin D) significantly increased best drive distance and tended to improve average driver distance ($p = 0.07$) more so than the placebo group. In addition, both groups experienced significant improvements in bench press strength while the SD also experienced significant improvements in peak power and peak velocity production after the first set of bench press throws while no such changes were observed in the placebo group. Supplementation was well tolerated and no safety concerns/side effects were noted.

Although this study was not designed to determine the mechanisms underpinning any observed changes with SD supplementation, one or more of the ingredients in the formula were likely responsible for the observed changes. For example, a number of previous investigations using creatine monohydrate at the dosage provided in this study (10 grams/day × first two weeks, 5 grams/day × last two weeks) have routinely reported improvements in strength, upper-body performance, power and overall exercise capacity [3,7]. Thus, even though we did

Table 3 Golf performance using repeated measures ANOVA

	Intervention			Comparison of change (p)		
	Pre	Post	Change	Effect size (*d*)	Within groups	Group × Time
Best 7 Iron Club Speed (miles/hour)						
PLA	86.7 ± 8.9	88.0 ± 4.6	1.39 ± 4.9	0.15	0.32	0.50
SD	92.1 ± 4.8	92.5 ± 5.2	0.44 ± 1.7	0.09	0.34	
Best 7 Iron Ball Speed (miles/hour)						
PLA	113.8 ± 12.9	115.4 ± 8.8	1.51 ± 7.5	0.11	0.79	0.44
SD	120.8 ± 6.3	120.5 ± 6.9	−0.25 ± 3.9	0.04	0.80	
Best Distance 7 Iron (yards)						
PLA	162 ± 24	169 ± 21	6.9 ± 13	0.31	0.08	0.93
SD	174 ± 15	181 ± 13	7.4 ± 18	0.53	0.14	
Best Driver Club Speed (miles/hour)						
PLA	104.5 ± 9.3	104.9 ± 6.5	0.45 ± 4.6	0.05	0.73	0.46§
SD	110.4 ± 5.1	110.1 ± 5.7	−0.31 ± 3.6	0.06	0.76	
Best Driver Ball Speed (miles/hour)						
PLA	147.5 ± 13.8	148.6 ± 9.5	1.1 ± 7.5	0.09	0.61	0.17§
SD	158.9 ± 6.6	159.1 ± 7.9	0.19 ± 7.6	0.03	0.93	
Best Driver Distance (yards)						
PLA	260.0 ± 30.4	258.8 ± 29.6	−1.2 ± 18.6	0.04	0.82	0.04§
SD	269.9 ± 18.5	283.5 ± 23.1	13.6 ± 29.0	0.75	0.10	

Values are mean ± SD. §= Group differences assessed using ANCOVA with respective baseline scores as the covariate due to significant difference between groups at baseline.

not collect muscle phosphagen data it is likely that the observed non-significant improvements in upper-body power and velocity primarily stemmed from the creatine monohydrate contained in SD. Future studies should utilize three groups to confirm this hypothesis (i.e. placebo vs. SD formula vs. creatine control).

Another potential candidate for performance enhancement in the SD formula is caffeine. As a dietary supplement, caffeine has successfully been used for years at doses of 3–6 mg/kg of body mass to improve both cognitive and physical aspects of exercise performance [10,11]. In the present study, no assessments of focus or concentration

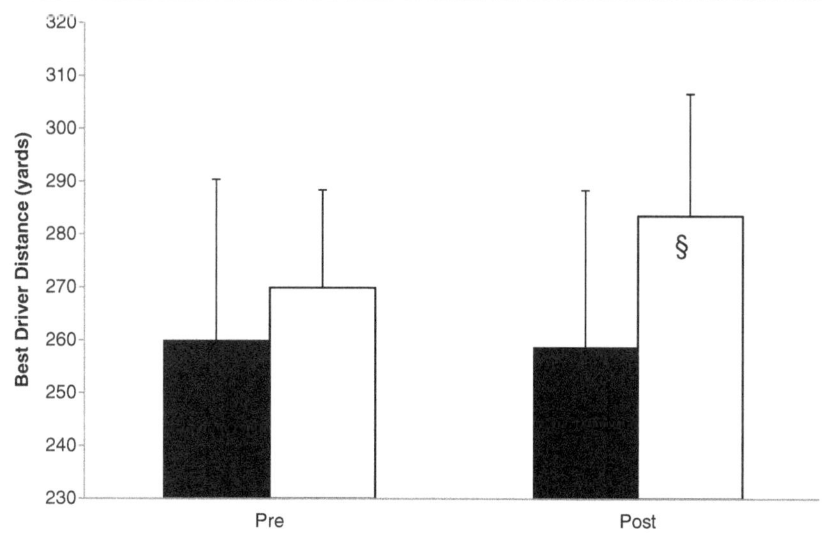

Figure 2 Best distance using driver for placebo = PLA (black bars) and Strong Drive = SD (white bars). § = Significant group differences using ANCOVA (p = 0.04) with respective baseline scores as the covariate due to significant differences between groups at baseline.

Table 4 Hemodynamic, whole blood and clinical chemistry markers of health and safety

	Intervention			Comparison of change (p)		
	Pre	Post	Change	Effect Size (*d*)	Within Groups	Group x Time
Resting Heart Rate (beats/min)						
PLA	67.5 ± 8.4	66.8 ± 7.2	−0.7 ± 6.3	0.09	0.70	0.81
SD	61.4 ± 7.4	60.1 ± 6.2	−1.3 ± 6.2	0.19	0.45	
Systolic Blood Pressure (mm Hg)						
PLA	133.3 ± 15.0	125.9 ± 12.3	−7.4 ± 13.2	0.54	0.07	0.76
SD	129.6 ± 11.0	123.7 ± 10.2	−5.9 ± 12.2	0.56	0.10	
Diastolic Blood Pressure (mm Hg)						
PLA	81.5 ± 6.5	79.5 ± 6.6	−1.9 ± 5.6	0.16	0.22	0.10
SD	80.0 ± 6.9	73.0 ± 9.6	−7.1 ± 9.1	0.85	0.01*	
White Blood Cell Count (x10^6/UL)						
PLA	5.6 ± 0.9	5.4 ± 1.4	−0.19 ± 1.4	0.13	0.62	0.55
SD	4.6 ± 1.4	4.7 ± 1.1	−0.14 ± 1.4	0.08	0.73	
Red Blood Cell Count (x10^6/UL)						
PLA	5.3 ± 0.4	5.2 ± 0.4	−0.06 ± 0.21	0.40	0.30	0.83
SD	5.0 ± 0.3	5.0 ± 0.3	−0.05 ± 0.09	0.00	0.07	
Hemoglobin (grams/dL)						
PLA	15.7 ± 1.0	15.5 ± 1.0	−0.24 ± 0.6	0.20	0.16	0.20
SD	14.6 ± 0.9	14.7 ± 0.7	−0.57 ± 0.6	0.12	0.72	
Hematocrit (%)						0.96
PLA	46.0 ± 2.9	45.6 ± 2.9	−0.45 ± 1.9	0.14	0.42	
SD	43.3 ± 1.7	42.8 ± 1.9	−0.42 ± 0.9	0.28	0.10	
Glucose (mg/dL)						0.10
PLA	93.0 ± 5.7	87.1 ± 7.0	−5.8 ± 7.1	0.90	0.01*	
SD	88.9 ± 8.2	90.6 ± 11.4	−1.9 ± 15.0	0.20	0.64	
Blood Urea Nitrogen (mg/dL)						0.35
PLA	15.4 ± 3.7	15.1 ± 4.3	−0.31 ± 2.4	0.07	0.65	
SD	18.7 ± 6.3	19.2 ± 6.4	- 0.5 ± 2.0	0.08	0.37	
Creatinine (mg/dL)						0.28
PLA	1.01 ± 0.17	1.02 ± 0.16	0.00 ± 0.09	0.00	0.76	
SD	1.08 ± 0.11	1.13 ± 0.12	0.05 ± 0.11	0.00	0.11	
BUN:Creatinine						0.57
PLA	15.1 ± 2.6	14.7 ± 3.9	−0.38 ± 2.1	0.12	0.52	
SD	17.2 ± 5.0	17.3 ± 6.1	−0.07 ± 2.1	0.02	0.90	
Sodium (mEq/L)						0.47
PLA	139.5 ± 1.6	140.4 ± 1.2	0.92 ± 1.4	0.64	0.04*	
SD	139.7 ± 1.5	140.1 ± 1.1	0.43 ± 2.0	0.30	0.44	
Potassium (mEq/L)						0.14
PLA	4.2 ± 0.26	4.5 ± 0.19	0.31 ± 0.36	1.18	0.01*	
SD	4.3 ± 0.32	4.4 ± 0.34	0.11 ± 0.33	0.39	0.25	
Chloride (mEq/L)						0.32
PLA	102.3 ± 2.1	102.0 ± 1.1	−0.31 ± 1.7	0.18	0.52	
SD	102.3 ± 1.9	101.4 ± 1.7	−0.93 ± 1.5	0.50	0.04*	

Table 4 Hemodynamic, whole blood and clinical chemistry markers of health and safety *(Continued)*

Carbon Dioxide (mmol/L)						0.11
PLA	24.1 ± 1.4	24.5 ± 1.8	0.46 ± 1.8	0.25	0.36	
SD	24.8 ± 2.2	26.4 ± 2.0	1.57 ± 1.7	0.76	0.005*	
Calcium (mg/dL)						0.31
PLA	9.63 ± 0.34	9.68 ± 0.39	−0.05 ± 0.33	0.28	0.62	
SD	9.49 ± 0.31	9.39 ± 0.22	−0.1 ± 0.40	0.39	0.37	
Total Protein (g/L)						0.69
PLA	7.39 ± 0.34	7.08 ± 0.39	−0.31 ± 0.36	0.85	0.01*	
SD	6.96 ± 0.28	6.70 ± 0.28	−0.26 ± 0.30	1.00	0.007*	
Albumin (g/dL)						0.72
PLA	4.64 ± 0.30	4.65 ± 0.27	−0.01 ± 0.25	0.33	0.91	
SD	4.60 ± 0.16	4.58 ± 0.14	−0.02 ± 0.15	0.00	0.61	
Globulin (g/dL)						0.27
PLA	2.75 ± 0.23	2.43 ± 0.26	−0.32 ± 1.7	1.18	<0.001*	
SD	2.36 ± 0.26	2.12 ± 0.23	−0.24 ± 0.19	1.18	<0.001*	
Albumin: Globulin						0.62
PLA	1.70 ± 0.20	1.93 ± 0.24	0.23 ± 0.15	1.00	<0.001*	
SD	1.99 ± 0.25	2.19 ± 0.26	0.20 ± 0.17	0.67	<0.001*	
Bilirubin (mg/dL)						0.94
PLA	0.62 ± 0.25	0.60 ± 0.27	−0.02 ± 0.13	0.00	0.67	
SD	0.65 ± 0.21	0.63 ± 0.31	−0.02 ± 0.25	0.39	0.75	
Alkaline Phosphatase (U/L)						0.89
PLA	74.0 ± 22.6	74.2 ± 24.4	0.15 ± 12.2	0.01	0.96	
SD	67.1 ± 13.8	66.8 ± 14.8	−0.4 ± 5.3	0.02	0.81	
Aspartate Aminotransferase, AST (U/L)						0.59
PLA	25.9 ± 15.3	24.7 ± 13.6	−1.23 ± 6.23	0.08	0.49	
SD	28.0 ± 10.2	27.8 ± 9.5	−0.21 ± 2.83	0.02	0.78	
Alanine Aminotransferase, ALT (U/L)						0.66
PLA	31.2 ± 16.9	29.0 ± 16.3	−2.15 ± 7.6	0.13	0.33	
SD	27.3 ± 11.7	23.9 ± 8.8	−3.4 ± 6.5	0.33	0.07	
Total Cholesterol (mg/dL)						0.55
PLA	186.2 ± 48.0	182.2 ± 46.2	−3.9 ± 26.8	0.08	0.61	
SD	166.3 ± 40.6	157.3 ± 35.9	−9.0 ± 15.9	0.23	0.053*	
Triglycerides (mg/dL)						0.34
PLA	116.0 ± 51.7	115.8 ± 78.7	−0.23 ± 55.3	0.00	0.99	
SD	92.0 ± 84.3	71.8 ± 36.6	−20.2 ± 50.6	0.31	0.16	
HDL Cholesterol (mg/dL)						0.36
PLA	47.5 ± 9.4	47.2 ± 11.6	−0.31 ± 6.0	0.03	0.86	
SD	53.1 ± 12.9	50.9 ± 10.5	−2.21 ± 4.6	0.19	0.10	
VLDL Cholesterol (mg/dL)						0.33
PLA	23.2 ± 10.3	23.2 ± 15.7	0.00 ± 11.2	0.00	1.00	
SD	18.4 ± 17.0	14.3 ± 7.3	−4.14 ± 10.2	0.31	0.15	
LDL Cholesterol (mg/dL)						0.90
PLA	115.5 ± 41.6	111.9 ± 40.5	−3.62 ± 23.6	0.09	0.59	
SD	94.7 ± 31.4	92.1 ± 32.7	−2.64 ± 14.4	0.08	0.51	

Table 4 Hemodynamic, whole blood and clinical chemistry markers of health and safety *(Continued)*

Vitamin D (as 25(OH)D, ng/mL)						0.46
PLA	21.5 ± 5.2	23.3 ± 5.0	1.78 ± 3.94	0.35	0.13	
SD	35.1 ± 29.0	40.9 ± 45.4	3.95 ± 19.0	0.15	0.27	
C-Reactive Protein (mg/L)						0.64
PLA	1.41 ± 0.90	1.19 ± 0.65	−0.22 ± 0.6	0.25	0.19	
SD	1.46 ± 1.57	1.03 ± 1.11	−0.43 ± 1.5	0.36	0.29	

Values are mean ± SD. *= Significant within group change via t-test.

were made to evaluate changes as a result of supplementation because of the relatively low dose of caffeine in the test product (i.e. 50 mg or ~ 0.6 mg/kg body mass for these subjects). In addition, the last dose of SD (or placebo) was taken 24-hours prior to day 30 testing. Thus, we consider it unlikely that the caffeine contained in the *coffea arabica* fruit extract (CoffeeBerry®) of SD played a major role in the results. It is worth mentioning we cannot completely discount the potential effects that other unique ingredients in CoffeeBerry® (e.g., various chlorogenic acids and plant phenolics), may have had on these results.

Finally, data surrounding boron and vitamin D continue to lend support towards these nutrients and their ability to mitigate pain [20] as well as improve bone [21] and muscle health [23]. Findings from the present study did not reveal improved outcomes associated with self-reported pain, fatigue or weakness levels as assessed before and after the four week supplementation period. We speculate that the primary reason for these findings was associated with the existing joint and bone health of our study participants. For example, our study participants were otherwise healthy, middle-aged men who golfed on a regular basis and as a result were maintaining a basic level of physical activity. When compared to the study participants in other published trials showing improvements in self-reported pain [19-21,24], participants from the present study were younger, healthier and had minimal baseline levels of pain. The lack of change found in serum levels of 25-hydroxy vitamin D as a result of supplementation was not entirely unexpected. Given the moderate dose (1,000 IU/day), the time of year the study was conducted (late Fall), and general latitude of the study location (Kent, OH = 41.15° N), it is our contention that the majority of supplemented vitamin D was quickly absorbed by peripheral tissues.

From an adverse event and/or clinical safety perspective, the SD supplement was well tolerated with no significant group × time interactive changes in any of the measured clinical markers (Tables 4 and 5). A few variables did experience significant within-group changes (e.g., diastolic blood pressure, glucose, sodium, potassium, carbon dioxide, albumin: globulin ratio, total protein and globulin, etc.), but in all such circumstances, both groups changes remained within clinical accepted normative values.

The strengths of the present study are that it was a double-blind, placebo-controlled investigation using a "free-living" approach. Thus, the findings are applicable to many consumers who golf but do not follow a rigid diet or exercise program. To date, extremely limited research is available exploring the potential impact of various nutritional agents on golf performance, with one of the only published accounts reporting an improvement in stress hormone levels and shot-making after phosphatidylserine supplementation [2]. The disadvantages of the present study primarily revolve around the pilot nature of the investigation and the lack of female subjects. The authors recognize that the relatively small number of subjects and short supplementation period (4 weeks) likely hindered the ability to uncover significant effects in some outcome measures, particularly since the participants were relatively young and healthy and were not required to follow a particular exercise training program or dietary regimen. It is also important to discuss other considerations related to our data and findings. For example, the positive outcome surrounding best drive distance is likely impacted by a number of other factors that we weren't able to be measured in our study design including, but not limited to: club head acceleration at the point of impact with the ball, club head deceleration through the zone of impact, rotational power, improved accuracy of club head placement relative the ball, club face angle at ball strike, and musculoskeletal range of motion. Two additional factors are upper-body strength and power that were measured in the present study by determining bench press 1RM and sagittal plane power development during bench press throws. The authors recognize that performance of the bench press exercise may be viewed by some as having very little carryover to golf swing performance, but these parameters were chosen due to their high reliability of measurement and as being valid and commonly used measures of maximal strength and power in the sports science literature. Additionally, it is important to highlight that Marta and colleagues indicate that the pectoralis major, deltoid, and latissimus dosi are the most active muscle groups during the golf swing movement, particularly during the acceleration phase [29]. A three-dimensional analysis of golf swing performance using two common clubs was

Table 5 Pain and quality of life data

	Intervention			Comparison of change (p)		
	Pre	Post	Change	Effect size (*d*)	Within groups	Group × Time
Worst Pain						
PLA	1.62 ± 2.60	1.38 ± 2.14	−0.23 ± 1.09	0.08	0.46	0.52
SD	0.79 ± 1.31	0.93 ± 1.33	0.14 ± 1.79	0.08	0.77	
Least Pain						
PLA	0.31 ± 0.63	0.31 ± 0.85	0.00 ± 0.58	0.00	1.00	0.50
SD	0.36 ± 0.74	0.14 ± 0.53	−0.21 ± 0.97	0.49	0.43	
Average Pain						
PLA	1.38 ± 1,89	1.15 ± 1.52	−0.23 ± 0.83	0.12	0.34	0.97
SD	0.79 ± 1.12	0.57 ± 1.09	−0.21 ± 1.53	0.18	0.61	
Pain Level Now						
PLA	0.69 ± 1.44	0.69 ± 1.32	0.00 ± 1.68	0.00	1.00	0.48
SD	0.43 ± 0.94	0.07 ± 0.27	−0.36 ± 0.74	0.45	0.10	
Relief						
PLA	13.8 ± 34.0	6.2 ± 22.2	−7.7 ± 27.7	0.26	0.34	0.53
SD	16.4 ± 33.9	18.6 ± 37.0	−2.1 ± 49.0	0.06	0.87	
Current Activity						0.88
PLA	0.54 ± 1.13	0.31 ± 0.85	−0.23 ± 1.4	0.20	0.55	
SD	0.50 ± 1.34	0.36 ± 0.74	−0.14 ± 1.7	0.10	0.75	
Current Mood						0.45
PLA	0.31 ± 0.75	0.15 ± 0.38	−0.15 ± 0.69	0.16	0.44	
SD	0.14 ± 0.53	0.21 ± 0.60	−0.07 ± 0.83	0.18	0.75	
Walking						0.08
PLA	0.38 ± 1.12	0.85 ± 1.81	−0.46 ± 0.97	0.27	0.11	
SD	0.21 ± 0.43	0.14 ± 0.53	−0.07 ± 0.47	0.22	0.58	
Normal Work						0.67
PLA	0.31 ± 0.63	0.23 ± 0.60	−0.07 ± 0.76	0.17	0.72	
SD	0.43 ± 0.94	0.21 ± 0.58	−0.21 ± 0.89	0.26	0.39	
Sleep Quality						0.48
PLA	0.46 ± 1.1	0.45 ± 1.1	0.00 ± 1.0	0.00	1.00	
SD	0.43 ± 1.1	0.14 ± 0.4	−0.29 ± 1.1	0.36	0.34	
Yale P1						0.26
PLA	5471 ± 4118	5954 ± 4705	- 483 ± 2436	0.11	0.49	
SD	6376 ± 6967	5175 ± 2238	−1200 ± 4755	0.22	0.36	
Yale P2						0.77
PLA	85.5 ± 34.3	64.3 ± 26.1	−21.2 ± 45.6	0.70	0.12	
SD	114.9 ± 57.6	86.5 ± 52.5	−28.4 ± 76.8	0.52	0.19	
PCS						0.35
PLA	52.6 ± 7.1	56.0 ± 2.8	3.4 ± 5.7	0.63	0.05	
SD	53.9 ± 4.3	55.5 ± 2.7	1.6 ± 4.0	0.45	0.17	
MCS						0.59
PLA	55.5 ± 4.2	53.6 ± 6.5	−1.87 ± 6.58	0.35	0.33	
SD	56.1 ± 5.1	55.3 ± 3.5	−0.82 ± 2.85	0.18	0.30	

Values are mean ± SD. No significant changes between or within groups were noted.

employed as a measurement method of golfing performance. While much more practical, this measurement method only reports on final performance and thus does not allow for a clearer understanding of what aspects of performance SD may have improved according to our findings, particularly as they relate to best drive distance. In this respect, it is important for the reader to understand other factors may have impacted our observed outcomes related to best driver distance.

Conclusions

This preliminary investigation yielded significantly greater improvements in best drive distance (~13.6 yards) and a tendency for average driver distance to improve in healthy male golfers consuming SD for four weeks. Careful interpretation of these data is encouraged due to their preliminary nature and need to be followed-up with a larger and longer investigation.

Competing interests

The authors declare that they have no competing or financial interests concerning the outcome of this investigation. The sponsor of this study, Purity Products (Plainview, NY) provided an independent research grant and donated the study product (SD) and placebo, but had no role in the collection, analyses, or interpretation of the data.

Authors' contributions

AWK provided medical oversight, subject screening, subject recruitment and assisted with data collection and manuscript preparation. TNZ and HLL designed the study, secured funding for project, assisted with data analysis and manuscript preparation. JES and SMH carried out subject recruitment, data collection, coordination of the study and compliance. RLA coordinated and assisted with all golf simulations and performance assessments. CMK assisted with data analysis and prepared the manuscript. All authors read and approved the final manuscript.

Acknowledgements

The authors would like to thank the subjects who participated in the study and the sponsor (Purity Products). The presentation of results of this study does not constitute endorsement by the any of the investigators, the universities they represent, The Center for Applied Health Sciences, or the journal in which it is published.

Author details

[1]The Center for Applied Health Sciences, 4302 Allen Road, Ste 120, Stow, OH 44224, USA. [2]Strength and Conditioning, Athletics Department, Kent State University, Kent, OH 44240, USA. [3]School of Sport, Recreation and Exercise Sciences, Lindenwood University, St. Charles, MO 63301, USA.

References

1. Smith MF. The role of physiology in the development of golf performance. Sports Med. 2010;40(8):635–55.
2. Jager R, Purpura M, Geiss KR, Weiss M, Baumeister J, Amatulli F, Schroder L, Herwegen H. The effect of phosphatidylserine on golf performance. J Int Soc Sports Nutr. 2007;4(1):23.
3. Buford TW, Kreider RB, Stout JR, Greenwood M, Campbell B, Spano M, Ziegenfuss T, Lopez H, Landis J, Antonio J. International Society of Sports Nutrition position stand: creatine supplementation and exercise. J Int Soc Sports Nutr. 2007;4:6.
4. Greenhaff PL. Muscle creatine loading in humans: Procedures and functional and metabolic effects. In: 6th International Conference on Guanidino Compounds in Biology and Medicine: 2001. Cincinnati, OH; 2001.
5. Greenhaff PL, Bodin K, Soderlund K, Hultman E. Effect of oral creatine supplementation on skeletal muscle phosphocreatine resynthesis. Am J Physiol. 1994;266(5 Pt 1):E725–30.
6. Hultman E, Soderlund K, Timmons JA, Cederblad G, Greenhaff PL. Muscle creatine loading in men. J Appl Physiol. 1996;81(1):232–7.
7. Kreider RB. Effects of creatine supplementation on performance and training adaptations. Mol Cell Biochem. 2003;244(1–2):89–94.
8. Kreider RB, Ferreira M, Wilson M, Grindstaff P, Plisk S, Reinardy J, Cantler E, Almada AL. Effects of creatine supplementation on body composition, strength, and sprint performance. Med Sci Sports Exerc. 1998;30(1):73–82.
9. Astorino TA, Roberson DW. Efficacy of acute caffeine ingestion for short-term high-intensity exercise performance: a systematic review. J Strength Cond Res. 2010;24(1):257–65.
10. Glade MJ. Caffeine-Not just a stimulant. Nutrition. 2010;26(10):932–8.
11. Goldstein ER, Ziegenfuss T, Kalman D, Kreider R, Campbell B, Wilborn C, et al. International society of sports nutrition position stand: caffeine and performance. J Int Soc Sports Nutr. 2010;7(1):5.
12. Davis JK, Green JM. Caffeine and anaerobic performance: ergogenic value and mechanisms of action. Sports Med. 2009;39(10):813–32.
13. Doherty M, Smith PM. Effects of caffeine ingestion on rating of perceived exertion during and after exercise: a meta-analysis. Scand J Med Sci Sports. 2005;15(2):69–78.
14. Einother SJ, Giesbrecht T. Caffeine as an attention enhancer: reviewing existing assumptions. Psychopharmacology. 2013;225(2):251–74.
15. Armstrong TA, Spears JW, Crenshaw TD, Nielsen FH. Boron supplementation of a semipurified diet for weanling pigs improves feed efficiency and bone strength characteristics and alters plasma lipid metabolites. J Nutr. 2000;130(10):2575–81.
16. Hooshmand S, Chai SC, Saadat RL, Payton ME, Brummel-Smith K, Arjmandi BH. Comparative effects of dried plum and dried apple on bone in postmenopausal women. Br J Nutr. 2011;106(6):923–30.
17. Scorei RI, Rotaru P. Calcium fructoborate–potential anti-inflammatory agent. Biol Trace Elem Res. 2011;143(3):1223–38.
18. Scorei R, Cimpoiasu VM, Iordachescu D. In vitro evaluation of the antioxidant activity of calcium fructoborate. Biol Trace Elem Res. 2005;107(2):127–34.
19. Miljukovic ND, Miljkovic DA, Ercegan GM. Osteoarthritis and Calcium Fructo Borate Supplementation: An Open-Label Pilot Study. Yugoslavia: University of Novi Sad; 2002.
20. Scorei R, Mitrut P, Petrisor I, Scorei I. A double-blind, placebo-controlled pilot study to evaluate the effect of calcium fructoborate on systemic inflammation and dyslipidemia markers for middle-aged people with primary osteoarthritis. Biol Trace Elem Res. 2011;144(1–3):253–63.
21. Price CT, Langford JR, Liporace FA. Essential Nutrients for Bone Health and a Review of their Availability in the Average North American Diet. Open Orthopaedics J. 2012;6:143–9.
22. Eglia L. Vitamin D and its role in skeletal muscle. Curr Opin Clin Nutr Metab Care. 2009;12(6):628–33.
23. Hamilton B. Vitamin D and human skeletal muscle. Scand J Med Sci Sports. 2010;20(2):182–90.
24. Sato Y, Iwamoto J, Kanoko T, Satoh K. Low-dose vitamin D prevents muscular atrophy and reduces falls and hip fractures in women after stroke: a randomized controlled trial. Cerebrovasc Dis. 2005;20(3):187–92.
25. Calvo MS, Whiting SJ, Barton CN. Vitamin D fortification in the United States and Canada: current status and data needs. Am J Clin Nutr. 2004;80(6 Suppl):1710S–6.
26. Cuka S, Dvornik S, Drazenovic K, Mihic J. Evaluation of the Dade Behring Dimension RxL clinical chemistry analyzer. Clin Lab. 2001;47(1–2):35–40.
27. Baechle TR, Earle RW. Essentials of Strength Training and Conditioning. Champaign, IL: Human Kinetics; 2000.
28. Alemany JA, Pandorf CE, Montain SJ, Castellani JW, Tuckow AP, Nindl BC. Reliability assessment of ballistic jump squats and bench throws. J Strength Cond Res. 2005;19(1):33–8.
29. Marta S, Silva L, Castro MA, Pezarat-Correia P, Cabri J. Electromyography variables during the golf swing: a literature review. J Electromyogr Kinesiol. 2012;22(6):803–13.
30. Hoffman JR, Ratamess NA, Kang J, Rashti SL, Faigenbaum AD. Effect of betaine supplementation on power performance and fatigue. J Int Soc Sports Nutr. 2009;6:7.

31. Stock MS, Beck TW, DeFreitas JM, Dillon MA. Test-retest reliability of barbell velocity during the free-weight bench-press exercise. J Strength Cond Res. 2011;25(1):171–7.
32. Weir JP. Quantifying test-retest reliability using the intraclass correlation coefficient and the SEM. J Strength Cond Res. 2005;19(1):231–40.
33. Kruskall LJ, Campbell WW, Evans WJ. The Yale Physical Activity Survey for older adults: predictions in the energy expenditure due to physical activity. J Am Diet Assoc. 2004;104(8):1251–7.

Dietary iron intervention using a staple food product for improvement of iron status in female runners

Ieva Alaunyte[1,2], Valentina Stojceska[1,3*], Andrew Plunkett[1] and Emma Derbyshire[1]

Abstract

Background: Adequate nutrient intake is critically important for achieving optimal sports performance. Like all athletes, female runners require a nutritionally balanced diet to maintain daily activities and a successful training regime. This study investigates the effects of cereal product based dietary iron intervention on iron status of recreational female runners (n = 11; 32 ± 7yr; 239 ± 153 minutes exercise/week, of which 161 ± 150 minutes running activity/week; VO_{2max} 38 ± 4 ml/kg/min).

Methods: Participants completed a 6-week dietary intervention study. They were asked to replace their usual bread with iron-rich Teff bread as part of their daily diet. During this period, their dietary habits were assessed by multiple pass 24-hr recalls; iron status was determined by venous blood analysis for serum transferrin, serum transferrin receptor, serum ferritin, total iron-binding capacity and transferrin receptor/ferritin log index.

Results: Pre-intervention a cohort of 11 female runners reported inadequate daily dietary iron intake of 10.7 ± 2.7 mg/day, which was associated with overall compromised iron status. Over a third of all participants showed depleted bodily iron stores (serum ferritin <12 μg/L). Pre-intervention macronutrient assessment revealed adequate energy, protein and fibre intakes, whilst total fat and saturated fat intake was above the recommendations at the expense of carbohydrate intake. A 6-week dietary intervention resulted in significantly higher total iron intakes (18.5 mg/day, $P < 0.05$) and improved iron tissue supply but not enlarged iron stores. Improvements in heamatological indices were associated with compromised baseline iron status, prolonged intervention period and increase in dietary iron intake.

Conclusion: Dietary iron interventions using a staple cereal product offer an alternative way of improving dietary iron intake and favourable affecting overall iron status in physically active females.

Keywords: Iron-deficiency, Athletes, Dietary intake, Ferritin

Background

Iron is an essential mineral for optimal physical performance [1]. It has a role in oxygen transport and energy production and serves as a functional component of haemoglobin and myoglobin. Additionally, iron is a crucial part of cytochromes, found in the electron transport system during production of ATP, hence, providing energy source for physical movement. Therefore, in order for the metabolism and oxygen transfer to take place efficiently during physical performance, there must be an adequate level of iron in the human body.

Considerable evidence suggests that nutritional iron deficiency has a negative impact not only on overall health and wellbeing [2] but also on exercise performance [3,4]; hence, improving overall iron status in athletes may enhance their athletic performance. Female athletes, especially runners, are at greater risk of iron deficiency due to increased iron loss in the gastrointestinal tract, sweat, urine and menstruation, and increased haemolysis during endurance training [1]. Furthermore, inadequate dietary iron intake, coupled with limited bioavailability of iron

* Correspondence: Valentina.Stojceska@brunel.ac.uk
[1]Department of Food and Tourism Management Old Hall Lane, Manchester Metropolitan University, Manchester M14 6HR, UK
[3]College of Engineering, Design and Physical Sciences, Brunel University, Uxbridge, Middlesex UB8 3PH, UK
Full list of author information is available at the end of the article

in the diet, may present even a greater risk of iron-deficiency in female athletes.

The effectiveness of conventional iron deficiency treatment of pharmacological doses of iron in supplement form is often questioned due to low compliance rates associated with the side effects such as nausea, stomach pain, constipation and diarrhoea [2]. Therefore, good nutritional practices to achieve adequate iron balance have been suggested as the first line of action in the prevention of iron deficiency in female athletes [3,5]. Although, iron-deficiency anaemia has been shown to have an adverse effect on performance [6,7], the evidence on iron deficiency in the absence of anaemia and the effect on athletic performance is conflicting. Whilst, some researchers reported significant improvements in performance and adaptation in endurance capacity of marginally iron-deficient females after the correction of iron status using iron supplements [8-10], others show no improvement or in fact little adverse effect of marginal iron depletion on exercise performance [11,12].

In addition to this, the research looking at the effects of dietary iron interventions on iron status and exercise performance in female athletes is very scarce. A longitudinal study conducted on swimmers investigated iron status and exercise performance during a 6-month period [13]. The authors reported no differences in iron status or performance scores between iron-rich diet and free choice diet participants. However, a four weeks iron-rich diet, which provided 18.2 mg/d, showed significant effects on serum ferritin concentration in rhythmic gymnasts [14]. Another study reported that a diet rich in iron (11.8 mg iron/day) was more effective in protecting iron status than were the supplements (50 mg ferrous sulphate/day) during 12 weeks of aerobic tests in previous sedentary women [15]. Additionally, the dietary intervention group also showed the highest improvement in their exercise tests. Another study on dietary intervention and iron status in athletes showed that a 4-week dietary advice counselling did not improve overall iron status [16]. However, the authors suggested that diet composition, in particularly the presence of enhancers of non-haem iron absorption, was the most predominant influence for iron absorption in this population. The most recent study investigated the effects of heme iron-rich food product consumption in women of reproductive age [17]. The authors concluded that dietary-based iron treatment using iron-rich crisp bread improved iron status similarly to iron supplements and provided fewer side effects.

The present study aimed to explore dietary iron intervention by the means of a staple food product and the effects of that on iron status in female runners.

Methods

Design

This study investigated the relationships between iron-rich food product incorporation into the daily diet and changes of iron status in physically active females during a 6-week intervention period. This study was conducted according to the guidelines laid down in the Declaration of Helsinki and all procedures involving human subjects were approved by the Ethics Committee of a UK Higher Education institution. Written consent was collected from all participants.

Participants

A total of 15 female subjects, recruited from local running clubs and leisure centers, expressed an interest in participating in the study. Participant's eligibility was tested by a screening questionnaire. The inclusion criteria included: age 18-45 years, engagement in purposeful physical activity, in particular running, for at least the previous 6 months at the level of at least 30 minutes a day 3 or more times a week, no muscoskeletal problems or recent injury, no heart conditions or complaints, no asthma, normal blood pressure, no-smokers, no current chronic diseases, regular menstrual cycles, no recent iron therapy, no blood donation or haemophilia, no current pregnancy or pregnant within the past year, no food allergies or intolerances, no recent history of eating disorders. After screening, 4 subjects dropped out due to the exclusion criteria (recent pregnancy, n = 1; Diabetes, n = 1) and compliance issues (missed their first appointment, n = 2).

Procedures

After pre-study screening, eligible subjects were assigned to a 6-week dietary intervention. During the intervention, study participants were asked to swap their usual bread with Teff bread per day (5.6 mg iron per 100 g), which was developed by the research team [18], and not to change any other of their dietary habits or exercise regimes.

All subjects were familiarised with the study's protocol a week prior to the intervention. Participants' current diet, exercise levels, anthropometric measurements, blood iron parameters and exercise performance were assessed on baseline (week 0), midpoint (week 3) and end (week 6) of the intervention. Subjects were also asked to keep a bread consumption log in order to record their compliance.

Anthropometric assessment

Subjects' height and weight were recorded at baseline (week 1), midpoint (week 3) and end (week 6) of the study using Seca 217 stadiometer (Cranlea, Birmingham, UK) and Seca 711 personal weighing machine (Cranlea, Birmingham, UK), respectively.

Dietary assessment

Dietary intakes and supplements usage were collected using multiple pass 24-hour diet recalls for each participant at baseline (week 1), midpoint (week 3) and end (week 6). The food records were analysed using NetWisp 3.0 (Tinuviel Software, Llanfechell, Anglesey, UK) diet analysis software. Missing food items' nutritional data were manually entered into the software by either locating food composition from product manufacturers' websites or the McCance and Widdowson's Composition of Foods integrated dataset (6th Summary, UK Nutrient Databank, 2002, UK).

Under-reporting was assessed by Goldberg cut-off limits [19]. Total energy was tested for under-reporting by applying the following formula: Basal metabolic rate (BMR) X 1.55. Test values below the cut-off limit were considered to represent underreporting. BMR for each participant was obtained by Henry equation [20].

Nutritional data were compared to the dietary reference values (DRVs) for energy [21], macro- and micronutrients [22]. Because carbohydrate requirements for athletes are higher than those in general population, carbohydrate recommendation intake was based on the American Dietetic Association (ADA), Dietitians of Canada (DC), and American College of Sports Medicine (ACSM) joint position statement recommendations [23].

Haematological assessment

Iron status was assessed from non-fasted blood samples taken at baseline (week 0) and completion of the intervention (week 6). To limit the possibility of an acute phase response to exercise affecting these results, samples were taken at least 12 hours after the last exercise session and at the same time of the day followed a controlled fluid and food intake [24].

The following blood indices were analysed: serum ferritin (sFer), serum transferrin (sTRF) and serum transferrin receptor (sTsfR). Because these serum iron status indicators are not immediately influenced by food intake [25], the subjects did not fast before having their blood taken. Serum was prepared from venous bloods by centrifugation after clotting and was stored at -20°C for determination of iron status indices. Serum ferritin (sFer) was measured by immunometry, using an electrochemiluminescence immunoassay (ECLIA) on Modular Analytics E170 (Roche Diagnostics GmbH, Mannheim, Germany). Serum transferrin was measured by immunoturbidimetric assay; and serum transferrin receptor (sTsfR) by particle-enhanced immunoturbidimetric assay, both using Cobas integra system (Roche Diagnostics GmbH, Mannheim, Germany). All serum samples were analysed concurrently at the completion of the study to eliminate variation in assay conditions. Reproducibility of the test kits was determined using human samples and controls in internal protocols. All analyses were performed at one point in time, therefore, coefficient of variance (CV) within run (n = 84 for sFer, n = 20 for sTRF and sTsfR) for the lower and upper range values were used.

Additional haematological indices were determined to obtain more comprehensive range of iron status indicators. Total iron binding capacity (TIBC) was calculated using the formula: TIBC (μmol/L) =25.1 × TRF (g/L) [26]. The upper threshold value of 1.5 was used for sTfR/log ferritin ratio (sTfR-F index) [27].

Statistical analysis

Statistical tests were carried out using SPSS 16.0 (SPSS Inc., Chicago, Illinois, US). A significance level of $P < 0.05$ was used.

The normality of dependent variables was tested by Shapiro-Wilk test for baseline values for subjects' age, BMI, training regime, iron status parameters, and exercise performance scores. The normal distribution, in terms of skewness and kurtosis, were assessed using 2 × standard deviation for both values. Log transformation was applied to variables that were not normally distributed. Boxplots were used to check for possible outliers.

Dietary confounders were assessed using baseline, midpoint and end means values applying repeated measures one-way ANOVA test.

Descriptive statistics and differences in mean values of investigated factors were tested by Pearson's where no account for possible confounders is needed and Partial Correlation with the presence of confounders and Paired-sample t-test to determine the statistical significance effect of pre- and post-intervention. These tests were applied for the haematological data at baseline and end.

Baseline dietary intakes for macro- and micronutrients were compared to dietary recommendations using One-sample t-test.

Results

Participants' characteristics

Characteristics of the participants are shown in Table 1. The mean age of participants was 32 years. The subjects were within the normal BMI range and engaged in regular exercise regime, mostly running.

Although the sample size was small (n = 11) the study employed stringent inclusion criteria and accounted for possible confounders, including dietary habits and training routine. The statistical tests for normality showed no significant anomalies for subjects' age, BMI, nutrients intakes, exercise and blood iron parameters, suggesting the present study had overall normal variables distribution. No case of dietary underreporting was evident in the sample.

Table 1 Characteristics of study participants

ID	Age (yrs)	BMI (kg/m^2)	Main sports participating*	Exercise regime (min/wk)	Running activity (min/wk)	VO_{2max} (ml/min/kg)	Compliance (bread slices/day)
1	44	20	R (l-d)	380	300	46	6.2
2	29	23	R	170	110	40	3.0
3	20	22	R, V	540	360	38	3.6
4	36	21	R	120	60	36	1.4
5	28	22	R, SW	120	60	35	2.5
6	39	21	R (l-d)	480	480	42	5.0
7	31	25	R	160	100	35	5.5
8	26	24	D, R	180	30	42	3.5
9	38	27	R	200	150	34	2.1
10	33	28	R	160	60	33	5.0
11	33	25	R (l-d)	120	60	33	5.4
Mean ± SD	**32 ± 7**	**23 ± 2**		**239 ± 153**	**161 ± 150**	**38 ± 4**	**2403 ± 392**

Key: *R-running, R (l-d)- long-distance running, V- volleyball, SW-swimming, D-dancing.

Adequacy of diets before intervention

Energy and nutrient intakes are presented in Figure 1. Female runners achieved the recommendations for total energy and protein. Fibre intakes were satisfactory. Total fat and saturated fatty acids intake was above the recommended value at the expense of carbohydrate intake, which was significantly lower than the recommendation. The intake of non-milk extrinsic sugars (NMES) was found to be above the recommended value of <10% total energy. Female runners exceeded the recommendations for Vitamin C, B-group vitamins, calcium and zinc. However, they did not meet recommendations for Vitamin A and showed significantly ($P < 0.001$) lower intake of iron compared to the recommendations (Figures 1 and 2).

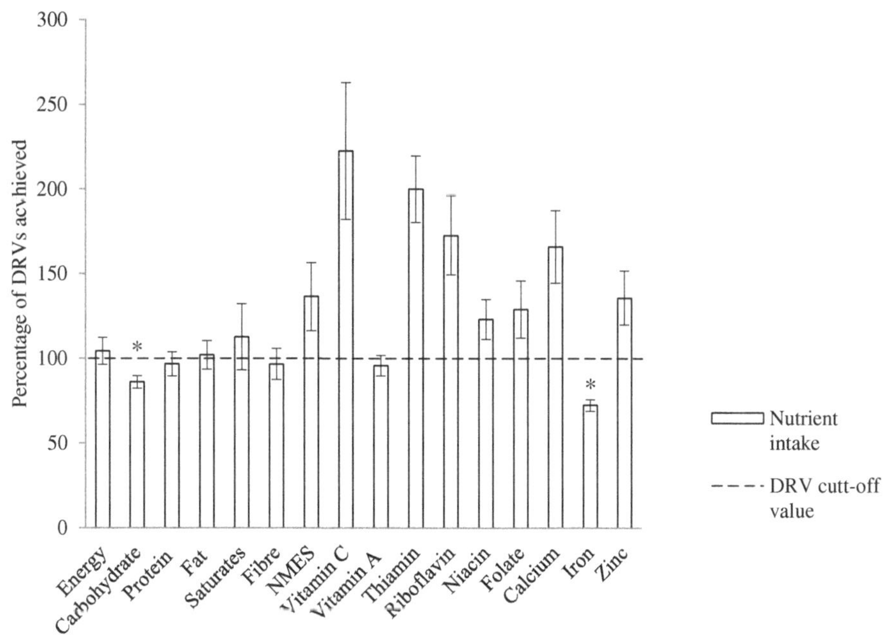

Figure 1 Comparison of mean daily energy, macro- and micro-nutrient intake of female runners and dietary reference values. Key: DRVs – Dietary Reference Values, TEI – total energy intake, NMES – non-milk extrinsic sugars. *represent significantly ($P < 0.001$) lower observed value compared to that of recommended intake. DRVs used: carbohydrate - 60% TEI [(Ref)], protein – 15% TEI [(Ref)], fat - <35% TEI [(Ref)], saturates - <10 TEI, fibre – 18g/day [(Ref)], NMES - <10% TEI, vitamin C – 40 mg/day, vitamin A - , thiamin - , riboflavin - , niacin - , folate, calcium – 700 mg/day, iron – 14.8 mg/day [(Ref)], zinc - .

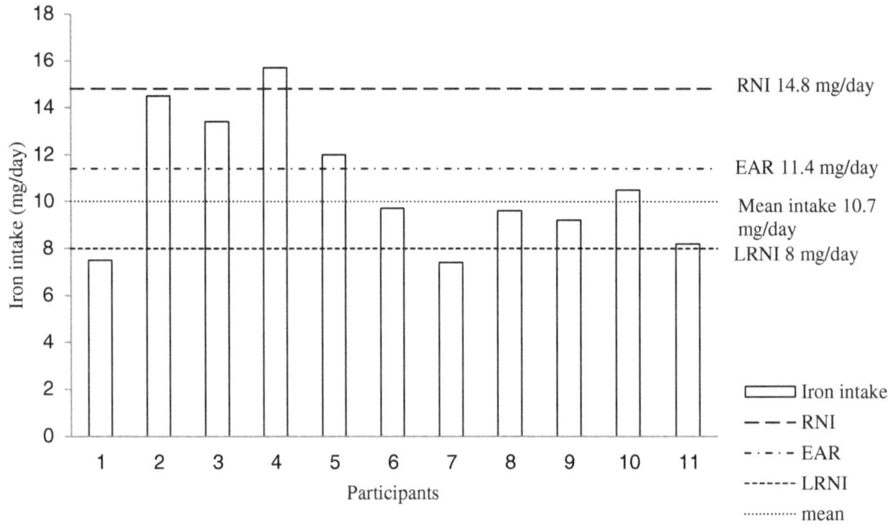

Figure 2 Comparison of individual daily dietary iron intake in female runners and dietary reference values. Key: LRNI - lower reference nutrient intake, EAR - estimated average requirements, RNI - reference nutrient intake.

Changes in nutrient intake and iron status during intervention

The intake of total dietary iron increased significantly, from 10.7 to 18.5 mg/day ($P < 0.05$) as a result of the intervention. Teff bread provided 7.0 ± 3.3 mg iron a day which contributed to 45% of the daily recommendation value for dietary iron throughout the intervention period. Teff bread also contributed to 15% of carbohydrate, 16% of protein, 5% of fat and 31% of fibre daily dietary reference values as presented in Table 2.

Although, haematological indices improved, there were no statistically significant differences observed in sTRF, sTsfR, sFer, TIBC and sTsfR-F index values before and after the intervention in the present study (Table 3).

Table 4 shows correlations between changes in iron indices during intervention period, baseline iron status and other intervention variables. The changes in iron status parameters were correlated with reduced baseline iron tissue supply. Because of compliance issues, the intervention period varied across this cohort (4 to 6 weeks). The prolonged intervention period was positively correlated to improved iron tissue supply (ΔsTRF and ΔsTsfR). In terms of dietary iron changes as a result of the intervention, a significant ($P < 0.05$) positive relationship was observed between increased dietary iron and enlarged iron stores (ΔsFer).

Discussion

Despite the increased interest in nutrition amongst athletes and the well documented importance of a balanced diet in athletic performance, research suggests that many athletes might be consuming diets that are less than optimal [28,29]. This trend also observed in the present study. The runners' diets provided inadequate amounts of carbohydrate, whilst their intake of total fat, saturated fat and NMES were above the national recommendations (Figure 1). Most of micronutrient intakes were observed to be above reference nutrient intake (RNI), with the exception of Vitamin A and iron. The baseline iron intake of the present study's cohort provided only 70% of RNI for

Table 2 Teff bread nutritional composition

Nutrients in Teff bread	Amount per 100 g	Total daily contribution to nutrients[1]	Percentage daily contribution to DRVs[1,2]
	Mean ± SD	Mean ± SD	Mean ± SD
Carbohydrate (g)	43.2 ± 2.32	54.1 ± 16.14	15 ± 5.9
Protein (g)*	11.0 ± 0.02	13.8 ± 4.11	16 ± 5.8
Fat (g)*	3.7 ± 0.16	4.6 ± 1.38	5 ± 1.9
Fibre (g)*	4.5 ± 0.32	5.6 ± 1.68	31 ± 9.3
Iron (mg)*	5.62 ± 0.22	7.0 ± 3.32	45 ± 19.0

Key: DRVs – Dietary Reference Values, TEI – total energy intake.
*experimentally determined as previously described [(Ref)].
[1]Based on reported consumption of average daily portion of 125 ± 37g of Teff bread by the participants.
[2]DRVs used: carbohydrate - 60% TEI [(Ref)], protein – 15% TEI [(Ref)], fat - <35% TEI [(Ref)], fibre – 18g/day [(Ref)], iron – 14.8 mg/day [(Ref)].

Table 3 Changes in haematological data pre- and post-intervention

Iron status parameter	Pre- intervention	Post-intervention	Change	Intrinsic error (lower-upper range values)*
Serum Transferrin (g/L)	3.21 ± 0.6	2.97 ± 0.4	- 5.4%	0.86 – 0.77%
Serum Transferrin Receptor (mg/L)	3.43 ± 1.8	2.96 ± 1.3	- 12.8%	0.76 – 1.1%
Serum Ferritin (μg/L)	29.64 ± 20.9	33.40 ± 18.8	+ 5.4%	3.8 – 2.1%
TIBC (μmol/L)	81.2 ± 14.7	76.2 ± 9.8	- 6.2%	N/A
sTfR-F index	3.66 ± 3.7	1.94 ± 2.2	- 16.7%	N/A

Key: *Intrinsic error was determined as coefficient of variance (CV) within run (n = 84 for sFer, n = 20 for sTRF and sTsfR) for the lower and upper reference range values for all direct measurement haematological indices.

iron [22]. This trend is in agreement with most of other researchers [30,31], who also reported most of macro- and micronutrient intakes to be above recommended values with the exception of iron. The mean intake iron in this study was 10.7 ± 2.7 mg/d. This corresponds to the other authors' reported iron intakes of 11.0-12.2 mg/d for female athletes' population [32,33] and in fact is similar to that of the general female population, which is reported to be at around 9.6 ± 3.0 mg/d [34]. In addition to this, the present study found that only 36% of runners reached estimated average requirement (EAR) of 11.4 mg/day, with 18% of them falling below the lower reference nutrient intake (LRNI) (Figure 2). This is similar to the levels (23%) reported for the general female population [34]. Taking into account that the iron requirement for female runners may be higher than general population [35], the baseline observations from the current study indicate that dietary iron intakes in this population are far from adequate.

Table 4 Relationships between incremental haematological data and intervention variables

Changes in haematological indices	% change	Correlations with	r value, *P* value
ΔsTRF (g/L)	-5.4	Baseline sTRF	r = - 0.7, *P* < 0.05
		Baseline sTsfR	r = - 0.8, *P* < 0.01
		Baseline TIBC	r = - 0.7, *P* < 0.05
		Baseline sTsfR-F index	r = - 0.8, *P* < 0.005
		No of days of intervention[1]	r = - 0.7, *P* < 0.05
ΔsTsfR (mg/L)	-12.8	Baseline sTsfR	r = - 0.8, *P* < 0.05
		Baseline sTRF	r = - 0.6, *P* < 0.05
		Baseline TIBC	r = - 0.6, *P* < 0.05
		Baseline sTsfR-F index	r = - 0.8, *P* < 0.005
		No of days of intervention*	r = - 0.6, *P* < 0.05
ΔsFer (μg/L)	+5.4	Δ sTsfR-F index	r = - 0.6, *P* < 0.05
		Δ dietary iron intake†	r = 0.8, *P* < 0.05

Key: sTRF - serum transferring, sTsfR - serum transferrin receptor, sFer - serum ferritin.
*partial correlations controlling for corresponding baseline haematological parameter.
†partial correlations controlling for changes in dietary calcium and vitamin C intake.
Δrepresents an incremental change.
*DRV cut-off value.

As a result of the intervention, the dietary iron intake increased to 18.5 ± 3 mg/d by the end of the study. However, the improvements in iron status were observed at a statistically non-significant level (Table 3). Nevertheless, within-subject variation, measured as coefficient of variance, showed that iron tissue supply parameters (sTRF and sTsfR) improved at a notably greater increment when compared to the intrinsic error. This indicates that the changes were due to the intervention. However, this was not observed in iron tissue parameters (sFer) which indicates the change must have been notably influences by the within-subject variation.

The lack of significant change in iron status in the current study may be attributed to several factors. One plausible explanation would be that mean serum ferritin baseline value showed iron-repletion state (sFer 29.64 ± 20.9 μg/L). Researchers have demonstrated an inverse relationship between iron absorption and serum ferritin [36]. Hence, it may be possible that the subjects in this study had sufficient iron stores at baseline, which would explain the lack of significant effect of increased dietary iron intake on overall iron status. The majority of other iron therapy research studies recruited iron-depleted female runners (sFer < 20 μg/L) and used pharmacological dosage of iron supplementation, hence, it is difficult to compare them to the findings from current study. A study using a heme iron-based crisp bread dietary intervention in women of reproductive age showed a significant improvement in serum ferritin after 12 weeks of daily 35 mg of dietary iron intake [17]. The baseline serum ferritin levels of 24 μg/L were reported in Hoppe *et al.* study which suggest that participants may have had depleted iron stores. A longitudinal study by Tsalis *et al.* demonstrated no change in sFer levels of swimmers after 5 months of dietary intervention (26 mg/day) and a decrease in sFer after 6 months [13]. The participants in Tsalis *et al.* study showed similar iron storage values to the present study (sFer > 30 μg/L). Hence, similar baseline iron status of these studies cohorts may explain the lack of iron therapy effect in both studies.

Another reason for the lack of notable changes in iron status might be due to the dietary iron bioavailability. However, researchers suggest that around two thirds of dietary non-haem iron was incorporated into the red blood cells (RBC) after 2 weeks of consumption in participants with sufficient iron stores [37]. Therefore, non-haem iron derived from an iron-rich bread product in this study during 6-week intervention period would have been sufficient for the iron uptake and utilisation. Nevertheless, cereal products provide a less absorbable form of non-haem iron compared to animal sources, which contain haem iron [38]. Therefore, the lack of the effect on iron status may suggest lower iron bioavailability in Teff bread used in the present study.

Finally, the increase in dietary iron intake by 7 mg/day might not have been sufficient to see notable changes in iron status, especially as most of studies showing iron status improvements used therapeutic supplementation dosages (100 mg elemental Fe/day) [8,9]. Ishizaki *et al.* suggested that 4-week dietary intervention of 15 mg of iron a day increased the activity of δ-ALAD, an enzyme participating in red blood cells (RBC) turnover; however, this intervention did not increase any other haematological indices [14]. The dosage of dietary iron supplementation in the present study (mean of 7 mg/day from Teff bread, total intake of 18.5 mg Fe/day) is similar to the total dietary treatment of 15 mg/day by Ishizaki *et al.*

Despite the lack of significant changes in haematological indices, the study findings showed some important correlations between baseline iron status and favourable outcomes of the intervention. The iron status of iron-depleted participants showed the greatest improvements in haematological parameters during the intervention (Table 4). This was indicated by the correlations between changes in tissue iron supply parameters (sTFR and sTsfR) and the highest initial values of these haematological indices, showing inadequate iron supply at baseline. This can be explained by the homeostatic body iron metabolism control as the absorption of dietary iron is increased with compromised iron status [39,40]. This is in agreement with the findings of the present study in which female runners with a compromised iron status pre-intervention improved their haematological indices the most.

The increment in iron storage was positively correlated with changes in dietary iron intake, even when controlling for initial iron status (Table 4). This suggests that iron stores were increased more in runners, who increased their dietary iron intake the most regardless of their baseline iron status. This also indicates that dietary iron was incorporated into body iron stores. Hence, even a modest increase in dietary iron (from 10.7 to 18.5 mg/day) can provide beneficial effects on storage iron level.

Conclusion

The present study revealed inadequate dietary iron intake in the cohort of female runners studied. In addition to this, over a third of the participants had serum ferritin levels that indicated an iron-deficiency state (serum ferritin <12μg/L). The dietary intervention showed significant improvements in total iron intake and a modest improvement in iron status.

Further research using larger groups of participants is needed to confirm if dietary intervention through a dietary change can significantly improve iron status and consequently exercise performance. Nevertheless, taking into account the research design and sample size limitations, the current study findings show a positive but modest improvement in iron status as a result of dietary iron intervention.

Availability of supporting data

All the data from this research are available on your request.

Competing interests

The authors declare that they have no competing interests.

Authors' contribution

VS supervised the whole project. IA, VS, ED and AP formulated the research questions and designed the study, IA and VS recruited participants, IA and ED conducted intervention studies. IA analyzed data and performed statistical analysis, IA wrote the manuscript. Other authors amended and approved the final manuscript. All authors read and approved the final manuscript.

Acknowledgment

This study was funded by the Department of Food & Tourism Management, Manchester Metropolitan University, UK (Studentship Registration Number RD/DO/09/32092).

Author details

[1]Department of Food and Tourism Management Old Hall Lane, Manchester Metropolitan University, Manchester M14 6HR, UK. [2]School of Health Sciences, Liverpool Hope University, Liverpool L16 9JD, UK. [3]College of Engineering, Design and Physical Sciences, Brunel University, Uxbridge, Middlesex UB8 3PH, UK.

References

1. Suedekum NA, Dimeff RJ: **Iron and the athlete.** *Curr Sports Med Rep* 2005, **4**:199–202.
2. Zimmermann MB, Hurrell R: **Nutritional iron deficiency.** *Lancet* 2007, **370**:511–520.
3. Beard J, Tobin B: **Iron status and exercise.** *Am J of Clin Nutr* 2000, **72**:594s–597s.
4. Di Santolo M, Stel G, Banfi G, Gonano F, Cauci S: **Anemia and iron status in young fertile non-professional female athletes.** *Eur J Appl Physiol* 2008, **102**:703–709.
5. Burke LM, Millet GE, Tarnopolsky MA: **Nutrition for distance events.** *J Sports Sci* 2007, **225**:S29–S38.
6. Edgerton VR, Ohira Y, Hettiarachchi J, Senewiratne B, Gardner GW, Barnard RJ: **Elevation of hemoglobin and work tolerance in iron-deficient subjects.** *J Nutr Sci Vitaminol* 1981, **27**:77–86.
7. Ohira Y, Edgerton VR, Gardner GW, Senewiratne B, Barnard RJ, Simpson DR: **Work capacity, heart-rate and blood lactate responses to iron treatment.** *Br J Haematol* 1979, **41**:365–372.

8. Friedmann B, Weller E, Mairbaurl H, Bartsch P: **Effects of iron repletion on red blood cell volume and exercise performance.** *Med Sci Sports Exerc* 2000, **32:**S75.
9. Lamanca JJ, Haymes EM: **Effects of iron repletion on VO2$_{max}$, endurance, and blood lactate in women.** *Med Sci Sports Exerc* 1993, **25:**1386–1392.
10. Brownlie T, Utermohlen V, Hinton PS, Haas JD: **Tissue iron deficiency without anemia impairs adaptation in endurance capacity after aerobic training in previously untrained women.** *Am J Clin Nutr* 2004, **79:**437–443.
11. Klingshirn LA, Pate RR, Bourque SP, Davis JM, Sargent RG: **Effect of iron supplementation on endurance capacity in iron-depleted female runners.** *Med Sci Sports Exerc* 1992, **24:**819–824.
12. Peeling P, Blee T, Goodman C, Dawson B, Claydon G, Beilby J, Prins A: **Effect of iron injections on aerobic-exercise performance of iron-depleted female athletes.** *Int J Sport Nutr Exerc Metab* 2007, **17:**221–231.
13. Tsalis G, Nikolaidis MG, Mougios V: **Effects of iron intake through food or supplement on iron status and performance of healthy adolescent swimmers during a training season.** *Int J Sports Med* 2004, **25:**306–313.
14. Ishizaki S, Koshimizu T, Yanagisawa K, Akiyama Y, Mekada Y, Shiozawa N, Takahashi N, Yamakawa J, Kawano Y: **Effects of a fixed dietary intake on changes in red blood cell delta-aminolevulinate dehydratase activity and hemolysis.** *Int J Sport Nutr Exerc Metab* 2006, **16:**597–610.
15. Lyle RM, Weaver CM, Sedlock DA, Rajaram S, Martin B, Melby CL: **Iron status in exercising women - the effect of oral iron therapy vs increased consumption of muscle foods.** *Am J Clin Nutr* 1992, **56:**1049–1055.
16. Anschuetz S, Rodgers CD, Taylor AW: **Meal composition and iron status of experienced male and female distance runners.** *J Exerc Sci Fit* 2010, **2010**(8):25–33.
17. Hoppe M, Brün B, Larsson MP, Moraeus L, Hulthén LMoraeus L, Hulthén LMoraeus L, Hulthén LMoraeus L, Hulthén L: **Heme iron-based dietary intervention for improvement of iron status in young women.** *Nutrition* 2013, **29:**89–95.
18. Alaunyte I, Stojceska V, Plunkett A, Ainsworth P, Derbyshire E: **Improving the quality of nutrient-rich Teff (*Eragrostis tef*) breads by combination of enzymes in straight dough and sourdough breadmaking.** *J Cereal Sci* 2012, **55:**22–30.
19. Goldberg GR, Black AE, Jebb SA, Cole TJ, Murgatroyd PR, Coward WA, Prentice AM: **Critical-evaluation of energy-intake data using fundamental principles of energy physiology. 1.Derivation of Cut off limits to identify under-recording.** *Eur J Clin Nutr* 1991, **45:**569–581.
20. Henry CJ: **Basal metabolic rate studies in humans: measurement and development of new equations.** *Public Health Nutr* 2005, **8:**1133–1152.
21. Scientific Advisory Committee on Nutrition (SACN): *Dietary Reference Values for Energy*; 2011. https://www.gov.uk/government/uploads/system/uploads/attachment_data/file/339317/SACN_Dietary_Reference_Values_for_Energy.pdf (assessed January 2014).
22. Department of Health Dietary Reference Values for Food, Energy and Nutrients for the United Kingdom: **Report of the Panel on Dietary Reference Values of the Committee on Medical Aspects of Food Policy.** London: H.M.S.O; 1991.
23. American Dietetic Association, Dietitians of Canada; American College of Sports Medicine: **American College of Sports Medicine position stand. Nutrition and athletic performance.** *Med Sci Sports Exerc* 2009, **41:**709–731.
24. Schwellnus M: *The Olympic Textbook of Medicine in Sport*. Oxford: Wiley-Blackwell; 2008.
25. Tobin B, Beard J: **Iron.** In *Sports Nutrition*. Edited by Wolinsky I, Driskell JA. Boca Raton: CRC Press; 1997.
26. Vernet M: **Immunochemical assay of transferrin and iron saturation in serum.** *Clin Chem* 1993, **39:**2352–2353.
27. Thomas C, Thomas L: **Biochemical markers and hematologic indices in the diagnosis of functional iron deficiency.** *Clin Chem* 2002, **48:**1066–1076.
28. Hinton PS, Sanford TC, Davidson MM, Yakushko OF, Beck NC: **Nutrient intakes and dietary behaviors of male and female collegiate athletes.** *Int J Sport Nutr Exerc Metab* 2004, **14:**389–405.
29. Papadopoulou SK, Papadopoulou SD, Gallos GK: **Macro- and micro-nutrient intake of adolescent Greek female volleyball players.** *Int J Sport Nutr Exerc Metab* 2002, **12:**73–80.
30. Berning J, Troup JP, Van Handel P, Daniels J, Daniels N: **The nutritional habits of young adolescent swimmers.** *Int J Sport Nutr Exerc Metab* 1991, **1:**240–248.
31. Hassapidou MN, Manstrantoni A: **Dietary intakes of elite female athletes in Greece.** *J Hum Nutr Diet* 2001, **14:**391–396.
32. Pate RR, Miller BJ, Davis JM, Slentz CA, Klingshirn LA: **Iron status of female runners.** *Int J Sport Nutr Exerc Metab* 1993, **3:**222–231.
33. Spodaryk K, Czekaj J, Sowa W: **Relationship among reduced level of stored iron and dietary iron in trained women.** *Physiol Res* 1996, **45:**393–397.
34. Public Health England: *National Diet and Nutrition Survey. Results from Years 1, 2, 3 and 4 (combined) of the Rolling Programme (2008/2009 – 2011/2012)*; 2014. https://www.gov.uk/government/uploads/system/uploads/attachment_data/file/310995/NDNS_Y1_to_4_UK_report.pdf (assessed May 2014).
35. Whiting SJ, Barabash WA: **Dietary reference intakes for the micronutrients: considerations for physical activity.** *Appl Physiol Nutr Metab* 2006, **31:**80–85.
36. Hulten L, Gramatkovski E, Gleerup A, Hallberg L: **Iron-absorption from the whole diet - relation to meal composition, iron requirements and iron stores.** *Eur J Clin Nutr* 1995, **49:**794–808.
37. Roughead ZK, Zito CA, Hunt JR: **Initial uptake and absorption of nonheme iron and absorption of heme iron in humans are unaffected by the addition of calcium as cheese to a meal with high iron bioavailability.** *Am J Clin Nutr* 2002, **76:**419–425.
38. Hallberg L: **Bioavailability of dietary iron in man.** *Annu Rev Nutr* 1981, **1:**123–147.
39. Beard J, Han O: **Systemic iron status.** *Biochim Biophys Acta* 2009, **1790:**584–588.
40. Frazer DM, Anderson GJ: **Iron imports. I. Intestinal iron absorption and its regulation.** *Am J Physiol Gastrointest Liver Physiol* 2005, **289:**G631–G635.

The effects of consuming a high protein diet (4.4 g/kg/d) on body composition in resistance-trained individuals

Jose Antonio*, Corey A Peacock, Anya Ellerbroek, Brandon Fromhoff and Tobin Silver

Abstract

Background: The consumption of dietary protein is important for resistance-trained individuals. It has been posited that intakes of 1.4 to 2.0 g/kg/day are needed for physically active individuals. Thus, the purpose of this investigation was to determine the effects of a very high protein diet (4.4 g/kg/d) on body composition in resistance-trained men and women.

Methods: Thirty healthy resistance-trained individuals participated in this study (mean ± SD; age: 24.1 ± 5.6 yr; height: 171.4 ± 8.8 cm; weight: 73.3 ± 11.5 kg). Subjects were randomly assigned to one of the following groups: Control (CON) or high protein (HP). The CON group was instructed to maintain the same training and dietary habits over the course of the 8 week study. The HP group was instructed to consume 4.4 grams of protein per kg body weight daily. They were also instructed to maintain the same training and dietary habits (e.g. maintain the same fat and carbohydrate intake). Body composition (Bod Pod®), training volume (i.e. volume load), and food intake were determined at baseline and over the 8 week treatment period.

Results: The HP group consumed significantly more protein and calories pre vs post ($p < 0.05$). Furthermore, the HP group consumed significantly more protein and calories than the CON ($p < 0.05$). The HP group consumed on average 307 ± 69 grams of protein compared to 138 ± 42 in the CON. When expressed per unit body weight, the HP group consumed 4.4 ± 0.8 g/kg/d of protein versus 1.8 ± 0.4 g/kg/d in the CON. There were no changes in training volume for either group. Moreover, there were no significant changes over time or between groups for body weight, fat mass, fat free mass, or percent body fat.

Conclusions: Consuming 5.5 times the recommended daily allowance of protein has no effect on body composition in resistance-trained individuals who otherwise maintain the same training regimen. This is the first interventional study to demonstrate that consuming a hypercaloric high protein diet does not result in an increase in body fat.

Keywords: Protein, Diet, Body composition, Exercise, Supplements

Introduction

Protein is the most important macronutrient vis-à-vis positive alterations in body composition. Previous work has suggested that protein intakes in the range of 1.2-2.0 grams per kilogram (kg) body weight per day (g/kg/d) are needed in active individuals [1-7]. In contrast, the US recommended daily allowance (RDA) for protein is 0.8 g/kg/d. The average protein intake for US adults is 91 grams daily or ~1.0 g/kg ideal body weight [8]. Thus, the average US adult consumes slightly more than the RDA; however, this level is inadequate for athletes or active individuals who engage in exercise/sport training for several hours per week. Nonetheless, consuming more than the RDA may be considered a 'high' intake of protein [9]. In a review by Tipton [10], the definition of a high protein diet may include intakes greater than 15-16% of total energy intake, intakes greater than the RDA or perhaps anything that exceeds 35% of total energy intake. Thus, there is disagreement as to what constitutes a 'high' protein diet. We would posit that using percentages as a means of defining 'low' or 'high'

* Correspondence: ja839@nova.edu
Exercise and Sports Sciences, Nova Southeastern University, 3532 S. University Drive, University Park Plaza Suite 3532, Davie, FL 33314, USA

protein intakes is misleading. If one were to consume the hypothetical low calorie diet (ex. 1000 kcal/d), a protein intake of 36% (of total kcals) would be 90 grams; in contrast, it would be 180 grams on a 2000 kcal/d. Thus, it is best to measure protein intake per unit body weight instead of as a percentage of total energy.

According to the Position Stand by the International Society of Sports Nutrition, intakes of 1.4-2.0 g/kg/d are needed for physically active individuals [7]. We would suggest that a 'high' protein intake is anything that exceeds 2.0 g/kg/d. However, little is known regarding the effects of protein intake exceeding 2.0 g/kg/d. A recent study compared low, normal and high protein diets [11]. However, even the high protein group was not 'high.' They consumed an average of 1.8 g/kg/d of protein. Certainly compared to the sedentary population, 1.8 g/kg/d is 'high;' however, 1.8 g/kg/d should be a baseline protein requirement for active individuals.

It is not clear if protein overfeeding will result in body fat gains. Certainly, overfeeding in general will promote body weight and fat mass gain [12]. Furthermore, the composition of meals during times of overfeeding will differentially affect body composition. Two weeks of overfeeding on candy versus peanuts showed that waist circumference increased only in the candy group despite the identical increase in caloric intake [12]. This suggests that overfeeding on sugar results in body fat gains in contrast to consuming a natural food comprised of unprocessed carbohydrate and fat. Furthermore, there may be no difference in overfeeding on fat or carbohydrate in terms of fat storage [13]. Presently, the effects of protein overfeeding in resistance-trained individuals is unknown. Therefore, the purpose of this investigation was to determine the effects of a high protein diet on body composition in resistance-trained men and women in the absence of changes in training volume.

Methods

Subjects

Forty resistance-trained subjects volunteered for this investigation. Subjects were unequally randomized to a control (CON n = 10) or high protein diet (HP n = 20) group. The purpose of unequal randomization was to take into account the loss of subjects from potential lack of compliance due to the high protein diet as well as gaining additional information on the treatment itself [14]. Participants were otherwise healthy resistance-trained men and women who had been resistance training regularly for the last 8.9 ± 6.7 years and an average of 8.5 ± 3.3 hours per week. Individuals in the control group were instructed to maintain the same dietary and training habits over the course of the study. On the other hand, the subjects in the high protein diet group were instructed to consume 4.4 grams of protein equal to 4.4 g/kg/d. All procedures involving human subjects were approved by Nova Southeastern University's Human Subjects Institutional Review Board in accordance with the Helsinki Declaration, and written informed consent was obtained prior to participation.

Food diary, workout Log, body composition

Subjects kept a daily diary of their food intake via a smartphone app (MyFitnessPal®). The use of mobile apps for diet self-monitoring have been previously used [15]. If they did not use the mobile app, subjects instead kept a paper diary and their daily food intake was measured via the Nutribase® program. In order to maintain a high protein diet, subjects consumed commercially available whey and casein protein powder (MusclePharm® and Adept Nutrition [Europa®]). Otherwise, the rest of their dietary protein was obtained from their normal food intake.

Height was measured using standard anthropometry and total body weight was measured using a calibrated scale. Body composition was assessed by whole body densitometry using air displacement via the Bod Pod® (COSMED USA, Concord, CA). All testing was performed in accordance with the manufacturer's instructions. Briefly, subjects were tested while wearing only tight fitting clothing (swimsuit or undergarments) and an acrylic swim cap. The subjects wore the exact same clothing for all testing. Thoracic gas volume was estimated for all subjects using a predictive equation integral to the Bod Pod® software. The calculated value for body density used the Siri equation to estimate body composition. Data from the Bod Pod® included body weight, percent body fat, fat free mass and fat mass. All testing was done with each subject at approximately the same time of day. Also, all subjects were required to keep a daily workout log showing the exercises with reps and sets performed. Volume load (repetitions × weight) was measured to ensure subjects did not alter their training regimen.

Statistical analysis

Data were analyzed utilizing a 2-way Analysis of Variance (ANOVA) with Tukey's test used for post-hoc analysis. Data are expressed as mean ± SD. A p value of <0.05 was considered significant.

Results

Forty subjects were initially recruited for this investigation. Ten subjects dropped out. Of the 10, three stated an inability to consume the protein needed for the study and one subject complained of gastrointestinal distress. Six did not provide a reason. Thirty healthy resistance-trained individuals participated in this study (mean ± SD; age: 24.1 ± 5.6 yr; height: 171.4 ± 8.8 cm; weight: 73.3 ± 11.5 kg; 11 female, 29 male). There were no differences between groups for any of the baseline measures (Table 1).

Table 1 Subject characteristics

	Age years	Height cm	Weight kg
Control n = 10 (2 female, 8 male)	22.0 ± 2.6	174.3 ± 8.2	76.4 ± 9.9
High Protein n = 20 (9 female, 11 male)	25.2 ± 6.3	170.0 ± 8.9	71.8 ± 12.2

Data are mean ± SD. There were no significant differences for any of the variables. *cm* centimeters, *kg* kilograms.

There were no statistically significant changes pre vs post or between groups for any of the body composition variables (Table 2).

There were no changes in training volume (Table 3). The dietary data are summarized in Table 4. There were no significant changes in the control group for any of the variables. There was a significant increase in total energy and protein intake in the high protein group. It should be noted that every subject in the high protein group consumed protein powder in order to meet the requirements for the study. Otherwise, it would be have virtually impossible or highly unlikely that one could consume a 4.4 g/kg/d via food alone.

Discussion

The key finding in the present study is that consuming a hypercaloric high protein diet has no effect on body composition in resistance-trained individuals. This is the first investigation in resistance-trained individuals to demonstrate that consuming a high protein hypercaloric diet does not result in a gain in fat mass. On average, they consumed 4.4 g/kg/d of protein which is more than five times the recommended daily allowance [16].

It should be noted that in previous studies, subjects that consumed a hypocaloric diet that is higher in protein and lower in carbohydrate, experienced more favorable alterations in body composition [17-20]. However, the effects of consuming extra calories above normal baseline intake coupled with changes in macronutrient content have not been fully elucidated. The current investigation found no changes in body weight, fat mass, or fat free mass in the high protein diet group. This occurred in spite of the fact that they consumed over 800 calories more per day for eight weeks. The high protein group consumed an extra 145 grams of protein daily (mean intake of 307 grams per day or 4.4 g/kg/d). This is the highest recorded intake of dietary protein in the scientific literature that we are aware of [21-30].

The results of the current investigation do not support the notion that consuming protein in excess of purported needs results in a gain in fat mass. Certainly, this dispels the notion that 'a calorie is just a calorie.' That is, protein calories in 'excess' of requirements are not metabolized by the body in a manner similar to carbohydrate. Recently, Bray et al. demonstrated that a relatively higher amount of protein does not contribute to an additional gain in fat mass [11]. In this investigation, subjects consumed a diet that exceeded their normal caloric intake by 954 kcal/d. Subjects were randomized into one of three groups: low protein (5% of total energy from protein), normal protein (15%) and high protein (25%). After a treatment period of eight weeks, fat mass increased in all three groups equally (~3.5 kg); however, lean body mass decreased by 0.7 kg in the low protein group in contrast to a gain in the normal (2.9 kg) and high protein (3.2 kg) group. According to the investigators, calories alone contributed to the increase in fat mass; however, protein contributed to gains in lean body mass but not fat mass [11]. Thus, eating extra calories will result in a gain in body fat; however, overfeeding on protein will also result in a gain in lean body mass perhaps due to an increase in muscle protein synthesis.

There are profound differences between the investigation by Bray et al. and the current one. For instance, the current investigation used highly trained subjects whereas the participants in the Bray et al. study did not exercise. What is intriguing is that subjects in the high protein group (Bray et al.) consumed 135 grams of protein daily (~1.8 g/kg/d) compared to their baseline intake of 93 grams (~1.2 g/kg/d). This is less than the amount of protein consumed at baseline for subjects in the current study (~1.9-2.3 g/kg/d). The gain in lean body mass experienced by the subjects in the Bray et al. study suggest that their initial protein intake was inadequate to begin with. Therefore, non-exercising subjects should consume protein at levels twice the recommended daily allowance while keeping carbohydrate

Table 2 Body composition

	Control			HP		
	Pre	Post	Change	Pre	Post	Change
BW (kg)	76.4 ± 9.9	77.2 ± 9.9	0.8 ± 1.6	71.8 ± 12.2	73.5 ± 12.5	1.7 ± 1.9
FFM (kg)	65.2 ± 11.7	66.5 ± 11.7	1.3 ± 2.0	59.5 ± 10.9	61.4 ± 11.6	1.9 ± 2.4
FM (kg)	11.2 ± 4.7	11.4 ± 5.0	0.3 ± 4.7	12.3 ± 7.0	12.0 ± 6.2	−0.2 ± 2.2
% BF	15.1 ± 6.9	14.2 ± 6.9	−0.9 ± 1.7	16.9 ± 8.3	16.3 ± 7.5	−0.6 ± 2.6

Data are mean ± SD. There were no significant differences for any of the variables. *BW* body weight, *FFM* fat free mass, *FM* fat mass,% *BF* percentage body fat, *HP* high protein.

Table 3 Training volume

	VL/day	
	Pre	Post
Control	37148 ± 40979	41847 ± 49022
HP	32481 ± 34193	34601 ± 34604

Data are mean ± SD. There were no significant differences for any of the variables. *HP* high protein, *VL* volume load (calculated as reps × weight).

and fat intake the same. This dietary strategy alone may promote gains in lean body mass.

On the other hand, the subjects in the current study were resistance-trained subjects who were instructed to not alter their training regimen. Thus, the lack of body composition changes in our group may be attributable to the fact that it is very difficult for trained subjects to gain lean body mass and body weight in general without significant changes in their training program.

An overfeeding study by Tchoukalova et al. demonstrated a gain in fat mass with no change in fat free mass [31]. In this investigation, all subjects consumed a diet that consisted of 50% carbohydrate, 15% protein, and 35% fat. Subjects were instructed to eat until they were 'more full than usual.' The extra calories were provided via the choice of an ice cream shake (402 kcal, 40% fat), a king-sized Snickers bar (510 kcal) (Mars Inc.), or Boost Plus (360 kcal/8 oz) (Nestle Nutrition). It is therefore not surprising that eight weeks of overfeeding on food that is largely comprised of carbohydrate would result in a fat mass gain. This is in agreement with other studies [11,12].

Table 4 Dietary intake

	Control		HP	
	Pre	Post	Pre	Post
Kcal	2295 ± 639	2052 ± 532	2042 ± 838	*#+2835 ± 865
CHO g	236 ± 56	227 ± 80	198 ± 100	226 ± 114
PRO g	149 ± 49	138 ± 42	162 ± 69	*#+307 ± 69
Fat g	79 ± 33	77 ± 30	79 ± 34	87 ± 30
	Control		HP	
	Pre	Post	Pre	Post
Kcal/kg/d	29.2 ± 6.3	26.2 ± 5.3	28.9 ± 10.8	*#+39.9 ± 9.9
CHO g/kg/d	3.0 ± 0.7	2.9 ± 0.9	2.8 ± 1.3	3.2 ± 1.6
PRO g/kg/d	1.9 ± 0.5	1.8 ± 0.4	2.3 ± 1.0	*#+4.4 ± 0.8
Fat g/kg/d	1.0 ± 0.4	1.0 ± 0.3	1.1 ± 0.4	1.2 ± 0.4
	Control		HP	
	Pre	Post	Pre	Post
CHO %	42.3 ± 8.0	43.1 ± 7.2	36.2 ± 9.9	29.6 ± 8.7
PRO %	26.7 ± 4.6	27.8 ± 5.7	30.5 ± 8.7	*#45.5 ± 9.9
Fat %	31.0 ± 8.5	28.9 ± 5.7	34.2 ± 9.6	27.0 ± 6.9

Data are mean ± SD. $P < 0.05$ *High Protein Post vs High Protein Pre. #High Protein Post vs Control Post. +High Protein Post vs Control Pre. *CHO* carbohydrate, *PRO* protein, *g* grams, *kg* kilograms, *d* days, *HP* high protein.

Carbohydrate overfeeding has been shown to elevate de novo lipogenesis; moreover, excess carbohydrate may be converted to fat via both hepatic and extrahepatic lipogenesis [13,32].

Norgan et al. had six young men overfeed for 42 days by 6.2 MJ/d (~1490 kcal) [33]. The composition of the overfed meals was 49% carbohydrate, 34% fat, and 17% protein. The mean increase in body weight, body fat and total body water was 6.03, 3.7, and 1.8 kg, respectively. They did not measure body composition per se; however, it would seem reasonable that part of that weight gain would lean body mass. The 17% protein intake in the Norgan et al. study is comparable to the 'normal' protein group in the Bray et al. investigation which demonstrated a gain in both fat and lean mass. However, it is in contrast with the current investigation which did not show any significant changes in either parameter.

One might suggest that the high thermic effect of protein may make it difficult to gain body weight during times of overfeeding. It has been shown that the greater the protein content of a meal, the higher the thermic effect [34]. Both young and old individuals experience an increase in resting energy expenditure after a 60 gram protein meal (17-21% increase) [35]. Also, the thermogenic response to a mixed meal (440 kcal of carbohydrate [glucose], fat, and protein) differs between lean and obese subjects [36]. In a study by Swaminathan et al., the thermic effect of fat was lower in obese (−0.9%) versus lean individuals (14.4%). In contrast, there was no difference in the thermic effect of glucose or protein. When subjects consumed a mixed meal, the thermogenic response was significantly less in the obese (12.9%) versus the lean individuals (25.0%) [36]. Another investigation found that the thermic effect of a 750 kcal mixed meal (14% protein, 31.5% fat, and 54.5% carbohydrate) was significantly higher in lean than obese individuals under conditions of rest, exercise and post-exercise conditions. According to the authors, "the results of this study indicate that for men of similar total body weight and BMI, body composition is a significant determinant of postprandial thermogenesis; the responses of obese are significantly blunted compared with those of lean men" [37].

The subjects in our study were lean, resistance-trained young men and women. Their baseline protein intake as ~2.0 g/kg/d. It has been previously demonstrated that a higher protein intake is associated with a more favorable body composition even in the absence of caloric restriction [38]. One might speculate that the thermic effect of consuming large amounts of dietary protein in trained subjects exceeds that of untrained but normal weight individuals.

It is unusual that despite no change in their training volume, the ~800 kcal increase in caloric intake had no effect on body composition. This is the first overfeeding study done on well-trained individuals; thus, one might speculate that their response differs from sedentary individuals. Although there was no significant change in the mean value for body weight, body fat, lean body mass or percent fat, the individual responses were quite varied. This may be due to the fact that other dietary factors were not controlled (e.g. carbohydrate intake). There was a mean increase in carbohydrate intake (~14%) in the high protein group. This was not significant due to the wide variation in intakes. Of the 20 subjects in the high protein group, 9 consumed more carbohydrate whereas 11 decreased or maintained the same intake. It is unclear if consuming protein only during the overfeeding period in the absence of fat or carbohydrate intake alterations would differentially impact body composition; however, we would speculate that protein overfeeding alone would likely have no effect on fat mass while promoting gains in lean body mass concurrent with a heavy resistance training regimen geared towards skeletal muscle hypertrophy.

Another factor that may have played a role in the current investigation is the type of protein consumed in the high protein group. Because of the difficulty in consuming 4.4 grams of protein per kg body weight daily, every subject in the high protein group acquired their additional protein calories primarily from whey protein powder. It has been shown that the thermic effect is greater with whey versus casein or soy protein [39]. Recently scientists demonstrated that consuming similar calories and protein during resistance training in initially untrained individuals resulted in greater gains in lean body mass in the whey supplemented group versus soy or carbohydrate [40]. Another investigation found that muscle protein synthesis after whey consumption was approximately 93% greater than casein and approximately 18% greater than soy. Furthermore, the same pattern held when measured post-exercise (whey > soy > casein) [41]. On the other hand, 48 grams of both whey and rice protein isolate consumed post resistance exercise improved indices of body composition and exercise performance similarly [42]. Thus, one might speculate that if the protein dose or intake is sufficiently high, it may not matter what that particular protein source may be.

Conclusion

This is the first investigation in resistance-trained individuals which demonstrates that a hypercaloric high protein diet does not contribute to a fat mass gain. Furthermore, there was no change in body weight or lean body mass. This is in contrast with other overfeeding studies which showed gains in body weight, fat mass and lean body mass; however, those investigations were performed in non exercise-trained individuals that were consuming a lower protein diet (in comparison to our study). It should be noted that the subjects in the current study did not alter their training. It would be intriguing to ascertain if a high protein diet concurrent with a heavy resistance bodybuilding training regimen would affect body composition (i.e. increase lean body mass and lower fat mass).

We did not measure blood indices to determine if any side effects (i.e. renal or hepatic function) occurred in the high protein group. A few subjects did complain of gastrointestinal distress as well as feeling 'hot' (i.e. their body temperature was chronically elevated). Future research should focus on trained subjects using a single source of protein during overfeeding. Furthermore, a heavy resistance program geared towards skeletal muscle hypertrophy in conjunction with protein overfeeding needs further investigation.

Competing interests

JA is the CEO of the International Society of Sports Nutrition. The protein powder was provided by MusclePharm® and Adept Nutrition (Europa® Sports Products brand); both are sponsors of the ISSN conferences.

Authors' contributions

JA (corresponding author) was responsible for the study design, the statistical analysis and the writing of the manuscript. AE and BF was involved in the execution of the measurements. CP and TS provided assistance in the study design, statistical analysis and editing of the manuscript. All authors read and approved the final manuscript.

Acknowledgement

We would like to thank Dr. Jordan Moon of MusclePharm® and Eric Hillman of Europa® Sports Products (Adept Nutrition) for kindly providing protein powder. Also, we would like to thank Jennie Von Doellen, Kat Fleming and Rachael Tutunick for helping with the data collection.

References

1. Lemon PW: **Do athletes need more dietary protein and amino acids?** *Int J Sport Nutr* 1995, **5**(Suppl):S39–S61.
2. Lemon PW, Tarnopolsky MA, MacDougall JD, Atkinson SA: **Protein requirements and muscle mass/strength changes during intensive training in novice bodybuilders.** *J Appl Physiol* 1992, **73**:767–775.
3. Lemon PW, Proctor DN: **Protein intake and athletic performance.** *Sports Med* 1991, **12**:313–325.
4. Lemon PW: **Protein and amino acid needs of the strength athlete.** *Int J Sport Nutr* 1991, **1**:127–145.
5. Lemon PW: **Protein and exercise: update 1987.** *Med Sci Sports Exerc* 1987, **19**:S179–S190.
6. Wilson J, Wilson GJ: **Contemporary issues in protein requirements and consumption for resistance trained athletes.** *J Int Soc Sports Nutr* 2006, **3**:7–27.
7. Campbell B, Kreider RB, Ziegenfuss T, La Bounty P, Roberts M, Burke D, Landis J, Lopez H, Antonio J: **International Society of Sports Nutrition position stand: protein and exercise.** *J Int Soc Sports Nutr* 2007, **4**:8.
8. Fulgoni VL 3rd: **Current protein intake in America: analysis of the National Health and Nutrition Examination Survey, 2003–2004.** *Am J Clin Nutr* 2008, **87**:1554S–1557S.
9. Westerterp-Plantenga MS: **How are normal, high- or low-protein diets defined?** *Br J Nutr* 2007, **97**:217–218.
10. Tipton KD: **Efficacy and consequences of very-high-protein diets for athletes and exercisers.** *Proc Nutr Soc* 2011, **70**:205–214.
11. Bray GA, Smith SR, de Jonge L, Xie H, Rood J, Martin CK, Most M, Brock C, Mancuso S, Redman LM: **Effect of dietary protein content on weight gain, energy expenditure, and body composition during overeating: a randomized controlled trial.** *JAMA* 2012, **307**:47–55.

12. Claesson AL, Holm G, Ernersson A, Lindstrom T, Nystrom FH: Two weeks of overfeeding with candy, but not peanuts, increases insulin levels and body weight. *Scand J Clin Lab Invest* 2009, **69**:598–605.
13. Lammert O, Grunnet N, Faber P, Bjornsbo KS, Dich J, Larsen LO, Neese RA, Hellerstein MK, Quistorff B: Effects of isoenergetic overfeeding of either carbohydrate or fat in young men. *Br J Nutr* 2000, **84**:233–245.
14. Dumville JC, Hahn S, Miles JN, Torgerson DJ: The use of unequal randomisation ratios in clinical trials: a review. *Contemp Clin Trials* 2006, **27**:1–12.
15. Turner-McGrievy GM, Beets MW, Moore JB, Kaczynski AT, Barr-Anderson DJ, Tate DF: Comparison of traditional versus mobile app self-monitoring of physical activity and dietary intake among overweight adults participating in an mHealth weight loss program. *J Am Med Inform Assoc* 2013, **20**:513–518.
16. Gregorio L, Brindisi J, Kleppinger A, Sullivan R, Mangano KM, Bihuniak JD, Kenny AM, Kerstetter JE, Insogna KL: Adequate dietary protein is associated with better physical performance among post-menopausal women 60–90 years. *J Nutr Health Aging* 2014, **18**:155–160.
17. Layman DK, Boileau RA, Erickson DJ, Painter JE, Shiue H, Sather C, Christou DD: A reduced ratio of dietary carbohydrate to protein improves body composition and blood lipid profiles during weight loss in adult women. *J Nutr* 2003, **133**:411–417.
18. Layman DK, Shiue H, Sather C, Erickson DJ, Baum J: Increased dietary protein modifies glucose and insulin homeostasis in adult women during weight loss. *J Nutr* 2003, **133**:405–410.
19. Tang M, Leidy HJ, Campbell WW: Regional, but not total, body composition changes in overweight and obese adults consuming a higher protein, energy-restricted diet are sex specific. *Nutr Res* 2013, **33**:629–635.
20. Layman DK, Evans E, Baum JI, Seyler J, Erickson DJ, Boileau RA: Dietary protein and exercise have additive effects on body composition during weight loss in adult women. *J Nutr* 2005, **135**:1903–1910.
21. Gordon MM, Bopp MJ, Easter L, Miller GD, Lyles MF, Houston DK, Nicklas BJ, Kritchevsky SB: Effects of dietary protein on the composition of weight loss in post-menopausal women. *J Nutr Health Aging* 2008, **12**:505–509.
22. Wycherley TP, Buckley JD, Noakes M, Clifton PM, Brinkworth GD: Comparison of the effects of weight loss from a high-protein versus standard-protein energy-restricted diet on strength and aerobic capacity in overweight and obese men. *Eur J Nutr* 2013, **52**:317–325.
23. Tang M, Armstrong CL, Leidy HJ, Campbell WW: Normal vs. high-protein weight loss diets in men: effects on body composition and indices of metabolic syndrome. *Obesity (Silver Spring)* 2013, **21**:E204–E210.
24. Pasiakos SM, Cao JJ, Margolis LM, Sauter ER, Whigham LD, McClung JP, Rood JC, Carbone JW, Combs GF Jr, Young AJ: Effects of high-protein diets on fat-free mass and muscle protein synthesis following weight loss: a randomized controlled trial. *FASEB J* 2013, **27**:3837–3847.
25. Wycherley TP, Moran LJ, Clifton PM, Noakes M, Brinkworth GD: Effects of energy-restricted high-protein, low-fat compared with standard-protein, low-fat diets: a meta-analysis of randomized controlled trials. *Am J Clin Nutr* 2012, **96**:1281–1298.
26. Soenen S, Bonomi AG, Lemmens SG, Scholte J, Thijssen MA, van Berkum F, Westerterp-Plantenga MS: Relatively high-protein or 'low-carb' energy-restricted diets for body weight loss and body weight maintenance? *Physiol Behav* 2012, **107**:374–380.
27. Toscani MK, Mario FM, Radavelli-Bagatini S, Wiltgen D, Matos MC, Spritzer PM: Effect of high-protein or normal-protein diet on weight loss, body composition, hormone, and metabolic profile in southern Brazilian women with polycystic ovary syndrome: a randomized study. *Gynecol Endocrinol* 2011, **27**:925–930.
28. Wycherley TP, Noakes M, Clifton PM, Cleanthous X, Keogh JB, Brinkworth GD: A high-protein diet with resistance exercise training improves weight loss and body composition in overweight and obese patients with type 2 diabetes. *Diabetes Care* 2010, **33**:969–976.
29. Morenga LT, Williams S, Brown R, Mann J: Effect of a relatively high-protein, high-fiber diet on body composition and metabolic risk factors in overweight women. *Eur J Clin Nutr* 2010, **64**:1323–1331.
30. Krebs NF, Gao D, Gralla J, Collins JS, Johnson SL: Efficacy and safety of a high protein, low carbohydrate diet for weight loss in severely obese adolescents. *J Pediatr* 2010, **157**:252–258.
31. Tchoukalova YD, Votruba SB, Tchkonia T, Giorgadze N, Kirkland JL, Jensen MD: Regional differences in cellular mechanisms of adipose tissue gain with overfeeding. *Proc Natl Acad Sci U S A* 2010, **107**:18226–18231.
32. Minehira K, Bettschart V, Vidal H, Vega N, Di Vetta V, Rey V, Schneiter P, Tappy L: Effect of carbohydrate overfeeding on whole body and adipose tissue metabolism in humans. *Obes Res* 2003, **11**:1096–1103.
33. Norgan NG, Durnin JV: The effect of 6 weeks of overfeeding on the body weight, body composition, and energy metabolism of young men. *Am J Clin Nutr* 1980, **33**:978–988.
34. Belko AZ, Barbieri TF, Wong EC: Effect of energy and protein intake and exercise intensity on the thermic effect of food. *Am J Clin Nutr* 1986, **43**:863–869.
35. Fukagawa NK, Bandini LG, Lim PH, Roingeard F, Lee MA, Young JB: Protein-induced changes in energy expenditure in young and old individuals. *Am J Physiol* 1991, **260**:E345–E352.
36. Swaminathan R, King RF, Holmfield J, Siwek RA, Baker M, Wales JK: Thermic effect of feeding carbohydrate, fat, protein and mixed meal in lean and obese subjects. *Am J Clin Nutr* 1985, **42**:177–181.
37. Segal KR, Gutin B, Nyman AM, Pi-Sunyer FX: Thermic effect of food at rest, during exercise, and after exercise in lean and obese men of similar body weight. *J Clin Invest* 1985, **76**:1107–1112.
38. Green KK, Shea JL, Vasdev S, Randell E, Gulliver W, Sun G: Higher dietary protein intake is associated with lower body fat in the Newfoundland Population. *Clin Med Insights Endocrinol Diabetes* 2010, **3**:25–35.
39. Acheson KJ, Blondel-Lubrano A, Oguey-Araymon S, Beaumont M, Emady-Azar S, Ammon-Zufferey C, Monnard I, Pinaud S, Nielsen-Moennoz C, Bovetto L: Protein choices targeting thermogenesis and metabolism. *Am J Clin Nutr* 2011, **93**:525–534.
40. Volek JS, Volk BM, Gomez AL, Kunces LJ, Kupchak BR, Freidenreich DJ, Aristizabal JC, Saenz C, Dunn-Lewis C, Ballard KD, Quann EE, Kawiecki DL, Flanagan SD, Comstock BA, Fragala MS, Earp JE, Fernandez ML, Bruno RS, Ptolemy AS, Kellogg MD, Maresh CM, Kramer WJ: Whey protein supplementation during resistance training augments lean body mass. *J Am Coll Nutr* 2013, **32**:122–135.
41. Tang JE, Moore DR, Kujbida GW, Tarnopolsky MA, Phillips SM: Ingestion of whey hydrolysate, casein, or soy protein isolate: effects on mixed muscle protein synthesis at rest and following resistance exercise in young men. *J Appl Physiol (1985)* 2009, **107**:987–992.
42. Joy JM, Lowery RP, Wilson JM, Purpura M, De Souza EO, Wilson SM, Kalman DS, Dudeck JE, Jager R: The effects of 8 weeks of whey or rice protein supplementation on body composition and exercise performance. *Nutr J* 2013, **12**:86.

An assessment of the nutritional intake of soccer referees

Cristian Martínez Reñón[1] and Pilar S Collado[2,3*]

Abstract

Objective: The present study aims to analyze the eating habits and attitudes of a group of soccer referees and linesmen.

Method: A nutritional study was undertaken of thirty-five soccer referees (aged between 18 and 50) refereeing at different levels, from the Spanish national third division down to the provincial second division. Through the use of a 3-day food diary and 24-hour recall, this study analyzed the intake and distribution of macro- and micro-nutrients and of dietary fiber consumed on different types of day (normal, training, and match days).

Results: There were no significant differences in calorie intake related to the three types of day (normal, training, and match days). This was true both of overall amounts (2371.1 kcal, 2479.7 kcal, and 2368.4 kcal, respectively) and amounts per unit of body weight (32.4 kcal/kg, 33.9 kcal/kg, and 32.4 kcal/kg, respectively). In respect of macro-nutrient intake, more specifically carbohydrates, the subjects consumed a diet with an insufficient amount of carbohydrates: 279 g, as against the 371 g (REC1) or 540 g (REC2) recommended according to physical activity levels. Slight increases were observed on game days, but were not statistically significant. Consideration of micro-nutrients showed that the quantities of three vitamins (B6, B12, and C) consumed were above the recommended amounts. However, this was not an issue, since the figures related to water-soluble vitamins. Finally, the amounts of minerals (Ca, Mg, and Fe) and fiber consumed were close to recommended values, regardless of the type of day being considered.

Conclusions: This study found that the group of referees investigated consumed a diet that did not have sufficient calories from carbohydrates, in view of their occupation. This poor nutritional status might interfere with the development of their sporting performance and ultimately increase the risk of injury. This implies a need to design and implement a diet and to introduce educational programs on nutrition for these sportspeople.

Keywords: Nutritional requirements, Dietary record, Soccer referees, Macro-nutrients, Analyses

Introduction

The link between nutritional habits and health has concerned mankind since the origin of the earliest societies and cultures. Scientific study of the relationship between eating habits and health began in the eighteenth century, when long sea journeys led sailors to have poor and monotonous diets that caused deficiency diseases [1]. Today, this concern is made evident by the increasing demand for nutritional information related to sport and physical activity. Interest in this matter is found in many areas, from elite athletes who are eager to win medals in the Olympics or other championships, down to individuals who practice sport simply to keep fit [2].

There is no such thing as a complete, perfect, and magical food [3]. The ideal formula would be based on choosing a variety of foodstuffs that, when combined, would provide a balance for the proper functioning of the metabolism. This balance must be adequate to meet the demands of concerted effort, for instance, a soccer game.

It is well known that food intake influences an athlete's training and thus, ultimately, his or her performance levels. For this reason, sportspeople who want to achieve a higher performance, regardless of their specialties,

* Correspondence: p.sanchez.collado@unileon.es
[2]Institute of Biomedicine (IBIOMED), University of Leon, Leon, Spain
[3]Department of Biomedical Sciences. Physiology, University of León, 24071 León, Spain
Full list of author information is available at the end of the article

ought to be interested in their own nutrition. Sports performance is linked to the proportions of basic nutrients in the daily diet. The attention that athletes pay to their diet should go beyond the day of a competition or match; their dietary concerns must embrace every day of their lives. It is true, nevertheless, that the food eaten before a competition or game merits particular attention [4].

Nowadays, there are organizations, for example the World Health Organization (WHO), that are firmly committed to evaluating different diets that are appropriate to specific areas. Their work informs the general population about these findings. Furthermore, since energy requirements differ for each sport, there are also many publications that consider the most appropriate nutritional recommendations for optimizing athletes' performance levels in such areas as getting the greatest benefit from training, improving recovery, or maintaining ideal weight and fitness, thus minimizing the risk of injury and illness [5]. However, there is still little specific literature related to nutrition for certain groups.

In spite of the fact that it affects all sporting groups and disciplines, sports nutrition has not received widespread attention in the literature. The group referred to in the present study was soccer referees and linesmen. Nevertheless, interest in nutrition with a view to improving performance in soccer in general is relatively recent [6,7]. Soccer is one of the most important sports worldwide. Although it is the players who attract the most attention in the soccer world, referees, linesmen, and other officials are of equal importance. As in all other sports, these individuals require an optimal fitness level so that they can react to the demands of the game in a satisfactory manner. Hence and as is the case with any other sport, it is necessary to consider the effects of certain aspects of their nutritional intake on their performance. Similarly to the demands made of soccer players, refereeing is characterized by cycles of short, high-intensity bursts of activity, essentially sprinting, combined with lower-intensity physical effort, such as medium- or light-intensity jogging [8]. In addition, attention must be paid to the category of soccer (in the sense of teams' playing standards) that each referee and linesman officiates, since physical and nutritional requirements will vary as categories change from less demanding (second division at provincial level) to more demanding (third division at national level).

Another factor that must be considered is the great distances that are run in a discipline such as soccer. Numerous studies that make use of GPS technology have shown that during soccer match participants travel distances of around 11,000 meters [9]. In soccer and in team sports in general, one of the most important factors in athletic performance is recovery from fatigue after training and competitions or games. This is especially the case for sports in which participants sometimes train and compete on the same day or on successive days, with little recovery time. The recovery process is influenced by numerous elements. One of the most important of these is nutrition, but its effectiveness depends on many variables, including the competition itself and the sex, training status, and nutritional status of the subjects [8,10].

In view of all the evidence discussed above, the present study aims to analyze the eating habits and attitudes of a group of soccer referees, and in so doing seeks to address the shortage of studies in the literature that investigate these aspects of referees' diets and compare them to recommended patterns. The intention in conducting the study was to demonstrate the importance of proper nutrition, both in general and for sportspeople at a particular level. More specifically, the aim was to compare the nutritional profiles of the referees studied with the values from two different sets of recommendations (aimed at sedentary individuals and high-level athletes), and also to assess the nutritional intake and eating patterns of referees according to the type of day (normal day, training day, or match day).

Methodology

Subjects

A qualitative descriptive epidemiological study of 35 soccer referees of different categories (from Spain's third division at national level down to the second division at a provincial level, roughly equivalent to county level) was undertaken. The inclusion criteria for the study included: being a soccer referee within one of the previously described categories; being 18 or older; and being free of injury at the time of the study. All subjects who participated in the study were active referees who had undergone a medical examination by their sports federation. Those taking any medication at the moment of the study were excluded. The average age of subjects was 25.9 years. All the referees had a day job that they combined with their refereeing duties. Participants were informed of the objective of the study in a talk that was given in order to explain what was going to be done, and they all submitted a signed consent form that had been specially prepared for the study. They were given the assurance that they could drop out of the study at any time should they so wish. The study followed the principles of the Declaration of Helsinki, and the local Ethics Committee of the University of Leon approved all procedures.

Dietary assessment

The subjects compiled a food diary, using forms provided for that purpose. These forms required them to record information about what they consumed each day: amounts, proportions of ingredients, methods of preparation, and so forth [11]. Each of these forms had an initial guidelines section to assist participants throughout the process, which lasted three days. Photographs of food models, measuring spoons, cups, bowls, and other prompts were called on to further improve the quality of the collected dietary data. Once the subject returned the 3-day food record, a trained researcher immediately checked through it and followed up with the athlete to request clarifications about specific items and/or obtain more detail if necessary.

All of the subjects in the group were also interviewed personally, by a trained research assistant, 24 hours they had submitted their forms. The aim of this interview was to rerecord the same information provided by the individual dietary records in order to perform a cross-check and thereby make the data used in the study more reliable.

The information about food, quantities, batches, and cooking processes collected from the participants by means of the dietary records and 24-hour recalls was manually analyzed on a daily basis and inputted. All the data were processed by the Nutriber V.1.1.1.R5 software package (produced by Funiber, Barcelona, Spain) in order to calculate individual diets. The combination of food diaries and recall after a twenty-four-hour period met the criteria for a simple, rapid, and inexpensive research method.

Determination of basal metabolism was by means of the Harris-Benedict equation [12]. This has been demonstrated to have good reliability and applicability in a number of studies [13]. For males, such as the participants in this study, the formula is:

$$66.473 + (13.7516 \times \textit{weight in kilograms}) + (5.0033 \times \textit{height in centimeters}) - (6.755 \times \textit{age in years})$$

Statistical analysis of the data

A Microsoft Office Excel 2007 spreadsheet was used to record and handle data and to produce graphs. The results were reported as mean values and standard error of the mean. In working out the Student's T-test of the sample, the statistical software package SPSS 17.0 was used. Values were taken as significant with $p < 0.05$ and highly significant with $p < 0.01$.

Results

Table 1 shows the characteristics of participants and their kilocalorie intakes and basal metabolic rates. Like the work done by Martínez Reñón et al. [14], in this nutritional study the sample was compared with the tables of recommended energy and nutrient intakes (RDI: Recommended Daily Intake) for the Spanish population as a whole [1]. Specifically, it was compared with two recommendations: REC1 (2,700 Kcal), for people of the same age and sex as the referees who undertake only light activity, and REC2 (3,600 Kcal), for people of the same age and sex as the referees who practice similar sports that require the same high levels of activity [1].

Table 1 General characteristics

Age	24.7 ± 9.9 years.
Height	178.5 ± 6.5 centimeters.
Weight	73.1 ± 8.2 kilograms.
Average intake	2408.8 ± 517.8 kilocalories.
Normal day average intake	2371.1 ± 519.1 kilocalories.
Training day average intake	2479.7 ± 430.7 kilocalories.
Game day average intake	2368.4 ± 584.7 kilocalories

An energy intake of 2,700 kcal is indicated by REC1 and one of 3,600 kcal by REC2. However, the total average energy intake of the subjects was 11% less than the first (the recommended intake for people with light activity), and 33.1% lower than the second (the recommendation for professional athletes of a similar age). The subjects were thus well below recommended energy intakes.

Calorie and macro-nutrient intakes are shown in Table 2, classified according to the type of day: normal (no training, with referees going about their usual trade or profession), training (which can possibly happen alongside continuing their normal occupations), and match days.

Table 2 Mean macro-nutrient intake values on the different types of day ± standard error of mean

	Normal	Training	Match
Energy			
Kcal	2371.1 ± 519.1	2479.7 ± 430.7	2368.4 ± 584.7
Kcal/kg	32.4 ± 7.6	33.9 ± 6.9	32.4 ± 5.3
Carbohydrates			
g	**278.9 ± 86.2**	**291.2 ± 54.0**	**300.6 ± 84.0**
Kcal	1115 ± 181	1164 ± 129	1202 ± 195
%	47.0	46.9	50.7
Proteins			
g	**125.8 ± 17.3**	**115.2 ± 40.0**	**118.5 ± 37.0**
Kcal	503.2 ± 178	460.8 ± 138.4	474.0 ± 113.6
%	21.2	18.5	20.0
Fats			
g	**100.2 ± 62.0**	**110.1 ± 35.0**	**97.6 ± 83.0**
Kcal	918.0 ± 121.6	990.1 ± 181.1	878.4 ± 161.9
%	38.7	39.8	36.8

The results show that calorie intakes did not vary from one type of day to another.

Figure 1 shows that relative to REC1 and REC2 the subjects' diets were low in carbohydrates, averaging 279 g, against the 371 g of REC1 and the 540 g of REC2. Similarly, they were high in protein, with an average of 125.8 g, compared to the 62.8 g of REC1 and 117.9 g of REC2. However, as can be seen in Table 2 and Figure 1, the type of day did have a small effect on carbohydrate intake, with a slight increase on match days. Nevertheless, this intake increase did not reach the values of either of recommendations REC1 and REC2.

Finally, with regard to fats, there were no significant differences from either of the recommendations, although the values noted did exceed the 30% of the total calorie intake suggested by REC1. There were no differences that were dependent on the type of day in the percentage values, which were 38.7%, 39.8% and 39.3% for normal, training, and match days respectively.

With regard to micro-nutrients, the vitamins that were assessed were B1, B2, B6, B12 and C. As with the macronutrients, intakes of vitamins and minerals were compared to RDI values. However, there was no need to make two separate comparisons with REC1 (low activity) and REC2 (high-performance athletes), since the recommended values for micro-nutrients are the same for both these populations (Table 3). Vitamin intake was therefore compared to REC1, and then subdivided according to the type of day involved.

The intake of B-complex vitamins (B1, B2, B6, and B12) can be seen from Table 3 to have been relatively high compared to the recommendations.

Of the individual vitamins, B6 showed a marked increase, at more than 50% higher than the recommended amount ($p < 0.05$). Most striking was vitamin B12, with stratospheric values of up to eight times the daily amount recommended for the "slightly active" population being recorded. Vitamin C intake was 60% higher than recommended total values.

Consideration of vitamin intakes according to the type of day showed that there were no significant differences among them. One interesting point was the figure for vitamin B12 on match days. This amounted to 19.3 milligrams, a level much higher than the recommended value.

The minerals analyzed were Ca, Mg, and Fe. The data for them are shown as milligrams (Table 3).

On average, the totals for all these minerals were either higher than recommended values or within the recommended range. For example, the mean amount of calcium (Ca), an essential mineral for bone production, lay close to the recommended range of 800 mg to 1,000 mg. The test subjects had an average daily intake of 1,138 mg of Ca, a figure somewhat on the low side, since the sample population was one performing moderate- to high- intensity activities.

The values for the intake of magnesium (Mg) were very similar to the quantities laid down in REC1 and REC2. In contrast, figures for iron (Fe) were more than 60% higher than the amounts suggested by REC1 and REC2.

A check on the quantities of minerals depending on the type of day showed no data of importance. This was because no differences were found between one type of day and another.

The data on fiber intakes recorded were very similar in terms of total amounts. The average quantity noted was 23.3 g, where recommended values would be around 25 g of fiber daily. When the figures were broken down by type of day, the differences were not statistically

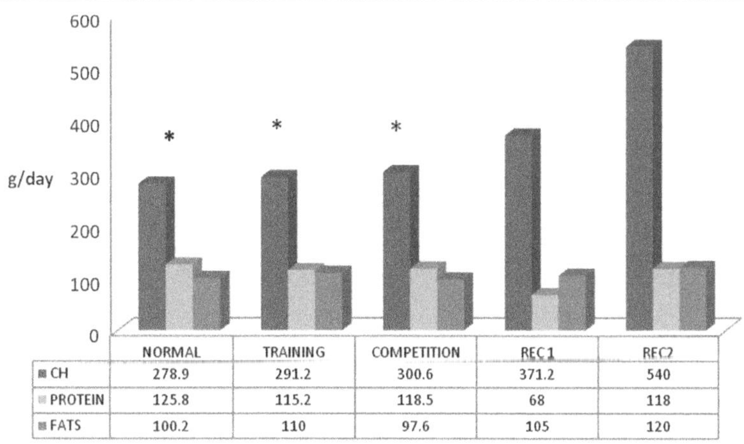

	NORMAL	TRAINING	COMPETITION	REC1	REC2
CH	278.9	291.2	300.6	371.2	540
PROTEIN	125.8	115.2	118.5	68	118
FATS	100.2	110	97.6	105	120

Figure 1 Relationships between mean values for macro-nutrient intakes and recommendations, depending on the type of day. *($p < 0.001$ versus REC2). REC1 = Recommendation for a person of the same age and sex undertaking light activity. REC2 = Recommendation for a person of the same age and sex undertaking a high level of activity.

Table 3 Relationship between mean values of intake of vitamins, minerals and fiber and its recommendation

		Total	Days			Recommendation
			Normal	Training	Competition	
Vitamins (mg)	B1	2.1±0.6	2.1±0.7	1.9±0.8	2.4±2.0	1.2
	B2	2.2±0.4	2.2±0.7	2.2±0.8	2.3±1.0	1.8
	B6	2.4±0.8*	2.6±1	2.3±0.9	2.2±0.9	1.1-1.8
	B12	16.9±1*	16.0±1.5	15.6±1.9	19.3±2.1	2
	C	141±11*	170±15	135±28	116±21	60
Minerals (mg)	Ca	1138±41	1161±44	1198±89	1057±149	800-1000
	Mg	376±122	389±151	383±126	356±80	350-400
	Fe	52.3±8.2*	50.1±12.7	62.4±16.1	44.5±5.4	10-15
Fiber (g)		23.3±2.4	22,2±2,7	28,5±3,8	19,2±3,1	25

*(p<0, 05 versus recommendation).

significant, all of them being close to the recommended amounts. Nonetheless, it is noteworthy that fiber intakes on training days averaged 28.5 g, while on normal days they were 22.3 g on average, and on match days the average fell to 19.2 grams.

Discussion

The importance of nutrition in professional refereeing, as in any sports activity, would seem to be more than clear. The nutritional requirements for each sport are specific and are related to the energy demands that the sport in question imposes [15]. The type, intensity, and duration of exercise affect the use of energy substrates. Thus, to satisfy the nutritional needs for different sports, in this case soccer it is necessary to develop adequate dietary plans. As was established by previous research, the requirements of a soccer referee are similar to those of a soccer player [16], and an adequate diet will positively influence the performance of these sportspeople. There is therefore a need to adjust the consumption of foods in the daily life of soccer referees so that they are be able to choose the right food at the right time in order to be efficient [17].

The importance of this can be seen in the fact that sportspeople who fail to observe these requirements may suffer an increased risk of injuries [18] and decreased performance [11]. It has been reported that approximately 25% of injuries occur in the last 15 to 20 minutes of a game, and this is because at that point energy reserves are coming to an end [19]. Nutritional management is therefore essential to achieve maximum performance in the practice of refereeing. There is widespread evidence that adjusting energy intake to energy expenditure is essential. The calorie intake of participants (kcal) in the present study was determined to be 2408 ± 518 kcal on average. This value is well below the recommendations established for sportspeople of the same age, sex, and level of activity, with the difference even more evident when compared with the requirements at a professional level. As already mentioned, an insufficient energy intake such that as found in the participants in the study can lead to a decrease in performance or an increase in the risk of injuries.

The results obtained were separated according to the type of day (normal, training, and match days). The participants kept their calorie-consumption levels more or less steady over the three sorts of day. Nonetheless, when the amount of macro-nutrients was considered, it was noticed that there was a slight increase, though not a significant upturn, in the consumption of carbohydrates on match days. It is thus evident that the intake of this type of nutrient did not conform to the recommendations. This should be regarded as an aspect requiring correction.

The recommended daily consumption of carbohydrates to maintain muscle glycogen stores over several days of intense training is between 500 g and 600 g, that is, between 60% and 70% of total energy intake [20]. However, in this study the amount of carbohydrates eaten fell well below these recommendations, to 33% less than the recommendation for athletes (REC2) and even to 11% less than the recommended intake for the group undertaking only light activity (REC1). A similar result was recorded in previous studies involving semi-professional soccer players, who were found to consume 40% less than the REC2 recommendation [14]. There is widespread evidence to suggest that an increase in carbohydrate intake can improve performance in various kinds of sports activity, including refereeing, which requires intermittent running at various intensities. Sportspeople who consume a diet rich in carbohydrates were found to be able to undertake 33% more high-intensity running during a game, and a diet with 65% carbohydrates was observed to improve performance when compared with alternatives in which carbohydrate consumption amounted to only 30% of the total diet [21-23]. A super-consumption of carbohydrates has shown noticeable benefits. However, this fact was not known to any of the participants [21-23].

When carbohydrates were analyzed by type of day, no significant differences were observed, with very similar carbohydrate intake values being obtained on all three sorts of day. One possible explanation for these results may be that the subjects did not have a good basic understanding of nutrition, and as a result their diet did not meet their daily needs.

Standard recommendations for the consumption of proteins are 0.80 g/kg/day. However, it is fully accepted that these amounts should be increased to between 1.4 g/kg/day and 1.7 g/kg/day, or in other terms 98 g/day to 119 g/day of proteins, for people who participate in intense physical activities [24]. The referees and linesmen in the sample had a greater consumption of proteins than the recommendation for adults, at 125.8 g/day. This may be of benefit to their performance, as the demands in relation to stamina and strength made upon them by their activity may be favorably affected by a protein intake that is above recommendations. This level of consumption may improve strength and provide amino acids to serve as a substrate for any increase in amino acid oxidation that may occur during training and games [25,26].

Finally, the preferred distribution of macro-nutrients indicates that the oils and fats consumed should provide between 20% and 30% of total calorie intake, even for sportspeople. In the present study all the referees' food diaries showed consumption falling within the recommended values. Although this type macro-nutrient helps to meet the increased energy demands of strenuous exercise, an increased consumption of lipids would not appear to be necessary [24].

With regard to micro-nutrient analysis, it is important to note that vitamins are structurally related organic compounds, but differ in their physiological action. However, they were studied together because their presence in the diet is essential for the body to carry out specific metabolic reactions [2].

In respect of vitamins and exercise, there appear to be no studies supporting vitamin supplementation for any kind for sports. This would make sense only in cases of vitamin deficiency caused by an unbalanced diet or some particular metabolic disorder. The vitamins investigated were the B-vitamin complex and vitamin C. Consumption similar to recommended daily amounts was noted for vitamins B1 and B2. In the case of vitamins B6, B12, and C, values above the recommended amounts were recorded. There were no significant differences when vitamins were examined by type of day and activity. This provides a possible explanation of these high values in the participants: they may be due to high protein intake in the case of the vitamins found in animal proteins, or to the consumption of large amounts of energy drinks on certain days, as these contain considerable amounts of vitamin B6 and B12.

The results recorded for vitamin C showed a consumption that was double recommended daily amounts. Vitamin C, or ascorbic acid, is important for the formation and maintenance of collagen and the synthesis of neurotransmitters [27]. The reason for these enhanced quantities of vitamin C may be that participants consumed foods with larger amounts of it in the hope of avoiding catching colds. Water-soluble vitamins like vitamin C are stored in the body to only an extremely limited extent, and are easily removed from it because of their solubility, meaning that excessive consumption is rarely dangerous.

In respect of other micro-nutrients in the study, the minerals investigated were sodium (Na), calcium (Ca), magnesium (Mg), and iron (Fe); consumption of all of these was indicated in milligrams. The average amounts for the minerals calcium and magnesium were close to those recommended for the population in general or even for those facing few physical demands, with calcium in the sample showing approximately recommended levels. In the case of iron, the values recorded were much higher than recommended. One of the possible explanations for the high levels of iron may be that this mineral is found in many of the foods that were recorded as being consumed in appreciable quantities, for example meat.

In conclusion, it may be stated that the information collected in this study provides a brief look at the eating habits and nutritional status of referees and linesmen, a little-studied group whose members are nevertheless are of great importance in sports, and who are increasingly required to have a high level of performance and fitness. The methodology employed is capable of extrapolation across various population sectors as a result of its wide applicability. It can be stated that the sportspeople studied had a nutritional status that was not entirely suited to their circumstances, as their diet contained fewer carbohydrates and more proteins than recommended. However, no serious nutrient deficiency was observed, indicating that their diet was varied. Education and awareness-raising about proper nutrient intakes is a day-to-day necessity for sportspeople of a certain level, whether in their own specific disciplines or in respect of others they may try where this need may become manifest [28]. Rigorous evidence relating to this aspect must be given special attention [29,30]. Because it is obvious that performance in training influences performance in competition, the implication is that there is a need to design and implement recommended diets and to introduce programs of education on nutrition for such sportspeople.

Competing interests
The authors declare that they have no competing interests.

Authors' contributions
CMR and PSC were involved in study design, data collection/analysis, manuscript`s preparation and gave final approval to the manuscript. Both authors read and approved the final manuscript.

Acknowledgements
We are grateful to Translation Service of the University of León for assistance language editing.

Author details
[1]Faculty of Sports Sciences (FCAFD), University of Leon, Leon, Spain.
[2]Institute of Biomedicine (IBIOMED), University of Leon, Leon, Spain.
[3]Department of Biomedical Sciences. Physiology, University of León, 24071 León, Spain.

References

1. Gil A. Tratado de nutrición. Madrid: Panamericana; 2010.
2. González J, Sánchez P, Mataix J. Nutrición en el deporte. Ayudas ergogénicas y dopaje. Madrid: Díaz de Santos; 2006.
3. González E. Guía de alimentación del jugador de fútbol. Madrid: Gymnos; 1999.
4. Von Post-Skagegard M, Samuelson G, Karlstrorm B, Mohsen R, Berglund L, Bratterby LE. Changes in food habits in healthy Swedish adolescents during the transition from adolescence to adulthood. Eur J Clin Nutr. 2002;56:532–8.
5. Varela G, Silvestre D. Nutrición, vida activa y deporte. Madrid, España: IM&C; 2010.
6. Reilly T, Williams AM. Science and soccer. London: Routledge; 2003.
7. Shephard RJ. Biology and medicine of soccer. An update. J Sports Sci. 1999;17:757–86.
8. Campbell B, Kreider RB, Ziegenfuss T, La Bounty P, Roberts M, Burke D, et al. International Society of Sports Nutrition position stands: protein and exercise. J Int Soc Sports Nutr. 2007;26:4–8.
9. Weston M, Castagna C, Franco M, Impellizzeri FM, Bizzini M, Williams AM, et al. Science and Medicine Applied to Soccer Refereeing. Sports Med. 2012;42 Suppl 7:615–31.
10. Bangsbo J. Energy demands in competitive soccer. J Sports Sci. 1994;12:S5–12.
11. Mielgo-Ayuso J, Collado PS, Urdampilleta A, Martínez-Sanz JM, Seco J. Changes induced by diet and nutritional intake in the lipid profile of female professional volleyball players after 11 weeks of training. J Int Soc Sports Nutr. 2013;10:55.
12. Roza AM, Shizgal HM. The Harris Benedict Equation reevaluated: resting energy requirements and the boy cell mass. Am J Clin Nutr. 1984;40:168–82.
13. Pierre J, Achamrah N, Grigioni S, Jocelyne C, Rimbert A, Folope V, Petit A, Déchelotte P, Coëffier M. Validity of predictive equations for resting energy expenditure according to the body mass index in a population of 1726 patients followed in a Nutrition Unit. Clin Nutr 2014, http://dx.doi.org/10.1016/j.clnu.2014.06.009.
14. Martínez-Reñón C, Collado PS. Nutritional study of a third division soccer team. Nutr Hosp. 2013;28 Suppl 2:319–24.
15. Iglesias E, García A, García P, Pérez J, Patterson A, García P. Is there relationship between the playing position of soccer players and their food and macronutrient intake? Appl Physiol Nutr Metab. 2012;37:1–8.
16. Bartha C, Petridis L, Hamar P, Puhl S, Castagna C. Fitness test results of hungarian and international-level soccer referees and assistants. J Strength Cond Res. 2009;23 Suppl 1:121–6.
17. Ono N, Kennedy E, Reeves S, Cronin L. Nutrition and culture in professional football. A mixed method approach. Appetite. 2012;58:98–104.
18. Panciera Y, Casamichana D, García JA, Robles FJ, Caro O, Wärnberg J. Evaluación de la Ingesta Nutricional de futbolistas en función de los puestos específicos de juego. [http://www.cartagena.es/files/115-19429-DOC_FICHERO/YAinaPanciera,etel.pdf]
19. Hawkins RD, Hulse MA, Wilkinson C, Hodson A, Gibson M. The association football medical research programmed: an audit of injuries in professional football. Br J Sports Med. 2001;35:43–7.
20. Clark K. Nutritional guidance to soccer players for training and competition. J Sports Sci. 1994;12:43–50.
21. Balsom PD, Wood K, Olsson P, Ekblom B. Carbohydrate intake and multiple sprint sports: with special reference to football (soccer). Int J Sport Med. 1999;20:48–52.
22. González-Gallego J, Villa J. Nutrición y ayudas ergogénicas en el deporte. Madrid: Síntesis; 2001.
23. Dorling J, Earnest C. Effect of carbohydrate mouth rinsing on multiple sprint performance. J Int Soc Sports Nutr. 2013;10:41.
24. Lemon PW. Protein requirements of soccer. J Sport Sci. 1994;12:17–22.
25. Umaña M. Nutrition for young soccer players. Int J Soccer Sci. 2005;3:13–22.
26. Figueiredo VC, Cameron-Smith D. Is carbohydrate needed to further stimulate muscle protein synthesis/hypertrophy following resistance exercise? J Int Soc Sports Nutr. 2013;10:42.
27. Sánchez JL, León P. Study of dietary habits of young sportsmen. Nutr Hosp. 2008;23 Suppl 6:619–29.
28. Molinero O, Márquez S. Use of nutritional supplements in sport: risks, knowledge and behavioral-related factors. Nutr Hosp. 2009;24 Suppl 2:128–34.
29. Pardo VP. La importancia de las vitaminas en la nutrición de personas que realizan actividad físico deportiva. Int J Med Sci Phys Act Sport. 2004;4 Suppl 16:233–42.
30. Márquez S, Garatachea N. Actividad física y salud. Madrid, España: Díaz de Santos; 2009.

Permissions

All chapters in this book were first published in JISSN, by BioMed Central; hereby published with permission under the Creative Commons Attribution License or equivalent. Every chapter published in this book has been scrutinized by our experts. Their significance has been extensively debated. The topics covered herein carry significant findings which will fuel the growth of the discipline. They may even be implemented as practical applications or may be referred to as a beginning point for another development.

The contributors of this book come from diverse backgrounds, making this book a truly international effort. This book will bring forth new frontiers with its revolutionizing research information and detailed analysis of the nascent developments around the world.

We would like to thank all the contributing authors for lending their expertise to make the book truly unique. They have played a crucial role in the development of this book. Without their invaluable contributions this book wouldn't have been possible. They have made vital efforts to compile up to date information on the varied aspects of this subject to make this book a valuable addition to the collection of many professionals and students.

This book was conceptualized with the vision of imparting up-to-date information and advanced data in this field. To ensure the same, a matchless editorial board was set up. Every individual on the board went through rigorous rounds of assessment to prove their worth. After which they invested a large part of their time researching and compiling the most relevant data for our readers.

The editorial board has been involved in producing this book since its inception. They have spent rigorous hours researching and exploring the diverse topics which have resulted in the successful publishing of this book. They have passed on their knowledge of decades through this book. To expedite this challenging task, the publisher supported the team at every step. A small team of assistant editors was also appointed to further simplify the editing procedure and attain best results for the readers.

Apart from the editorial board, the designing team has also invested a significant amount of their time in understanding the subject and creating the most relevant covers. They scrutinized every image to scout for the most suitable representation of the subject and create an appropriate cover for the book.

The publishing team has been an ardent support to the editorial, designing and production team. Their endless efforts to recruit the best for this project, has resulted in the accomplishment of this book. They are a veteran in the field of academics and their pool of knowledge is as vast as their experience in printing. Their expertise and guidance has proved useful at every step. Their uncompromising quality standards have made this book an exceptional effort. Their encouragement from time to time has been an inspiration for everyone.

The publisher and the editorial board hope that this book will prove to be a valuable piece of knowledge for researchers, students, practitioners and scholars across the globe.

List of Contributors

Satoko Takeda
Graduate School of Comprehensive Human Sciences, University of Tsukuba, Ibaraki, Japan

Jong-Hoon Park
Center for Disease Biology and Integrative Medicine, University of Tokyo, Tokyo, Japan
Department of Physical Education, Konkuk University, Seoul, South Korea

Eriko Kawashim
Yokohama Research Center, JNC Corporation, Yokohama, Japan

Ikuko Ezawa
Japan Women's University, Tokyo, Japan

Naomi Omi
Graduate School of Comprehensive Human Sciences, University of Tsukuba, Ibaraki, Japan
Faculty of Health and Sport Sciences, University of Tsukuba, Ibaraki, Japan
Institute of Health and Sports Sciences, Graduate School of Comprehensive Human Sciences, University of Tsukuba, Tsukuba, Ibaraki 305-8574, Japan

Dona L Tomlin
School of Exercise Science, Physical and Health Education, University of Victoria, Victoria, BC, Canada

Shannon K Clarke
School of Exercise Science, Physical and Health Education, University of Victoria, Victoria, BC, Canada

Meghan Day
BC Ministry of Health, 4th Floor, 1520 Blanshard Street, Victoria, BC, Canada

Heather A McKay
Centre for Hip Health and Mobility, Vancouver Coastal Health Research Institute, VGH Campus. 302 - 2647Willow Street, Vancouver, BC, Canada

Patti-Jean Naylor
School of Exercise Science, Physical and Health Education, University of Victoria, Victoria, BC, Canada

Ryan P Lowery
Department of Health Sciences and Human Performance, The University of Tampa, Tampa, FL, USA

Jordan M Joy
Department of Health Sciences and Human Performance, The University of Tampa, Tampa, FL, USA

Joshua E Dudeck
Department of Health Sciences and Human Performance, The University of Tampa, Tampa, FL, USA

Eduardo Oliveira de Souza
Laboratory of Neuromuscular Adaptations to Strength Training, School of Physical Education and Sport, University of São Paulo, São Paulo, Brazil

Sean A McCleary
Department of Health Sciences and Human Performance, The University of Tampa, Tampa, FL, USA

Shawn Wells
Dymatize® Enterprises, LLC. & Dymatize® Nutrition Sport Performance Institute (DNSPI), Dallas, Texas, USA

Robert Wildman
Dymatize® Enterprises, LLC. & Dymatize® Nutrition Sport Performance Institute (DNSPI), Dallas, Texas, USA

Jacob M Wilson
Department of Health Sciences and Human Performance, The University of Tampa, Tampa, FL, USA

Shawn M Talbott
SupplementWatch, 648 Rocky Knoll, Draper, UT 84020, USA

Julie A Talbott
SupplementWatch, 648 Rocky Knoll, Draper, UT 84020, USA

Mike Pugh
MonaVie, 10855 S River Front Parkway, South Jordan, UT 84095, USA

Brad Jon Schoenfeld
Department of Health Science, Lehman College, Bronx, NY, USA

Alan Albert Aragon
California State University, Northridge, CA, USA

James W Krieger
Weightology, LLC, Issaquah, WA, USA

Song-Gyu Ra
Graduate School of Comprehensive Human Sciences, University of Tsukuba, Tsukuba, Ibaraki 305-8574, Japan
Research Fellow of the Japan Society for the Promotion of Sciences, Chiyoda-ku, Tokyo 102-0083, Japan

Teruo Miyazaki
Joint Research Center, Tokyo Medical University Ibaraki Medical Center, Ami, Ibaraki 300-0395, Japan

Keisuke Ishikura
Sports Research and Development Core, University of Tsukuba, Tsukuba, Ibaraki 305-8574, Japan

Hisashi Nagayama
School of Health and Physical Education, University of Tsukuba, Tsukuba, Ibaraki 305-8574, Japan

Shoichi Komine
Graduate School of Comprehensive Human Sciences, University of Tsukuba, Tsukuba, Ibaraki 305-8574, Japan

Yoshio Nakata
Faculty of Medicine, University of Tsukuba, Tsukuba, Ibaraki 305-8574, Japan

Seiji Maeda
Faculty of Health and Sport Sciences, University of Tsukuba, Tsukuba, Ibaraki 305-8574, Japan

Yasushi Matsuzaki
Division of Gastroenterology and Hepatology, Department of Internal Medicine, Tokyo Medical University Ibaraki Medical Center, Ami, Ibaraki 300-0395, Japan

Hajime Ohmori
Faculty of Health and Sport Sciences, University of Tsukuba, Tsukuba, Ibaraki 305-8574, Japan

Zhifang Zhao
Department of Physiology, School of Basic Medical Science, Ningxia Medical University, Yinchuan 750004, China

Yan Luo
Department of Physiology, School of Basic Medical Science, Ningxia Medical University, Yinchuan 750004, China

Guanghua Li
Department of Physiology, School of Basic Medical Science, Ningxia Medical University, Yinchuan 750004, China

Lingqin Zhu
Department of Physiology, School of Basic Medical Science, Ningxia Medical University, Yinchuan 750004, China

Yin Wang
Department of Physiology, School of Basic Medical Science, Ningxia Medical University, Yinchuan 750004, China

Xuehong Zhang
Department of Pediatrics, General Hospital of Ningxia Medical University, Yinchuan 750004, China

Rodrigo Vitasovic Gomes
School of Physical Education and Sport, University of São Paulo, Av Prof Mello Moraes 65, São Paulo, SP 05508-030, Brazil

Caroline Dario Capitani
School of Applied Sciences, University of Campinas, Av Pedro Zacaria, 1300, Limeira, SP 13484-350, Brazil

Carlos Ugrinowitsch
School of Physical Education and Sport, University of São Paulo, Av Prof Mello Moraes 65, São Paulo, SP 05508-030, Brazil

Michael Christopher Zourdos
Department of Exercise Science and Health Promotion, Florida Atlantic University, 777 Glades Road, FH 11 Boca Raton, FL 33431, USA

Jaime Fernandez-Fernandez
Sports Research Centre, Miguel Hernandez University, Avda. Universidad s/n, Elche, Alicante 03202, Spain

Alberto Mendez-Villanueva
ASPIRE Academy for Sports Excellence, Al Waab, Doha 22287, Qatar

Marcelo Saldanha Aoki
School of Arts, Sciences and Humanities, University of São Paulo, Av Arlindo Bettio, 1000, São Paulo 03828-000, Brazil

Michel B Araújo
Laboratory of Nutrition, Metabolism and Exercise, Department of Physical Education, Universidade Estadual Paulista (UNESP), 24ª avenue n° 1515, P.O. Box 199, Bela Vista, Rio Claro, São Paulo, Brazil

Leandro P Moura
Laboratory of Nutrition, Metabolism and Exercise, Department of Physical Education, Universidade Estadual Paulista (UNESP), 24ª avenue n° 1515, P.O. Box 199, Bela Vista, Rio Claro, São Paulo, Brazil

Roberto C Vieira Junior
Post-Graduation Program - Graduation in Bioscience of Faculty of Nutrition from Federal University of Mato Grosso, UFMT, Cuiabá, Mato Grosso, Brazil

Marcelo C Junior
Laboratory of Nutrition, Metabolism and Exercise, Department of Physical Education, Universidade Estadual Paulista (UNESP), 24ª avenue n° 1515, P.O. Box 199, Bela Vista, Rio Claro, São Paulo, Brazil

Rodrigo A Dalia
Laboratory of Nutrition, Metabolism and Exercise, Department of Physical Education, Universidade Estadual Paulista (UNESP), 24ª avenue n° 1515, P.O. Box 199, Bela Vista, Rio Claro, São Paulo, Brazil

Amanda C Sponton
Laboratory of Nutrition, Metabolism and Exercise, Department of Physical Education, Universidade Estadual Paulista (UNESP), 24ª avenue n° 1515, P.O. Box 199, Bela Vista, Rio Claro, São Paulo, Brazil

Carla Ribeiro
Laboratory of Nutrition, Metabolism and Exercise, Department of Physical Education, Universidade Estadual Paulista (UNESP), 24ª avenue n° 1515, P.O. Box 199, Bela Vista, Rio Claro, São Paulo, Brazil

Maria Alice R Mello
Laboratory of Nutrition, Metabolism and Exercise, Department of Physical Education, Universidade Estadual Paulista (UNESP), 24ª avenue n° 1515, P.O. Box 199, Bela Vista, Rio Claro, São Paulo, Brazil

Antti A Mero
Department of Biology of Physical Activity, University of Jyväskylä, P.O. Box 35, Jyväskylä 40351, Finland

Petri Hirvonen
Department of Biology of Physical Activity, University of Jyväskylä, P.O. Box 35, Jyväskylä 40351, Finland

Janne Saarela
Department of Biology of Physical Activity, University of Jyväskylä, P.O. Box 35, Jyväskylä 40351, Finland

Juha J Hulmi
Department of Biology of Physical Activity, University of Jyväskylä, P.O. Box 35, Jyväskylä 40351, Finland

Jay R Hoffman
Sport and Exercise Science, University of Central Florida, Orlando, Florida, USA

Jeffrey R Stout
Sport and Exercise Science, University of Central Florida, Orlando, Florida, USA

Jason M Cholewa
Department of Kinesiology, Recreation, and Sport Studies, Coastal Carolina University, Conway, SC, USA

Monika Wyszczelska-Rokiel
Department of Environmental Chemistry, University of Lodz, Pomorska 163, 90-236, Lodz, Poland, USA

Rafal Glowacki
Department of Environmental Chemistry, University of Lodz, Pomorska 163, 90-236, Lodz, Poland, USA

Hieronim Jakubowski
Institute of Bioorganic Chemistry, Polish Academy of Sciences, Poznan, Department of Biochemistry and Biotechnology, Life Sciences University, Poznan, NJ, Poland UNDMJ-New Jersey Medical School, Newark, NJ, USA

Tracey Matthews
Department of Exercise Science and Sport Studies, Springfield College, Springfield, MA, USA

Richard Wood
Department of Exercise Science and Sport Studies, Springfield College, Springfield, MA, USA

Stuart AS Craig
DuPont Nutrition & Health, Tarrytown, NY, USA

Vincent Paolone
Department of Exercise Science and Sport Studies, Springfield College, Springfield, MA, USA

James Ackerman
Health and Exercise, School of Medical Sciences, University of New South Wales, Sydney, Australia

Tom Clifford
Department of Exercise Science, University of Portsmouth, Portsmouth, UK

Lars R McNaughton
Department of Sport and Physical Activity, Edge Hill University, Ormskirk, UK

David J Bentley
Human Exercise Performance Laboratory, School of Medical Sciences, University of Adelaide, Adelaide 5005, South Australia

Eric T Trexler
Department of Exercise and Sport Science, University of North Carolina at Chapel Hill, 209 Fetzer Hall, CB# 8700, Chapel Hill, NC 27599-8700, USA

Abbie E Smith-Ryan
Department of Exercise and Sport Science, University of North Carolina at Chapel Hill, 209 Fetzer Hall, CB# 8700, Chapel Hill, NC 27599-8700, USA

Layne E Norton
BioLayne LLC, Tampa, FL, USA

Cainara Lins Draeger
VP Research Institute, Rua Pedro Morganti, 103 - Vila Mariana, PO Box 04020-070, São Paulo, SP, Brazil

Andréia Naves
VP Research Institute, Rua Pedro Morganti, 103 - Vila Mariana, PO Box 04020-070, São Paulo, SP, Brazil

Natália Marques
VP Research Institute, Rua Pedro Morganti, 103 - Vila Mariana, PO Box 04020-070, São Paulo, SP, Brazil

Ana Beatriz Baptistella
VP Research Institute, Rua Pedro Morganti, 103 - Vila Mariana, PO Box 04020-070, São Paulo, SP, Brazil

Renata Alves Carnauba
VP Research Institute, Rua Pedro Morganti, 103 - Vila Mariana, PO Box 04020-070, São Paulo, SP, Brazil

Valéria Paschoal
VP Research Institute, Rua Pedro Morganti, 103 - Vila Mariana, PO Box 04020-070, São Paulo, SP, Brazil

Humberto Nicastro
VP Research Institute, Rua Pedro Morganti, 103 - Vila Mariana, PO Box 04020-070, São Paulo, SP, Brazil

Thapanee Roengrit
Department of Physiology, Faculty of Medicine, Khon Kaen University, Khon Kaen 40002, Thailand
The Exercise and Sport Sciences Research and Development Group, Khon Kaen University, Khon Kaen 40002, Thailand

Panakaporn Wannanon
Department of Physiology, Faculty of Medicine, Khon Kaen University, Khon Kaen 40002, Thailand
The Exercise and Sport Sciences Research and Development Group, Khon Kaen University, Khon Kaen 40002, Thailand

Piyapong Prasertsri
Faculty of Allied Health Sciences, Burapha University, Chonburi 20130, Thailand
The Exercise and Sport Sciences Research and Development Group, Khon Kaen University, Khon Kaen 40002, Thailand

Yupaporn Kanpetta
Exercise and Sport Sciences Program, Graduate School, Khon Kaen University, Khon Kaen 40002, Thailand
The Exercise and Sport Sciences Research and Development Group, Khon Kaen University, Khon Kaen 40002, Thailand

Bung-orn Sripanidkulchai
Faculty of Pharmaceutical Sciences, Khon Kaen University, Khon Kaen 40002, Thailand
The Center for Research and Development of Herbal Health Products, Khon Kaen University, Khon Kaen 40002, Thailand

Naruemon Leelayuwat
Department of Physiology, Faculty of Medicine, Khon Kaen University, Khon Kaen 40002, Thailand
The Exercise and Sport Sciences Research and Development Group, Khon Kaen University, Khon Kaen 40002, Thailand

Jose Antonio
Exercise and Sports Sciences, Nova Southeastern University, 3532 S. University Drive, University Park Plaza Suite 3532, Davie, FL 33314, USA

Victoria Ciccone
Exercise and Sports Sciences, Nova Southeastern University, 3532 S. University Drive, University Park Plaza Suite 3532, Davie, FL 33314, USA

Giuseppe Potrick Stefani
Laboratório de Fisiologia - UFCSPA/Porto Alegre, Rua Sarmento Leite, 245, 900050-170 Porto Alegre, RS, Brazil

Ramiro Barcos Nunes
Laboratório de Fisiologia - UFCSPA/Porto Alegre, Rua Sarmento Leite, 245, 900050-170 Porto Alegre, RS, Brazil

André Zuanazzi Dornelles
Laboratório de Fisiologia - UFCSPA/Porto Alegre, Rua Sarmento Leite, 245, 900050-170 Porto Alegre, RS, Brazil

Jadson Pereira Alves
Laboratório de Fisiologia - UFCSPA/Porto Alegre, Rua Sarmento Leite, 245, 900050-170 Porto Alegre, RS, Brazil

Marcella Ody Piva
Laboratório de Poluição Atmosférica e Estresse Oxidativo - UFCSPA/Porto Alegre, Porto Alegre, RS, Brazil

Marlise Di Domenico
Laboratório de Poluição Atmosférica e Estresse Oxidativo - UFCSPA/Porto Alegre, Porto Alegre, RS, Brazil

Cláudia Ramos Rhoden
Laboratório de Poluição Atmosférica e Estresse Oxidativo - UFCSPA/Porto Alegre, Porto Alegre, RS, Brazil

Pedro Dal Lago
Laboratório de Fisiologia - UFCSPA/Porto Alegre, Rua Sarmento Leite, 245, 900050-170 Porto Alegre, RS, Brazil
Programa de Pós Graduação em Ciências da Reabilitação - UFCSPA/Porto Alegre, Porto Alegre, RS, Brazil

Jay R Hoffman
Institute of Exercise Physiology and Wellness, Sport and Exercise Science, University of Central Florida, Orlando, FL, USA

Geva Landau
Israel Defense Force, Medical Corps, Tel Hashomer, Israel

Jeffrey R Stout
Institute of Exercise Physiology and Wellness, Sport and Exercise Science, University of Central Florida, Orlando, FL, USA

Matan Dabora
Israel Defense Force, Medical Corps, Tel Hashomer, Israel

Daniel S Moran
Israel Defense Force, Medical Corps, Tel Hashomer, Israel
School of Health Science, Ariel University, Center of Samaria, Ariel, Israel

Nurit Sharvit
Israel Defense Forces, Combat Fitness Branch, Netanya, Israel

Mattan W Hoffman
Israel Defense Force, Medical Corps, Tel Hashomer, Israel

Yuval Ben Moshe
Israel Defense Force, Medical Corps, Tel Hashomer, Israel

William P McCormack
Institute of Exercise Physiology and Wellness, Sport and Exercise Science, University of Central Florida, Orlando, FL, USA

Gil Hirschhorn
Israel Defense Force, Medical Corps, Tel Hashomer, Israel

Ishay Ostfeld
Israel Defense Force, Medical Corps, Tel Hashomer, Israel

Muqing Yi
Center for Sports Nutrition, National Institute of Sports Medicine, 1st Anding Road, Chaoyang District, Beijing 100029, China

Jinde Fu
Center for Sports Nutrition, National Institute of Sports Medicine, 1st Anding Road, Chaoyang District, Beijing 100029, China

Lili Zhou
Center for Sports Nutrition, National Institute of Sports Medicine, 1st Anding Road, Chaoyang District, Beijing 100029, China

Hong Gao
Center for Sports Nutrition, National Institute of Sports Medicine, 1st Anding Road, Chaoyang District, Beijing 100029, China

Chenguang Fan
Chinese Baiyi Cycling Team, Fengtai District, Beijing 100072, China

Jing Shao
Center for Sports Nutrition, National Institute of Sports Medicine, 1st Anding Road, Chaoyang District, Beijing 100029, China

Baohua Xu
Center for Sports Nutrition, National Institute of Sports Medicine, 1st Anding Road, Chaoyang District, Beijing 100029, China

Qirong Wang
Center for Sports Nutrition, National Institute of Sports Medicine, 1st Anding Road, Chaoyang District, Beijing 100029, China

Juntao Li
Center for Sports Nutrition, National Institute of Sports Medicine, 1st Anding Road, Chaoyang District, Beijing 100029, China

Guangwei Huang
Almond Board of California, Modesto, CA 95354, USA

Karen Lapsley
Almond Board of California, Modesto, CA 95354, USA

Jeffrey B Blumberg
Antioxidants Research Laboratory, Jean Mayer USDA Human Nutrition Research Center on Aging, Tufts University, Boston, MA, USA

C-Y Oliver Chen
Antioxidants Research Laboratory, Jean Mayer USDA Human Nutrition Research Center on Aging, Tufts University, Boston, MA, USA

Zali Yager
College of Education, Victoria University, Melbourne, Australia

Jennifer A O'Dea
Faculty of Education and Social Work, University of Sydney, Sydney, Australia

Igor Z Zubrzycki
Jędrzej Śniadecki Academy of Physical Education and Sport ul, Kazimierza Górskiego 1, Gdańsk 80-336, Poland
School of Health and Applied Sciences, Polytechnic of Namibia, Private Bag 13388, 13 Storch Street, Windhoek, Namibia

Zbigniew Ossowski
Jędrzej Śniadecki Academy of Physical Education and Sport ul, Kazimierza Górskiego 1, Gdańsk 80-336, Poland

Stanislaw Przybylski
Jędrzej Śniadecki Academy of Physical Education and Sport ul, Kazimierza Górskiego 1, Gdańsk 80-336, Poland

Magdalena Wiacek
Jędrzej Śniadecki Academy of Physical Education and Sport ul, Kazimierza Górskiego 1, Gdańsk 80-336, Poland

Anna Clarke
Department of Microbiology and Biochemistry, University of Fort Hare, P/B X1314, Alice 5700, South Africa

Bartosz Trabka
Jędrzej Śniadecki Academy of Physical Education and Sport ul, Kazimierza Górskiego 1, Gdańsk 80-336, Poland

Jonathan Furlong
Department of Kinesiology Exercise Physiology Core Laboratory, University of Virginia, 203 Memorial Gymnasium, Charlottesville 22904, Virginia, USA

Corey A Rynders
Department of Human Movement Sciences, Human Performance Laboratory, Old Dominion University, Norfolk, VA, USA

Mark Sutherlin
Department of Kinesiology Exercise Physiology Core Laboratory, University of Virginia, 203 Memorial Gymnasium, Charlottesville 22904, Virginia, USA

James Patrie
Department of Kinesiology Exercise Physiology Core Laboratory, University of Virginia, 203 Memorial Gymnasium, Charlottesville 22904, Virginia, USA

Frank I Katch
Department of Kinesiology Exercise Physiology Core Laboratory, University of Virginia, 203 Memorial Gymnasium, Charlottesville 22904, Virginia, USA

Jay Hertel
Department of Kinesiology Exercise Physiology Core Laboratory, University of Virginia, 203 Memorial Gymnasium, Charlottesville 22904, Virginia, USA

Arthur Weltman
Department of Kinesiology Exercise Physiology Core Laboratory, University of Virginia, 203 Memorial Gymnasium, Charlottesville 22904, Virginia, USA

Karolina Łagowska
Department of Human Nutrition and Hygiene, Dietetic Division, University of Life Sciences, Wojska Polskiego 28 str, 60-637 Poznań, Poland

Karina Kapczuk
Department of Perinatology and Gynecology, Division of Gynecology, Karol Marcinkowski University of Medical Sciences in Poznań, Polna 33 str, 60-535 Poznań, Poland

Zbigniew Friebe
Department of Perinatology and Gynecology, Division of Gynecology, Karol Marcinkowski University of Medical Sciences in Poznań, Polna 33 str, 60-535 Poznań, Poland

Joanna Bajerska
Department of Human Nutrition and Hygiene, Dietetic Division, University of Life Sciences, Wojska Polskiego 28 str, 60-637 Poznań, Poland

Eric R Helms
Sport Performance Research in New Zealand (SPRINZ) at AUT Millennium Institute, AUT University, 17 Antares Place, Mairangi Bay, Auckland 0632, New Zealand

Alan A Aragon
California State University, Northridge, CA, USA

Peter J Fitschen
Division of Nutritional Sciences, University of Illinois, Urbana, IL, USA

Tim N Ziegenfuss
The Center for Applied Health Sciences, 4302 Allen Road, Ste 120, Stow, OH 44224, USA

Scott M Habowski
The Center for Applied Health Sciences, 4302 Allen Road, Ste 120, Stow, OH 44224, USA

Robert Lemieux
Strength and Conditioning, Athletics Department, Kent State University, Kent, OH 44240, USA

Jennifer E Sandrock
The Center for Applied Health Sciences, 4302 Allen Road, Ste 120, Stow, OH 44224, USA

A William Kedia
The Center for Applied Health Sciences, 4302 Allen Road, Ste 120, Stow, OH 44224, USA

Chad M Kerksick
School of Sport, Recreation and Exercise Sciences, Lindenwood University, St. Charles, MO 63301, USA

Hector L Lopez
The Center for Applied Health Sciences, 4302 Allen Road, Ste 120, Stow, OH 44224, USA

Ieva Alaunyte
Department of Food and Tourism Management Old Hall Lane, Manchester Metropolitan University, Manchester M14 6HR, UK
School of Health Sciences, Liverpool Hope University, Liverpool L16 9JD, UK

Valentina Stojceska
Department of Food and Tourism Management Old Hall Lane, Manchester Metropolitan University, Manchester M14 6HR, UK
College of Engineering, Design and Physical Sciences, Brunel University, Uxbridge, Middlesex UB8 3PH, UK

Andrew Plunkett
Department of Food and Tourism Management Old Hall Lane, Manchester Metropolitan University, Manchester M14 6HR, UK

Emma Derbyshire
Department of Food and Tourism Management Old Hall Lane, Manchester Metropolitan University, Manchester M14 6HR, UK

Jose Antonio
Exercise and Sports Sciences, Nova Southeastern University, 3532 S. University Drive, University Park Plaza Suite 3532, Davie, FL 33314, USA

Corey A Peacock
Exercise and Sports Sciences, Nova Southeastern University, 3532 S. University Drive, University Park Plaza Suite 3532, Davie, FL 33314, USA

Anya Ellerbroek
Exercise and Sports Sciences, Nova Southeastern University, 3532 S. University Drive, University Park Plaza Suite 3532, Davie, FL 33314, USA

Brandon Fromhoff
Exercise and Sports Sciences, Nova Southeastern University, 3532 S. University Drive, University Park Plaza Suite 3532, Davie, FL 33314, USA

Tobin Silver
Exercise and Sports Sciences, Nova Southeastern University, 3532 S. University Drive, University Park Plaza Suite 3532, Davie, FL 33314, USA

Cristian Martínez Reñón
Faculty of Sports Sciences (FCAFD), University of Leon, Leon, Spain

Pilar S Collado
Institute of Biomedicine (IBIOMED), University of Leon, Leon, Spain
Department of Biomedical Sciences. Physiology, University of León, 24071 León, Spain